Hepatitis C Choices, 4th Edition (
A Service of the Caring Ambassador

MW00712125

For faster processing, please print and complete <u>all</u> fields.

Name:_____

Street Address:_____

City:_____   State:_____   Zip Code:_____

E-mail address:_____

Daytime phone:_____

Fax number:_____

Check one: ___ ordering for personal use   ___ordering for organizational use

If ordering for an organization, please complete the following:

Your Job Title:_____

Organization:_____

Is your organization: __ for profit   __ not for profit

Please check the populations served by your organization. Check all that apply.

__ people with hepatitis C

__ people at risk for hepatitis C

__ people with HIV/AIDS

__ people seeking help for substance abuse

__ people seeking help for sexually-transmitted disease concerns

__ other
   (please describe):_____

Order Amount and Donation Options

(Please fill out a separate form if you want books shipped to more than one location.)

The Caring Ambassadors Program offers a Book Matching Program.

By adding a $20 donation to your book order, we will use your donation to make <u>Hepatitis C Choices</u> available to libraries, public health clinics, and individuals who are otherwise unable to pay for the book.

Number of books requested: ___ x $24.99 per book = $_____
Book Matching Donation   ___ x $20.00 per book = $_____
Additional donation to Caring Ambassadors Hepatitis C Program: $_____
                                    TOTAL ENCLOSED $_____

I don't need a book, but please accept my donation to the Caring Ambassadors Hepatitis C Program in the amount of $_____.

Please enclose a check made payable to: **Caring Ambassadors Program.**

Mail your completed order form to:
Caring Ambassadors Program
604 E. 16th Street, Suite 201
Vancouver, WA 98663

Please allow 3-6 weeks for delivery.

For additional information about the **Caring Ambassadors Hepatitis C Program**,
please visit us online at www.HepCChallenge.org, or call us at (360) 816-4186.

Hepatitis C Choices
4th Edition

Diverse Viewpoints and Choices for Your Hepatitis C Journey

Hepatitis C Choices, 4th Edition

Tina M. St. John, MD and Lorren Sandt, Editors

Contributing Authors
(in alphabetical order)
Terry Baker
Misha Cohen, OMD, LAc
Stewart Cooper, MD
Randy Dietrich
Gregory T. Everson, MD
Sylvia Flesner, ND
Robert G. Gish, MD
Peter Hauser, MD
Randy Horwitz, MD, PhD
David W.Indest, PsyD
Jessica Irwin, PAC
Julia Jernberg, MD
Joyce S. Kobayashi, MD
Douglas R. LaBrecque, MD
Lark Lands, PhD
Shri K. Mishra, MD, MS
Sharon D. Montes, MD
Julie Nelligan, PhD
J. Lyn Patrick, ND
Bharathi Ravi, BAMS
Aparna Roy, M.D., MPH
Lorren Sandt
Kathleen B. Schwarz, MD
Tina M. St. John, MD
Amy E. Smith, PAC
Diana L. Sylvestre, MD
Norah Terrault, MD, MPH
Sivarama Prasad Vinjamury, MD
Qing Cai Zhang, MD (China), LAc
Susan L. Zickmund, PhD

Dedication

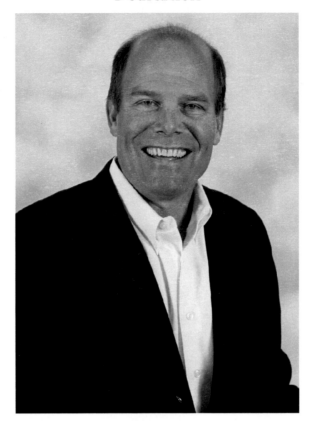

Randy Dietrich

The Caring Ambassadors Hepatitis C Program dedicates the 4th edition of Hepatitis C Choices to program founder, Randy Dietrich. Randy established the Caring Ambassadors Hepatitis C Program in 1999 after being diagnosed with chronic hepatitis C.

After years of learning about hepatitis C and diligently fine-tuning his health, Randy made the decision to undergo interferon-based therapy in 2007. Randy is now considered cured of hepatitis C. While he is personally free of hepatitis C, Randy's dedication to the hepatitis C community remains steadfast. Randy inspires and calls us all to remain committed to working for improved health and wellness of all people living with hepatitis C.

Without Randy's dedication and commitment, the Caring Ambassadors Hepatitis C Program and this book would not exist. Thank you Randy — this world is truly a better place because of you.

Acknowledgements

The Caring Ambassadors Hepatitis C Program is profoundly grateful to the members of the Hepatitis C Medical Team and the other contributing authors. We are proud of the way these dedicated professionals from many different healthcare disciplines have listened to one another, worked together, and become a team — a team dedicated to providing better healthcare to all people living with hepatitis C. Without their willingness to open their minds to treatment options other than their own, this book would not have been possible.

The process of keeping Hepatitis C Choices current is perpetually ongoing. We are profoundly grateful to the authors of the book for their dedication, generosity, time, and expertise. Without their commitment to this project, we would be unable to offer this important resource to the hepatitis C community.

Like a family, the Caring Ambassadors Hepatitis C Program has a core of support upon which it stands and draws on for strength. Hepatitis C Choices would not be possible without the love, generosity, and hard work of the Possehl Family, the Dietrich Family, and Republic Financial Corporation. Thank you for all you do for the Caring Ambassadors Program and for the community.

Last but not least, the Caring Ambassadors Hepatitis C Program acknowledges the hepatitis C community —the people who bravely face the challenges of living with hepatitis C, the loved ones who offer them steadfast support and comfort, the healthcare providers who work to alleviate hepatitis C-related suffering, and the advocates who work tirelessly to provide hope, support, and improve the future for those with chronic hepatitis C. We are proud to work side-by-side with you. Thank you for your feedback, which helps us better focus each new edition of Hepatitis C Choices to meet the community's needs.

The Hepatitis C Choices authors are personally grateful to the following people for their support.

Sharon Bahrych, RN, NP	Ingrid Park
Kay Lewis, Jon, and Tara Baker	Meera Y. Patel
Carla Carwile	Gail Rando
Tom Daws	Kevin Sandt
Linda Catherine, Brad, and Todd Everson	Audrey Spolaric
Heather French Henry	Hope Reidun St. John
Jian Gao, MD	Tracy Swan
Erick Ingraham	George Webb
Judy LaBrecque	Andrew Weil, MD
Nancy Legato	Carla Wilson
Ken Moore	Margaret Wilson

Thanks to our sponsors for their generous support.

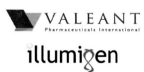

Hepatitis C Choices, 4th Edition
Table of Contents

PART 3: OTHER TOPICS FOR PEOPLE LIVING WITH HEPATITIS C

APPENDICES

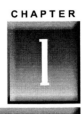

How to Use Choices

Organization of *Hepatitis C Choices*

Each person with *hepatitis C* is unique, and each reader of *Hepatitis C Choices* is also unique. Recognizing that your informational needs are personal and may change over time, *Hepatitis C Choices* has been written so that each chapter can be read and understood on its own.

Many people find that reading the entire book provides the most benefit. But for any of a number of reasons, this may be hard to do. If reading the book cover to cover seems overwhelming, we encourage you to read those parts of *Hepatitis C Choices* that are most relevant to your immediate questions and needs. Then come back to other chapters as needed.

You may find medical words in the book that are new to you. These words are italicized. The definitions of these words are in the *Glossary* at the back of the book. Becoming familiar with these words will help you better understand hepatitis C. It might also help you communicate more easily with your healthcare providers. Foreign words also appear in italics. These words are explained in the text but do not appear in the *Glossary*.

Part 1: Information for Everyone with Hepatitis C
These chapters contain information for all people affected by *chronic hepatitis* C. The authors consider this information very important for anyone with chronic hepatitis C regardless of your treatment goals.

Part 2: Hepatitis C Treatment and Management Approaches
These chapters cover treatment options for chronic hepatitis C. Each chapter presents the author's professional view of chronic hepatitis C, and its management and treatment.

Some treatment options have been evaluated in *clinical trials* or other research studies to determine their effectiveness. We have included information about the evidence to support the use of a given treatment if available. This information may come from healthcare providers' personal experience (*anecdotal* evidence), or from formal studies such as *controlled clinical trials*. Overall, evidence from clinical trials is considered to be stronger than anecdotal evidence.

Part 3: Other Topics for People Living with Hepatitis C
These chapters cover topics of concern to specific populations affected by chronic hepatitis C, and other issues of interest to people living with hepatitis C.

Also included in the Appendices are other important documents including:

- matrix showing how chronic hepatitis C is diagnosed
- matrix showing management options for chronic hepatitis C
- additional information about topics covered in the chapters
- a *Resource Directory* for people living with chronic hepatitis C

Purpose of *Hepatitis C Choices*

Hepatitis C Choices was written with several purposes in mind:

- to provide information about chronic hepatitis C to help you make decisions about your treatment and lifestyle
- to provide a balanced view of the currently available treatment options from western medicine and *complementary and alternative medicine* (CAM)
- to help you communicate more effectively with your healthcare providers
- to help you become empowered to be the best *advocate* for your own healthcare

Making Informed Decisions

Potentially life-changing decisions are one aspect of having a serious illness such as chronic hepatitis C. Each of us is unique in how we make decisions. Some people want to know everything they possibly can about their disease. They want to make all their own treatment decisions. Other people prefer to have their healthcare providers make treatment decisions based on their knowledge and expertise. Some prefer having a friend or family member seek out and sort through information. Many use a combination of approaches.

Each person with chronic hepatitis C has his or her own treatment goals. Some consider getting rid of the virus to be their most important goal. Others top priority is enjoying the best possible quality of life. Many have a list of goals with some being more important than others are. Many people make lifestyle changes, while others do not make such choices for personal reasons.

We urge you to identify your personal strengths and limitations. Decide what makes up an acceptable quality of life for you. Knowing these things will help you make healthcare decisions that best suit your personality.

We hope *Hepatitis C Choices* will help you understand your disease and some of the healthcare options available to you. Knowledge empowers you to ask the necessary questions to become your own best advocate. When your questions have been asked and answered, you and your healthcare providers will be in the best possible situation to determine the best treatment approach for you.

Knowing Your Options

You have the right to advocate for yourself to receive the best possible treatment regardless of the source of payment for your healthcare.

In the past, people with chronic hepatitis C often found they had few treatment options and limited opportunity to participate in their own healthcare decisions. Increasingly, healthcare providers and the public are interested in changing this legacy. Being an informed consumer and knowing your rights are particularly important when you are looking for healthcare that is not only of good quality, but also fits your personal needs. This is even more important if you intend to combine or integrate several healing approaches in your hepatitis C treatment plan.

Regaining Control

The day before your hepatitis C diagnosis, you were probably able to say what you hoped to be doing in the near future. The day after your diagnosis, you may have felt that something else had suddenly taken control of your life.

The process of regaining control begins with learning about your disease and your treatment options. Many people newly diagnosed with chronic hepatitis C are relieved to find that it may not be necessary to make an immediate decision about treatment. If your hepatitis C has not progressed significantly <u>and</u> you stop drinking *alcohol*, you may never have to make a decision about aggressive therapy.

Some people with chronic hepatitis C stay healthy by making lifestyle changes in addition to not drinking alcohol. For some, lifestyle changes such as eating a healthier diet, taking vitamins and/or supplements, and exercising regularly have a profound effect on their health and well-being. Others choose homeopathy, naturopathy, traditional Chinese medicine, and/or other CAM disciplines to maintain their general health and keep the virus in check.

> **Regardless of your current disease status, drinking and hepatitis C infection are a dangerous mix. You should not drink alcohol in any form.**

How you go about maintaining your health, and whomever you decide to consult for your healthcare is up to you. However, we urge you to gather information about the different treatment options you are considering. This will help you make informed decisions about what options are best suited to your treatment goals and personality.

Some Additional Thoughts

The decision to begin any treatment is a big step. Only you know if you are ready to take that step. The purpose in creating *Hepatitis C Choices* was not to advocate for one treatment approach over another, but to encourage you to carefully look at all of your options.

Chronic hepatitis C is often a progressive disease, so your options may change over time. The healthcare provider you choose to see is not nearly as important as having a consistent approach to follow your disease. It is important to realize that unless your blood and liver are examined periodically, you cannot know if your disease is progressing.

We encourage you to decide on your treatment goals and discuss all your options and concerns with your healthcare providers. It is often helpful to get a second opinion, or even a third. Choosing healthcare providers you are comfortable speaking with will help you work together as a team. Making decisions that are right for you will make your choices easier to incorporate into your life.

> **It is very important to inform each of your healthcare providers about all of the treatment approaches you are using. This is particularly important if you choose an integrative medicine approach that involves healthcare providers or treatments from several different medical disciplines.**

Hepatitis C Choices was created to help you become the best possible advocate for your own healthcare. We hope it provides useful information to help you make treatment and lifestyle choices that are right for you. However, this book is only a guide, a collection of reference materials. We strongly encourage you to continue to explore your treatment and lifestyle options, and to gather as much information as you need. Doing so can help you make the best possible decisions for your healthcare and your life.

An Important Note to the Reader

This book was created to provide information about a wide variety of approaches to the treatment and management of chronic hepatitis C. The Caring Ambassadors Hepatitis C Program and the authors of *Hepatitis C Choices* believe access to good information leads to better decisions. However, this book is not a substitute for medical advice. It is critical that you consult your healthcare provider about any matter concerning your health, particularly with regard to new or changing *symptoms* that may require medical attention.

Each chapter and section of the book has been authored independently. Therefore, each chapter reflects the unique approach to the treatment of hepatitis C of its author, based on his or her medical discipline and experience. For this reason, an author is responsible only for the accuracy of the information presented in his or her chapter or section. No author can confirm the accuracy of the information presented in any other chapter or section.

Most of the contributors to *Hepatitis C Choices* are members of the Caring Ambassadors Hepatitis C Medical Team. Others are guest authors invited by the Caring Ambassadors Hepatitis C Program. The unifying characteristic of the Hepatitis C Medical Team is a willingness to listen and evaluate the diverse viewpoints and treatment options available to people with chronic hepatitis C. *Hepatitis C Choices* evolved from a consensus within the Hepatitis C Medical Team that a single resource describing the various modalities of treatment available would be useful to people with hepatitis C. Cooperation and open discussion are key components of the interaction among members of the Hepatitis C Medical Team, though individual members remain aligned with their own discipline.

Be aware that the only treatment proven through controlled clinical trials to show sustained *clearance* of the hepatitis C virus (as detected by *HCV* RNA testing of the blood) is *interferon-based antiviral* therapy. Recent studies of pegylated interferon plus *ribavirin* report overall *sustained responses* in 50% to 60% of those treated. In other words, 50% to 60% of people receiving this treatment remain virus-free and are considered *cured*.

We strongly encourage anyone who has significant *fibrosis* on *liver biopsy* to be followed closely for evidence of disease progression. This should include a medical history, physical examination, and laboratory tests. People with *cirrhosis* need to be monitored for *clinical* and biochemical deterioration, and considered for referral to a liver transplant center. If *liver failure* occurs, liver transplantation counseling should be sought immediately. Regular screening for the development of *liver cancer* (*hepatocellular carcinoma*) should be part of any ongoing hepatitis C management plan.

The choice of treatment for hepatitis C is a personal one. What is right for one person may not be so for another. What is right for you will depend on the status of your disease, the health of your liver, your age, lifestyle, treatment goals, and many other factors. We encourage you to carefully assess the information provided here and elsewhere, and to work with your healthcare providers to choose treatment approaches that meet your individual needs and goals.

Overview of Hepatitis C

Robert G. Gish, MD

Introduction

Hepatitis C virus (*HCV*) infection is a leading cause of chronic liver disease across the globe. HCV is estimated to affect 4 to 5 million people in the United States and 180 million people worldwide.[1-4] The estimated number of HCV-infected people in the United States is based on population surveys. The prevalence of hepatitis C in high-risk populations has not been thoroughly studied. Therefore, many hepatitis C experts believe the true number of people infected with HCV is higher than the stated estimates.[3]

> **At least 1 out of every 50 people in the United States has been infected with the hepatitis C virus.**

Nearly two decades after the discovery of HCV, our knowledge about the natural history of *chronic hepatitis* C is still limited. Studies have provided varying estimates of the risk of disease progression with chronic hepatitis C. Typically, chronic hepatitis C is slowly progressive.

An estimated 15% to 45% of people infected with HCV clear the virus from their body without treatment. Another 25% have no *symptoms*, and have consistently normal levels of *liver enzymes* called aminotransferases. This means that approximately 40% to 70% of people infected with HCV either recover or do not develop symptoms.[5] These facts indicate there are people whose *immune systems* are capable of getting rid of HCV. However, for reasons we do not yet understand, others' immune systems allow the virus to persist, leading to potentially serious consequences.

> **Unlike many chronic viruses, hepatitis C is potentially curable with antiviral treatment.**

The Course of Chronic Hepatitis C

Several factors influence the course of chronic hepatitis C. The most significant of these factors include:

- **Age at infection** — Persons infected after age 40 may have disease that is more progressive.[6-9]

- **Alcohol consumption** — *Alcohol* has serious negative effects on people infected with HCV.[8]

- **Sex** — Overall, women (especially those under age 50) do significantly better than men[10,11] with less severity of infection.[12] Women also appear to *spontaneously clear* the hepatitis C virus more frequently than men do.[13-15]

- **Coinfection with *hepatitis B* virus (*HBV*) and/or human immunodeficiency virus (HIV)** — Coinfection with one or both of these viruses leads to faster hepatitis C disease progression.[16] Rapid progression is also seen in people with organ transplants taking immunosuppressant medications.

- ***Fatty liver*** — The presence of fat in the liver is associated with higher degrees of *fibrosis*.[17]

- ***Iron*** — Increased iron in the liver can accelerate progression of HCV or lead to decreased *interferon* response or cure.[18-20]

> **Hepatitis C genotype and viral load do <u>not predict disease progression.</u>**

Viral characteristics such as HCV type (*genotype*) and *viral load* (the amount of virus present in the blood) do not seem to affect the course of the disease. However, these factors are used to determine the length of treatment, and to predict the chance of treatment response.[6]

HCV was once thought to affect only the liver. We now know it can affect nearly any organ in the body. In other words, hepatitis C is a systemic disease. As you read *Chapter 5, Signs and Symptoms that May be Associated with Hepatitis C*, you may find some of the symptoms you thought were caused by something else may actually be caused by HCV. This is important because knowing why you are having a symptom is often the first step in making it less troublesome.

How Hepatitis C Is Diagnosed

Screening: Hepatitis C Antibody Tests

Hepatitis C is diagnosed with a blood test. Most people are initially tested for *HCV antibodies* in the blood. The immune system produces *antibodies* to foreign objects such as viruses and bacteria. When someone is infected with HCV, the body begins producing antibodies specifically designed to search out and destroy HCV.

An HCV antibody test is not currently included in most routine physicals. A doctor generally orders the test only if liver disease is suspected, or if the patient has a history of potential exposure to the hepatitis C virus. Hepatitis C screening is routinely performed on all donated blood.

HCV antibody tests are not always completely accurate. This is especially true in people with a weakened immune system. People with a weakened immune system might not produce enough antibodies to be detected by the antibody test. People with normal immune systems also sometimes have a negative antibody test despite being infected with HCV. This is because in some people, HCV antibodies might not be detected for up to one year after the initial infection.[21] If there is any doubt about the results of the HCV antibody test, people are given another test that detects the HCV virus itself in the blood.

Confirming Hepatitis C: Viral Testing

A diagnosis of current infection with the hepatitis C virus is usually confirmed by testing for the presence of the virus itself in the blood. This type of testing is known as nucleic acid testing or NAT. Different NAT methods are used by different laboratories. Examples of these methods include *polymerase chain reaction (PCR)*, *transcription mediated amplification (TMA)*, and *branched chain deoxyribonucleic acid (b-DNA)*.[22]

Most doctors believe NAT is the most effective way to confirm a diagnosis of HCV. Other tests, such as the *recombinant immunoblot assay (RIBA)*, were originally designed for the blood banking industry, but are sometimes used to confirm an HCV diagnosis.[23]

Anyone suspected of having HCV should have liver *enzyme* tests (*ALT* and *AST*) to check for liver damage. Blood tests for liver function should also be performed. The initial work up for hepatitis C should start with a complete history and physical examination. Initial blood tests typically include:

HCV genotype	*BUN* and *creatinine*	*TSH*	*electrolytes*
PT-INR	*total protein* and *albumin*	*urinanalysis*	uric acid
CBC with differential	AST, ALT, Alk Phos, *GGT*	ron, *TIBC*, and *ferritin*	*glucose*
total bilirubin	uric acid	total *cholesterol* and *triglycerides*	HDL, LDL, VLDL

For more information on laboratory tests, see *Chapter 6, Laboratory Tests and Procedures*.

Acute Phase Hepatitis C

The first six months after being infected with HCV is called *acute phase hepatitis C*. After infection, there is a period of 7 to 8 weeks before there is a rise in liver enzymes. HCV antibodies are usually detectable in the blood 3 to 12 weeks after infection. The virus itself is usually detectable in the blood within 1 to 3 weeks after infection.[24,25]

Most people acutely infected with HCV are *asymptomatic* meaning they do not have any symptoms of disease. However, 25% to 35% of infected people experience a mild illness with vague and *nonspecific* symptoms.

Fifteen percent to 45% of people infected with HCV appear to clear the virus on their own without developing any *secondary condition* or result from the infection. Experts believe clearing the virus is at least partially related to the amount of virus in the initial infection.[26-29] Other factors are also likely to be involved. The process of *spontaneous clearance* is not well understood, and is an area of active medical research.

> **Patients diagnosed with acute hepatitis C infection and rising viral levels are often considered candidates for immediate treatment with interferon and ribavirin.**

If your body does not rid itself of HCV within six months after infection, you are considered to be in the chronic phase of hepatitis C.

Chronic Phase Hepatitis C Infection

The course of chronic phase hepatitis C is usually that of slow disease progression. Most people have no physical *signs* or symptoms of HCV infection during the first 10 to 20 years after infection. Some have only vague, mild symptoms that come and go without presenting much difficulty.

The rate of disease progression in chronic hepatitis C differs from one person to another. The rate at which a person's hepatitis C will progress cannot be accurately determined by the liver enzyme levels, viral load, or HCV genotype.[30,31] It has been noted that people with normal liver enzymes and low viral load usually have milder liver disease with lower-grade liver *inflammation*. However, even these people occasionally develop *fibrosis* or *cirrhosis*. The inability to accurately predict disease progression makes it difficult for healthcare providers to identify people who are most likely to benefit from treatment.

Why Liver Biopsies Are Performed and How They Are Used

Many healthcare providers believe a *liver biopsy* to be the best way to identify those most likely to have progressive hepatitis C disease. This is the group of people most likely to gain the greatest benefit from curative treatment.

A liver biopsy gives your healthcare provider a great deal of information about your liver including:

- the amount of inflammation present
- the presence and amount of fibrosis (scarring)
- the presence and amount of cirrhosis
- the presence and amount of fat
- other causes of chronic liver disease such as too much iron or medication toxicity
- the need for *liver cancer* screening

A liver biopsy can also help your healthcare provider decide if and when an evaluation for a liver transplant is needed. Your healthcare provider uses the information from a liver biopsy to help predict the rate of your disease progression, and to determine whether you are likely to benefit from treatment. Studies have shown that hepatitis C progresses slowly in people with mild liver inflammation and no fibrosis. For people with fibrosis, hepatitis C is generally more rapidly progressive.[12]

A number of new tests are being developed to measure the amount of scar tissue in the liver has without a liver biopsy. These tests are called as noninvasive liver fibrosis tests and include specific products such as FibroSURE™, *FIBROSpect*™, and FibroScan™. To date, none of these tests have been approved for use in the United States by the Food and Drug Administration, although applications are pending. The decision whether to use a noninvasive liver fibrosis test is something each patient should decide carefully with his/her doctor. As treatments become more effective, the role of liver biopsy and other tests to assess liver fibrosis in the management of hepatitis C may change.

> **Liver biopsy remains the "gold standard" for determining disease status in hepatitis C patients.**

Your healthcare provider will consider a number of factors before suggesting a change from monitoring hepatitis C to treating with curative intent therapy. These factors typically include age, general health, likelihood of response to treatment, and other illnesses you may have such as *HIV*, heart disease, kidney disease, and others. Other considerations are also taken into account such as the length of therapy required, cost, frequency of monitoring, past medical history, side effects, and your ability to take the medication as directed. Your healthcare provider should discuss all *contraindications* to any therapy he or she recommends to you.

For more information about liver biopsy results, see *Chapter 4.1, Liver Disease Progression*.

HCV Genotype

The hepatitis C family of viruses is divided into groups called genotypes. There are 6 known genotypes and more than 90 subtypes of the hepatitis C virus.[32] The types are numbered 1 through 6, and the subtypes are labeled a, b, c, and so on, in order of their discovery.

Presently, *genotype testing* is used to determine the duration of *interferon-based treatment*, to help healthcare providers advise people about their potential treatment response, and for research purposes. Genotype testing is an important part of standard, western medical care for people with HCV infection who are being counseled about interferon-based treatment. The reason is that researchers have found certain strains of HCV are more likely to respond to interferon-based treatment than others are. Further, some strains respond more quickly than others do and require a shorter treatment interval. Therefore, it is very important to know the genotype and subtype of HCV with which you are infected. If you are infected with one of the strains that is hard to treat, your healthcare provider may advise a longer than normal course of treatment to see if you might eventually respond.

You may hear the term *quasispecies* in relation to HCV genotype. Quasispecies occur because HCV mutates freely, causing diverse genetic strains in each infected person. The longer you have been infected with HCV, the more likely you are to have a number of quasispecies of HCV in your body. One small study found changes in quasispecies were associated with levels of the liver enzyme ALT during the acute phase of infection. This finding suggests that the formation of quasispecies might be related to the severity of HCV infection.[33] Additional research is need to clarify the role of quasispecies in hepatitis C disease management and treatment.

Researchers are working to discover why different HCV genotypes respond differently to interferon-based treatment. Currently, genotypes 1a and 1b account for 65% to 75% of chronic HCV in the United States. While genotypes 1a and 1b experience the lowest response rate to interferon-based treatment, you should not allow your genotype alone to deter you from treatment. People with all genotypes have cleared the virus. Remember, your genotype does not determine how your disease will progress.

The *sustained response* rate for genotype 1 following treatment with *pegylated* interferon and *ribavirin* is approximately 40%.[34,35] However, for patients who adhere to a full year of treatment at full dose, the viral response rate or "cure" can be up to 50%.[36] With genotype 2 or 3, response rates with pegylated interferon plus ribavirin can increase from an average of 70% to 80% up to 90% with strict adherence and full dose therapy.[37-40]

The duration of interferon-based therapy varies depending on genotype, and is another area of ongoing medical research. See *Chapter 8, Western (Allopathic) Medicine* for additional information on duration of interferon-based therapy.

No studies are available to date showing that genotype influences symptom or disease response to *complementary and alternative medicine (CAM)* treatments. Further, there are no data to date proving that CAM therapies cure HCV disease (that is, clear the virus from the body).

Liver Failure

Liver failure is a common cause of death in the United States, claiming more than 30,000 lives each year.[41] Hepatitis C is a common cause of liver failure and is a very serious, growing public health problem.[42] While the number of new HCV infections has declined in the United States, it is believed that the number of people who will develop complications of advanced liver disease will increase over the next 10 to 20 years.[42,43] Approximately 20% to 30% of people with chronic hepatitis C will develop cirrhosis over a 20 to 30 year period. Ten percent of those who develop cirrhosis will eventually progress to end-stage liver disease.[44,45,46]

It is important to remember that a diagnosis of cirrhosis is not a death sentence! Even if you have a cirrhotic liver, unless you develop complications, you can live a long, productive life. Nonetheless, people with cirrhosis should discuss the need for liver cancer screening with their medical practitioners.

Liver Transplantation

Liver failure due to chronic hepatitis C is the most common reason for liver transplantation in the United States. There are currently almost 17,000 people waiting for a liver transplant in this country, but only about 6,000 livers are available for transplant each year.[47]

Evidence to date shows that all patients with chronic HCV infect their new liver shortly after transplantation. *Clinical trials* are currently underway to try to interrupt this process.[48,49] However, at this time, HCV infection of a transplanted liver is expected, and therefore, ongoing disease monitoring and discussion about treatment must take place for all liver transplant patients.[50,51]

Liver transplant patients must take medicines called antirejection drugs to keep the body from rejecting the new organ. Antirejection drugs suppress the immune system. This can cause HCV disease to progress faster than it would otherwise. Your healthcare provider will work closely with you to decide if you should consider using *antiviral* therapy after your liver transplant.

It is very important to talk with your healthcare providers about all treatments and/or supplements you are taking or are considering taking. This information is important in making recommendations regarding liver transplantation.

How Hepatitis C Is Transmitted

Blood-to-Blood Contact

HCV is transmitted from one person to another through blood-to-blood contact. In other words, a person is infected with the hepatitis C virus only if their blood system comes into contact with another person's HCV-infected blood. Blood-to-blood contact occurs in a variety of ways, some very obvious and others you may not have considered.

Examples of blood-to-blood contact that can lead to HCV transmission include:

- receiving blood or blood products prior to 1992
- sharing drug paraphernalia, even once
- being stuck by a used blood needle
- being on kidney dialysis
- having a tattoo or body piercing done in an unsterile environment
- having sexual activity that involves contact with blood
- having a job that exposed you to blood
- sharing personal care items (razors, toothbrushes, nail clippers, etc.) with others
- having been incarcerated
- having been in combat in the military

Pregnancy and Breast Feeding

The Centers for Disease Control and Prevention (CDC) report that the risk of transmission of HCV from an infected mother to her infant at birth is approximately 4% (that is, the baby is infected in 4 out of every 100 births to mothers with chronic hepatitis C). In mothers who have both HCV and HIV, the risk of transmitting hepatitis C to the baby goes up to approximately 19%. There is currently no medication to prevent the transmission of hepatitis C from a mother to her baby.

CDC states that there is no evidence that hepatitis C is spread through breast milk. However, nursing mothers should consult with their doctor if there are breaks in the skin and/or bleeding of the nipples associated with breastfeeding.

Sexual Intercourse and Other Sexual Activity

Hepatitis C is rarely transmitted through sexual intercourse though it does occur. Among the general population, a rate of sexual transmission of 3% or less is considered accurate by most experts.[52] However, increased levels of risk have been reported[53,54] in association with:

- multiple sexual partners
- activity that involves blood-to-blood exposure
- the presence of a sexually transmitted infection
- coinfection with HIV have been reported to be important factors in new hepatitis C infections. CDC states there is no evidence of HCV transmission associated with oral sex.

In general, most experts agree that sexual transmission of HCV through intercourse plays a role in the ongoing spread of the disease, but that this route of transmission is uncommon overall.

If you have any questions about the sexual transmission of hepatitis C, talk with your doctor. All people, regardless of health challenges, are sexual beings and your doctor understands that sexual health is an important component of your overall health.

Summary

The decision to begin any hepatitis C treatment is a big step. Only you know if you are ready to take that step. Once you have decided on your treatment goals, discuss all of your options and concerns with your healthcare providers. It is often helpful to get a second opinion, or even a third. Choosing healthcare providers you are comfortable speaking with will help you work together as a team.

> **Making treatment decisions that fit your goals, personality, and lifestyle will make your choices easier to incorporate into your life.**

Taking steps to enhance your general health by doing things such as eating a healthy diet, stopping all alcohol consumption, and attaining a normal body weight are important parts of your treatment plan. Exercise, spiritual practices, massage, acupuncture, herbs, and other complementary therapies can all have a role in attaining better health.

We know a great deal about hepatitis C. However, there is even more we do not yet know. Good *clinical* research is needed in all areas of hepatitis C management including western medicine, naturopathy, traditional Chinese medicine, Ayurveda, homeopathy, nutritional support, and other complementary therapies. This research will lead to the next advances in the care of those living with hepatitis C.

Therapy for hepatitis C is evolving rapidly. As a result, treatment recommendations are likely to change every few years. We anticipate new approaches in the near future that will improve the effectiveness of treatment for those living with HCV.

References

1. Alter MJ, Kruszon-Morgan D, Nainan OV, et al. The prevalence of hepatitis C virus infection in the United States, 1988 through 1994. *N Engl J Med*. 1999;341(8):556-562.
2. Alter MJ. Epidemiology of hepatitis C. *Hepatology*. 1997;26(3 Suppl 1):62-65S.
3. Gish RG, et al. Management of hepatitis C virus in special populations: patient and treatment considerations. *Clin Gastroenterol Hepatol* 2005; 3(4):311-318.
4. World Health Organization Available at: http://www.who.int/vaccine_research/diseases/viral_cancers/en/index2.html. Accessed July 24, 2008
5. EASL: International Consensus Conference on Hepatitis C Consensus Statement. *J Hepatol*. 1999;30:956-961.
6. Amarapurkar D. Natural history of hepatitis C virus infection. *J Gastroenterol Hepatol*. 2000;15(Suppl E):105-110.
7. Lucidarme D, Dumas F, Arpurt JP, et al. Rapid progress of cirrhosis in hepatitis C: the role of age at the time of viral contamination. *Presse Med*. 1998;27(13):608-611.
8. Bortolotti F, Faggion S, Con P. Natural history of chronic viral hepatitis in childhood. *Acta Gastroenterol Belg*. 1998;61(2):198-201.
9. Hutlin Y. et al. Global Burden of Disease (GBD) for Hepatitis C. *J Clin Pharmacol*. 2004; 44; 20
10. Datz C, Cramp M, Haas T, et al. The natural course of hepatitis C virus infection 18 years after an epidemic outbreak of non-A, non-B hepatitis in a plasmapheresis centre. *Gut*. 1999;44(4):563-567.
11. Poynard T, Bedossa P, Opolon P. Natural history of liver fibrosis progression in patients with chronic hepatitis C. The OBSVIRC, METAVIR, CLINIVIR, and DOSVIRC groups. *Lancet*. 1997;349(9055):825-832.
12. Kuboki M, Shinzawa H, Shao L, et al. A cohort study of hepatitis C virus (HCV) infection in an HCV epidemic area of Japan: age and sex-related seroprevalence of anti-HCV antibody, frequency of viremia, biochemical abnormality and histological changes. *Liver*. 1999;19(2):88-96.
13. Alric L, Fort M, Izopet J, et al. Study of host- and virus-related factors associated with spontaneous hepatitis C virus clearance. *Tissue Antigens*. 2000;56(2):154-158.
14. Inoue G, Horiike N, Michitaka K, Onji M. Hepatitis C virus clearance is prominent in women in an endemic area . *J Gastroenterol Hepatol*. 2000;15(9):1054-1058.
15. Yamakawa Y, Sata M, Suzuki H, Noguchi S, Tanikawa K. Higher elimination rate of hepatitis C virus among women. *J Viral Hepat*. 1996;3(6):317-321.
16. Alberti A, Chemello L, Benvegnù L. Natural history of hepatitis C. *J Hepatol*. 1999;31(Suppl 1):17-24.
17. Hourigan LF, Macdonald GA, Purdie D, et al. Fibrosis in chronic hepatitis C correlates significantly with body mass index and steatosis. *Hepatology*. 1999;29(4):1215-1219.
18. Eisenbach C, Gehrke SG, Stremmel W. Iron, the HFE gene, and hepatitis C. *Clin Liver Dis* 2004; 8(4):775-viii.
19. Fujita N. et al. Hepatic oxidative DNA damage correlates with iron overload in chronic hepatitis C patients. *Free Radic Biol Med*. 2007 Feb 1;42(3):353-62.
20. Fujita N. et al. Comparison of hepatic oxidative DNA damage in patients with chronic hepatitis B and C. *J Viral Hepat*. 2008 Jul;15(7):498-507.
21. Gretch DR. Diagnostic tests for hepatitis C. *Hepatology*. 1997;26(3 Suppl 1):43-47S.
22. de Medina M, Schiff ER. Hepatitis C: diagnostic assays. *Semin Liver Dis*. 1995;15(1):33-40.
23. Atrah HI, Ahmed MM. Hepatitis C virus seroconversion by a third generation ELISA screening test in blood donors. *J Clin Path*.

1996;49:254-255.

24. Dienstag JL. Non-A, non-B hepatitis. I. Recognition, epidemiology and clinical features. *Gastroenterology.* 1983; 85(2):439-462.

25. Marcellin P. Hepatitis C: the clinical spectrum of the disease. *J Hepatol.* 1999;31(Suppl 1):9-16.

26. Barrett S, et al. The natural course of hepatitis C virus infection after 22 years in a unique homogenous cohort: spontaneous viral clearance and chronic HCV infection. *Gut* 2001 Sep 2001;423-430.

27. Afdhal NH. The natural history of hepatitis C. *Semin Liver Dis* 2004; 24 Suppl 2:3-8.

28. Heller T, Rehermann B. Acute hepatitis C: a multifaceted disease. *Semin Liver Dis* 2005; 25(1):7-17.

29. Zhang M, et al. Correlates of spontaneous clearance of hepatitis C virus among people with hemophilia. *Blood* 2005.

30. Seeff LB. Natural history of hepatitis C. *Hepatology.* 1997;26(3 Suppl 1):21-28S.

31. Hoofnagle JH. Hepatitis C: the clinical spectrum of disease. *Hepatology.* 1997;26(3 Suppl 1):15-20S.

32. Stuyver L, Wyseur A, van Arnhem W, Hernandez F, Maertens G. Second-generation line probe assay for hepatitis C virus genotyping. *J Clin Microbiol* 1996;34:2259-2266.

33. Yuki N, Hayashi N, et al. Relation of disease activity during chronic hepatitis C infection to complexity of hypervariable region 1 quasispecies. *Hepatology.* 1997;25(2):439-444.

34. Shepherd J, et al.Pegylated interferon alpha-2a and -2b in combination with ribavirin in the treatment of chronic hepatitis C: a systematic review and economic evaluation. *Health Technol Assess.* 2004 Oct;8(39):iii-iv, 1-125.

35. Siebert U, et al. Effectiveness and cost-effectiveness of initial combination therapy with interferon/peginterferon plus ribavirin in patients with chronic hepatitis C in Germany: a health technology assessment commissioned by the German Federal Ministry of Health and Social Security. *Int J Technol Assess Health Care.* 2005 Winter;21(1):55-65.

36. Reddy KR, et al.Impact of ribavirin dose reductions in hepatitis C virus genotype 1 patients completing peginterferon alfa-2a/ribavirin treatment. *Clin Gastroenterol Hepatol.* 2008 Mar;6(3):367.

37. McHutchison JG, Gordon SC, Schiff ER, et al. Interferon alfa-2b alone or in combination with ribavirin as initial treatment for chronic hepatitis C. *N Engl J Med.* 1998;339(21):1485-1492.

38. McHutchison JG, Fried MW. Current therapy for hepatitis C: pegylated interferon and ribavirin. *Clin Liver Dis.* 2003;7(1):149-161.

39. Fried MW, Shiffman ML, Reddy KR, et al. Peginterferon alfa-2a plus ribavirin for chronic hepatitis C virus infection. *N Engl J Med.* 2002;347(13):975-982.

40. Manns MP, McHutchison JG, Gordon SC, et al. Peginterferon alfa-2b plus ribavirin compared with interferon alfa-2b plus ribavirin for initial treatment of chronic hepatitis C: a randomised trial. *Lancet.* 2001;358(9286):958-965.

41. Hsiang-Ching Kung, Ph.D. et al. National Vital Statistics Volume 56, Number 10 April 24, 2008 Deaths: Final Data for 2005

42. Wise, M. et al. Changing trends in hepatitis C related mortality in the United States. *Hepatology*, Vol 47, No 4, 2008:1128

43. Takahashi M, Yamada G, Miyamoto R, et al. Natural course of chronic hepatitis C. *Am J Gastroenterol.* 1993;88(2):240-243.

44. National Institutes of Health Consensus Development Conference Panel. Statement: management of hepatitis C. *Hepatology.* 1997;26(Suppl 1):2-10S.

45. Yano M, Kumada H, Kage M, et al. The long-term pathological evolution of chronic hepatitis C. *Hepatology.* 1996;23(6):1334-1340.

46. Di Bisceglie AM. Hepatitis C and hepatocellular carcinoma. *Hepatology.* 1997;26(Suppl 1):34-38S.

47. Organ Procurement Transplantation Network. Available at: http://www.optn.org/latestData/rptData.asp. Accessed July 8, 2008

48. Nudo CG. et al. Effect of pretransplant hepatitis C virus RNA status on posttransplant outcome. *Transplant Proc.* 2008 Jun;40(5):1449-55

49. Lodato F. et al. Peg-interferon alfa-2b and ribavirin for the treatment of genotype 1 hepatitis C recurrence after liver transplantation. *Aliment Pharmacol Ther.* 2008 Jun 11.[Epub ahead of print]

50. Triantos C, et al.Liver transplantation and hepatitis C virus: systematic review of antiviral therapy. *Transplantation* 2005; 79(3):261-268.

51. Gruener NH, Jung MC, Schirren CA. Recurrent hepatitis C virus infection after liver transplantation: natural course, therapeutic approach and possible mechanisms of viral control. *J Antimicrob Chemother* 2004; 54(1):17-20.

52. Cavalheiro N. Sexual transmission of hepatitis C. *Rev Inst Med trop S Paulo* [serial online]. 2007; 49(5): 271-277.

53. Wang CC, et al. Acute hepatitis C in a contemporary US cohort: modes of acquisition and factors influencing viral clearance. *J Infect Dis.* 2007;196(10):1474-82.

54. Terrault NA. Sexual activity as a risk factor for hepatitis C. *Hepatology* 2002; 36(5 Suppl):S99-S105.

ALCOHOL AND HEPATITIS C

Douglas R. LaBrecque, MD and Lorren Sandt

Introduction

The three most important factors associated with rapid progression of *chronic hepatitis* C are age over 40 years, male gender, and *alcohol* consumption.[1,2,3] You cannot change your age or sex, but you <u>can</u> eliminate alcohol.

> **Eliminating alcohol is the single most important lifestyle change you can make to decrease your risk for developing complications from chronic hepatitis C.**

"But I Only Drink Beer"

Most people in the United States who drink alcohol do so socially. You may be used to having a glass of wine with dinner or a mixed drink at a party. However, if you have *hepatitis* C, <u>any</u> consumption of alcohol is potentially damaging to your liver. Whether alcohol is consumed in a drink, cough syrup, or another nonprescription product, alcohol is an enemy to people infected with the hepatitis C virus (*HCV*). Alcohol should be <u>completely</u> avoided.

The primary cause of liver damage from alcohol is the alcohol itself. It makes no difference whether the alcohol is contained in beer, wine, or hard liquor. A twelve--ounce can of beer contains the same amount of alcohol as a four-ounce glass of wine or a one-ounce shot of hard liquor. That means drinking a six-pack of beer is the same as having six shots or six mixed drinks. "Doubles" obviously double the amount of alcohol you are consuming. Expensive drinks are just as damaging as cheap ones.

What We Have Learned About Alcohol and HCV

Several studies have shown that a frighteningly high number of people suffering from alcoholism also have hepatitis C. The numbers range from 11% to 36%. Compare this to the 1.8% HCV infection rate in the general population.[4,5] Among alcoholics with liver disease, as many as 51% are infected with HCV. This is 4 to 10 times more frequent than in alcoholics without liver disease.[6-11]

Studies have shown that alcohol abuse (4 to 5 drinks per day) accelerates the progression of liver damage and *fibrosis* associated with chronic HCV.[1,6,12-21] In a study of 6,664 people in France, excessive alcohol intake doubled the risk of developing *cirrhosis* and increased the rate of fibrosis progression by 34% per year.[22]

Research has clearly shown that the severity of liver disease in alcoholics increases in the presence of HCV. In a study from Italy, the incidence of cirrhosis was ten times higher in alcoholics who had HCV than in alcoholics who did not.[23] Another study found the survival rate for alcoholics who had *HCV antibodies* was lower than for alcoholics who did not have HCV infection.[24] In addition, several studies have found a significantly increased risk of developing *liver cancer* among heavy alcohol drinkers who also have HCV.[25-28]

Some studies have shown an association between increasing levels of HCV with increasing alcohol consumption, and reduction of *viral load* when alcohol is avoided. These findings suggest that alcohol may have an effect on HCV *replication* (viral reproduction).[29-31] However, a recent review article reported that this association is inconsistent.[32]

Alcoholics have an increase in the number and complexity of HCV *quasispecies*.[34] This may explain why alcoholics tend to have a lower response rate to HCV *antiviral* therapy than nonalcoholics. Several studies have shown a decreased rate of *viral clearance* among people who drink alcohol compared to those who do not drink. Studies have shown an even lower frequency of achieving a *durable response*.[35-39] This decreased response rate to antiviral therapy continues for up to six months after eliminating all alcohol intake. Most experts recommend at least six months of *abstinence* from alcohol before attempting *interferon-based therapy*. Other effects of alcohol may contribute to the greater severity of HCV disease in those who consume it. Some of these effects are listed below.

- possible changes in *gene* expression
- reduction in the *immune system*'s ability to respond to and fight off viruses
- inhibition of the liver's ability to regenerate and repair itself
- stimulation of fibrosis development in the liver
- increased *iron* deposition in the liver

Most of the studies discussed above clearly show increased liver damage suffered by people with HCV who have more than 4 to 5 drinks of alcohol per day.[20,40-42] Other studies show liver damage with as little as <u>one</u> drink per day. Currently, the amount of alcohol consumption that is considered safe for healthy individuals is one drink per day for women and two for men. However, no amount of alcohol can be considered safe if you are infected with HCV.[20,43] People with HCV are strongly urged to eliminate <u>all</u> alcohol consumption.

How Alcohol Damages The Liver

Alcohol is a poisonous chemical that the liver has to break down. As the liver breaks down alcohol, byproducts such as *acetaldehyde* are formed. Some byproducts produced by the breakdown of alcohol are more toxic to the body than alcohol itself.[44]

Inflammation is the body's response to tissue damage or infection. Long-term alcohol use abnormally prolongs the inflammatory process. This leads to an overproduction of *free radicals*, molecules that can destroy healthy liver tissue and interfere with some of its important functions such as energy production. Alcohol can also interfere with the production of *antioxidants*. Antioxidants are one of the body's natural defenses against free radical damage. This combination of alcohol effects can lead to liver damage.[45]

Cytokines are produced by liver cells and the immune system in response to infection or cell damage. Alcohol use increases cytokine levels.[46] Cirrhosis development involves the interaction of certain cytokines and specialized liver cells such as *stellate cells*. In a normal liver, stellate cells function as storage depots for *vitamin A*. When activated by cytokines, stellate cells divide rapidly to increase in number. Activated stellate cells lose their vitamin A stores and begin to produce scar tissue. They also constrict blood vessels, reducing the delivery of oxygen to liver cells.[47,48] Acetaldehyde, a byproduct of alcohol break down, may activate stellate cells, directly causing liver scarring without *inflammation*.[49, 50]

Normal scar formation is part of the wound healing process. Cell death and inflammation caused by alcohol can result in abnormal liver scarring. Scarring may distort the liver's internal structure and interfere with liver function. Scarring in the liver is called fibrosis. Fibrosis that progresses to the point of distorting the structure of the liver is called cirrhosis.

Women, Alcohol, and Hepatitis C

Studies show that women are more susceptible to the damaging effects of alcohol than men are. More alcoholic women die from cirrhosis than alcoholic men.[51] The reason for this difference between men and women is not entirely clear. However, there appears to be several contributing factors.

- Men generally have greater body mass and fluid content than women do. This means women have higher concentrations of alcohol in their blood than men do have after consuming the same amount of alcohol.[46, 52-56]

- Women's livers appear to *metabolize* alcohol at a faster rate than men's do, most likely because women's livers are larger compared to their body size than those of men.[57,58]

- Estrogens (female *hormones*) may add to the effects of alcohol in women's livers.[59]

About Alcohol Use

For most people, drinking alcohol is an occasional social activity. For others, drinking alcohol becomes a chronic, progressive disorder called alcoholism. The hallmark of alcoholism is a strong need to drink despite negative consequences including serious health or social problems. Like many diseases, alcoholism has a predictable course and recognizable symptoms. The occurrence of alcoholism is influenced by genetic and environmental factors. We continue to learn more about these factors everyday.

We do not yet have a *cure* for alcoholism. However, alcoholism is a treatable disorder. Alcoholism is a lifelong problem. Even an alcoholic who has been sober for many years may still be at risk of relapsing and should avoid all alcoholic beverages.

Alcoholism has little to do with what kind of alcohol you drink, how long you have been drinking, or even how much alcohol you drink. The defining characteristic of alcoholism is the uncontrollable need for alcohol. This description helps us understand why most alcoholics cannot just "use a little willpower" to stop drinking. He or she is usually in the grip of a powerful craving for alcohol. This craving can feel as strong as the need for food or water. While some people are able to recover on their own, the majority of alcoholics need outside help. With support and treatment, many people with alcoholism are able to stop drinking and rebuild their lives. Cutting down on drinking does not work for an alcoholic. Stopping alcohol use completely is necessary for successful recovery. This is especially important for people living with chronic hepatitis C.

Even individuals who are determined to stay sober may suffer one or more slips or *relapses* before achieving long-term sobriety. Relapses are very common and do not signify failure. Nor do they mean a person cannot eventually recover from alcoholism. Every day a recovering alcoholic stays sober prior to a relapse is extremely valuable time. This time is important for both the individual and his or her family. Sober time also gives the liver an opportunity to repair itself. If a relapse occurs, it is very important to try to stop drinking again and to get whatever additional support is needed to *abstain* from drinking.

Help for Alcohol Abuse

Acknowledging you need help for an alcohol problem is difficult. Many alcoholics do not begin to deal with their alcoholism until a significant life-changing or life-threatening event occurs. Recovering alcoholics often refer to this as "hitting bottom." The event that represents hitting bottom is different for each person. It depends on your personality and life circumstances. While it is not necessary to hit bottom in order to begin the recovery process, it is often the case. This is because denial is very prevalent in alcoholism. Denial is a coping strategy whereby people avoid dealing with difficult situations by denying that they exist. It is difficult for a person in denial to recognize and understand the effects alcohol has on him or her. This is also true for family members and friends who are frequently in denial with regard to a loved one's alcoholism.

Many people find the following quiz on drinking helpful. It may help you recognize whether alcohol is a problem in your life.

- Do you drink alone when you feel angry or sad?

- Does your drinking ever make you late for work?

- Does your drinking worry your family?

- Do you ever drink after telling yourself you won't?

- Do you ever forget what you did while you were drinking?

- Do you get headaches or have a hangover after you have been drinking?

If you answered yes to one or more of these questions, you may have a problem with alcohol.

Many people feel uncomfortable discussing their drinking habits even with a healthcare provider or a personal or spiritual advisor. This often stems from some common misconceptions in our society about alcoholism. There is a myth in our society that an alcohol problem is a sign of moral weakness. As a result, you may feel that to seek help is to admit a shameful defect in your character. Unfortunately, family and friends may support your denial for the same reason. The truth is that alcoholism is a disease. It is no more a sign of weakness than is asthma or diabetes.

Moving Forward

Even if alcohol is taking a significant negative toll on your life, it can be very difficult to begin taking steps to address the problem. This is because what lies ahead is unknown. However, eliminating alcohol from your life has an enormous payoff. It is a chance for a healthier, more rewarding life.

Because alcohol has a tremendous impact on the health of people with chronic hepatitis C, your healthcare provider will probably ask you several questions about your alcohol use. If your healthcare provider determines that you are not alcohol dependent but are involved in a pattern of alcohol abuse, he or she can assist you in the following ways.

- Help you examine the benefits of stopping an unhealthy drinking pattern.

- Help you set a drinking goal for yourself. Some people choose to abstain from alcohol. Others prefer to limit the amount they drink. *Appendix I* contains a worksheet to help you cut down on your drinking. Remember, with hepatitis C, the goal is no alcohol.

- Help you examine situations that trigger unhealthy drinking patterns and develop new ways of handling those situations so you can achieve your drinking goal.

- Recommend a specialist and/or treatment program if you are having difficulty eliminating alcohol from your life.

Your healthcare provider may determine you are dependent on alcohol. He or she may recommend that you see a specialist in diagnosing and treating alcoholism. As hard as this may be to hear, try to understand that your healthcare provider is doing his/her best to help you be well. Ask your provider to explain your treatment choices.

Your healthcare provider may delay HCV treatment if he or she determines you have an alcohol problem. Studies have proven that interferon-based therapy is much less effective in people who drink alcohol than in those who do not drink.[60, 61] For this reason, many healthcare providers will not offer treatment of any kind for chronic hepatitis C until all alcohol use has been stopped for at least six months.[39]

The nature of treatment for alcohol abuse depends on the severity of the problem. It also depends on the resources available in the community. Treatment may include detoxification. Detoxification is the process of safely getting alcohol out of your system. Treatment for alcoholism may involve one or more of the following components: prescription medications, individual counseling, and group counseling. Promising counseling techniques teach recovering alcoholics to identify situations and feelings that trigger the urge to drink. This can help you find new ways to cope with stressful situations that do not include alcohol use. Treatment for alcoholism may be provided in a hospital, residential treatment setting, or on an outpatient basis.

Involvement of friends and family members is important to the recovery process. Many programs offer brief marital counseling and family therapy as part of the treatment process. Some programs also link individuals with vital community resources such as legal assistance, job training, childcare, and parenting classes.

Treatment for alcoholism may require a combination of social support and drug therapy. When faced with the anxiety and fears associated with hepatitis C, you may feel the urge to turn to alcohol. Remember, you are not alone. Reach out and get help to remain alcohol-free.

A few of the common treatment options available for eliminating alcohol from your life are outlined below. Research has shown that no single treatment option is superior to another. Data from a large *clinical trial* that examined the efficacy of different treatment approaches for alcoholism found that the quality of care is more important than the structure of the treatment delivery.[62]

BRIEF INTERVENTIONS

Many people with alcohol-related problems receive counseling from primary care doctors or nurses in a few office visits.[63] This form of treatment is known as brief intervention. It generally consists of straightforward information about the negative consequences of alcohol consumption.

It also gives practical advice on strategies for eliminating alcohol from your life. Information is provided about community resources to achieve alcohol moderation or abstinence.[64,65] Most brief interventions are designed to help people at risk for developing alcohol-related problems. They are also used to help people without alcoholism reduce alcohol consumption.

Alcohol-dependent people are encouraged to enter specialized treatment programs where the goal is complete abstinence.[64]

STRUCTURED OUTPATIENT THERAPY

Structured outpatient treatment for alcohol abuse usually spans several months. It typically involves educational lectures, group therapy, and one-on-one counseling. The objectives and activities of outpatient treatment typically include a combination of the following:

- develop an understanding of substance abuse and addiction
- identify how alcohol has affected the participant's life
- instill greater self-awareness
- identify and understand factors that contribute to alcohol abuse
- learn effective communication skills
- understand factors that contribute to relapse and how to prevent them
- begin participation in a community-based support program such as Alcoholics Anonymous (AA)

INPATIENT THERAPY

Residential or inpatient treatment takes place in a dormitory-like setting. Clients often share a room and live in the facility for at least 30 days. Some clients stay for several months depending on individual circumstances and needs. Programs vary from one facility to another, but many are based on 12-step program principles such as those of AA. The social setting allows people who are facing a similar challenge to share experiences and support one another. Typically, clients attend lectures, meetings, group therapy, and individual therapy throughout the day.

In a residential facility, a client's physical and mental status can be closely monitored. The temporary protection of a residential treatment facility provides clients a safe place to begin rebuilding their lives without the distractions of work or other pressures. An essential component of residential treatment is making plans for how to maintain sobriety after leaving the facility.

Some facilities offer part-time residential treatment for clients who cannot or do not choose to take time off work. Clients continue to attend work, but spend the rest of their time in the treatment facility. These programs typically last 30 to 60 days.

Sober-living homes are another residential treatment option. Clients who have been through full-time residential treatment may transition to a sober-living home after completing their primary program. Clients live in the facility for an extended period while working on rebuilding their lives. This type of facility is often useful for people who have been through treatment in the past, but have relapsed after returning to their usual environment.

COUPLES THERAPY
Evidence indicates that involvement of a nonalcoholic partner in a treatment program can improve participation by the person with alcoholism. This support increases the likelihood that the alcoholic person will change his or her drinking behavior after treatment ends.[66] There are different approaches to couples therapy. Most of these include shared activities, and learning communication and conflict resolution skills.[67] Partners of people in treatment for alcohol abuse or dependence are often encouraged to also discontinue drinking alcohol. It can be quite difficult for an alcoholic to abstain if his or her partner continues to drink.

MOTIVATIONAL ENHANCEMENT THERAPY
Motivational enhancement therapy (MET) was developed in the late 1990's for a large clinical trial called Project MATCH sponsored by the National Institute on Alcohol Abuse and Alcoholism. MET continues to be used as a successful treatment approach for alcoholism. It begins with the assumption that the responsibility and capacity for change lie within the individual.[68,69] Therapy begins by providing individualized feedback about the effects of the person's drinking. The therapist and client explore the benefits of abstinence. Together, they review treatment options and design a plan to implement treatment goals.

PHARMACOTHERAPY
Medications are available for blocking alcohol-brain interactions that might promote alcoholism. People with HCV should not take any of these medications before speaking to a healthcare provider because taking one of these medications may be harmful to the liver. Your healthcare provider will review the drugs available and determine if any are appropriate for you.

SELF-HELP PROGRAMS
Self-help groups are the most commonly used programs for alcohol-related problems.[70] Alcoholics Anonymous is the most widely known of these self-help groups. AA describes itself as a "worldwide fellowship of men and women who help each other to stay sober." It offers a 12-step program that has been effective for many people seeking to eliminate alcohol from their lives. Alcoholics can become involved with AA before entering professional treatment for alcoholism, as a part of it, or as aftercare. The AA approach is well known, but the program has not been studied in clinical trials.[71] This is due to an essential requirement of the program that people remain anonymous. In AA, only first names are used.

The benefits of AA may be partially due to the replacement of the participant's social network of drinking friends with a fellowship of AA members who can provide motivation and support for maintaining abstinence.[70,72] AA's approach often results in the development of new coping skills. Many of these skills are similar to those taught in more structured treatment settings. These skills can lead to reduced alcohol consumption.[70,73]

Most treatment programs for alcoholism include AA meetings. AA is generally recognized as an effective support program for recovering alcoholics. However, not everyone responds to AA's style and message. If AA is not for you, other recovery programs are available. Even those who are helped by AA find it usually works best in combination with other forms of treatment. This may include individual counseling and/or medical care.

The Final Word

No studies have ever determined a safe amount of alcohol to drink. If you have HCV, the authors of this book strongly recommend you eliminate <u>all</u> alcohol from your life. You will live better and longer!

Note: Much of the information in this chapter was obtained from the National Institute on Alcohol Abuse and Alcoholism (NIAAA). For additional information, visit the NIAAA Internet site at www.niaaa.nih.gov.

Resources

For more information on alcohol abuse and alcoholism, contact the following organizations.

Al-Anon Family Group Headquarters

1600 Corporate Landing Parkway
Virginia Beach, VA 23454-5617
Internet address: www.al-anon.alateen.org
Al-Anon headquarters provides referrals to local Al-Anon groups, which are support groups for spouses and other significant adults in an alcoholic person's life. They also provide referrals to Alateen groups, which offer support to children of alcoholics.
Locations of Al-Anon or Alateen meetings worldwide can be obtained by calling the toll-free number, (888) 425-2666, Monday through Friday, 8 AM to 6 PM (EST).
Informational materials can be obtained on line or by calling (757) 563-1600

Alcoholics Anonymous (AA) World Services

Box 459
New York, NY 10163
(212) 870-3400
Internet address: www.alcoholics-anonymous.org
This organization makes referrals to local AA groups and provides informational materials about the AA program. Many cities and towns also have a local AA office listed in the telephone directory.

Faces and Recovery

1010 Vermont Ave. #708
Washington, DC 20005
 (202) 737-0690
Internet address: www.facesandvoicesofrecovery.org
Faces & Voices of Recovery is a national campaign of individuals and organizations joining together with a united voice to *advocate* for public action to deliver the power, possibility and proof of recovery. Faces & Voices of Recovery is governed by a diverse group of recovery advocates from around the country and supports local recovery advocacy by increasing access to research, policy, organizing and technical support; facilitating relationships among local and regional groups; improving access to policymakers and the media; and providing a national rallying point for recovery advocates.

National Council on Alcoholism and Drug Dependence (NCADD)

244 East 58th Street 4th Floor
New York, NY 10022
(800) NCA-CALL
Internet address: www.ncadd.org
Operators provide telephone numbers of local NCADD affiliates that can provide information on local treatment resources. Educational materials on alcoholism are available via the toll-free number above.

National Institute on Alcohol Abuse and Alcoholism (NIAAA)

5635 Fishers Lane, MSC 9304

Bethesda, MD 20892-9304

(301) 443-3860

Internet address: www.niaaa.nih.gov

NIAAA is part of the National Institutes of Health. NIAAA's mission is to provide leadership in the national effort to reduce alcohol-related problems. The NIAAA Internet site has an abundance of information about alcohol-related problems in both Spanish and English.

Substance Abuse Treatment Facility Locator

(800) 662–4357

Internet address: www.findtreatment.samhsa.gov/

Offers alcohol and drug information and treatment referral assistance. (This service is provided by the Substance Abuse and Mental Health Services Administration, U.S. Department of Health and Human Services.)

References

1. Wiley TE, McCarthy M, Breidi L, McCarthy M, Layden TJ. Impact of alcohol on the histological and clinical progression of hepatitis C infection. *Hepatology*. 1998;28(3):805-809.
2. Poynard T, Bedossa P, Opolon P. Natural history of liver fibrosis progression in patients with chronic hepatitis C. *Lancet*. 997;349(9055):825-832.
3. Zeuzem S. Heterogeneous virologic response rates to interferon-based therapy in patients with chronic hepatitis C: who responds less well? *Ann Intern Med*. 2004;140(5):370-81.
4. Regev A, Jeffers LJ. Hepatitis C and alcohol. *Alcohol Clin Exp Res*. 1999;23(9):1543-1551.
5. Schiff ER. The alcoholic patient with hepatitis C virus infection. *Am J Med*. 1999;107(6B):95-99S.
6. Ohta S, Watanabe Y, Nakajima T. Consumption of alcohol in the presence of hepatitis C virus is an additive risk for liver damage. *Prev Med*. 1998;27(3):461-469.
7. Caldwell SH, Jeffers LJ, Ditomaso A, et al. Antibody to hepatitis C is common among patients with alcoholic liver disease with and without risk factors. *Am J Gastroenterol*. 1991;86(9):1219-1223.
8. Pares A, Barrera JM, Caballeria J, et al. Hepatitis C virus antibodies in chronic alcoholic patients: association with severity of liver injury. *Hepatology*. 1990;12(6):1295-1299.
9. Coelho-Little ME, Jeffers LJ, Bernstein DE, et al. Hepatitis C virus in alcoholic patients with and without clinically apparent liver disease. *Alcohol Clin Exp Res*. 1995;19(5):1173-1176.
10. Mendenhall CL, Seeff L, Diehl AM, et al. Antibodies to hepatitis B virus and hepatitis C virus in alcoholic hepatitis and cirrhosis: their prevalence and clinical relevance. *Hepatology*. 1991;14(4 Pt 1):581-589.
11. Mendenhall CL, Moritz T, Rouster S, et al. Epidemiology of hepatitis C among veterans with alcoholic liver disease. *Am J Gastroenterol*. 1993;88(7):1022-1026.
12. Corrao G, Arico S. Independent and combined action of hepatitis C virus infection and alcohol consumption on the risk of symptomatic liver cirrhosis. *Hepatology*. 1998;27(4):914-919.
13. Pessione F, Degos F, Marcellin P, et al. Effect of alcohol consumption on serum hepatitis C virus RNA and histological lesions in chronic hepatitis C. *Hepatology*. 1998;27(6):1717-1722.
14. Ostapowicz G, Watson KJ, Locarnini SA, Desmond PV. Role of alcohol in the progression of liver disease caused by hepatitis C virus infection. *Hepatology*. 1998;27(6):1730-1735.
15. Khan MH, Thomas L, Byth K, et al. How much does alcohol contribute to the variability of hepatic fibrosis in chronic hepatitis C? *J Gastroenterol Hepatol*. 1998;13(4):419-426.
16. Kondili LA, Tosti ME, Szklo M, et al. The relationships of chronic hepatitis and cirrhosis to alcohol intake, hepatitis B and C, and delta virus infection: a case-control study in Albania. *Epidemiol Infect*. 1998;121(2):391-395.
17. Frieden TR, Ozick L, McCord C, et al. Chronic liver disease in central Harlem: the role of alcohol and viral hepatitis. *Hepatology*. 1999;29(3):883-888.
18. Nevins CL, Malaty H, Velez ME, Anand BS. Interaction of alcohol and hepatitis C virus infection on severity of liver disease. *Dig Dis Sci*. 1999;44(6):1236-1242.
19. Loguercio C, Di Pierro M, Di Marino MP, et al. Drinking habits of subjects with hepatitis C virus-related chronic liver disease: prevalence and effect on clinical, virological and pathological aspects. *Alcohol Alcohol*. 2000;35(3):296-301.
20. Monto A, Patel K, Bostrom A, et al. Risks of a range of alcohol intake on hepatitis C-related fibrosis. Hepatology. 2004;39(3):826-34.
21. Bellentani S, Saccoccio G, Costa G, et al. Drinking habits as cofactors of risk for alcohol induced liver damage. *Gut*. 1997;41(6):845-50.
22. Roudot-Thoraval F, Bastie A, Pawlotsky JM, Dhumeaux D. Epidemiological factors affecting the severity of hepatitis C virus- related liver disease: a French survey of 6,664 patients. *Hepatology*. 1997;26(2):485-490.
23. Bellentani S, Tiribelli C, Saccoccio G, et al. Prevalence of chronic liver disease in the general population of northern Italy: the Dionysos Study. *Hepatology*. 1994;20(6):1442-1449.

24. Takase S, Tsutsumi M, Kawahara H, et al. The alcohol-altered liver membrane antibody and hepatitis C virus infection in the progression of alcoholic liver disease. *Hepatology.* 1993;17(1):9-13.

25. Donato F, Tagger A, Chiesa R, et al. Hepatitis B and C virus infection, alcohol drinking, and hepatocellular carcinoma: a case-control study in Italy. Brescia HCC Study. *Hepatology.* 1997;26(3):579-584.

26. Mori M, Hara M, Wada I, et al. Prospective study of hepatitis B and C viral infections, cigarette smoking, alcohol consumption, and other factors associated with hepatocellular carcinoma risk in Japan. *Am J Epidemiol.* 2000;151(2):131-139.

27. Khan KN, Yatsuhashi H. Effect of alcohol consumption on the progression of hepatitis C virus infection and risk of hepatocellular carcinoma in Japanese patients. *Alcohol Alcohol.* 2000;35(3):286-295.

28. Noda K, Yoshihara H, Suzuki K, et al. Progression of type C chronic hepatitis to liver cirrhosis and hepatocellular carcinoma - its relationship to alcohol drinking and the age of transfusion. *Alcohol Clin Exp Res.* 1996;20(1 Suppl):95-100A.

29. Oshita M, Hayashi N, Kasahara A, et al. Increased serum hepatitis C virus RNA levels among alcoholic patients with chronic hepatitis C. *Hepatology.* 1994;20(5):1115-1120.

30. Cromie SL, Jenkins PJ, Bowden DS, Dudley FJ. Chronic hepatitis C: effect of alcohol on hepatitic activity and viral titre. *J Hepatol.* 1996;25(6):821-826.

31. Zhang T, Li Y, Lai JP, et al. Alcohol potentiates hepatitis C virus replicon expression. *Hepatology.* 2003;38(1):57-65.

32. Anand BS, THornby J. Alcohol has no effect on hepatitis C virus replication: a meta-analysis. *J. Gut.* 2005 Oct;54(10):1468-72.

33. Cesario K, et al. Excessive Alcohol Consumption is associated with high viral load in patients with chronic hepatitis C infection. DDW 2005 Abstract presentation M1218.

34. Sherman KE, Rouster SD, Mendenhall C, Thee D. Hepatitis C RNA quasispecies complexity in patients with alcoholic liver disease. *Hepatology.* 1999;30(1):265-270.

35. Ohnishi K, Matsuo S, Matsutani K, et al. Interferon therapy for chronic hepatitis C in habitual drinkers: comparison with chronic hepatitis C in infrequent drinkers. *Am J Gastroenterol.* 1996;91(7):1374-1379.

36. Okazaki T, Yoshihara H, Suzuki K, et al. Efficacy of interferon therapy in patients with chronic hepatitis C. Comparison between non-drinkers and drinkers. *Scand J Gastroenterol.* 1994;29(11):1039-1043.

37. Tabone M, Sidoli L, Laudi C, et al. Alcohol abstinence does not offset the strong negative effect of lifetime alcohol consumption on the outcome of interferon therapy. *J Viral Hepat.* 2002;9(4):288-94.

38. Loguercio C, Di Pierro M, Di Marino MP, et al. Drinking habits of subjects with hepatitis C virus-related chronic liver disease: prevalence and effect on clinical, virological and pathological aspects. *Alcohol Alcohol.* 2000;35(3):296-301.

39. National Institutes of Health Consensus Development Conference Statement: Management of hepatitis C 2002 (June 10-12, 2002). *Gastroenterology.* 2002;123(6):2082-99.

40. Hezode C, Lonjon I, Roudot-Thoraval F, Pawlotsky JM, Zafrani ES, Dhumeaux D. Impact of moderate alcohol consumption on histological activity and fibrosis in patients with chronic hepatitis C, and specific influence of steatosis: a prospective study. *Aliment Pharmacol Ther.* 2003;17(8):1031-7.

41. Hutchinson SJ, Bird SM, Goldberg DJ. Influence of alcohol on the progression of hepatitis C virus infection: a meta-analysis. *Clin Gastroenterol Hepatol.* 2005 Nov;3(11):1150-9.

42. Delarocque-Astagneau E, et al. Past excessive alcohol consumption: a major determinant of severe liver disease among newly referred hepatitis C virus infected patients in hepatology reference centers, France 2001. *Ann Epidemiol.* 2005 Se:15(8):551-7

43. Westin J, Lagging LM, Spak F, et al. Moderate alcohol intake increases fibrosis progression in untreated patients with hepatitis C virus infection. *J Viral Hepat.* 2002;9(3):235-41.

44. Ma X, Svegliati-Baroni G, Poniachik J, et al. Collagen synthesis by liver stellate cells is released from its normal feedback regulation by acetaldehyde-induced modification of the carboxyl-terminal propeptide of procollagen. *Alcohol Clin Exp Res.* 1997;21(7):1204-1211.

45. McClain C, Shedlofsky S, Barve S, Hill D. Cytokines and alcoholic liver disease. *Alcohol Health Res World.* 1997;21(4):317-320.

46. Lands WE. Cellular signals in alcohol-induced liver injury: a review. *Alcohol Clin Exp Res.* 1995;19(4):928-938.

47. Maher J, Friedman S. Pathogenesis of hepatic fibrosis. In: Hall P (Ed.). *Alcoholic Liver Disease: Pathology and Pathogenesis.* London, England. Oxford University Press. 1995.

48. Lieber CS. Hepatic and other medical disorders of alcoholism: from pathogenesis to treatment. *J Stud Alcohol.* 1998;59(1):9-25.

49. Lieber CS. Alcoholic liver disease: new insights in pathogenesis lead to new treatments. *J Hepatol.* 2000;32(1 Suppl):113-128.

50. Kurose I, Higuchi H, Kato S, Miura S, Ishii H. Ethanol-induced oxidative stress in the liver. *Alcohol Clin Exp Res.* 1996;20(1 Suppl):77-85A.

51. Gavaler J, Arria A. Increases susceptibility of women to alcoholic liver disease: Artifactual or real? In: Hall P (Ed.). *Alcoholic Liver Disease: Pathology and Pathogenesis.* London, England. Oxford University Press. 1995.

52. Tuyns AJ, Pequignot G. Greater risk of ascitic cirrhosis in females in relation to alcohol consumption. *Int J Epidemiol.* 1984;13(1):53-57.

53. Nicholls P, Edwards G, Kyle E. Alcoholics admitted to four hospitals in England. II. General and cause-specific mortality. *Q J Stud Alcohol.* 1974;35(3):841-855.

54. Patwardhan RV, Desmond PV, Johnson RF, Schenker S. Impaired elimination of caffeine by oral contraceptive steroids. *J Lab Clin Med.* 1980;95(4):603-608.

55. Johnson RD, Williams R. Genetic and environmental factors in the individual susceptibility to the development of alcoholic liver disease. *Alcohol Alcohol.* 1985;20(2):137-160.

56. Frezza M, di Padova C, Pozzato G, et al. High blood alcohol levels in women. The role of decreased gastric alcohol dehydrogenase activity and first-pass metabolism. *N Engl J Med.* 1990;322(2):95-99.

57. Taylor JL, Dolhert N, Friedman L, et al. Alcohol elimination and simulator performance of male and female aviators: a preliminary report. *Aviat Space Environ Med.* 1996;67(5):407-413.

58. Kwo PY, Ramchandani VA, O'Connor S, et al. Gender differences in alcohol metabolism: relationship to liver volume and effect of adjusting for body mass. *Gastroenterology.* 1998;115(6):1552-1557.

59. Li T, Beard J, Orr W, et al. Gender and ethnic differences in alcohol metabolism. *Alcohol Clin Exp Res.* 1998;22(3):771-772.

60. Mochida S, Ohnishi K, et al. Effect of alcohol intake on the efficacy of interferon therapy in patients with chronic hepatitis C as evaluated by

multivariate logistic regression analysis. *Alcohol Clin Exp Res.* 1996;20(95):371-377A.

61. Chang A. The impact of past alcohol use on treatment response rates in patients with chronic hepatitis C. *Aliment Pharmacol Ther.* 2005 Oct 15;22(8):701-6

62. Anon. Matching Alcoholism Treatments to Client Heterogeneity: Project MATCH posttreatment drinking outcomes. *J Stud Alcohol.* 1997;58(1):7-29.

63. Fleming M, Manwell LB. Brief intervention in primary care settings. A primary treatment method for at-risk, problem, and dependent drinkers. *Alcohol Res Health.* 1999;23(2):128-137.

64. Alcohol Alert No. 43. Brief intervention for alcohol problems. National Institute on Alcohol Abuse and Alcoholism. Bethesda, Maryland. 1999.

65. DiClemente CC, Bellino LE, Neavins TM. Motivation for change and alcoholism treatment. *Alcohol Res Health.* 1999;23(2):86-92.

66. Steinglass P. Family Therapy: Alcohol. In: Galanter M, Kleber H, (Eds.). *The American Psychiatric Press Textbook of Substance Abuse Treatment.* American Psychiatric Press. Washington, DC. 1999.

67. O'Farrell TJ. Marital and family therapy in alcoholism treatment. *J Subst Abuse Treat.* 1989;6(1):23-29.

68. Matching Alcoholism Treatments to Client Heterogeneity: Project MATCH posttreatment drinking outcomes. *J Stud Alcohol.* 1997;58(1):7-29.

69. Miller WR, Zweben A, DiClemente CC, Rychatrik R. *Motivational Enhancement Therapy Manual.* NIH Pub. No. 94-3723. National Institutes of Health. Rockville, Maryland. 1995.

70. Humphreys K, Mankowski ES, Moos RH, Finney JW. Do enhanced friendship networks and active coping mediate the effect of self-help groups on substance abuse? *Ann Behav Med.* 1999;21(1):54-60.

71. Tonigan JS, Toscova R, Miller WR. Meta-analysis of the literature on Alcoholics Anonymous: sample and study characteristics moderate findings. *J Stud Alcohol.* 1996;57(1):65-72.

72. Longabaugh R, Wirtz PW, Zweben A, Stout RL. Network support for drinking, Alcoholics Anonymous and long-term matching effects. *Addiction.* 1998;93(9):1313-1333.

73. Morgenstern J, Labouvie E, McCrady BS, et al. Affiliation with Alcoholics Anonymous after treatment: a study of its therapeutic effects and mechanisms of action. *J Consult Clin Psychol.* 1997;65(5):768-777.

UNDERSTANDING HEPATITIS C DISEASE

Lorren Sandt

LIVER DISEASE PROGRESSION

Introduction

Throughout this book, you will often read that *chronic hepatitis* C and its treatments affect each person differently. The broad range of variability observed between persons living with hepatitis C is especially true of disease progression. There is no accurate way to predict the course of chronic hepatitis C in an individual person.

This chapter provides information about possibilities that *might* happen. Remember, none of the situations discussed in this chapter will necessarily happen to you. However, it is important to be aware of the possibilities so that if any of them do occur, you will be prepared and better able to make good decisions.

About the Liver

The liver is the largest internal organ of the body. In a normal adult, the liver weighs 3½ to 4 pounds (1,300 to 1,500 grams). It accounts for about 2.5% of the total weight of the body. The liver is wedge-shaped (see Figure 1). It measures approximately 7 inches (14 cm) across by 5½ inches (18 cm) along its diagonal.

The liver is divided into two main lobes, the right and the left. The right lobe is slightly larger than the left and extends down the right side of the rib cage. The left lobe extends from the right lobe to about the middle of the abdomen. There are also two minor lobes of the liver, the caudate and quadrate lobes. *Fibrous* ligaments separate the lobes. All lobes of the liver perform the same functions. The entire liver is enclosed in a fibrous sheath called Glisson's capsule.

Figure 1. Anatomy of the Liver*

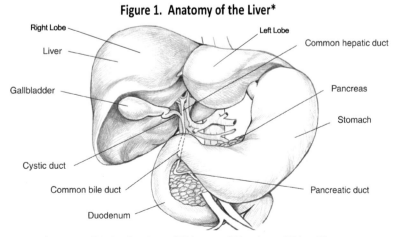

*Courtesy of National Institute of Diabetes and Digestive and Kidney Diseases

Figure 2. Placement of the Liver in the Body

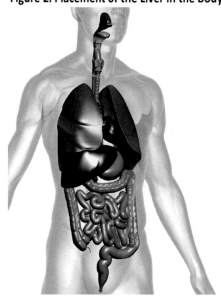

The liver is located on the right side of the abdominal cavity just below the lungs and diaphragm, the muscle that separates the chest cavity from the abdominal cavity (see Figure 2). The liver is packed so tightly into the abdomen that the right kidney, parts of the large and small intestines, and the stomach actually leave impressions on its surface. Even the ribs and muscle bands of the diaphragm make indentations on the surface of the liver.

Approximately 25% to 30% of the blood coming from the heart goes to the liver. Although there are no *lymph nodes* in the liver itself, it produces over ⅓ of the body's *lymphatic fluid*. The fluid drains into *lymph channels* and lymph nodes in the abdomen.

The hepatitis C virus (*HCV*) enters the body through the blood stream. It is carried by the blood to the liver where it infects *hepatocytes* (liver cells). HCV reproduces in liver cells. Studies suggest HCV is also reproduced in cells of the blood and bone marrow.

Once diagnosed with hepatitis C, you will have many tests to determine the status of your disease. For detailed information on the tests you may have and why, see *Chapter 6, Laboratory Tests and Procedures*.

Checking blood levels of the *liver enzymes* such as *alanine aminotransferase* (*ALT*) and *aspartate aminotransferase* (*AST*) is one way to tell if liver cells are dying. When liver cells die, ALT and AST are released into the blood. After an abnormal amount of liver cell death, ALT and AST levels rise over a period of 7 to12 days and then slowly return to normal. If liver cells continue to die in abnormally high numbers over time, ALT and AST levels remain elevated.

ALT and AST levels provide information about liver damage, but do not provide information about how much liver repair is taking place. Studies show that liver enzyme levels do not predict disease outcome. You can have normal liver enzyme levels and still have liver damage.

Liver enzymes also provide no information about how well the liver is functioning.[1, 2] Your liver can maintain its many functions despite a remarkable amount of damage. Therefore, it is important to look at the results of other test such as *albumin*, *bilirubin*, *prothrombin time*, and *platelet* count to determine how well your liver is functioning.

> Liver enzymes such as AST and ALT reflect liver damage but not liver function.
> Liver enzymes do not predict disease outcome.

Stages of Disease Progression

Like other liver diseases, HCV disease progresses in *stages*. The usual progression is from *inflammation* to *fibrosis* to *cirrhosis* (see Figure 3). Cirrhosis can progress to end-stage liver disease and/or can give rise to *liver cancer*.

Figure 3. Chronic Hepatitis C Disease Progression

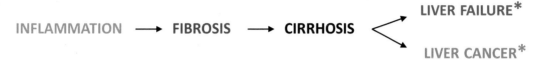

Inflammation

Inflammation is the body's normal response to injury or infection. When the liver is inflamed, there is an overabundance of special cells called inflammatory cells in the liver. Inflammation is labeled chronic when it persists for prolonged period of time.

Chronic inflammation can lead to changes in liver structure, slowed blood circulation, and the death of liver cells (*necrosis*). Prolonged liver inflammation can eventually cause scarring, which is called fibrosis. By controlling liver inflammation, you can potentially control progression to fibrosis.

Fibrosis

Fibrosis is the harmful outcome of chronic inflammation. Fibrosis is scar tissue that forms as a result of chronic inflammation and/or extensive liver cell death. Your healthcare provider uses the amount of fibrosis in your liver as one way of evaluating how quickly your hepatitis C appears to be progressing. Knowledge of approximately when you were initially infected with HCV is a great help in determining your rate of disease progression.

The best way to accurately determine the amount of fibrosis in the liver is to have a *liver biopsy*. No other test can give you and your healthcare providers the important information that is learned from a liver biopsy.

Cirrhosis

When fibrosis becomes widespread and progresses to the point that the internal structure of the liver is abnormal, fibrosis has progressed to cirrhosis. Cirrhosis is the result of long-term liver damage caused by chronic inflammation and liver cell death. The most common causes of cirrhosis include viral hepatitis, excessive intake of *alcohol*, inherited diseases, and *hemochromatosis* (abnormal handling of iron by the body).

Cirrhosis leads to a reduction in blood supply to the liver. The loss of healthy liver tissue and reduced blood supply can lead to abnormalities in liver function. Even when liver disease has progressed to cirrhosis, it may still be possible for the damage to be at least partially reversed if the underlying cause can be eliminated. Cirrhosis progression can usually be slowed or even stopped with effective treatment.

People are often surprised to learn that you can have cirrhosis of the liver and not know it. The onset of cirrhosis is usually silent with few specific *symptoms* to signal this development in the liver.

As scarring (fibrosis) and liver cell destruction continue, some of the following *signs* and symptoms may occur:

- loss of appetite
- nausea and/or vomiting
- weight loss
- change in liver size
- gallstones
- generalized, persistent itching (*pruritus*)
- *jaundice*

> **Despite the seriousness of cirrhosis, large numbers of people live many, many years with cirrhosis without symptoms and without progressing to liver failure.**

Once cirrhosis develops, it is very important to avoid further progression of the disease. Consumption of alcohol in any form, including such things as certain mouthwashes and cough medicines, must be <u>completely</u> avoided by people with cirrhosis.

If you have cirrhosis, this may be a time to reevaluate your treatment goals. If you have not had *interferon-based therapy*, you may want to consider it or other available treatments that aim to rid the body of HCV. It may also be time to look into other means of improving your liver health.

Liver Cancer

Most people with HCV never develop liver cancer. Nonetheless, people with HCV are at an increased risk for liver cancer. The presence of cirrhosis and/or having been infected with HCV for more than 20 years further increases the level of risk. The development of liver cancer (*hepatocellular carcinoma*) is most commonly seen in people who have cirrhosis,[3] but rare cases of this cancer have been reported in HCV patients without cirrhosis.[4] The reported risk for the development of liver cancer among HCV-positive patients with cirrhosis is 1% to 2% per year.[5]

Liver cancer screening remains controversial in the United State because there are no large scale *clinical trials* to prove that such testing improves overall liver cancer survival rates. However, liver cancer screening among people with chronic hepatitis C is widely accepted and practiced by most *hepatologists* and *gastroenterologists*.

Liver cancer is life threatening, so do not delay telling your healthcare provider about any changes in your symptoms. If you have cirrhosis, you need to be followed closely by a healthcare provider who will monitor you with the appropriate liver cancer screening tests such as liver *ultrasonography* and/or *alfa-fetoprotein* levels.

Liver Biopsy for Determining Disease Progression

Scoring Inflammation and Fibrosis

The most accurate way to check the severity of liver disease is with a biopsy. A liver biopsy is a test in which small pieces of liver tissue are removed and examined under a microscope. The three main things that will be looked for are inflammation, fibrosis, and cirrhosis. The biopsy report may also reveal other *histological* and *pathological* findings such as the presence of lymphoid nodules, damage to small *bile* ducts, and/or the presence of fat.

Many people are surprised to learn it is possible to have normal liver enzymes and still have cirrhosis. (See *Chapter 6, Laboratory Tests and Procedures* for additional information about liver enzymes.) Remember, a liver biopsy is the only way to know with certainty whether cirrhosis has developed.

Liver Biopsy Scoring and Grading

When you receive the results of your liver biopsy, you will hear the terms inflammatory *grade* and fibrotic *stage*. Healthcare providers use these terms to indicate the amount of injury to the liver. Three different methods are used for scoring liver biopsies. This can cause confusion for both patients and healthcare providers. Be aware that the scoring systems are also subject to interpretation by the doctor in the laboratory who examines your biopsy. The three most commonly used scoring systems for liver biopsies in the U.S. are described below.

KNODELL SCORING SYSTEM (ALSO KNOWN AS THE ORIGINAL HAI [HISTOLOGY ACTIVITY INDEX])

This was the first scoring system established to specifically assess the changes (inflammation and fibrosis) seen with chronic hepatitis. It was introduced in 1981 and remains the most commonly used scoring system.[6] The system uses three categories to describe the amount of inflammation and liver cell death present, and a fourth category to assess the fibrosis (which is reported on a scale of 0 to 4).

The tricky part of interpreting a Knodell Score is that the three inflammatory grading numbers and the fibrosis staging number are added together into a single final score. This "problem" is overcome by examining each of the four individual numbers reported instead of just the final score.

ISHAK SCORING SYSTEM (ALSO KNOWN AS THE MODIFIED HAI)

The Ishak scoring system is a modification of the Knodell HAI system. It is reported to be more sensitive and accurate in assessing fibrosis than the original HAI system. Fibrosis staging is scored from 0 to 6 (instead of 0 to 4). The Ishak scoring system is frequently used in the *clinical* research setting because of its detail.

METAVIR SCORING SYSTEM

The METAVIR scoring system was first introduced by a study group out of France in 1996. The METAVIR system has the advantage of being somewhat simpler than the Ishak system to use, but that simplicity is also considered by some to be its greatest disadvantage because it lacks the detailed specificity of other systems. The METAVIR scoring system gives an inflammation score (0 to 4) and a fibrosis score (also 0 to 4).

Two other systems currently in use to describe the histological activity seen on liver biopsies are the Scheuer system and the Batts-Ludwig system. If your biopsy is reported with either of these systems, talk with your doctor to get the results explained to you in terms you can both understand and use in your decision-making process.

Interpreting Your Liver Biopsy Results

A few key factors will help you understand your liver biopsy report.

- What system did the laboratory use to grade each of your biopsies?
    - A score for a given biopsy characteristic in one system does <u>not</u> mean the same thing in the other systems.
- The scores for all the characteristics of the tissue sample are added together for a final score, except as specified in the notes under the table for that system (see Tables 1-5).
    - If you have had more than one biopsy, you need to look at changes in both the individual characteristics and changes in the overall score.
- A final score from one biopsy may have the same score as that of a follow-up biopsy, but the scores for individual characteristics may have changed. This means your situation could actually be better or worse depending on the individual characteristic scores.

Ask your healthcare provider to explain the results of your liver biopsy thoroughly. Ask for an explanation of the individual scores as well as the final score. Your report should contain a description of the inflammatory grade and fibrotic stage. Ask to speak with the laboratory that evaluated your liver biopsy if your healthcare provider is unable to provide this information.

A liver biopsy is an invasive test that you are unlikely to want or need frequently. It is very important to understand the results of your liver biopsy so you can use this information to help you make decisions about your healthcare. Tables 1 through 5 compare the Knodell (Orginal HAI), the Ishak (Modified HAI), and the METAVIR liver biopsy scoring systems. They are presented here courtesy of David Kleiner, MD at the National Cancer Institute.

Table 1. Comparison of Liver Biopsy Scoring Systems – Periportal Necroinflammatory Changes

Score	Knodell/Original HAI[a(7)]	Ishak/Modified HAI[(8)]	METAVIR[b(9)]
0	None	Absent	Absent
1	Mild piecemeal necrosis	Mild (focal, few portal areas)	Focal alteration of the periportal plate in some portal tracts
2		Mild/Moderate (focal, most portal areas)	Diffuse alteration of the periportal tract in some portal tracts or focal
3	Moderate piecemeal necrosis (involves less than 50% of the circumference of most portal tracts)	Moderate (continuous around <50% of tracts or septae)	Diffuse alteration of the periportal plate in all portal tracts
4	Marked piecemeal necrosis (involves more than 50% of the circumference of most portal tracts)	Severe (continuous around >50% of tracts or septae)	

[a]The periportal component of the Knodell HAI has been split into a periportal piecemeal necrosis and a bridging/confluent necrosis component for better comparison to the other scoring systems. In order to recreate the original scale, the bridging/confluent necrosis component should be added to the periportal piecemeal necrosis component.
[b]The periportal component of the METAVIR score is used with the focal necrosis score to determine overall inflammatory activity.

Table 2. Comparison of Liver Biopsy Scoring Systems – Bridging and Confluent Necrosis

Score	Knodell/Original HAI[a(7)]	Ishak/Modified HAI[(8)]	METAVIR[b(9)]
0	Absent	Absent	Absent
1		Focal confluent necrosis	Present
2	Bridging necrosis (more than two such bridges)	Zone 3 necrosis in some areas	
3		Zone 3 necrosis in most areas	
4		Zone 3 necrosis + occasional portal-central bridging necrosis	
5		Zone 3 necrosis + multiple portal-central bridging necrosis	
6	Multilobular necrosis	Panacinar or multiacinar necrosis	

[a] The periportal component of the Knodell HAI has been split into a periportal piecemeal necrosis and a bridging/confluent necrosis component for better comparison to the other scoring systems. In order to recreate the original scale, the bridging/confluent necrosis component should be added to the periportal piecemeal necrosis component.
[b]The METAVIR score for bridging necrosis is not used in the overall activity determination by this system and is provided only for comparison with other scales.

Table 3. Comparison of Liver Biopsy Scoring Systems – Focal (Spotty) Lobular Necrosis and Hepatocellular Apoptosis

Score	Knodell/Original HAI[a(7)]	Ishak/Modified HAI[(8)]	METAVIR[b(9)]
0	None	Absent	Less than one necroinflammatory focus per lobule
1	Mild (acidophilic bodies, ballooning degeneration, and/or scattered foci of hepatocellular necrosis in less than 1/3 of lobules/nodules)	One focus or less per 10x field	At least one necroinflammatory focus per lobule
2		2 - 4 foci per 10x field	Several necroinflammatory foci per lobule or confluent/bridging necrosis
3	Moderate (involvement of 1/3 to 2/3 of lobules/nodules)	5 - 10 foci per 10x field	
4	Marked (involvement of more than 2/3 of lobules/nodules)	More than 10 foci per 10x field	

Table 4. Comparison of Liver Biopsy Scoring Systems – Portal Inflammation

Score	Knodell/Original HAI[(7)]	Ishak/Modified HAI[(8)]	METAVIR[b(9)]
0	No portal inflammation	None	Absent
1	Mild (sprinkling of inflammatory cells in less than 1/3 of portal tracts)	Mild, some or all portal areas	Presence of mononuclear aggregates in some portal tracts
2		Moderate, some or all portal areas	Mononuclear aggregates in all portal tracts
3	Moderate (increased inflammation in 1/3 to 2/3 of portal tracts)	Moderate/marked, all portal areas	Large and dense mononuclear aggregates in all portal tracts
4	Marked (dense packing of inflammatory cells in more than 2/3 of portal tracts)	Marked, all portal areas	

[a] The METAVIR score for bridging necrosis is not used in the overall activity determination by this system and is provided only for comparison with other scales.

Table 5. Comparison of Liver Biopsy Scoring Systems – Fibrosis

Score	Knodell/Original HAI[a(7)]	Ishak/Modified HAI[8]	METAVIR[b(9)]
0	No fibrosis	No fibrosis	No fibrosis
1	Fibrosis portal expansion	Fibrosis expansion of some portal areas, with or without short fibrous septa	Stellate enlargement of portal tracts without septae formation
2		Fibrosis expansion of most portal areas, with or without short fibrous septa	Enlargement of portal tracts with rare septae formation
3	Bridging fibrosis (portal-portal or portal-central linkage)	Fibrosis expansion of most portal areas, with occasional portal to portal bridging	Numerous septae without fibrosis
4	Cirrhosis	Fibrosis expansion of portal areas, with marked bridging (portal to portal as well as portal to central)	Cirrhosis
5		Marked bridging with occasional nodules (incomplete cirrhosis)	
6		Cirrhosis, probable or definite	

Table 6 shows how the HAI inflammation scores relate to the grade of histological injury. In the HAI system, the various inflammation scores are added together. These numbers are directly related to the descriptive grade of inflammation.

Table 6. Relationship of Aggregate Inflammation Scores to Grade of Activity[(10)]

Sum of inflammation Scores in HAI or Modified HAI systems	Description of Activity
0	None
1-4	Minimal
5-8	Mild
9-12	Moderate
13-18	Marked

Other Liver Biopsy Findings

FATTY LIVER (STEATOSIS OR STEATOHEPATITIS)

Fatty liver is a general term indicating the accumulation of fat in liver cells. *Steatosis* is the presence of fat in liver cells without inflammation. *Steatohepatitis* is the presence of fat in liver cells with inflammation. You may hear other terms to describe fatty liver, depending on your medical condition.

- *NAFL – nonalcoholic fatty liver*
- *NAFLD – nonalcoholic fatty liver disease*
- *NASH – nonalcoholic steatohepatitis*

Fatty liver is emerging as a major medical problem. Obesity affects up to 35%[11] of adults in the U.S. population and 17% to 33% have NAFLD.[12] Approximately one-third of people with NAFLD will have progressive liver disease.[13]

For the hepatitis C patient, fatty liver is another factor that may accelerate in the progression of fibrosis.[14] A liver biopsy can determine both the presence of fat in the liver and the level of fibrosis. This information will allow your healthcare provider to counsel you about your risk of progressive liver disease.

Alcohol consumption can increase the amount of fat in the liver and is the most common cause of fatty liver. The association between fatty liver and alcohol is another very important reason for you to refrain from drinking <u>any</u> alcohol. However, not all cases of fatty liver are caused by alcohol use. Diabetes and high *triglycerides* are also associated with fatty liver and should be managed closely by your healthcare provider.

The liver must *metabolize* any fat that is not eliminated through the intestinal tract. If you eat excessive amounts of fat, the amount that goes to your liver may be too much for it to metabolize. Excess fat that is not metabolized begins to accumulate in the liver. This accumulation of fat can cause inflammation. Inflammation can lead to scarring, which may eventually lead to decreased liver function. Therefore, it is important not to have excessive amounts of fat in your diet. It is particularly important to limit your intake of animal fat because animal fat is especially difficult for the liver to metabolize. See *Chapter 15, Nutrition and Hepatitis C* for suggested dietary guidelines.

Achieving or maintaining your ideal body weight (a *body mass index [BMI]* of approximately 20 to 25) and limiting the amount of fat in your diet are important for your liver health. Your BMI is calculated by taking your weight (in kilograms) and dividing by your height (in meters) squared. A free BMI calculator is available on the Internet at www.nhlbisupport.com/bmi/bmicalc.htm. Normal body weight not only helps your liver but can also improve your energy level, reduce *hypertension*, and lower your risk of heart disease. Regular exercise can help you maintain a normal body weight and avoid the development of fatty liver.

If you are considering interferon-based therapy, obesity may play a role in your response. One study showed an 80% decrease in *sustained response* to interferon therapy in obese patients compared to those with normal body weight.[15] Your doctor may suggest weight loss before beginning interferon-based therapy if you are significantly above your ideal body weight. Healthcare providers have also begun to *advocate* for individualized weight-based dosing of *pegylated interferon* alfa-2b (PegIntron®) plus *ribavirin* to improve the chance for response to treatment One large study showed that heavier patients were much more likely to achieve an SVR with weight-based ribavirin dosing versus flat-dosed ribavirin (64% versus 25%).[16]

People with fatty liver often have high *blood sugar* and *lipids* such as *cholesterol* and *triglycerides*. If you have a fatty liver, your healthcare provider should monitor you for the development of these problems.

Some medications and other substances can cause fatty liver. Be sure to review all of your medications with your healthcare provider and avoid the following, if possible.

- alcohol
- amiodarone (anti-arrhythmia medicine)
- methotrexate (arthritis medicine)
- high doses of *vitamin A*
- tetracycline (antibiotic)
- cortisone (steroid medicine)
- prednisone (steroid medicine)

Systemic Complications of Hepatitis C

Although the effects of HCV on the liver are most visible, the virus can affect other body systems and organs. This results in *extrahepatic* (outside the liver) conditions or manifestations of *chronic hepatitis* C.

Many *autoimmune* diseases occur as secondary diagnoses after a primary diagnosis of chronic hepatitis C or in association with hepatitis C. Some examples of these diseases include:

- type 2 diabetes
- mixed *cryoglobulinemia*
- *thyroiditis*
- *erythema nodosum*
- erythema multiforme
- *glomerulonephritis*
- *hypothyroidism*
- *lichen planus*
- polyarteritis
- *urticaria*
- *porphyria cutanea tarda*
- *polymyalgia*
- B cell lymphoma
- Mooren corneal ulcers

There is much controversy regarding the true cause of the many so-called HCV-related conditions that have been reported. Some of them probably are related to hepatitis C. Others probably are not, and occurred by chance in a few individuals unrelated to HCV. Many studies on this topic come from clinics that treat only specific diseases, which may skew the study findings.

The way HCV produces extrahepatic conditions and the true prevalence of these conditions is the subject of ongoing research. The link to type 2 diabetes has been studied by numerous groups and it appears that HCV causes *insulin* resistance.[17-20] In other HCV-related extrahepatic conditions, HCV stimulates the *immune system* to produce *autoimmune antibodies, antibodies* against the body's own tissues. This appears to be the mechanism for HCV-related *thyroid* and blood disorders.

We are hopeful that ongoing research will help clarify both the mechanism of these potentially debilitating conditions and new treatments to help alleviate the suffering caused by them.

Summary

The question of whether it is the virus or the person infected by the virus that determines how HCV disease will progress is an active area of medical research. At this point, several personal factors and several viral factors have been identified that may influence the rate of HCV disease progression.

Personal factors related to disease progression include some variables you can control. The consumption of alcohol can markedly affect disease progression. The amount of fat in one's diet, and body weight can also influence disease progression and treatment outcomes. Your environment, diet, exercise plan, lifestyle, and support system may all be important factors that could affect the course of your HCV infection.

In terms of viral characteristics, the existence of multiple *quasispecies* can accelerate disease progression. HCV *genotype* affects response to interferon-based therapy and is therefore an important factor in halting disease progression by *viral clearance*.

Progression of chronic hepatitis C in any given person cannot be predicted. The majority of people will not progress to cirrhosis. However, the seriousness of this disease for people with advanced cirrhosis is beyond question. If you follow the progression of your disease with all the tests available to you, you will be in a better position to make informed decisions about your treatment options.

We are confident that ongoing research will improve the ability to predict disease progression and intervene more effectively.

References

1. Datz C, Cramp M, Haas T, Dietze O Nitschko H. The natural course of hepatitis C virus infection 18 years after an epidemic outbreak of non-A, non-B hepatitis in a plasmapheresis centre. *Gut.* 1999;44(4):563-567.
2. Persico M, Persico E, Suozzo R, et al. Natural history of hepatitis C virus carriers with persistently normal aminotransferase levels. *Gastroenterology.* 2000;118(4):760-764.
3. El-Serag HB. Epidemiology of hepatocellular carcinoma. *Clin Liver Dis.* 2001;5:87-107.
4. De Mitri MS, Poussin K, Baccarini P, et al. HCV-associated liver cancer without cirrhosis. *Lancet.* 1995;345:413-415.
5. Fattovich G, Giustina G, Degos F, et al. Effectiveness of interferon alfa on incidence of hepatocellular carcinoma and decompensation in cirrhosis type C. *J Hepatol.* 1997;27:201–205.
6. Brunt EM. Grading and staging the histopathological lesions of chronic hepatitis: the Knodell histology activity index and beyond. *Hepatology.* 2000;31:241-6.
7. Knodell R, Ishak K, Black W, et al. Formulation and application of a numerical scoring system for assessing histological activity in asymptomatic chronic active hepatitis. *Hepatology.* 1981;1(5):431-435.
8. Ishak K, Baptista A, Bianchi L, et al. Histological grading and staging of chronic hepatitis. *J Hepatol.* 1995;22(6):696-699.
9. The French METIVIR Cooperative Study Group. Intraobserver and interobserver variations in liver biopsy interpretation in patients with chronic hepatitis C. *Hepatology.* 1994;20(1 Pt 1):15-20.
10. Desmet V, Gerber M, Hoofnagle J, et al. Classification of chronic hepatitis: diagnosis, grading and staging. *Hepatology.* 1994;19(6):1513-1520.
11. Ogden CL, Carroll MD, McDowell MA, Flegal KM. Obesity among adults in the United States – no change since 2003—2004. NCHS data brief no 1. Hyattsville, MD: National Center for Health Statistics, 2007.
12. Farrell GC, Larter CZ. Nonalcoholic fatty liver disease: from steatosis to cirrhosis. *Hepatology.* 2006 Feb;43(2 Suppl 1):S99-S112.
13. Duvnjak M, et al. Pathogenesis and management issues for non-alcoholic fatty liver disease. *World J Gastroenterol.* 2007 Sep 14;13(34):4539-50.
14. Castera L, Hezode C, Roudot-Thoraval F, et al. Worsening of steatosis is an independent factor of fibrosis progression in untreated patients with chronic hepatitis C and paired liver biopsies. *Gut.* 2003;52:288-292.
15. Bressler B, Guindi M, Tomlinson G, Heathcote J. . High body mass index is an independent risk factor for nonresponse to antiviral treatment in chronic hepatitis C. *Hepatology.* 2003;38:639-644.
16. Jacobson I, Brown Jr. R, Freilich B, et al. Weight based ribavirin dosing (WBD) increases sustained viral response (SVR) in patients with chronic hepatitis C (CHC): final results of the WIN-R study, a U.S. community-based trial. *Hepatology.* 2005;42(suppl 1):749A.
17. Delgado-Borrego A, Liu YS, Jordan SH, et al. Prospective study of liver transplant recipients with HCV infection: evidence for a causal relationship between HCV and insulin resistance. *Liver Transpl.* 2008 Feb;14(2):193-201.
18. Albert L, et al, High Prevalence of Glucose Abnormalities in Patients With Hepatitis C Virus Infection. *Diabetes Care* Volume 27, Number 5, May 2004
19. Hui JM, Sud A, Farrell GC, et al. Insulin resistance is associated with chronic hepatitis C virus infection and fibrosis progression [corrected]. *Gastroenterology.* 2004 Feb;126(2):634.
20. Shintani Y, Fujie H, Miyoshi H, et al. Hepatitis C virus infection and diabetes: direct involvement of the virus in the development of insulin resistance. *Gastroenterology.* 2004 Mar;126(3):840-8

UNDERSTANDING HEPATITIS C DISEASE

Lorren Sandt

PROMOTING LIVER HEALTH

Introduction

The human body is amazingly resilient. It can recover from devastating trauma and disease. It continues to function with missing or malfunctioning limbs. The body even adapts to the loss of some organs and the severely limited function of others. However, the human body cannot survive for more than 24 hours without a liver. The liver is an incredibly complex organ. It is involved in more than 500 body functions. Your liver is responsible for such things as detoxifying drugs and *alcohol*, making vital substances such as *proteins*, and processing nearly every class of nutrient.

Many things we do or are exposed to can increase the work our livers must do to keep us healthy and alive. Alcohol, environmental pollutants, food preservatives and additives, drugs, and other *toxic* substances can challenge the liver's ability to function effectively. *Hepatitis C* infection makes these challenges even more difficult for the liver.

One way to help your liver perform its best despite *HCV* infection is to reduce other challenges to the liver. This chapter discusses some ways to accomplish this in your own life.

The Healing Power of a Positive Attitude

How do you meet the demands of a disease like hepatitis C and live a full life? A positive, healing attitude helps many people meet this challenge head-on.

Negative feelings may drain your body of the energy needed for healing. Without qualities such as endurance, integrity, honor, and self-esteem, healing the physical body is a difficult task. It has been said, "If you *believe* you can, you probably can. If you *believe* you won't, you most assuredly won't. Belief is the ignition switch that gets you off the launching pad."[1]

For many people with a life-changing illness, a positive attitude is not just a cliché, it is what gets them through the day. Consider positive thinking as the process of creating thoughts that produce and focus energy, which in turn brings about positive outcomes. Positive thinking is a powerful healing tool. We all have access to it, but few of us put it into full use.

One research study of cancer patients who had a spontaneous *remission* found only one factor common to each person they examined. Everyone in the study had changed his or her attitude prior to remission and, in some way, had found hope. Each had become more positive in his or her approach to the disease.[2]

Acceptance of reality is the first step toward taking responsibility for and controlling one's life. Each of our lives is influenced by a number of outside factors, many of which we cannot control. Your attitude, however, reflects the ways in which you respond to what is happening to you. And your attitude is completely within your control.

> **How you adapt to situations and the actions you take can affect your health and may influence your recovery.**

Some believe that every thought you have produces a reaction in each cell in your body, from the top of your head to the tips of your toes. They believe the body is constantly reacting to thoughts, whether those thoughts are based on real situations or your imagination. According to this belief, your body becomes an obedient servant of your mind, reacting with the emotional intensity that you associate with your thoughts. Pleasant thoughts produce pleasant feelings; unpleasant thoughts produce unpleasant feelings.

How do you begin to practice having a positive attitude? Every time your life is not going according to plan or presents you with a challenge, try thinking of it as an opportunity. Challenges and disappointments can be opportunities to try new approaches, to amass more know-how, and to exercise your brainpower.

There is so much we still do not know about the human body and how it works. We are only beginning to discover the powerful interactions between our minds and bodies. When you consider the miracle of the human body, it is not hard to believe that it is capable of contributing to its own healing.

Lifestyle Changes and Personal Habits

Changing your lifestyle and personal habits to reduce the effects of *chronic hepatitis* C may be one of the hardest things you do in your life. Try to remember that you are not alone in facing these difficult tasks. Ask for help if you need it. It is much easier to address problems you may experience if you have support and proper medical care.

Sleep

Our society tends to focus on health issues. We spend billions of dollars on *nutritional supplements* and pills. We try to keep ourselves physically fit and mentally stable. We exercise and strive for more quality time with our families. But we often overlook the most fundamental aspect of good health – sleep. Many professionals consider sleep to be the most fundamental practice associated with good health. Sleep enhances immune function, and *immune system* activity enhances sleep.[3]

Getting enough sleep in our fast-paced world is not always easy. We all experience situations that can keep us up around the clock, if we allow it to happen. While adequate sleep is crucial for everyone, it is particularly vital for those living with a long-term disease such as hepatitis C.

Ambitious schedules are not the only enemy of sleep. Anxiety and/or *depression* are experienced by many people with *chronic hepatitis* C. These problems are often associated with sleeping difficulties. Lack of sleep often intensifies anxious and/or depressed feelings creating a vicious cycle. It is important to get the help you need to end this cycle, and to ensure yourself a healthy amount of sleep.

A large study from the United Kingdom showed that decreased amounts of sleep over time was associated with a significantly increased risk of cardiovascular death.[4] However, the amount of sleep needed varies from one person to another. The same study mentioned above also found that people who significantly increase their nightly sleep over prolonged periods of time also have increased mortality rates due to non-cardiac causes.

Listening to your own body is the best way to know if you are getting adequate sleep. If you require a jolt of *caffeine* every morning to awaken fully, feel uncharacteristically irritable, fall asleep during tasks, or otherwise feel tired throughout the day, you may not be getting sufficient sleep. One way to determine how much sleep you need is to keep an activity diary for a month. Keep track daily of the quantity and quality of your sleep, your daytime activities, and your mood. By looking at the patterns in your diary, it will become clear what amount of sleep is best for you.

Exercise: Staying Active

Many people do not realize the central role of exercise in maintaining good health. People who exercise regularly not only feel better, but also often respond more positively to medical treatment.[5] Exercise boosts the immune system. Several studies have shown that exercise can enhance specific immune function. They have shown increased *natural killer cell* activity and increased speed and magnitude of *antibody* response.[6, 7] A recent study showed that exercise can also alleviate depression. They found the optimal benefit on depression occurs when 17.5 calories per kilogram of body weight is expended per week.[8] As an added bonus, exercise gives us self-esteem and confidence by providing a sense of accomplishment and a feeling of independence. Remember, exercise is anything that causes you to be physically active. Everyday activities such as housework, gardening, raking leaves, and walking the dog all "count" as exercise because they are forms of physical activity.

Exercise causes the *pituitary gland* to release substances called *endorphins*. Endorphins remain in the body for hours and have a number of effects. They improve mood, relieve pain, increase *red blood cell* production, and reduce the amount of cortisol in the blood. Increased red blood cell production provides better *oxygenation* to the body tissues. Better oxygenation helps us feel more energetic and leads to better brain function. Cortisol is a hormone linked to stress and depression. Reduced levels of cortisol may lead to reduced stress and better mood.

For someone living with hepatitis C, the key to exercise is moderation. Moderate exercise performed regularly boosts the *immune system* and increases resistance to disease. However, extreme exercise such as marathon running causes immediate suppression of the immune system. Extreme forms of exercise may be particularly harmful if you have *cirrhosis*.

HCV increases your risk of *osteoporosis*, a weakening of the bones. To counter this risk, some experts advise people with liver disease to incorporate weight-bearing exercises into their exercise routine because weight bearing strengthens bones. Weight training also reduces the amount of fat in the liver.[5] In advanced liver disease, the body may use its own muscle tissue as a source of energy. Moderate exercise may help counter and/or reduce the impact of this muscle destruction. By building strong bones and muscles, you can build up a reserve to help fight off some of the physical complications of liver disease.

It is important to drink plenty of water before, during, and after any type of exercise to prevent *dehydration*. Many people like to have a massage after their workout. If you have a massage after exercising, it is especially important to drink plenty of water to flush out the toxins released into the blood by the massage.

Review your exercise program with your healthcare provider to make sure your routine is healthy for you. It is also important to listen to what your body tells you. There may be days, or even weeks or months, during which you may not be able to engage in your normal exercise routine. When you are not up to your normal routine, you may want to consider other gentle forms of exercise such as *qi gong, tai chi*, or yoga. See *Chapter 13, Mind-Body Medicine and Spiritual Healing* for more information on these forms of exercise.

Weight Management

Exercise can be an effective tool for weight management. Maintaining or achieving your ideal body weight has several benefits for people living with HCV. Researchers in Australia reported that weight loss improved the *fibrosis, ALT, insulin* and triglyceride status in people with HCV.[9] Although this was a small study, the results suggested significant benefits associated with weight loss. The *grade* of *steatosis* (fat in the liver) decreased in all seven patients, and the fibrosis score was reduced in three of the seven patients.

People with high BMIs have a higher incidence of *fatty liver*.[10] This is important because fatty liver has been shown to increase the risk of fibrosis progression in untreated HCV-positive patients, especially those with *genotype* 3.[11-13] HCV-infected patients with significant amounts of liver fat have lower response rates to *interferon-based therapy* than those without fatty liver disease.[14-16] One study showed that obesity lowered the chance of a *sustained response* to *antiviral* therapy, independent of the amount of fatty liver.[17] See *Chapter 15, Nutrition and Hepatitis C* for more information about how to achieve and/or maintain your ideal weight.

Sexual Activity

When first diagnosed with hepatitis C, many people become fearful about continuing their sex life. What is normal is different for everyone, but according to a study by researchers at Wilkes University, sexual activity can benefit your immune system.[18] The arousal, desire, excitement, and physical release of sexual activity may enhance the ability of the immune system to ward off illness.

Many people find thinking of themselves as sexual beings, regardless of whether or not they participate in sexual activity, helps them develop a greater ability to enjoy life. The feelings we have when we are sexually aware are sufficient to alleviate a variety of physical and emotional ills. Being or feeling sexual can be good for your self-esteem. It can help ward off depression. As a form of physical exercise, sexual activity helps trigger endorphin release creating a more positive attitude. Sexual activity allows you to relax and, at least for a time, to forget about some of your troubles. Your sexuality can go a long way toward enhancing the healing process and creating an environment for a better functioning immune system.

Sexual expression often becomes a concern for people living with hepatitis C. There is an almost universal concern about passing the virus on to others through sexual activity. Sexual transmission of HCV has been a hot-button issue for both the hepatitis C and public health communities. The Centers for Disease Control and Prevention (CDC) has stated that "sexual transmission of HCV is possible but inefficient." CDC further noted in 2006 that, "Additional data are needed to determine whether sexual transmission of HCV might be increased in the context of *HIV* infection or other STDs."[19]

CDC's recommendations state that people with HCV who have one long-term sexual partner do not need to change their sexual practices. People with HCV who are not in *monogamous* relationships are cautioned to practice safe sex. This means using latex condoms correctly and consistently with every sexual encounter. Practicing safe sex prevents the transmission of HCV to others, and protects you from being exposed to other HCV genotypes. It also helps you avoid other sexually-transmitted diseases such as HIV, *hepatitis B*, and gonorrhea.

If it is applicable to your situation, talk with your healthcare provider about whether you should avoid certain sexual practices such as rough sex, "high risk" sexual activities, and sex while menstruating.[20]

Stress

Stress does not cause disease directly, but it can contribute to disease. Stress can suppress the immune system, which may cause you to be more vulnerable to disease. Hepatitis C can be a frightening diagnosis. Your stress may be compounded by the fact that you may never know how, when, or where the infection occurred since most people are not diagnosed until well after the initial infection.

Stress-reduction techniques such as warm baths, yoga, *meditation*, visualization, and/or keeping a journal can help soothe your soul and thereby strengthen your immune system. Asking questions and trying to understand as much as you can about hepatitis C can also go a long way toward reducing your stress level. Without knowledge, you run the risk of having your decisions controlled by fear and misinformation.

Regardless of how well-informed you are, there will be times when fear and stress dominate your thought processes. These feelings make it difficult to concentrate on the important issues you need to focus on to make informed decisions about your health and ultimately, your life. It is in those times of fear and stress when it most important to realize you are not alone.

Many people turn to friends, loved ones, and personal advisors during times of stress. If you do not already have a trusted support network of friends, advisors, and mentors, you may want to consider developing such a network. If you choose to pursue this option, seek out people with whom you can openly share your experiences and feelings. Look for people with whom you can speak freely, and from whom you can gain information and insight.

You may also want to consider pursuing individual counseling with a mental health professional or clergy member. These people can further help you adjust to the new realities of your life with hepatitis C. Your physical, mental, and emotional health can all benefit when you share your voice with others, exchange ideas and concepts, and engage in thought-provoking discussions. You can gain much useful information from others who are facing similar circumstances. However, try to keep in mind that each person's experiences are different.

Stressful situations may cause people to seek an escape from their troubles. This leads some people to turn to alcohol or drugs. Drugs and alcohol are very dangerous for people with hepatitis C. Be very cautious about taking any drug (legal or not). Drugs have the potential to seriously complicate the situation for a person living with HCV. Similarly, people with HCV should not drink any alcohol because alcohol is known to increase the liver damage done by chronic HCV infection.

If you are feeling overwhelmed by your situation, we strongly urge you to ask for help. **You are not alone!** Many people are available to help make your situation more manageable and tolerable.

Prescription Medicines and Over-The-Counter Drugs

Some prescription medicines and over-the-counter drugs have toxic effects on the liver. Many over-the-counter compounds contain *acetaminophen* (also known as APAP). Acetaminophen taken in quantities over the recommended or prescribed amount can cause *liver failure*, even in people with a healthy liver. A partial list of common brand name products that contain acetaminophen is shown below. Always read the label to see if the medication you are about to take contains acetaminophen.

Anacin® Aspirin Free
Excedrin P.M.®
Excedrin® Extra-Strength
Excedrin® Migraine
Genapap®
Goody's® Extra Strength Tablets
Tylenol® (all varieties)
Tylenol® Arthritis Pain Extended Relief Caplets®
Vanquish®

Many over-the-counter combination remedies and prescription pain medicines also contain acetaminophen. Some common examples include:

Allerest®
Dristan®
Endocet®
Lorcet-HD®
Lortab®
Midol®
Pamprin®
Percocet®
Percodan®
Percogesic®
Roxicet®
Sinarest®
Sinutab®
Sudafed® Sinus & Headache
Tylox®
Vicodin®

If you are considering taking acetaminophen, discuss it with your healthcare provider first to determine if it is safe for you. The same advice holds true for any medicinal product you are considering taking.

> **Always ask your healthcare provider before taking a new product to make sure it is not toxic to the liver.**

The Physician's Desk Reference (PDR) is available at most local libraries. It provides information about prescription drugs. However, the PDR is written for healthcare professionals and contains technical language that can be quite difficult to understand. Several books written for people with hepatitis C contain excellent lists of prescription drugs about which people with hepatitis C need to be aware. Two examples are *The Hepatitis C Handbook* and *The Hepatitis C Help Book*. See *Appendix IV* for a list of some prescription and over-the-counter medicines that can be harmful to the liver.

Street Drugs and Other Recreational Drugs

People with hepatitis C need to be very cautious about taking drugs of any kind. Nearly all drugs are metabolized by the liver. Some drugs are *hepatotoxic* meaning they have the potential to directly damage the liver. Many other drugs suppress the immune system even if they are not directly hepatotoxic. For example, marijuana is not hepatotoxic but it is *immunosuppressive* and *carcinogenic*.

Immunosuppression makes the body more susceptible to infections. Carcinogens induce chemical changes in the body that can eventually lead to cancer. People with hepatitis C are already at increased risk for *hepatocellular carcinoma* (*liver cancer*). Using carcinogenic drugs adds to this risk. A recent study showed that daily marijuana (cannabis) smoking is significantly associated with fibrosis progression during chronic hepatitis C.[21]

The liver damage caused by HCV can prevent the liver from effectively *metabolizing* and processing drugs. This may cause the effects of drugs to be intensified, increasing the possibility of an overdose.

Even if you already have HCV, you can still be infected with other *quasispecies* of the virus. This can make it more difficult to treat your infection. If you are an intravenous drug user, do not share any equipment. Take every precaution possible to keep a sterile environment to avoid transmitting HCV to someone else. One microscopic drop of blood containing HCV can change another person's life forever.

Tobacco

We know the far-reaching dangers of tobacco use including lung cancer, head and neck cancer, mouth cancer, emphysema, chronic bronchitis, and other conditions. Tobacco contains much more than nicotine, the addictive substance that hooks people into long-term use. Tobacco contains many naturally occurring carcinogens. During the manufacturing process, many other chemicals are added to all forms of tobacco including cigarettes, cigars, pipe tobacco, and chew. Many of these chemical additives are also carcinogens.

Hepatitis C infection and smoking are independent risk factors for liver cancer. Therefore, combining these two risk factors increases your risk for liver cancer. Keeping your body free of tobacco is one important way to help preserve your liver health.

Toxic Chemicals

Every chemical we are exposed to has the potential to stress the liver. Repeated exposure to the following highly toxic chemicals should be rigorously avoided.[22]

> benzene
> carbon monoxide
> carbon tetrachloride and other dry cleaning fluids
> chlorine
> dioxin
> exhaust fumes
> fluoride and fluorine

organophosphorous *pesticides*
paints
petroleum-based chemicals such as gasoline and diesel fuel
radioactive substances
solvents

Vaccines

In general, people with chronic hepatitis C should be vaccinated against *hepatitis A* and hepatitis B. The exceptions would be people who have already had (or currently) have these viruses. There are other exceptions as well, but this is a very important topic to discuss with your doctor.

Protecting yourself against hepatitis A and hepatitis B will prevent the potentially serious complications that may occur if you are infected with more than one of the hepatitis viruses.

Talk with your doctor about whether you need to be vaccinated against hepatitis A and hepatitis B as soon as possible. At the same time, discuss whether you need to be immunized against other infectious diseases as well such as pneumonia and influenza.

Summary

Regular exercise, adequate sleep, and a positive attitude can help promote liver health. Avoiding addictive substances and environmental toxins will also help keep your liver healthy. Behaviors that enhance your immune system should be practiced every chance you get. Anything you can do to promote the health of your liver will help you live a longer, healthier life with hepatitis C.

For more tips on promoting your overall health, see *Chapter 13, Mind-Body Medicine*.

References

1. Waitley D. *The Psychology of Winning.* New York, New York. Simon & Schuester. 1995.
2. Pearsall P. *Superimmunity: Master Your Emotions and Improve Your Health.* New York, New York. McGraw-Hill. 1987.
3. Hobson, A. *Chemistry of Conscious States.* Cambridge, Mass. MIT Press. 1999.
4. Ferrie JE, Shipley MJ, Cappuccio FP, et al. A prospective study of change in sleep duration: associations with mortality in the Whitehall II cohort. *Sleep.* 2007;30(12):1659-66.
5. Palmer M. *Hepatitis and Liver Disease; What you Need to Know.* Venore, TN. Avery. 2000.
6. Fairey AS, Courneya KS, Filed CJ, et al. Randomized controlled trial of exercise and blood immune functioni in postmenopausal breast cancer survivors. *J Appl Physiol.* 2005 Apr;98(4):1534-40
7. Kohut ML, Senchina DS. Reversing age-associated immunosenescence via exercise. *Exerc Immunol Rev.* 2004;10:6-41
8. Dunn AL, Trivedi MH, Kampert JB, et al. Exercise treatment for depression: efficacy and dose response. *Am J Prev Med.* 2005 Jan;28(1):1-8
9. Hickman IJ, Jonsson JR, Prins JB, et al. Modest weight loss and physical activity in overweight patients with chronic liver disease results in sustained improvements in alanine aminotransferase, fasting insulin, and quality of life. *Gut.* 2004 Mar;53(3):413-9
10. Solis-Herruzo JA, Perez-Carreras M, Rivas E, et al. Factors associated with the presence of nonalcoholic steatohepatitis in patients with chronic hepatitis C. *Am J Gastroenterol.* 2005 May;100(5):1091-8
11. Castera L, Hezode C, Roudot-Thoraval F, et al. Worsening of steatosis is an independent factor of fibrosis progression in untreated patients with chronic hepatitis C and paired liver biopsies. *Gut.* 2003;52(2):288-292.
12. Gordon A, McLean CA, Pedersen JS, et al. Hepatic steatosis in chronic hepatitis B and C: predictors, distribution and effect on fibrosis. *J Hepatol.* 2005 Jul;43(1):38-44
13. Younossi ZM, McCullough AJ, Ong JP, et al. Obesity and non-alcoholic fatty liver disease in chronic hepatitis C. *J Clin Gastroenterol.* 2004 Sep;38(8):705-9
14. Harrison SA. Steatosis and chronic hepatitis C infection: mechanisms and significance. *Clin Gastroenterol Hepatol.* 2005 Oct;3(10 Suppl 2):S92-6.
15. Harrison SA, Brunt EM, Qazi RA, et al. Effect of significant histologicic steatosis or steatohepatitis on response to antiviral therapy in patients with chronic hepatitis C. *Clin Gastroenterol Hepatol.* 2005 Jun;3(6):604-9.
16. Antunez I, Aponte N, Fernandez-Carbia A, et al. Steatosis as a predictive factor for treatment response in patients with chronic hepatitis C. *P R Health Sci J.* 2004 Jun:23(2 Suppl):57-60.

17. Bressler B, Guindi M, Tomlinson G, Heathcote J. High body mass index is an independent risk factor for nonresponse to antiviral treatment in chronic hepatitis C. *Hepatology*. 2003;38:639-644.
18. Charnetski CJ, Brennan FX. The effect of sexual behavior on immune system function. Eastern Psychological Association Convention. Providence, Rhode Island. 1999. Available at:http:// www.altmedicine.com/Article.asp?ID=1867. Accessed August 25, 2008
19. Workowski K, Berman S. Sexually Transmitted Diseases Treatment Guidelines, 2006 *MMWR*, August 4, 2006 / 55(RR11);1-94
20. Recommendations for prevention and control of hepatitis C virus (HCV) infection and HCV-related chronic disease. *MMWR*. 1998;47(No. RR19);1-39.
21. Hezode C, Roudot-Thoraval F, Nguyen S, et al. Daily cannabis smoking as a risk factor for progression of fibrosis in chronic hepatitis C. *Hepatology*. 2005 Jul:42(1):63-71.
22. Dolan M. *The Hepatitis C Handbook, 2nd Ed*. Berkeley, California. North Atlantic Books. 1999.

Signs and Symptoms That May Be Associated with Hepatitis C

CHAPTER 5

Tina M. St. John, MD

Introduction

Hepatitis C affects different people in different ways. Your experience with hepatitis C will be as unique as you are. This chapter reviews the most common *signs* and *symptoms* experienced by people with *chronic hepatitis* C. At first glance, the mere length of the chapter may appear overwhelming. But keep in mind, this is just a list of possibilities. Many people with hepatitis C have no symptoms.

If you have any of the signs or symptoms described in this chapter, it is important not to assume they are a result of having hepatitis C. Your healthcare provider can determine if they are associated with your hepatitis C. Many symptoms come and go on their own. For troublesome and/or persistent problems, there are things you and your healthcare provider can do to either make them go away, or make them easier to live with.

You may be wondering what the difference is between a sign and a symptom. A sign is an abnormality detected by your healthcare provider during an examination. A symptom is something you, as a person with hepatitis C, experience because of the virus. Signs and symptoms are discussed together because sometimes a sign is also a symptom. Fever is a good example of something that is both a sign and a symptom. Your healthcare provider can take your temperature and detect a fever, so it is a sign. But if you have a fever, you experience its discomfort, so fever is also a symptom.

There are three sections following this introduction. The first section briefly explains how the hepatitis C virus causes disease. The second section reviews possible signs and symptoms that people with hepatitis C who do not have *cirrhosis* may experience. The last section reviews additional signs and symptoms that people with hepatitis C who have cirrhosis may experience.

How the Hepatitis C Virus Causes Disease

According to current understanding, the hepatitis C virus (*HCV*) causes disease in two general ways. The first is by infecting cells. Once inside the cell, the virus directly damages or kills the cell. This mechanism is called *cytopathic* damage. The second way the hepatitis C virus causes damage is by provoking an immune response. The *immune system* is your body's way of protecting itself from invading agents such as viruses and bacteria. An overactive or misdirected immune response can damage infected cells and the normal surrounding tissues. This mechanism is called *immunopathic* damage.

When HCV was first discovered, experts thought the virus infected only liver cells. However, research has revealed that HCV also infects parts of the immune system, specifically the *lymphatic system* and *peripheral blood mononuclear cells*.

Experts now understand that hepatitis C is not just a liver disease, but is a systemic disease, meaning it can affect nearly any organ of the body. As you read the list of possible signs and symptoms associated with hepatitis C infection, you may find some of the symptoms you have been experiencing that you thought were caused by something else may actually be caused by hepatitis C. This is important because knowing why you are having a symptom is often the first step in alleviating the symptom, or making it less troublesome.

Signs and Symptoms of Hepatitis C Without Cirrhosis

The possible signs and symptoms of hepatitis C without cirrhosis involve every organ system of the body. Although some of these symptoms can be quite uncomfortable, most of them do not indicate that your liver disease is getting worse. New symptoms should always be discussed with your healthcare provider so you can work together to keep your life with hepatitis C as active, productive, and enjoyable as possible. The lists are presented in alphabetical order to make it easier to look up those signs and symptoms of interest to you.

Generalized Signs and Symptoms

ARTHRALGIA

Arthralgia is pain in the joints. Frequent sites of joint pain are the hips, knees, fingers, and spine, although any joint can be a source of pain. Arthralgia associated with hepatitis C can be migratory, meaning the discomfort moves from one location to another over time. You may have pain in your hip one day and in your knee the next. This symptom usually comes and goes, and is rarely present all the time.

If you experience joint pain, it is important to talk with your healthcare provider before taking anything to treat the pain because some over-the-counter pain medicines such as *acetaminophen* are potentially harmful to the liver. See *Appendix IV* for a list of substances that may injure the liver.

FATIGUE

Fatigue is feeling tired. Nearly all people with hepatitis C experience fatigue at one time or another. The fatigue may be mild and relieved by naps or going to bed early. However, fatigue can be severe, feeling like near exhaustion even after a full night of sleep. Fatigue experienced by people with hepatitis C may also be accompanied by feelings of anger, hostility, and *depression*. These feelings may persist even after the fatigue has passed.

FEVER, CHILLS, AND NIGHT SWEATS

Many people with the hepatitis C virus (HCV) experience fevers from time to time. The fevers are usually low, typically less than 101 degrees Fahrenheit. As the fever comes down, you may experience chills and sweating. You may have fevers only at night. If this happens, you may wake up with your bedclothes and/or your sheets wet with sweat. This experience is called night sweats.

FLUID RETENTION

Fluid retention occurs when your body holds on to more water than it needs. The extra water leaks into the tissues. You may notice swelling of your feet, ankles, fingers, and/or face. People with fluid retention often have frequent urination, especially at night.

FLU-LIKE SYNDROME

People with hepatitis C can experience periodic flu-like syndromes. These episodes usually last a few days, rarely more than a week. The most common symptoms are fever, chills, headache, fatigue, and/or muscle aches.

LYMPHADENOPATHY

Lymphadenopathy is swelling of the *lymph nodes*. Lymph nodes are normally about the size of a pea. Because HCV infects the lymphatic system, it frequently causes the lymph nodes to swell. The lymph nodes of the armpits, groin, and neck are relatively close to the skin surface, and are usually examined to see if you have lymphadenopathy. If you have lymphadenopathy, it may or may not be painful when you press on the swollen lymph nodes.

MYALGIA

Myalgia is muscle pain or aching. This symptom is typically experienced as a generalized feeling. However, some people report pain in only one area of the body. Myalgia tends to come and go, and is rarely present all the time. If you experience muscle aches or pain, it is important to talk with your healthcare provider before taking anything to treat the pain because some over-the-counter pain medicines are potentially harmful to the liver.

PRURITUS

Pruritus is the medical word for itching. People with hepatitis C sometimes have pruritus. Often, it is limited to the palms of the hands and/or the soles of the feet. However, some people have generalized pruritus, meaning they itch all over.

SLEEP DISTURBANCES

Insomnia is difficulty sleeping. It occurs in different forms. You may have trouble falling asleep, or you may wake up often during the night. Some people report having unusually vivid, intense, and/or frightening dreams. Such dreams can contribute to insomnia.

SPIDER NEVI

Spider nevi are small, red, spider shaped spots on the skin. They are usually less than ½ inch around. They are most commonly seen on the face and chest, but can occur anywhere on the skin. Spider nevi are painless and do not itch.

WEAKNESS

People with hepatitis C sometimes experience a sense of weakness. This symptom can vary from mild to severe, and tends to come and go.

Abdominal and Digestive System Signs and Symptoms

ABDOMINAL PAIN

You may experience episodes of abdominal pain if you have hepatitis C. Pain on the right side just below the ribs is likely to be from the liver. People usually report this pain as being short, sharp, or stabbing. More constant, cramping pain closer to the middle of chest, but under the ribs, can be due to gall bladder problems that may accompany hepatitis C. You may experience pain elsewhere in the abdomen.

If you experience any new pain in the abdomen, it is important for you to tell your healthcare provider right away so the source of the pain can be determined.

APPETITE CHANGES AND WEIGHT LOSS

People with hepatitis C often report changes in appetite. You may find you no longer want the foods you once enjoyed. Many people find they are particularly put off by fatty foods and alcohol. For some, foods at room temperature or served cold are more appealing than hot foods. The distaste for alcohol is actually good for you because alcohol increases the damage done to the liver by HCV. People with hepatitis C should not drink any *alcohol* including beer, wine, wine coolers, and mixed drinks.

If changes in your appetite are causing weight loss, discuss this with your healthcare provider because good nutrition is particularly important for people with hepatitis C.

BLOATING

Bloating is usually described as a feeling of fullness in the abdomen. You may notice your clothes seem tight around your waist. This bloating may or may not be accompanied by weight gain. Talk with your doctor about any new bloating you experience.

DIARRHEA

Diarrhea can be experienced as unusually loose stools or an increase in the frequency of bowel movements, with or without a change in the consistency of the stool. Persistent diarrhea, especially if accompanied by weight loss, should be discussed with your doctor right away.

INDIGESTION AND HEARTBURN

Indigestion is typically experienced as an uncomfortable feeling of fullness in the stomach. It is often accompanied by queasiness and burping of a mixture of gas and stomach contents. When this occurs, you may notice a burning feeling in your throat and/or a sour taste in your mouth. Heartburn is experienced as pain or burning in the chest under the breastbone. It, too, may be accompanied by burping of gas and stomach contents. Both indigestion and heartburn can be brought on by and last longer after a fatty meal.

JAUNDICE

Jaundice is a yellowish discoloration of the skin and/or the whites of the eyes. It is caused by a yellow substance in the blood called *bilirubin*. The liver normally breaks down bilirubin. If the liver is not working normally, bilirubin can build up in the blood and begin to stain the skin.

NAUSEA

Nausea is the feeling that you may vomit. Although it is usually not accompanied by vomiting, nausea can be a very uncomfortable and debilitating symptom. If you are experiencing nausea, talk with your healthcare provider because there are many ways to treat this symptom.

Cognitive, Mood, and Nervous System Signs and Symptoms

COGNITIVE CHANGES

Cognition is your ability to think clearly and to concentrate. Some people with hepatitis C notice changes in their cognitive ability. This can take several different forms. You may find you cannot concentrate for long periods of time, or may notice your thought processes seem slower than usual. You may have a hard time coming up with words you want to say, or may just feel mentally tired. These cognitive changes are sometimes called "brain fog." Like other symptoms of hepatitis C, these cognitive changes often come and go. Always discuss cognitive changes with your doctor as they may or may not be related to hepatitis C.

DEPRESSION

Hepatitis C does not directly cause depression, but concerns about the disease and changes it may cause in your life can lead to depression. Some of the symptoms of depression include:

- sleeping more or less than usual
- eating more or less than usual
- hopelessness
- helplessness
- irritability
- lack of interest in your usual activities
- feelings of sadness and/or despair most of the time

If you have one or more of these symptoms, you may have depression. Depression can seriously interfere with your quality of life and make it difficult for you to take care of yourself. Depression is nothing to be ashamed of, and it can be treated. If you have any of the symptoms of depression, talk to your healthcare provider right away.

DIZZINESS

Some people experience dizziness as feeling as if they are going to faint. Others experience dizziness as disorientation, or feeling as if the world is spinning around them. Both of these symptoms have been reported by people living with hepatitis C. If you are experiencing dizziness, talk with your healthcare provider because this can be not only troublesome but also dangerous.

HEADACHES

Headaches are common and may be part of your experience with hepatitis C. The pain can range from minor to severe. If you are having headaches, talk to your healthcare provider before taking any medicines for your headaches because some over-the-counter pain medicines can be harmful to your liver.

MOOD SWINGS

Some people with hepatitis C report sudden mood swings. Mood swings may be related to depression, anxiety, or the medications you are taking.

NUMBNESS OR TINGLING

A number of people with hepatitis C have numbness or tingling in their extremities (arms, legs, fingers, or toes). Most people with numbness or tingling feel it in their fingers and toes, but it may extend into the arms and legs. Numbness is a decreased sense of feeling. In its most severe form, the affected areas have no feeling. Tingling can be painful. People describe painful tingling as feeling like being stuck with pins. This symptom tends to come and go.

VISUAL CHANGES

A number of visual changes can accompany hepatitis C infection. You may find you are not seeing as clearly as you once did. Peripheral vision, the ability to see things that are at the sides of your view, can also be diminished. Some people report seeing small specks called "floaters" moving across their view. This can occur when the eyes are open or closed. Any sudden changes in vision should be reported to your doctor right away.

Another symptom you may experience is dryness of the eyes, or feeling as if there is something scratchy in your eyes. All of these symptoms can come and go.

Other Signs and Symptoms

BLOOD SUGAR ABNORMALITIES

Hepatitis C can cause *blood sugar* abnormalities, either high or low. High blood sugar causes symptoms such as extreme thirst, frequent urination, fatigue, and weight loss. Low blood sugar causes light-headedness, dizziness, nausea, and weakness. The symptoms of low blood sugar are worst when you have not eaten for several hours, and are relieved by eating or drinking something. If you are having any of the symptoms of either high or low blood sugar, tell your healthcare provider right away.

CHEST PAIN

Hepatitis C can cause chest pain, usually a form of heartburn. However, chest pain can also be a symptom of serious heart or lung disease. If you have chest pain, contact your healthcare provider immediately.

MENSTRUAL AND MENOPAUSAL CHANGES

Women with hepatitis C have reported menstrual changes such as irregular periods, spotting, or increased premenstrual symptoms. Menopausal women may experience an increase in menopausal symptoms such as hot flashes and mood swings.

PALPITATIONS

A heart *palpitation* is involuntarily becoming aware of your heart beating. Palpitations occur in different forms. You may feel your heart is beating harder or faster than usual, or that it is beating irregularly. If you have palpitations, you need to tell your healthcare provider immediately so he or she can make sure you are not having a problem with your heart.

SEXUAL CHANGES

Some people with hepatitis C have a decreased interest in sexual activity. Decreased sexual response and lack of intensity of sexual response have also been reported. Sexual changes can be quite upsetting. If you are experiencing sexual changes, talk with your healthcare provider, and your spouse or partner. There are things that you, your healthcare provider, and your partner can do to help you have a satisfying sex life.

Signs and Symptoms of Hepatitis C With Cirrhosis

Approximately 20% to 40% of people with chronic hepatitis C go on to develop liver cirrhosis over a period of 10 to 40 years. Because blood cannot flow well through a cirrhotic liver, blood backs up in the vessels leading to the liver. This back up leads to an increase in pressure in those blood vessels, a condition known as *portal hypertension*. Many of the signs and symptoms of cirrhosis are related to portal hypertension. The liver has many functions, so there are a number of things that can go wrong when the liver is not functioning normally. Abnormal liver function causes the other signs and symptoms of hepatitis C with cirrhosis.

ASCITES
Portal hypertension can cause fluid to leak from the blood vessels leading to the liver. This fluid builds up in the abdomen and is called *ascites*. Ascites causes the abdomen to become *distended* or enlarged. This can be experienced as bloating or a feeling of persistent fullness in the gut.

BLEEDING PROBLEMS
The liver produces many of the substances needed for normal blood clotting. A cirrhotic liver may not produce enough of these substances for normal clotting. If you have a cirrhotic liver and begin bleeding for any reason, it may be difficult to get the bleeding stopped.

BONE PAIN
Cirrhosis can lead to a deficiency in *vitamin D*. This can cause softening of the bones and bone pain. This pain is most often felt in the legs, hips, and spine.

BRUISING
Cirrhosis can lead to a deficiency in vitamin K and low levels of clotting factors in the blood. This can lead to easy bruising. If you are experiencing easy bruising, tell your healthcare provider because this symptom can often be reversed with appropriate treatment.

CAPUT MEDUSAE
Caput medusae refers to enlarged, visible veins that start at the navel and spread out and up over the abdomen. They are caused by portal hypertension.

GASTROESOPHAGEAL VARICES
Gastroesophageal varices are another complication of portal hypertension. Varices are enlarged, fragile veins found where the esophagus (the tube that takes food from your mouth to your stomach) meets the stomach. These veins can burst and bleed.

If you have cirrhosis and begin to vomit blood, you must call an ambulance and get to an emergency room as soon as possible to get the bleeding stopped.

GLOSSITIS
Glossitis is a sore tongue. If you have glossitis, your tongue will be redder than usual and will be sensitive to salty and sour foods, and carbonated beverages.

HEMORRHOIDS
Hemorrhoids are enlarged, fragile veins found around the anus (the opening through which your bowel movements pass). Hemorrhoids can be a complication of portal hypertension. Hemorrhoids may bleed occasionally. If the bleeding persists or is frequent, be sure to discuss it with your healthcare provider.

HEPATIC ENCEPHALOPATHY
Hepatic encephalopathy is one of the most serious complications of cirrhosis. It can occur in an acute form that devel-

ops over a period of days to weeks, or it can occur in a chronic form that develops over a period of months to years. A number of different symptoms may indicate hepatic encephalopathy, but all of them indicate abnormalities of the nervous system. Early symptoms include euphoria (feeling unusually happy for no apparent reason), depression, confusion, slurred speech, or abnormal sleeping patterns.

If these symptoms are not treated, they can progress to severe confusion, incoherent speech, tremors, and rigidity. It is urgent for these symptoms to be treated or you could fall into a coma. With the acute form of hepatic encephalopathy, treatment will usually reverse all of the symptoms. However, with the chronic form, some of the symptoms may not be reversible.

MELANOSIS
Melanosis is a gradual darkening of those areas of skin that are exposed to the sun. The skin tends to get darker over time.

NIGHT BLINDNESS
Cirrhosis can lead to a deficiency in *vitamin A*. This can lead to episodes of night blindness (poor vision in the dark). If this occurs, be certain to talk about it with your healthcare provider because this symptom is often reversible.

SHORTNESS OF BREATH
Shortness of breath can develop as a complication of portal hypertension. Some people experience this symptom only at night; others experience it during the day as well. If you are having shortness of breath, discuss it with your healthcare provider.

STEATORRHEA
Steatorrhea is the passing of fat in your bowel movements. The presence of fat in the stool makes the stool smell particularly bad and causes it to float in the toilet bowl. Steatorrhea is usually accompanied by an increased amount of stool and intestinal gas.

XANTHELASMA
Xanthelasmas are small deposits of fat just under the surface of the skin around your eyes. They appear as small, raised, yellowish bumps on the skin.

XANTHOMA
Xanthomas are small deposits of fat just under the surface of the skin over your joints and/or tendons. They appear as small, raised, yellowish nodules.

Summary

The experience of living with hepatitis C is quite different from one person to another. It is also variable for each person over time. There will probably be days when you feel great. At other times, you may feel overwhelmed by signs and symptoms associated with hepatitis C. And there will likely be still other times when you feel somewhere in between these two states. Below are a few things you may find helpful to keep in mind about your signs and symptoms as you learn to live with hepatitis C.

- Discuss your signs and symptoms with your healthcare provider. There are many ways to treat the signs and symptoms associated with hepatitis C, so there is no need to suffer in silence.

- Always tell your healthcare provider if you experience a new sign or symptom. Doing this will help them in their efforts to help you feel your best.

- Keep all of your healthcare providers informed about what treatments, medicines, and supplements you are using to manage your hepatitis C. Different treatments may interact with one another and cause side effects you may experience as new signs or symptoms.

- Do not panic if you start to experience new signs or symptoms. Although many of the signs and symptoms associated with hepatitis C can be troubling, they do not necessarily mean your liver disease is getting worse.

References

1. Dolan, M. *The Hepatitis C Handbook*, 2nd ed. Berkeley, California: North Atlantic Books; 1999.
2. Fauci A, Braunwald E, Isselbacher K, Wilson J, Martin J, Kasper D, Hauser S, Longo D, eds. *Harrison's Principles of Internal Medicine*. 14th ed. New York, New York: McGraw Hill Companies; 1998.
3. Mandell G, Bennett J, Dolin R, eds. *Principles and Practice of Infectious Diseases*. 4th ed. New York, New York: Churchill Livingstone; 1995.

LABORATORY TESTS AND PROCEDURES

Tina M. St. John, MD

Introduction

Chronic hepatitis C is a complex disease. The course and *symptoms* vary from one person to another.

The liver is one of the most important organs of the body. It performs many jobs including:

- production of *proteins*, *cholesterol*, *bile*, *heme*, and other substances
- regulation of fats in the body
- activation of *vitamins* and drugs
- detoxification of harmful chemicals

With all of these important jobs, many things can potentially go wrong if the liver is damaged. Further complicating the disease is the fact that, although the *hepatitis C virus* (*HCV*) primarily infects the liver, it can affect any organ system of the body.

Laboratory testing is one tool healthcare providers use to find out how HCV is affecting your body. A number of tests are available. This chapter describes some of the most common laboratory tests used to diagnose and/or monitor chronic hepatitis C.

Your healthcare provider will consider your symptoms and disease status in deciding what tests you need and when they should be done. Therefore, you should not look at this list as tests that should be done, but rather as a list of tests that may be helpful in specific situations.

Other tests are available that are not listed here. If your healthcare provider orders a test you are not familiar with, ask him or her what the test is and why it is being done. If you are considering *interferon-based therapy*, be sure to read, "What You Need to Know Regarding Therapy" in *Chapter 8.2, Initial Treatment Options* for a complete list of recommended tests before, during, and after treatment.

What Is Normal?

Each testing laboratory has its own range of normal values for each test. A laboratory's normal range means that the majority of people in good health tested by that laboratory have values within this range. Your test results will be compared to the laboratory's normal range. If you have had the same test before, the new result will be compared to previous results. This allows your healthcare provider to look for changes over time. It is important for you and your healthcare provider to know what laboratory is conducting your tests to ensure that appropriate comparisons are being made.

We suggest that you request copies of your laboratory test results for your own files. This can help you better understand and track your disease process.

Liver Enzymes and Liver Function Tests

You will probably hear your healthcare providers talk about *liver enzymes* and *liver function tests* (LFTs). These two broad categories of tests give your healthcare providers different information about what is happening in your liver. Liver enzymes are proteins inside liver cells. When liver cells are damaged, liver enzymes are released into the blood. Therefore, liver enzyme tests indicate how much damage is occurring to your liver. Examples of liver enzymes that are frequently monitored in chronic hepatitis C include *AST, ALT, GGT*, and *alkaline phosphatase*.

Although liver enzymes indicate how much damage is being done to the liver cells, they do not tell your healthcare provider how much repair is taking place. Unlike many other organs, the liver has a remarkable ability to repair itself. This is important when considering liver enzymes because, although there may be ongoing damage to liver cells, the liver may be able to repair this damage without a decrease in function.

Liver function tests give your healthcare providers information about how well the liver is performing its many jobs. Because the liver has so many different jobs, there are many different liver function tests, each indicating how well the liver is performing a specific job. Examples of LFTs commonly monitored in chronic hepatitis C include *bilirubin, albumin*, and *platelet* count.

Viral Load Testing

HCV *viral load* testing determines how much of the virus is present in the blood. Viral load is one factor your doctor takes into consideration when estimating your chance of success with interferon-based therapy. If you are already on treatment, the test is used to check your response to the medications.

There are different methods used to perform viral load testing including *PCR, b-DNA*, and *TMA*. These methods are described later in the chapter. Viral testing methods are often referred to collectively as molecular testing or nucleic acid testing (NAT). Most laboratories buy their testing materials from companies that produce hepatitis C viral testing kits. However, some large laboratories have developed their own testing materials and procedures.

Although it is not necessary for you to understand the technical differences between the various methods of molecular testing, you do need to be aware of the fact that different methods often give different results. Sometimes these differences are quite large. Therefore, when you have HCV viral load testing, you need to be aware of what type of test was used and where the test was performed. Without this information, it is almost impossible to interpret the meaning of changes in viral load.

In addition to the type of viral load test used, you also need to be aware of how the test result is reported. When HCV viral load tests were first developed, the results were reported as the number of copies per mL (copies/mL) or equivalents per mL (equiv/mL). To simplify and standardize reporting, the World Health Organization developed a standard unit for reporting the results of HCV viral load tests. The current reporting standard for viral load testing is International Units per mL (IU/mL).

If your viral loads have been reported in different units over time, you may be confused about what is happening with your viral load. Below are two mathematical conversions to help you.

If PCR was used
To convert IU/mL into copies/mL, take the result in IU/mL and multiply by 2.7.
        Example: 1,000,000 IU/mL x 2.7 = 2,700,000 copies/mL
To convert copies/mL into IU/mL, take the result in copies/mL and divide by 2.7.
        Example: 2,700,000 copies/mL ÷ 2.7 = 1,000,000 IU/mL

If TMA was used
To convert IU/mL into copies/mL, take the result in IU/mL and multiply by 5.2.
        Example: 1,000,000 IU/mL x 5.2 = 5,200,000 copies/mL
To convert from copies/mL into IU/mL, take the result in copies/mL and divide by 5.2.
        Example: 5,200,000 copies/mL ÷ 5.2 = 1,000,000 IU/mL

HCV viral loads do not reflect liver disease status nor disease progression.

HCV viral loads fluctuate within a very broad range. These fluctuations are typical of untreated, chronic hepatitis C. Therefore, many healthcare providers do not monitor HCV viral load in people who are not on interferon-based therapy. However, if you are considering interferon-based therapy or are on such treatment, your HCV viral load becomes important.

HCV viral load is measured before and during interferon-based therapy because it is used to determine response to treatment. Research has shown that those people who experience a *sustained viral response* to interferon-based therapy have a significant drop in HCV viral load by week 12 of treatment (an early viral response or EVR). More recently, researchers have been studying a new time point in predicting the probability of sustained viral response to interferon-based therapy. This new time point has been dubbed rapid viral response or RVR and describes a significant drop in HCV viral load by week 4 of treatment.

HCV Viral Response Terms

EVR: Early Viral Response
> Greater than or equal to 100-fold drop in HCV viral load by week 12 of interferon-based treatment.

RVR: Rapid Viral Response
> Greater than or equal to 100-fold drop in HCV viral load by week 4 of interferon-based treatment.

SVR: Sustained Viral Response
> Undetectable hepatitis C virus for at least 24 weeks after therapy is completed.

Healthcare providers often discuss viral load changes using the term "logs." The term "log" refers to the mathematical notation called logarithms. Although there are many log scales, when used to discuss viral load, the scale being referred to is log10 or log base 10. While this may seem complicated, the use of logs is just a shorthand way of talking about viral load changes.

1-log change is a 10-fold change in viral load
> Examples:
> 1,000 copies /mL to 10,000 copies/mL is a 1-log increase in viral load
> → (1,000 x 10 = 10,000)
>
> 50,000,000 copies/mL to 5,000,000 copies/mL is a 1-log decrease in viral load
> → (50,000,000 ÷ 10 = 5,000,000)

2-log change is a 100-fold change in viral load
> Examples:
> 1,000 copies/mL to 100,000 copies/mL is a 2-log increase in viral load
> → (1,000 x 100 = 100,000)
>
> 8,500,000 copies/mL to 85,000 copies/mL is a 2-log decrease in viral load
> → (8,500,000 ÷ 100 = 85,000)

3-log change is a 1,000-fold change in viral load

Examples:

1,000 copies/mL to 1,000,000 copies/mL is a 3-log increase in viral load
→ (1,000 x 1,000 = 1,000,000)

250,000,000 copies/mL to 250,000 copies/mL is a 3-log decrease in viral load
→ (250,000,000 ÷ 1,000 = 250,000)

If you have questions about a change in your viral load, talk with your healthcare provider. He or she can explain what your test results mean.

Sample Laboratory Report

Following is a sample laboratory report. The tests on the sample report are described in the next section of this chapter.

The Testing Laboratory
100 The Road
Anytown, OH 00000

Patient: John Doe   **Sex:** M   **DoB:** 12/01/55

TEST	RESULT	NORMAL RANGE (see note below)
WBC	7.2	5-10 thousand/mm^3
RBC	4.80	4.70-6.10 million/ mm^3
Hemoglobin	13.6 L	14.0-18.0 g/dL
Hematocrit	41.6 L	42.0-52.0%
Platelet Count	260	140-440 thousand/ mm^3
PT	11.9	10.0-12.5 seconds (0.9-1.1 INR)
Fibrinogen	385	150-450 mg/dL
Sodium	141	140-148 mmol/L
Potassium	3.9	3.6-5.2 mmol/L
Chloride	104	100-108 mmol/L
Carbon Dioxide	24.5	21.0-32.0 mmol/L
Albumin	3.4	3.4-5.0 g/dL
Total Protein	6.2 L	6.4-8.2 g/dL
Glucose	85	70-110 mg/dL
Cholesterol, Total	216 H	<200 mg/dL
BUN	10	7-18 mg/dL
Creatinine	0.8	0.6-1.3 mg/dL
Bilirubin, Total	0.18	0.00-1.00 mg/dL
AST	42 H	15-37 IU/L
ALT	78 H	30-65 IU/L
GGT	46	5-85 IU/L
Alk Phos	74	50-136 IU/L
Ethanol	0	None detected
Ammonia	18	11-35 µmol/L
Ferritin	149	15-200 ng/mL
AFP	12	<25 ng/mL
HCV Antibodies	positive*	negative
HCV RNA	650,000*	undetectable
HCV Genotype	1b	--------
ANA	negative	negative
Cryoglobulins	negative	negative

IMPORTANT NOTE: This laboratory report is only an example. The units and normal ranges reported by your testing laboratory may be different. Please see your own laboratory reports to find if your test values are within *your* laboratory's normal range.

Laboratory Test List

The laboratory tests described below are in alphabetical order. For each test, you will see:

- the name of the test
- other names for the test (if applicable)
- what the test is
- why the test is used in people with chronic hepatitis C

Be aware that there are other uses for many of the tests listed, but only their role in hepatitis C is described here.

AFP – see *alfa-fetoprotein*

alanine aminotransferase (ALT)

Other Names

alanine transaminase, previously called *glutamate pyruvate transaminase* (*GPT* or *SGPT*)

What?

alanine aminotransferase (*ALT*) is an enzyme found inside liver cells. It is also found in other cells such as those of the heart and pancreas. The liver contains large amounts of ALT.

Why Test?

Testing the blood for ALT is one way of telling if liver cells are dying. When liver cells die, ALT is released into the blood. ALT levels rise over a period of 7 to 12 days, and then slowly return to normal. When there is ongoing liver cell death, ALT levels remain elevated. Your ALT level tells your healthcare provider how much ongoing damage is occurring in your liver. However, an elevated ALT level does not necessarily mean your liver disease is getting worse because this test cannot determine how much repair is occurring and how many new liver cells are being produced.

albumin

What?

Albumin is the most abundant protein in the blood. It is made in the liver.

Why Test?

In advanced *cirrhosis*, the liver begins to fail at its many jobs. Since albumin is made in the liver, a failing liver may not make enough albumin. Measuring albumin is one way of testing how well a cirrhotic liver is making proteins.

alcohol

What?

Alcohol is the intoxicating substance in beer, wine, and hard liquor. It may also be found in over-the-counter medications such as cough syrups, and in certain mouthwashes and other products.

Why Test?

Alcohol is toxic to the liver. People with hepatitis C should not consume any alcohol. Research has shown that even small amounts of alcohol may worsen the damage done to your liver by the hepatitis C virus. Your blood alcohol should always be zero.

alfa-fetoprotein (AFP)

What?

Alfa-fetoprotein (AFP) is a substance normally found in only trace amounts in the body. High amounts may indicate the presence of a *tumor*.

Why Test?

People with chronic hepatitis C are at increased risk for *liver cancer*. Alfa-fetoprotein is a tumor marker for liver cancer, meaning an abnormally high amount may indicate the presence of a cancerous liver tumor. Elevated alfa-fetoprotein does not always indicate the presence of liver cancer. However, it is often used to screen for the disease in people with HCV.

alkaline phosphatase (ALP or alk phos)
What?

ALP is an enzyme found in nearly every tissue of the body. The highest concentrations of ALP are found in the liver, bones, intestines, kidneys, and the placentas of pregnant women. In normal adult men and non-pregnant adult women, most of the alkaline phosphatase in the blood comes from the liver and bones.

Why Test?

Testing the blood for ALP is one way to know if the bile ducts of the liver are working normally. When liver cells die, scarring takes place. Scarring may cause blockage of the bile ducts slowing bile flow through the liver. This condition is called *cholestasis*. Cholestasis causes the liver to make more ALP. Some of this ALP is released into the blood. ALP is also elevated when bile flow is blocked outside the liver. A common cause of this type of blockage is gallstones.

alkaline phosphatase isoenzymes (ALP isoenzymes)
What?

ALP from different tissues differs chemically. The ALP isoenzyme test measures the different forms of ALP.

Why Test?

If the ALP is elevated in the blood, it is important to know what tissue(s) it came from. The test for ALP isoenzymes measures how much ALP is from the liver and how much is from other tissues. Elevated ALP from the liver usually indicates a blockage of bile flow either inside or outside the liver.

ALT – see *alanine aminotransferase*

aminopyrine clearance test
What?

Aminopyrine is a chemical used to determine how well the liver is *metabolizing* and detoxifying substances.

Why Test?

Two of the liver's many important jobs are to metabolize drugs and detoxify foreign chemicals. The a*minopyrine clearance test* is used to determine how well the liver is performing these jobs. A single test does not give much useful information, but comparing a series of tests over time can show if liver function is decreasing.

ammonia
What?

Ammonia is a chemical normally found in very low levels in the blood. It comes from the normal breakdown of proteins in the body.

Why Test?

One potential complication of cirrhosis and *portal hypertension* is a condition called *hepatic encephalopathy*. See *Chapter 5, Signs and Symptoms That May be Associated with Hepatitis C* for an explanation of hepatic encephalopathy. Ammonia levels are high in hepatic encephalopathy and testing for ammonia can help make the diagnosis.

anti-HCV antibodies
Other Names

HCV antibodies, hepatitis C screening test, HCV-EIA

What?

After being exposed to the hepatitis C virus, the body develops several different *antibodies* to the virus. The anti-HCV test detects these antibodies.

Why Test?

The presence of HCV antibodies indicates a person has been exposed to HCV. Several different tests are available to detect HCV antibodies. Depending on the test used, there are differences in how soon HCV antibodies can be detected in the blood after exposure to the virus. If this screening test is positive, a second test called a confirmatory test is usually performed to test for the hepatitis C virus itself. The presence of the hepatitis C virus in the blood confirms current infection with the virus. The *anti-HCV antibody* test cannot tell whether you currently have the hepatitis C virus in your body. It only determines whether you have been exposed to the virus.

anti-liver-kidney microsomal antibodies (anti-LKM)
What?
Anti-liver-kidney microsomal antibodies (*anti-LKM*) are a type of *autoantibody*. Normally, the body makes antibodies only against foreign substances such as bacteria and viruses. *Autoantibodies* are abnormal antibodies that act against your own cells.
Why Test?
More than half of all people with chronic hepatitis C have one or more autoantibodies in their blood. This is important to know because autoantibodies can cause additional symptoms and disease.

anti-nuclear antibodies (ANA)
What?
Anti-nuclear antibodies (ANA) are a type of autoantibody. Normally, the body makes antibodies only against foreign substances such as bacteria and viruses. Autoantibodies are abnormal antibodies that act against your own cells.
Why Test?
More than half of all people with chronic hepatitis C have one or more autoantibodies in their blood. This is important to know because autoantibodies can cause additional symptoms and disease.

anti-smooth muscle antibodies (anti-SMA)
What?
Anti-smooth muscle antibodies (*anti-SMA*) are a type of autoantibody. Normally, the body makes antibodies only against foreign substances such as bacteria and viruses. Autoantibodies are abnormal antibodies that act against your own cells.
Why Test?
More than half of all people with chronic hepatitis C have one or more autoantibodies in their blood. This is important to know because autoantibodies can cause additional symptoms and disease.

APTT – see *partial thromboplastin time*

aspartate aminotransferase (AST)
Other Names
aspartate transaminase, previously called *glutamate oxaloacetate transaminase* (*GOT* or SGOT)
What?
Aspartate aminotransferase (AST) is an enzyme found in liver cells. It is also found in other cells such as those of the heart and muscles. The largest amounts of AST are found in the heart and liver.
Why Test?
Testing the blood for AST is one way of telling if liver cells are dying. When liver cells die, AST is released into the blood. AST levels rise over a period of 7 to 12 days, and then slowly return to normal. When there is ongoing liver cell death, AST levels remain elevated. Your AST level tells your healthcare provider how much ongoing damage is occurring in your liver. However, an elevated AST level does not necessarily mean your liver disease is getting worse because this test cannot determine how much repair is occurring and how many new liver cells are being produced.

AST – see *aspartate aminotransferase*

AST/ALT Ratio
What?
This is not a laboratory test per se, but rather a calculation based on the AST and ALT test results. The AST result is divided by the ALT result to get the ratio.
Why Test?
In patients with viral hepatitis, elevations in ALT are typically equal to or greater than AST elevations. This results in an AST/ALT ratio less than or equal to 1. Conversely, ALT is typically elevated to a lesser degree than AST in alcoholic liver disease and cirrhosis. This results in an AST/ALT greater than 1. Following the AST/ALT ratio over time is one of the many pieces of information doctors use in monitoring for the development of cirrhosis.

bicarbonate (HCO$_3$)

Other Names
total carbon dioxide

What?
Bicarbonate is a charged particle called an *electrolyte*. It is one of four major electrolytes in the body.

Why Test?
Electrolytes perform many important jobs in the body. Two of the most important jobs are regulating the amount of water in your body and keeping your blood pH normal. Some people with hepatitis C hold more water in their bodies than they need. This can cause abnormal bicarbonate levels. This is more likely in people with cirrhosis than in those without cirrhosis.

bile acids

What?
Bile acids are a group of chemicals produced by the breakdown of *cholesterol*.

Why Test?
Blood bile acid levels are a sensitive indicator of liver and gall bladder function. Abnormal bile acid levels suggest abnormal functioning of the liver and/or gall bladder.

bilirubin, conjugated

Other Names
direct bilirubin

What?
Bilirubin is a yellow chemical produced during the normal breakdown of red blood cells. Bilirubin is normally processed by the liver into other substances that can be eliminated from the body. There are two forms of bilirubin in the body, conjugated (direct) bilirubin and unconjugated (indirect) bilirubin. *Conjugated bilirubin* is bilirubin that is attached to another chemical called glucuronic acid in a process called conjugation. Conjugation takes place inside liver cells. Conjugated bilirubin is excreted in the bile. Normally, conjugated bilirubin makes up less than 10% of the total bilirubin.

Why Test?
If the total bilirubin in the blood is high, it is important to know how much of it is conjugated because this tells your healthcare provider what process in the liver is not working normally. High amounts of conjugated bilirubin usually means the bile flow is blocked either inside or outside the liver. Problems inside the liver such as hepatitis, *fibrosis*, and cirrhosis can cause increased conjugated bilirubin. Problems outside the liver such as gallstones can also cause increased conjugated bilirubin. A high level of conjugated bilirubin in the blood can also be detected in the urine.

bilirubin, total

What?
Bilirubin is a yellow chemical produced during the normal breakdown of red blood cells. Bilirubin is normally processed by the liver into other substances that can be eliminated from the body.

Why test?
Testing the blood for bilirubin is one measure of how well the liver is working. When the liver is not working normally, bilirubin can build up in the body. If bilirubin levels get very high, the skin and/or the whites of the eyes will become yellow, a condition called *jaundice*. However, bilirubin levels can be elevated without jaundice.

bilirubin, unconjugated

Other Names
indirect bilirubin

What?
Bilirubin is a yellow chemical produced during the normal breakdown of red blood cells. Bilirubin is normally processed by the liver into other substances that can be eliminated from the body. There are two types of

bilirubin in the body, conjugated (direct) bilirubin and unconjugated (indirect) bilirubin. Conjugated bilirubin is bilirubin that is attached to another chemical called glucuronic acid in a process called conjugation. Conjugation takes place inside liver cells. Conjugated bilirubin is excreted in the bile. *Unconjugated bilirubin* has not undergone the conjugation process. Normally, unconjugated bilirubin makes up over 90% of the total bilirubin.

Why Test?
If the total bilirubin in the blood is high, it is important to know how much of it is unconjugated because this tells your healthcare provider what process in the liver is not working normally. In hepatitis, fibrosis, and cirrhosis, high amounts of unconjugated bilirubin signify the liver is not conjugating bilirubin normally causing it to build up in the blood.

blood urea nitrogen (BUN)
What?
Blood urea nitrogen (BUN) is a chemical produced by the liver in the process of breaking down proteins.
Why Test?
BUN is normally eliminated from the body in the urine. BUN is most commonly measured to check how well the kidneys are working. When the kidneys are not working normally, BUN increases. Some people with advanced cirrhosis and *liver failure* develop a condition called hepatorenal syndrome. With this syndrome, the kidneys begin to fail because the liver is failing. BUN is one test used to check for hepatorenal syndrome in people with cirrhosis and liver failure.

In the absence of kidney failure, BUN is often lower than normal in people with cirrhosis and liver failure. This is because the failing liver does not metabolize proteins normally, and as a result, lower than normal amounts of BUN are produced. Because of this, BUN is one test that can be used to see how well the liver is performing one of its many jobs in people with cirrhosis and liver failure, but no kidney failure.

branched DNA test for HCV (b-DNA)
What?
The *branched DNA test* for HCV (b-DNA) is used to check for the presence of the virus in the blood.
Why Test?
HCV viral load testing is used to predict possible response to interferon-based therapy, and to monitor for response during such therapy. The b-DNA test is one form of HCV viral load testing. In order for a b-DNA test to be positive, there has to be a certain amount of virus in the blood. For this reason, a negative b-DNA test is reported as "undetectable," not zero. The b-DNA test for HCV is not as sensitive as the *HCV PCR* test, another test used to check viral load. This means the b-DNA test cannot detect as low a viral load as the HCV PCR test.

See "Viral Load Testing" at the beginning of this chapter for additional information on the use and interpretation of HCV viral load tests.

BUN – see *blood urea nitrogen*

caffeine metabolism
What?
Caffeine is the stimulating chemical in coffee, black teas, colas, chocolate, and other foods. Caffeine is processed (metabolized) by the liver.
Why Test?
Caffeine *metabolism* decreases as liver function decreases. Therefore, caffeine metabolism is one way to evaluate liver function. The rate of caffeine metabolism is markedly decreased in people with cirrhosis. Caffeine metabolism can be evaluated by checking the fasting caffeine level in the blood, measuring the release of radiolabeled carbon dioxide in the breath after a dose of labeled caffeine is administered, or measuring the rate of elimination of caffeine from the blood after a loading dose is administered.

calcium
What?
Calcium is a charged particle called an electrolyte. It is needed for many important functions of the body including bone formation and muscle activity.

Why Test?

People with cirrhosis can have lower than normal *vitamin D* levels because it is not being absorbed normally in the intestines. When the level of vitamin D is too low, the amount of calcium in the blood also drops. Many different symptoms can occur if your calcium is too low. If cirrhosis has led to development of hepatorenal syndrome in which both the kidneys and the liver fail, the blood calcium can become elevated, which can cause other problems.

CBC – see *complete blood count*

chloride (Cl)

What?

Chloride (Cl) is a charged particle called an electrolyte. It is one of the four major electrolytes in the body.

Why Test?

Electrolytes perform many important jobs in the body. Two of the most important jobs are regulating the amount of water in your body and keeping your blood pH normal. Some people with hepatitis C hold more water in their bodies than they need. This can cause abnormal chloride levels. This is more likely in people with cirrhosis than in those without cirrhosis.

cholesterol

What?

Cholesterol is a *lipid* or fat that is both absorbed from the food we eat and manufactured by the liver. Most of the circulating blood cholesterol comes from the liver, not from what we eat.

Why Test?

The liver is responsible for both production and breakdown of cholesterol. The liver breaks down cholesterol and excretes it into the bile. Blockage of bile flow either inside or outside the liver increases the amount of cholesterol in the blood. The more obstructed the bile flow, the higher the amount of cholesterol in the blood. Cirrhosis can block bile flow in the liver, and gallstones can block bile flow outside of the liver. Both of these situations can occur with chronic hepatitis C infection.

complete blood count (CBC)

What?

A *complete blood count (CBC)* is a group of tests indicating the concentration and characteristics of cells circulating in the blood. A CBC typically includes the following tests: *RBC* count, *WBC* count, *hemoglobin*, *hematocrit*, and platelet count. Other tests may also be included.

Why Test?

See individual tests for an explanation of the role of each test in chronic hepatitis C.

conjugated bilirubin – see *bilirubin, conjugated*

coproporphyrin

What?

Coproporphyrin is a substance produced in the liver and bone marrow during the process of making a chemical called heme. Heme is the chemical that binds oxygen to red blood cells.

Why Test?

Since the liver is one of two sites for heme production, liver cell damage can interfere with the production of heme. When heme production is abnormal, the substances used to make heme build up in the blood. Coproporphyrin is used to determine how well the liver is performing its job of making heme.

creatinine

What?

Creatinine is a waste product of muscle cell metabolism. Creatinine is excreted by the kidneys in the urine.

Why Test?

Creatinine is most commonly measured to check how well the kidneys are working. When the kidneys are not working normally, blood creatinine increases. Some people with advanced liver cirrhosis and liver failure develop a condition called hepatorenal syndrome. With this syndrome, the kidneys begin to fail because the liver is failing. Creatinine is one test used to check for hepatorenal syndrome in people with cirrhosis and liver failure.

cryoglobulins

What?

Cryoglobulins are *immunoglobulins* that are joined together.

Why Test?

Some people with hepatitis C develop cryoglobulins in their blood, a condition called *cryoglobulinemia*. It is important to know if someone has cryoglobulinemia because it can cause kidney damage and problems with other organ systems.

direct bilirubin – see *bilirubin, conjugated*

enzyme immunoassay (EIA)

What?

Enzyme immunoassay (*EIA*) is a common testing method used to screen for anti-HCV antibodies in the blood.

Why Test?

EIA is a rapid, economical method of screening for the presence of anti-HCV antibodies. A *RIBA* test is often used to confirm a positive EIA test for anti-HCV antibodies. For additional information about the significance of a positive test result, see anti-HCV antibodies.

ferritin

What?

Ferritin is a protein found in the liver, spleen, and intestine. It binds *iron*.

Why Test?

Ferritin is measured to check for iron overload in the body. High amounts of ferritin in the blood signify an overabundance of iron in the body. This is important because iron overload is often seen with chronic hepatitis C. This condition must be treated because iron overload worsens the damage done to the liver by the hepatitis C virus.

fibrinogen

What?

Fibrinogen is a protein produced by the liver. It is to the main protein used to form blood clots to stop bleeding.

Why Test?

A cirrhotic, failing liver may be unable to produce normal amounts of fibrinogen. Measuring fibrinogen is one way of telling how severely the liver is failing. Testing the amount of fibrinogen in the blood is also important because, if the level gets very low, a person may not be able to form a blood clot if he or she begins to bleed for any reason.

FIBROSpect™

What?

FIBROSpect™ is a proprietary set of blood tests used together to differentiate no/mild liver fibrosis from severe fibrosis.

Why Test?

Liver biopsy remains the most certain method of determining the presence and degree of liver fibrosis. However, some people are hesitant to have a liver biopsy because it is an invasive test and has an associated risk of rare but serious complications. While FIBROSpect™ is not a substitute for liver biopsy, it can possibly provide some useful information for people who cannot or do not wish to have a liver biopsy.

FibroSURE™

Other Names

HCV FibroSURE™

What?

FibroSURE™ is a proprietary set of blood tests used together to differentiate no/mild liver fibrosis from severe fibrosis.

Why Test?

Liver biopsy remains the most certain method of determining the presence and degree of liver fibrosis. However, some people are hesitant to have a liver biopsy because it is an invasive test and has an associated risk of rare but serious complications. While FibroSURE™ is not a substitute for liver biopsy, it can possibly provide some useful information for people who cannot or do not wish to have a liver biopsy.

gamma-glutamyl transferase (GGT)

Other Names

GGTP, glutamyl *peptide*

What?

Gamma-glutamyl transferase (GGT) is an enzyme found in all cells of the body except muscle cells.

Why Test?

GGT is elevated in all forms of liver disease. It is highest when bile flow is blocked either inside or outside the liver.

genotyping

What?

There are many different strains of the hepatitis C virus. A *genotyping* test tells what strain of the virus a person has.

Why Test?

Genotyping is currently used to determine the required length and potential response to interferon-based therapy. There are 6 common *HCV genotypes*. Researchers have discovered that certain genotypes are more likely to respond to treatment than others are. Future studies will hopefully uncover why this occurs. This may allow researchers to develop more effective treatments for HCV.

GGT – see *gamma-glutamyl transferase*

GGTP – see *gamma-glutamyl transferase*

glucose

What?

Glucose is another name for *blood sugar*.

Why Test?

People with chronic hepatitis C can have blood sugar abnormalities, either too high or too low. A glucose test is done to see if your blood sugar level is abnormal.

glutathione

What?

Glutathione is an *amino acid* found throughout the body.

Why Test?

Glutathione protects cells from a type of injury called oxidative damage. Scientists believe oxidative damage is one of the key ways HCV damages liver cells. This damage is done by agents called *free radicals*. Glutathione prevents free radicals from causing damage to cells. Measuring the amount of glutathione in the blood is one way your healthcare providers can tell how capable your liver is of preventing and/or repairing liver damage.

HCV polymerase chain reaction (HCV PCR)

Other Names

PCR, RT-PCR, reverse transcription polymerase chain reaction

What?

HCV PCR checks for the presence of HCV in the blood. The test detects the genetic material of the virus (***HCV RNA***).

Why Test?

HCV viral load testing is used to predict possible response to interferon-based therapy, and to monitor for response during such therapy. The PCR test is one form of HCV viral load testing. The HCV PCR test is also used to confirm the diagnosis of current HCV infection in someone who has tested positive on a hepatitis C antibody screen.

There are two types of HCV PCR tests. The first is a qualitative test. A qualitative HCV PCR test does not measure the amount of virus in the blood, but rather determines if there is detectable virus in the blood. The second type of test is called a quantitative test. It is used to measure the amount of detectable HCV in the blood. The amount of detectable virus is called the viral load.

A certain amount of virus must be present in the blood to be detected using PCR. For this reason, a negative PCR test is reported as "undetectable," not zero. See "Viral Load Testing" at the beginning of this chapter for additional information on the use and interpretation of HCV viral load tests.

HCV transcription mediation amplification (HCV TMA)

What?
HCV TMA is used to measure the amount of detectable HCV in the blood.

Why Test?
HCV viral load testing is used to predict possible response to interferon-based therapy, and to monitor for response during such therapy. The TMA test is one form of HCV viral load testing. The HCV TMA test is also used to confirm the diagnosis of current HCV infection in someone who has tested positive on a hepatitis C *antibody* screen. A certain amount of virus must be present in the blood to be detected using TMA. For this reason, a negative TMA test is reported as "undetectable," not zero. See "Viral Load Testing" at the beginning of this chapter for additional information on the use and interpretation of HCV viral load tests.

hematocrit (HCT)

What?
A h*ematocrit* (*HCT*) test measures the percentage of the blood made up by red blood cells.

Why Test?
Liver disease can lead to a shortage of red blood cells, a condition called *anemia*. The hematocrit is used to test for anemia.

hemoglobin (HGB)

What?
Hemoglobin is the protein inside red blood cells that carries oxygen.

Why Test?
Liver disease can lead to a shortage of hemoglobin. The hemoglobin test is used to check if there is enough hemoglobin in the blood.

immunoglobulins (Igs)

What?
Immunoglobulins are a group of proteins that act as antibodies. Antibodies are one of the two arms of the *immune system*.

Why Test?
When the Igs are tested in the laboratory, the different proteins of the group are separated and each is measured. The test shows how much of each type of protein is present. Different patterns may point to different problems in the liver. For example, one pattern may indicate liver cell damage, while a different pattern indicates that cirrhosis has developed.

indirect bilirubin – see *bilirubin, unconjugated*

INR – see *prothrombin time*

iron (Fe)

What?
Iron is a metal found in red blood cells. It helps red blood cells carry oxygen to all the cells of the body.

Why Test?

The liver is one of the main places in the body where iron is stored. When liver cells are damaged, iron is released into the blood. Therefore, the amount of iron in the blood is one way to check how much damage is being done to liver cells by HCV. Iron overload worsens the damage done to the liver by HCV.

lactate dehydrogenase (LDH)

What?

Lactate dehydrogenase (*LDH*) is an enzyme found in many cells of the body. It is highly concentrated in red blood cells, liver, heart, and muscle cells.

Why Test?

Elevated LDH is one indicator of liver cell damage. However, since it is found in many other cell types, it is usually tested in combination with other liver enzymes.

LIPA assay – see *genotyping*

liver biopsy

What?

A liver biopsy is a surgical procedure to remove two or three tiny pieces of the liver using a long needle that is inserted into the liver through the skin of the abdomen. The samples are stained and looked at under a microscope.

Why Test?

A liver biopsy is the only way to be certain what is happening in the liver as a result of hepatitis C infection. The three main things that will be looked for are *inflammation* (the presence of inflammatory cells in the liver), fibrosis (scar tissue that forms when liver cells are destroyed by the virus), and cirrhosis (widespread damage to the liver resulting in abnormal liver structure and function). See *Chapter 4.1, Liver Disease Progression* for additional information about liver biopsy and the interpretation of the results.

5'-nucleotidase (5'NT)

Other Names

5'-ribonucleotide phosphohydrolase (NTP)

What?

5'-nucleotidase (*5'NT*) is an enzyme found in many tissues throughout the body including the liver.

Why Test?

5'NT is increased 2 to 6 times the normal amount when bile flow is blocked either inside or outside the liver. Hepatitis, fibrosis, and cirrhosis can block bile flow inside the liver. Gallstones can block bile flow outside the liver.

partial thromboplastin time (PTT)

Other Names

activated partial thromboplastin time, APTT

What?

A *partial thromboplastin time* is a test to see how quickly blood is able to form a clot.

Why Test?

The liver produces many of the proteins needed for clot formation. People with cirrhosis and liver failure may not be able to produce normal amounts of these proteins. The *PTT* is one indicator of the liver's ability to make proteins. It is also important to know if someone cannot form blood clots normally because he or she may not be able to stop bleeding once it starts.

PCR – see *HCV polymerase chain reaction*

platelet count

What?

Platelets are small pieces of cells circulating in the blood. Platelets help form blood clots to halt bleeding.

Why Test?
Liver disease can cause a shortage of platelets. The platelet count is used to test for such a shortage, which can lead to easy bruising and uncontrollable bleeding.

polymerase chain reaction – see *HCV polymerase chain reaction*

porphyrins
What?
Porphyrins are a group of substances produced in the liver and bone marrow during the process of making a chemical called heme. Heme is the chemical that binds oxygen to red blood cells.
Why?
Since the liver is one of two sites for heme production, liver cell damage can interfere with the production of heme. When heme production is abnormal, the substances used to make heme build up in the blood. Testing for porphyrins is a check on how well the liver is performing its job of making heme.

potassium (K)
What?
Potassium is a charged particle called an electrolyte. It is one of the four major electrolytes in the body.
Why Test?
Electrolytes perform many important jobs in the body. Two of the most important jobs are regulating the amount of water in your body and keeping your blood pH normal. Some people with hepatitis C hold more water in their bodies than they need. This can cause abnormal potassium levels. This is more likely in people with cirrhosis than in those without cirrhosis.

prealbumin – see *transthyretin*

prothrombin time (PT)
Other Names
INR (International Normalized Ratio), PT/INR
What?
Prothrombin time (PT) is a test to see how quickly the blood is able to form a clot.
Why Test?
The liver produces many of the proteins needed for clot formation. People with cirrhosis and liver failure may not be able to produce normal amounts of these proteins. The PT is one indicator of the liver's ability to make proteins. It is also important to know if someone cannot form blood clots normally because he or she may not be able to stop bleeding once it starts.

PT test reporting is often in the form of a ratio called the International Normalized Ratio or INR. The World Health Organization devised this system to standardize the reporting of PT test results so that no matter what laboratory checks the prothrombin time, the result should be the same.

PT – see *prothrombin time*

PTT – see *partial thromboplastin time*

RBC – see *red blood cell count*

recombinant immunoblot assay (RIBA)
What?
RIBA is a sensitive testing method used to detect the presence of anti-HCV antibodies in the blood.
Why Test?
The RIBA test is most often used to confirm a positive result on an EIA (enzyme immunoassay) screening test for anti-HCV antibodies. There are currently three generations of RIBA tests for HCV denoted RIBA-1, RIBA-2, and RIBA-3. For additional information about the significance of a positive test result, see anti-HCV antibodies.

red blood cell count (RBC)

What?

Red blood cells carry oxygen from the air we breathe to all of the organs and tissues of the body.

Why Test?

Liver disease can lead to a shortage of red blood cells, a condition called anemia. The red blood cell count is used to test for anemia.

retinol – see *vitamin A*

rheumatoid factor (RF)

What?

Rheumatoid factor is a type of autoantibody. Normally, the body makes antibodies against foreign substances such as bacteria and viruses. Autoantibodies are abnormal antibodies that act against your own cells.

Why Test?

More than half of all people with chronic hepatitis C have one or more autoantibodies in their blood. This is important to know because autoantibodies can cause additional symptoms and disease.

RIBA – see *recombinant immunoblot assay*

sodium

What?

Sodium is a charged particle called an *electrolyte*. It is one of four major electrolytes in the body.

Why Test?

Electrolytes perform many important jobs in the body. Two of the most important jobs are regulating the amount of water in your body and keeping your blood pH normal. Some people with hepatitis C hold more water in their bodies than they need. This can cause abnormal sodium levels. This is more likely in people with cirrhosis than in those without cirrhosis.

T3 – see *triiodothyronine*

T4 – see *thyroxin*

thyroid stimulating hormone (TSH)

Other Names

thyrotropin

What?

Thyroid stimulating hormone (*TSH*) is produced by the *pituitary gland*. It acts on the thyroid gland to cause it to produce the two thyroid hormones.

Why Test?

Some people with hepatitis C develop thyroid problems. Measuring the TSH along with the thyroid hormone levels tells your healthcare provider if the thyroid gland is working normally.

thyroxin (T4)

What?

Thyroxin is one of two hormones produced by the thyroid gland.

Why Test?

Some people with hepatitis C develop thyroid problems. Measuring the thyroxin in the blood is one way to test whether the thyroid gland is working normally.

TIBC – see *total iron binding capacity*

TMA – see *HCV transcription mediation amplification*

total bilirubin – see *bilirubin, total*

total iron binding capacity (TIBC)

What?

The total iron binding capacity (TIBC) is a measurement of how much iron the blood is able to capture.

Why Test?

TIBC is one test used to check the amount of iron in the body. The more iron there is in the body, the lower the TIBC. An abnormally low TIBC means there is too much iron in the body. This is important because iron overload can be seen with chronic hepatitis C. This condition must be treated because iron overload worsens the damage done to the liver by HCV.

total protein (TP)

What?

Total protein is a measure of all proteins in the blood.

Why Test?

The liver produces many of the proteins found in the blood. Measuring the total protein in the blood is one way of testing how well the liver is performing its job of producing proteins.

transthyretin

Other Names

prealbumin

What?

Transthyretin is a small protein made by the liver. It is used to make the larger protein called albumin.

Why Test?

Transthyretin is a sensitive indicator of how well the liver is able to produce proteins. The lower the transthyretin level in the blood, the poorer the liver is performing its job of making proteins.

triiodothyronine (T3)

What?

Triiodothryonine is one of two hormones produced by the thyroid gland.

Why Test?

Some people with hepatitis C develop thyroid problems. Measuring triiodothyronine is one way to test whether the thyroid gland is working normally.

TSH – see *thyroid stimulating hormone*

unconjugated bilirubin – see *bilirubin, unconjugated*

viral load – see *HCV polymerase chain reaction* and *branched DNA test for HCV*

vitamin A

Other Names

retinol, retinoic acid

What?

Vitamin A is a fat-soluble vitamin.

Why Test?

Absorption of vitamin A from the intestines requires bile. If bile is not being made and secreted normally, the body may not be able to absorb as much vitamin A as it needs. In extreme cases, this can result in night blindness, dry skin, and brittle hair and nails.

vitamin D

Other Names

ergocalciferol, cholecalciferol

What?

Vitamin D is a fat-soluble vitamin.

Why Test?

Absorption of vitamin D from the intestines requires bile. If bile is not being made and secreted normally, the body may not be able to absorb as much vitamin D as it needs. Further, liver cells convert absorbed vitamin D into its active form. In cirrhosis and liver failure, the liver may not perform this job normally. In extreme cases, vitamin D deficiency can result in softening of the bones and bone pain.

vitamin E

Other Names

alfa-tocopherol

What?

Vitamin E is a fat-soluble vitamin.

Why Test?

Absorption of vitamin E from the intestines requires bile. If bile is not being made and secreted normally, the body may not be able to absorb as much vitamin E as it needs. In extreme cases, vitamin E deficiency can cause a shortage of red blood cells and muscle loss.

vitamin K

Other Names

phylloquinone, antihemorrhagic factor

What?

Vitamin K is a fat-soluble vitamin.

Why Test?

Absorption of vitamin K from the intestines requires bile. If bile is not being made and secreted normally, the body may not be able to absorb as much vitamin K as it needs. Vitamin K is required for the production of proteins needed for blood clotting. Vitamin K deficiency can lead to easy bruising and bleeding problems.

WBC – see *white blood cell count*

white blood cell count

Other Names

WBC count

What?

White blood cells protect your body against infections. They are part of the body's *immune system*. There are several different kinds of white blood cells including *neutrophils*, *lymphocytes*, and *macrophage*s.

Why Test?

An elevated white blood cell count often accompanies acute infection. Changes in your white blood cell count may indicate a change in your hepatitis C disease status.

Summary

Laboratory tests and procedures give a great deal of useful information to your healthcare providers. They can provide information about how well the liver is performing its many jobs, and how much damage HCV is doing to your liver. In deciding what tests you need, your healthcare provider considers several factors, such as:

- How have you been feeling?
- Are you having any new signs or symptoms?
- What treatments or medicines are you taking?
- Where are you in your treatment plan?

Since the answers to these questions are different for each person and may differ from one medical visit to the next, there is no one group of laboratory tests that is considered standard for people living with hepatitis C.

If you have questions about why you need a certain test or what the results mean, ask your healthcare provider. Understanding your laboratory tests can help you understand how your body is responding to HCV and the management plan you have chosen.

References

1. Burtis CA, Ashwood ER, eds. *Tietz Textbook of Clinical Chemistry*. 3rd ed. Philadelphia, Pennsylvania: W.B. Saunders Company; 1999.
2. Cotran RS, Kumar V, Robbins SL, Schoen FJ, eds. *Robbins Pathological Basis of Disease*. 5th ed. Philadelphia, Pennsylvania: W.B. Saunders Company; 1994.
3. Dolan M. *The Hepatitis C Handbook*. 2nd ed. Berkeley, California: North Atlantic Books; 1999.
4. Fauci AS, Braunwald E, Isselbacher KJ, Wilson JD, Martin JB, Kasper DL, Hauser SL, Longo DL, eds.. *Harrison's Principles of Internal Medicine*. 14th ed. New York, New York: McGraw-Hill Companies; 1998.
5. Mandell GL, Bennett JE, Dolin R eds. *Principles and Practice of Infectious Diseases*. 4th ed. New York, New York: Churchill Livingstone Inc.; 1995.

THE IMMUNE SYSTEM AND THE HEPATITIS C VIRUS

Tina M. St. John, MD

MEET THE IMMUNE SYSTEM

Introduction

The *immune system* is the body's defense against infections. Think of the immune system as the body's army, protecting it from invaders. Just as the army has soldiers trained to perform different jobs, the immune system also has many types of cells performing different jobs. The cells of the immune system circulate through every tissue of the body.

When the body is infected with the *hepatitis C* virus (*HCV*), the immune system swings into action. The immune systems of approximately 15% to 45% of people infected with HCV are able to rid their bodies of the virus. This is called spontaneous *clearance*. However, 55% to 85% of people infected with HCV are unable to clear the virus and become chronically infected. In immunology terms, chronic infection is called "persistence."

Among those who are chronically infected, the immune system appears to have a role in the rate of disease progression and liver damage caused by HCV. Therefore, the interaction between the hepatitis C virus and the immune system is at the core of HCV disease and its treatment.

This chapter provides a brief introduction to the immune system, and how it relates to chronic hepatitis C. At first glance, the concepts in this chapter may seem very complex. Many of the terms are likely to be new to you. However, reading this information may help you better understand some of the logic behind current hepatitis C treatment and research.

What Is the Immune System?

Every day, you are exposed to millions of germs or *microbes* including bacteria, viruses, fungi, and molds. Many of these microbes are harmless, but others can cause diseases ranging from the common cold to life-threatening infections such as pneumonia. The skin is the body's first line of defense against infections. It prevents most of the microbes we encounter from entering the body.

> **The immune system is the body's defense against those disease-causing microbes that get by our exterior defenses and enter the body.**

The immune system runs through every tissue of the body. The primary parts of the immune system include the lymphatic vessels, *lymph nodes*, the *thymus gland*, the spleen, and the bone marrow (see Figure 1). Immune system cells and tissues are located throughout the body. Solitary immune system cells travel through the body via the blood and *lymphatic systems*, much like soldiers on patrol.

Figure 1. Immune System Tissues*

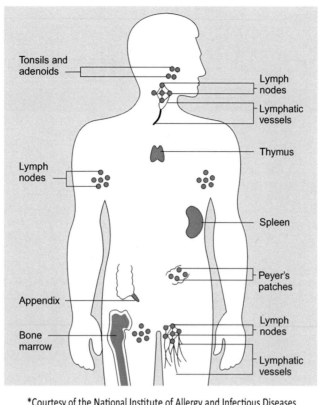

Tonsils and adenoids

Lymph nodes

Lymphatic vessels

Thymus

Lymph nodes

Spleen

Peyer's patches

Appendix

Lymph nodes

Bone marrow

Lymphatic vessels

*Courtesy of the National Institute of Allergy and Infectious Diseases

Cells of the Immune System

The immune system has many different types of cells performing different jobs. The names of these cells can be confusing. Some of the most important cells of the immune system are listed in Figure 2. *White blood cells* called *lymphocytes* are the main "soldiers" of the immune system.

There are two main groups of lymphocytes, *T cells* and *B cells*. T cells are grouped according to the jobs they perform and include *T helper cells*, *T suppressor cells*, *cytotoxic T cells*, and *memory T cells*. Similarly, B cells are grouped according to their function. *Plasma cells* and *memory B cells* are two types of B cells. A third type of lymphocyte called a natural killer or *NK cell* is also important in the immune system. The specific jobs performed by different types of lymphocytes are discussed throughout the chapter.

Identification of Invaders: Immune Recognition

Just as a soldier must be able to determine a friend from an enemy, the immune system must be able to recognize when a potentially harmful invader enters the body. In other words, the immune system must be able to distinguish between things that are supposed to be in the body ("self") versus things that are invaders ("non-self").

The immune system has a complex surveillance system to identify invaders. Some researchers believe HCV's ability to "hide" from the immune system may explain, at least in part, how HCV is able to live in the body without being destroyed in those people with chronic infections.[1, 2]

The cells of the body and invading microbes each have many *proteins* on their surface. The combination of proteins on the surface of a cell or an invader enables the immune system to tell friend (self) from invader (non-self). Think of the surface proteins on cells as coats. All the cells of the body (self cells) have red coats. One day, an immune cell

Figure 2. Lymphocytes of the Immune System

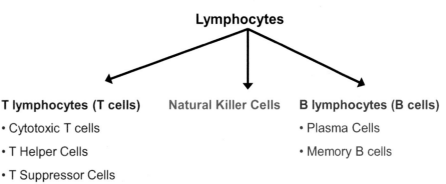

encounters a microbe in a green coat. The immune cell quickly recognizes that anything <u>not</u> in a red coat is an invader, and sounds the alarm to notify the rest of the immune system that an invader has made its way into the body. How HCV is able to subvert this critical recognition is the subject of much research, as is discussed in great detail in *Chapter 7.2, Immunology Takes on Hepatitis C.*

Beyond distinguishing self from invader, surface proteins <u>specifically</u> identify cells and microbes. Think of surface proteins as a labeling system. Surface proteins are "read" by the immune system. For example, Figure 3 shows a cartoon of the surface proteins of a measles virus and a hepatitis C virus. The circles and triangles on the outside of the viruses represent their surface proteins. The surface proteins of the measles virus and the hepatitis C virus are different. The immune system reads this difference. The combination of the measles surface proteins tells the immune system, "I am a measles virus." The surface proteins of HCV tell the immune system, "I am a hepatitis C virus." Thus, the immune system can not only detect the presence of an invader, it can also tell one type of invader from another because of their different surface proteins.

A surface protein that is recognized by the immune system and leads to *antibody* production is called an *antigen* or *immunogen*. Detection of foreign antigens is the primary way the immune system is alerted to the presence of invading microbes.

Figure 3. Surface Antigens on Measles and Hepatitis C Viruses

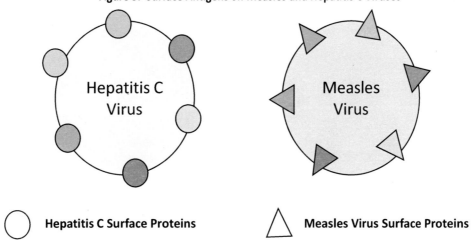

What is an Antibody?

Antibodies are substances produced by the immune system that interact with microbes to kill them. *Immunoglobulin* is another term you may hear used for antibodies.

Antibodies are most effective against bacteria and viruses that live outside of cells (*extracellular* microbes). The immune cells that produce antibodies are special lymphocytes called *activated B cells* or plasma cells.

Several steps are required for the production of antibodies.

1. A white blood cell called a *macrophage* ingests (eats) an invading microbe. The microbe is digested by the macrophage (see Figure 4). Some of the microbe's digested proteins (antigens) are displayed by the macrophage on its surface to alert other cells of the immune system that an invader is present.

Figure 4. Macrophage Digesting Microbe and Displaying Antigen

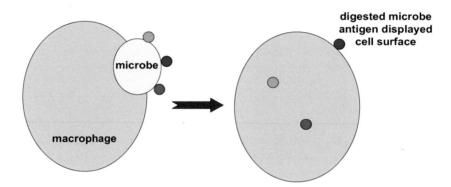

2. Lymphocytes called B cells also process and display the invader's proteins on their surfaces (see Figure 5).

Figure 5. B Cell Digesting Microbe and Displaying Antigen

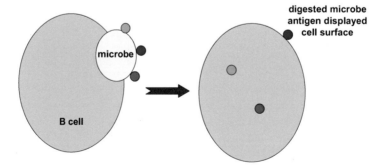

3. When an immune cell called a T helper cell sees the same protein on the surface of a B cell <u>and</u> a macrophage, it sandwiches itself between the two other immune cells (see Figure 6). The formation of this bridge complex stimulates the B cell to begin dividing, making more copies of itself. The resulting group of activated B cells produces antibodies against the invading microbe's displayed proteins (antigens).

Figure 6. T Helper Cell Activates B Cell Causing B Cell Expansion and Antibody Production

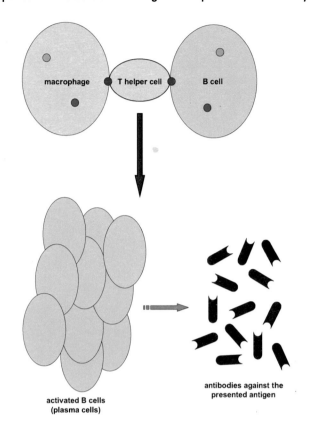

The antibodies produced against an invader attach to antigens on its surface. The presence of antibodies on the surface of the invader serves as a "red flag" to the rest of the immune system and marks the invader for destruction. The killing takes place in one of two ways. The antibodies may cause leaks in the outer coat of the microbe; the leaky invader cannot recover and dies. More commonly, antibodies on the surface of the invader alert the killer cells of the immune system to ingest (eat) and destroy the invader.

Antigen-antibody interactions are very specific. Antibodies produced in response to a specific antigen normally react only with that antigen. Antigen-antibody interactions are often likened to a lock and key. A given lock can only be "activated" by a matching key. Similarly, a given antibody only reacts with its matching antigen.

In certain conditions, the immune system mistakes self antigens for foreign antigens. As a result, the immune system produces antibodies against self. These abnormal antibodies are called *autoantibodies*. Disease states caused by autoantibodies include:

- systemic lupus erythematosis (SLE)

- *autoimmune* hepatitis

- autoimmune *thyroiditis*

- rheumatoid arthritis

Examples of specific autoantibodies include *anti-liver-kidney microsomal antibodies (anti-LK)*, *anti-nuclear antibodies (ANA)*, *anti-smooth muscle antibodies (anti-SMA)*, and rheumatoid factor (RF).

More than half of all people with chronic hepatitis C have one or more autoantibodies in their blood. This is important because autoantibodies may cause additional symptoms and disease. Your doctor may test your blood for autoantibodies if you are having unexplained signs or symptoms. See *Chapter 6, Laboratory Tests and Procedures* for additional information about these tests.

Cell-Mediated Immunity

Cell-mediated immunity is another tactic the body uses to defend itself against invaders through the direct actions of specific immune cells. Two important types of cells in the cell-mediated immune response are cytotoxic T cells and *natural killer cells* (NK cells).

Cytotoxic T cells are specific in their destructive action. They kill only cells that display the antigens they are programmed to seek-and-destroy. In contrast, natural killer cells are not very selective. An NK cell may kill any of a number of different cells. Both NK cells and cytotoxic T cells kill their targets directly and almost immediately after binding to them. Think of this as "the kiss of death" because once an immune system killer cell binds to an invader, that invader is doomed to die.

Cell-mediated immunity defends the body against fungi, parasites, cancer cells, foreign tissue (transplanted organs), and viruses that live inside cells (*intracellular* viruses) such as the hepatitis C virus. Specific actions of the cell-mediated branch of the immune system in response to HCV infections are discussed in *Chapter 7.2, Immunology Takes on Hepatitis C.*

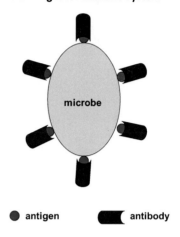

Figure 7. Antibody Tags Microbe Marking It for Immune System

microbe

● antigen ▬◖ antibody

The Immune Response to Hepatitis C

Since the discovery of the hepatitis C virus in 1992, researchers have focused on trying to unravel the mysteries of how the immune system responds to HCV. Much has been learned, but there remain more questions than answers. For example:

- Why do some people spontaneously clear the virus while others develop chronic infection?

- How does the virus "outwit" the complex and sophisticated immune system?

- How does the interaction of the virus and the immune system cause liver damage?

These questions are easy to pose, but the answers are very complicated. Many highly skilled researchers continue to work diligently to find answers to these and other questions. This section provides an overview of some basic information scientists have discovered about the immune response to the hepatitis C virus. Each of these topics is explored in detail in *Chapter 7.2, Immunology Takes on Hepatitis C.*

Antibody Response to Hepatitis C

In a person with a normal immune system, HCV infection quickly leads to the production of antibodies against the virus. Anti-HCV antibodies are usually detectable in the blood within 3 to 12 weeks after infection. These antibodies persist even in people who spontaneously clear the virus. The presence of these antibodies is the basis for hepatitis C screening tests, which detect anti-HCV antibodies. The presence of anti-HCV antibodies in the blood indicates exposure to the virus, but does not indicate whether the virus is still present in the body.

While HCV circulates in the blood of an infected person, the virus spends most of its life inside liver cells. Once inside, HCV "hijacks" the liver cell's production equipment in order to produce more copies of itself. The rate at which a virus is able to make copies itself is called its *replication rate*. HCV has an extremely high replication rate with 10^{12} (that is 1,000,000,000,000) virus particles produced each day in an infected person.[3, 4]

With so many copies of the virus being made each day, there is some variation in the virus particles produced. Think of the *replication* process as a very rapid assembly line of HCV production. With the assembly line running at such a high rate of speed, the viruses produced are not perfect copies of the original. Therefore, as an HCV infection persists, several slightly different versions of the virus emerge. The process leading to these slight variations is called *mutation*, and the variant viruses produced are called *quasispecies*. Research findings suggest that the production of HCV quasispecies may contribute to HCV's ability to persist in the body. It appears that some HCV quasispecies are not recognized by the immune system as invaders. As such, these quasispecies are not attacked by the immune system.

The fact that HCV is predominantly an intracellular virus also appears to help it survive even in the face of a strong antibody response from the immune system. Recall that antibodies work best against invaders that live outside of cells. With HCV living primarily inside liver cells, most virus particles are able to escape antibody destruction. In the end, it appears that an antibody response alone is unable to rid the body of HCV. For a thorough review of this topic including the latest research findings, see *Chapter 7.2, Immunology Takes on Hepatitis C.*

Cell-Mediated Immune Response to Hepatitis C

Since HCV is an intracellular virus, the cell-mediated branch of the immune system is the predominant responder to HCV infection. Studies have proven that HCV lives inside the liver cells of an infected person. Some evidence suggests that HCV may also live inside specific types of immune cells.[5, 6]

The cell-mediated immune response to HCV is complex, and we have much yet to learn. However, several theories exist about the role of cell-mediated immunity in hepatitis C that have sufficient supporting evidence to warrant mentioning.

LIVER INJURY

The word "hepatitis" means inflammation of the liver. Indeed, liver cell injury and death are the features of HCV infection that threaten health. Some experts believe the liver injury associated with chronic HCV is caused by an ongoing but relatively low level, cell-mediated immune attack on the liver. It is believed that cytotoxic T cells attack and kill infected liver cells in an attempt to rid the body of HCV.[7, 8] If this theory is correct, it follows that while the attack of the cytotoxic T cells is at least partially responsible for the slowly progressive liver damage seen in chronic hepatitis C, it is at the same time inadequate to rid the body of the virus.

Research suggests that an individual's T cell response to HCV infection may play an important role in whether the virus is spontaneously cleared or becomes chronic. A strong initial T cell response has been associated with *viral clearance*, while a weak initial response that builds in strength over time has been linked to chronic infection.[9]

EARLY T HELPER CELL RESPONSE AND VIRAL PERSISTENCE

T helper cells are members of the T lymphocyte family of white blood cells. T helpers are also sometimes called *CD4 cells*. There are two types of T helper cells, Th1 and Th2. Th1 cells are cell-mediated immunity helpers. Th2 cells are *humoral immunity* helpers.

Research suggests that a person's T helper cell response in the first few months after HCV infection may be an important factor in whether the infection becomes chronic.[10, 11] A strong, sustained Th1 response appears to be important in spontaneous clearance of HCV. Scientists continue to explore the details of this important finding.

CYTOTOXIC T LYMPHOCYTES AND VIRAL PERSISTENCE

Cytotoxic T lymphocytes (CTLs or *CD8 cells*) are targeted killers of infected cells. When a virus invades a cell, some of the virus' proteins are displayed on the surface of the infected cell. The displayed virus proteins are "red flags" to the CTLs. CTLs attach to cells bearing the "I'm infected with a virus" red flag and deliver "the kiss of death." With HCV, infected liver cells are killed to stop additional HCV production and release of new viruses. The seek-and-destroy mission of CTLs is specific. That is to say, an anti-hepatitis C CTL will only bind to and kill a cell with HCV proteins displayed on its surface

Figure 8. Anti-HCV Cytotoxic T Lymphocytes Destroy Infected Liver Cells

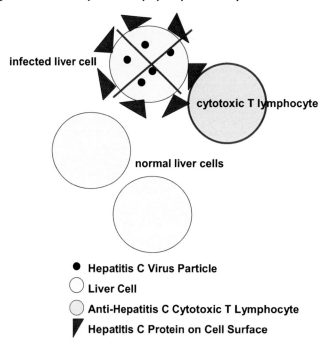

infected liver cell

cytotoxic T lymphocyte

normal liver cells

● **Hepatitis C Virus Particle**
○ **Liver Cell**
○ **Anti-Hepatitis C Cytotoxic T Lymphocyte**
▮ **Hepatitis C Protein on Cell Surface**

(those with the HCV "red flag"). Thus, only HCV infected cells are killed by anti-HCV CTLs (see Figure 8). A strong and prolonged anti-HCV CTL response appears to be important in spontaneous clearance of HCV.[12, 13, 14] Weak and/or limited CTL responses have been suggested as possible factors in the development of chronic HCV infection. Some evidence suggests that *interferon-based therapy* may act, at least in part, by enhancing the body's cytotoxic T cell response to HCV.[15, 16]

A person's *genetic* makeup strongly influences how he or she responds to immune system challenges. Researchers continue to study exactly how genetic factors affect an individual's immune response to HCV infection. Each of these topics and other cutting edge immunology research findings are discussed in detail in *Chapter 7.2, Immunology Takes on Hepatitis C.*

Extrahepatic Immune Syndromes and Chronic Hepatitis C

HCV lives primarily in the liver, and many of the symptoms of the disease are related to liver damage. However, approximately 38% of people with *chronic hepatitis* C also have immunologic disorders.[17] Although the association between HCV and *extrahepatic* (outside the liver) immune syndromes is accepted by most experts, the interaction between chronic hepatitis C and immunologic disorders such as *cryoglobulinemia*, kidney disease, Sjögren's syndrome, and *neuropathy* is not completely understood. Immune syndromes most often develop during the course of long-standing hepatitis C, and most frequently occur in people whose liver disease has progressed to *cirrhosis*.

Cryoglobulinemia

Cryoglobulins are abnormal immunoglobulins (antibodies). Cryoglobulins can get stuck and block tiny blood vessels causing symptoms. The location of the blocked vessels determines what symptoms a patient experiences.
The portion of people with hepatitis C who also have cryoglobulinemia has been reported from <1% to almost 60% in various studies conducted throughout the world.[17] Differences in the quality of the tests used to detect cryoglobulins may be responsible for some of this wide variation. Regardless of the portion of HCV patients affected, the association

between chronic hepatitis C and cryoglobulinemia is strong. Although some people with cryoglobulinemia do not experience symptoms, others experience one or more of a range of signs and symptoms as shown in Table 1. The signs and symptoms are listed from most to least common. The best treatment for symptoms caused by HCV-associated cryoglobulinemia is to rid the body of the virus. Nearly all symptoms gradually resolve with viral clearance.

Lymphoma

A recent analysis examining the results of 23 separate studies concluded that chronic hepatitis C increases the risk for development of *non-Hodgkin's lymphoma* greater than 5-fold compared to those without HCV.[18] Non-Hodgkin's lymphoma (NHL) is a form of lymphatic system cancer. Although it is unclear precisely how HCV enhances the risk of developing NHL, the presence of the increased risk is certain.

Table 1. Common Signs and Symptoms Associated with Cryoglobulinemia

Symptom	Description/Notes
Weakness	Approximately 2/3 of people with cryoglobulinemia experience this symptom.
Kidney disease	Several kidney disorders can be seen with cryoglobulinemia. The most common is membranoproliferative glomerulonephritis (MPGN). In some cases, people are initially diagnosed with MPGN and unsuspected chronic hepatitis C is diagnosed in the process of trying to uncover the cause for this disorder. Approximately ¼ of people with cryoglobulinemia have kidney involvement.
Neuropathy	Neuropathy is numbness, tingling, or other abnormal sensations in the hands and feet. These sensations make work their way up the arms or legs over time. Neuropathy is experienced by approximately ¼ of people with cryoglobulinemia.
Raynaud's phenomenon	Raynaud's phenomenon describes intermittent episodes when the arteries of the fingers or toes suddenly go into spasm causing the skin to become very pale, cold, and numb. Attacks are usually brought on by exposure to the cold or emotional stress. This phenomenon is experienced by approximately ¼ of people with cryoglobulinemia.
Skin disorders	Purpura (dark red to purple lesions on the skin) are the most common skin manifestation of cryoglobulinemia. These lesions usually appear on the lower legs, but can be present elsewhere. Around 20% of people with cryoglobulinemia have associated skin disorders.
Sjögren's syndrome	Sjögren's syndrome is a drying of the normally moist membranes of the eyes, mouth, and upper airway. This syndrome affects approximately 20% of people with cryoglobulinemia.
Joint disease	Approximately 15% of people with cryoglobulinemia experience joint pain that may be confused with rheumatoid arthritis.

Summary

The interaction between the immune system and the hepatitis C virus is a complex mystery that we are just beginning to unravel. Ongoing research will continue to provide insights into the interactions between hepatitis C and the immune system. A detailed review is presented in *Chapter 7.2, Immunology Takes on Hepatitis C*. With each new discovery, we come one step closer to new methods to intervene in the hepatitis C disease process.

References

1. Wang H, Eckels DD. Mutations in immunodominant T cell epitopes derived from the nonstructural 3 protein of hepatitis C virus have the potential for generating escape variants that may have important consequences for T cell recognition. *J Immunol.* 1999;162(7):4177-83.
2. Pavio N, Lai MM. The hepatitis C virus persistence: how to evade the immune system? *J Biosci.* 2003;28(3):287-304.
3. Zeuzem S, Schmidt JM, Lee JH, von Wagner M, Teuber G, Roth W K. Hepatitis C virus dynamics in vivo: effect of ribavirin and interferon alfa on viral turnover. *Hepatology.* 1998;28:245-52.
4. Neumann AU, Lam NP, Dahari H, et al. Hepatitis C viral dynamics in vivo and the antiviral efficacy of interferon-alpha therapy. *Science.* 1998;282:103-7.
5. Lanford RE, Chavez D, Chisari FV, Sureau C. Lack of detection of negative-strand hepatitis C virus RNA in peripheral blood mononuclear cells and other extrahepatic tissues by the highly strand-specific rTth reverse transcriptase PCR. *J Virol.* 1995;69:8079-83.
6. Cribier B, Schmitt C, Bingen A, Kirn A, Keller F. In vitro infection of peripheral blood mononuclear cells by hepatitis C virus. *J Gen Virol.* 1995;76:2485-91.
7. Reiser M, et al. Serum interleukin 4 and interleukin 10 levels in patients with chronic hepatitis C virus infection. *J Hepatol.* 1997;26(3):471-8.
8. He XS, Rehermann B, et al. Quantitative analysis of hepatitis C virus-specific CD8(+) T cells in peripheral blood and liver using peptide-MHC tetramers. *Proc Natl Acad Sci U S A.* 1999;96(10):5692-7.
9. Ferrari C, Penna A, et al. Antiviral cell-mediated immune responses during hepatitis B and hepatitis C virus infections. *Recent Results Cancer Res.* 1998;154:330-6.
10. Diepolder HM, Zachoval R, Hoffmann RM, Wierenga EA, Santantonio T, et al. Possible mechanism involving lymphocyte response to non-structural protein 3 in viral clearance in acute hepatitis C virus infection. *Lancet.* 1995;346:1006–7.
11. Missale G, Bertoni R, Lamonaca V, Valli, A, Massari M, et al. Different clinical behaviors of acute hepatitis C virus infection are associated with different vigor of the anti-viral cell-mediated immune response. *J Clin Invest.* 1996;98:706–14.
12. Lechner F, Wong DK, Dunbar PR, Chapman, R, Chung RT, et al. Analysis of successful immune responses in persons infected with hepatitis C virus. *J Exp Med.* 2000;191:1499–512.
13. Shoukry NH, Grakoui A, Houghton M, Chien DY, Ghrayeb J, et al. Memory CD8+ T cells are required for protection from persistent hepatitis C virus infection. *J Exp Med.* 2003;197:1645–55.
14. Thimme R, Oldach D, Chang KM, Steiger C, Ray SC, Chisari FV. Determinants of viral clearance and persistence during acute hepatitis C virus infection. *J Exp Med.* 2001;194:1395–406.
15. Cramp ME, Rossol S, Chokshi S, Carucci P, Williams R, Naoumov NV. Hepatitis C virus-specific T-cell reactivity during interferon and ribavirin treatment in chronic hepatitis C. *Gastroenterology.* 2000;118:346–55.
16. Kamal SM, Fehr J, Roesler B, Peters T, Rasenack JW. Peginterferon alone or with ribavirin enhances HCV-specific CD4 T-helper 1 responses in patients with chronic hepatitis C. *Gastroenterology.* 2002;123:1070–83.
17. Mayo, MJ. Extrahepatic manifestations of hepatitis C infection. *Am J Med Sci.* 2002;325:135-48.
18. Matsuo K, Kusano A, Sugumar A, Nakamura S, Tajima K, Mueller NE. Effect of hepatitis C virus infection on the risk of non-Hodgkin's lymphoma: A meta-analysis of epidemiological studies. *Cancer Sci.* 2004;95(9):745-52.

THE IMMUNE SYSTEM AND THE HEPATITIS C VIRUS

Stewart Cooper, MD

IMMUNOLOGY TAKES ON HEPATITIS C

Introduction

Humans protect themselves from viral infections with specialized cells that interact with and destroy most viruses that pose a threat. The specialized cells that work together to detect and destroy foreign viruses and bacteria are collectively called the *immune system*. The science of immunology studies how this highly efficient system works.

Because the immune system typically protects against infection and kills viruses, it is unusual that it is unable to clear the *hepatitis C* virus (*HCV*) when infected. Most people infected with HCV experience persistent infection whereby the virus evades, subverts, and/or weakens the immune system and survives for the life of the infected person. Such chronic infection with HCV often results in liver damage, which can lead to *cirrhosis*, *liver failure*, *liver cancer*, and/or premature death.

Approximately 5 million Americans and at least 180 million people worldwide are chronically infected with HCV, with a significant proportion developing progressive liver disease. This makes HCV the most common reason in the western hemisphere for liver transplantation.

Clearly, the stakes are high for conducting research that leads to the development of a vaccine to protect against HCV. The basic approach to begin this work is to unravel the type of *immunity* that naturally overcomes HCV then to design vaccines and/or therapies aimed at stimulating and amplifying that immunity. Strategies could conceivably involve stimulating specific immune cell types, such as *lymphocytes*, and/or blocking natural influences that decrease the body's response to infection with HCV. In other words, we are looking for a way to firmly push the immune system's "on" button while blocking all attempts to trigger the "off" button. My intent here is to introduce you to aspects of the immune system that seem central to this endeavor at the present time.

At the outset, it is essential to recognize that some fundamental questions relating to the immunology of hepatitis C remain unanswered. For example:

- How is HCV cleared from the body naturally, and in response to *interferon-based therapy*?
- Can the immune response itself contribute to the progression of liver disease?

In this chapter, the focus will be on current immunological knowledge and future research directions that show promise for improving the prevention and treatment of hepatitis C.

On a personal note, I hope this chapter will be of interest to a broad readership, including people currently infected by and recently exposed to HCV, and those living with and caring for people suffering this still much too silent epidemic. My aim is that attentive information seekers will:

- understand the logical basis of immunological studies
- derive a sense of where immunologists currently are in this arena of research
- procure adequate knowledge to follow the gist and implications of immunological research as it unravels
- be stimulated to ask questions and thereby contribute to the research endeavor

Like all fields of medical research, this one will be greatly enriched and even accelerated by more public interest and participation. I believe the latter will be encouraged by better understanding of the key scientific questions and obstacles. My principal assignment, therefore, is to translate the concepts, discoveries, and jargon of everyday science into something palatable for non-specialists. Any failure to achieve this rests solely with the author, who will always welcome questions, comments, and suggestions. I will begin with a preamble to provide some context and basic grounding.

Background Information

HCV Persistence Versus Clearance

A virus that is not cleared from the body by the immune system is said to persist. Persistence is unusual for viruses like HCV, which are made of a short single strand of RNA (a close but distinct chemical relative of *DNA*). The most infamous RNA virus, *HIV*, ultimately persists by inserting itself among the infected person's *genes* where it permanently avoids detection by the immune system. We do not believe HCV hides from the immune system in this way.

The viral and patient (called the host) factors that are responsible for the persistence of HCV have yet to be fully explained. However, it is clear that the fate of hepatitis C (whether it is cleared or persists) is nearly always determined during the early (acute) phase of infection, that is, within the first 6 months after exposure.[1] Although it can sometimes take longer, most people who naturally (spontaneously) clear HCV from their body experience this *clearance* within the first 6 months of infection.

Timeframes are important in HCV infection. Natural clearance of HCV by the immune system prevents disease progression and returns liver health. Therefore, early HCV infection has become the focus of intense attention for some immunologists, including this author. If we understand the type of immunity that allows people with *acute hepatitis* C to clear infection, we can devise methods of stimulating the same type of protective immune response in others. That is, we can make a vaccine.

HCV Clearance Has Been Difficult to Study

Acute hepatitis C has been difficult to study because it is rarely diagnosed. Curiously, most people have few or no symptoms with acute hepatitis C. In the absence of symptoms, people feel well and are unaware they've been infected. As a result, very few doctors are likely to see even one case of acute hepatitis C per year.

This situation has severely limited research regarding the predictors and rate of *viral clearance* in natural HCV infection. In recent years, researchers have begun studying special groups of people to gain a window into early HCV infection: those who experience high rates of new HCV infections.

INJECTION DRUG USERS EXPERIENCE A HIGH RATE OF ACUTE HCV INFECTION

While modern blood-supply screening practices have reduced the number of new HCV infections in the West, cases continue to arise particularly among injection drug users (IDU's). In recent years, diligent work by scientists who analyze the incidence, spread, and control of diseases in populations has defined study groups (called cohorts) of IDU's who experience a high incidence of acute hepatitis C. These precious cohorts now provide an unprecedented opportunity to investigate acute HCV infection.

A Smoldering Immune Response May Underpin Liver Disease Progression

While unraveling the details of successful immune responses is of great interest to aspiring HCV vaccine developers, the details of host immunity in people with *chronic hepatitis* C may provide clues for halting the progression of liver scarring (*fibrosis*).

For chronically infected people, interactions between the immune system and HCV-infected liver cells may determine the amount and rate of liver fibrosis and therefore the rate of liver disease progression. In this regard, the liver injury associated with persistent HCV may be similar to that incurred in chronic *hepatitis B* virus (*HBV*) infection. Like HBV, HCV probably causes little or no liver damage if ignored by host immune cells. When HCV stimulates but defeats waves of immune attack, the immune system may actually cause liver injury.

Certain immune defense strategies—which may be genetically influenced—might be particularly damaging. Some people with hepatitis C seem particularly prone to form scar tissue. A variety of other factors may further contribute to the cascade of events that leads to liver injury and scarring, such as alcohol consumption and, conceivably, stress and diet. To complicate the plot further, each contributing factor may have immunological effects.

Liver Damage Is Not Universal

A central question is why liver inflammation converts to scar tissue only in some people. It will be important to work out the immune defense tactics deployed in these ill-fated battles, with the intent of distinguishing pathways that promote liver fibrosis. The eventual goal is to develop therapies aimed at blocking, dampening, or diverting harmful interactions. Thus, in the chronic setting, the immune response might be more detrimental to the person infected than to the virus. Passive coexistence with HCV may prove more harmonious than unsuccessful attempts at eviction.

Successful Interferon-based Therapy May Need a Healthy Immune System

An accumulating body of evidence suggests that in order to work, *interferon-α* (*IFN*) and *ribavirin* probably need to boost a critical arm of the immune system. Therefore, studying the components of natural HCV immunity could also hold implications for understanding the mechanism of viral clearance in response to IFN and ribavirin. A possible role for the immune system in treatment-induced HCV clearance will be discussed later in the chapter.

Thorough study of the immunology of hepatitis C will undoubtedly require further collaboration between doctors and scientists from different disciplines. In this chapter, I will review what is known about the immune response to HCV and for reasons described previously, I will pay particular attention to the way in which the immune system interacts with the virus during the acute phase of infection.

A coherent discussion of these issues is not possible without initially devoting some attention to the hepatitis C virus itself.

Hepatitis C Virology For Beginners

What Is HCV Made Of?

To understand the concepts of HCV immunity, it is helpful to appreciate the basic structure of the virus. HCV is a relatively small virus made from *ribonucleic acid* (*RNA*) genetic materials, not DNA, which is the building material of human genes.[2] The entire genetic component (the *genome*) of HCV is made of a single strand of RNA of only 9,600 units. By comparison, the average length of a single human gene is 27,000 units.

Each RNA genetic unit (called a base because of its chemical property) is made up of a sugar unit (ribose) fused to a molecule of either guanine (G), adenine (A), cytosine (C) or uracil (U) arranged in specific sequence.
Each sequence of 3 bases constitutes a code that usually specifies a particular *amino acid*. For example, AUG specifies the amino acid called methionine. Each set of 3 bases is called a codon. A series of codons specifies a series of amino acids.

Amino acids are the individual units that when strung together build *proteins*. In nature, the vast majority of proteins are assembled from only 20 amino acids that are arranged in diverse combinations, as genetically instructed. The structure of a particular protein is determined by the specific sequence of amino acids that are strung together.

HCV has ten major proteins (see Figure 1). The structure of all ten individual HCV proteins is determined by the specific sequence of bases in the HCV RNA. The ten HCV proteins taken together are called the HCV polyprotein.

Figure 1. Schematic of the HCV Polyprotein

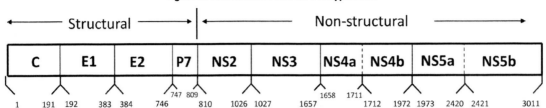

Letters indicate the names of the individual HCV proteins. Numbers indicate the amino acid coordinates of each protein. Shown here are the protein coordinates of HCV-1, the 'prototype' strain discovered by Choo and associates.[2]

C=Core, the capsid protein.

E=Envelope proteins, which participate in the viral outer structure – possibly with P7, a protein of unknown function.

NS=Non-structural proteins.

> NS2 forms a *protease* in conjunction with NS3.
> NS3 possesses 3 different *enzyme* activities.
> NS4, like NS5, comprises two proteins, each denoted "a" and "b".

HCV Is a Virus With a Highly Variable Structure

Remarkably, HCV seems to change its genetic and protein sequences with relative ease. This is an important concept and I will devote some time to it.

The act of switching one genetic building block (a base) to another is called a *mutation*. In general, RNA viruses like HCV have much higher rates of mutation than DNA viruses.

Recall that HCV possesses a single strand of RNA. In a liver cell, this positive sense or (+) strand is copied into a complementary (-) strand, which acts as the blueprint for making more (+) strands. However, this process is error prone. On average each daughter HCV RNA strand will possess at least one different base from its parent and siblings. This is depicted in Figure 2.

We estimate that approximately one trillion *replications* of HCV occur each day in a single person infected with HCV. Because mutations occur largely at random, this huge number of replications implies that every single base in the HCV RNA strand can theoretically undergo mutation daily. In reality, many mutations will not lead to a fully functioning virus because they injure some aspect of the lifecycle. Nevertheless, many capable mutant viruses emerge to face the host's immune defenses. The consequences are worth thinking about, which I will develop later in the chapter. For detail seekers, excellent reviews can be found in reference number 3 and 4.

The main point is that no one infected with HCV is infected with merely a single virus, but instead with a mixture of related viral sequences. Remarkably, the HCV sequences in a single person can exhibit a greater percentage of genetic difference than that distinguishing major mammalian species, for example, such as a human and a chimpanzee. Scientists describe these circulating families of close viral relatives as *quasispecies*.[5] In essence, each infected person harbors a group of HCV quasispecies, not a single entity.

Genetic diversity results in diversity among the encoded proteins, which creates the basic material on which natural selection can operate when a population is placed under environmental pressure. This holds true for all living things. In comparison to humans and other animal species however, RNA viruses play out the evolutionary game by producing remarkable numbers of genetically diverse offspring in relatively brief timeframes. This creates a rich opportunity for natural selection to operate quickly. Thus it is notable that many of the observed amino acid mutations in HCV proteins are clustered at sites targeted by the immune system, indicating they have not emerged merely by chance. Chance would not favor clustered mutations. We know that these mutations can disrupt the viral targets of immune attack, which in scientific jargon are called *epitopes*.[6, 7] The important point is that if mutation alters the structure of an epitope, the mutant virus is liberated from that source of immune attack.

Figure 2. HCV Replication Is Error-Prone

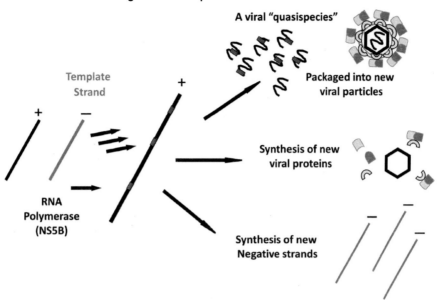

Following entry into a liver cell, HCV starts reproducing. The positive-stranded HCV genome (+) makes a complementary negative strand (-), shown in blue. New (+) strands are synthesized by the viral enzyme RNA *polymerase* using the negative strand as a template. Each daughter (+) strand is likely to contain at least one mutation compared with the parental strands. These new (+) strands are used to manufacture more negative strands and new viral proteins that fold around the (+) strands to make new virus particles. To reflect the differences in HCV RNA sequence even in single individuals, the infecting virus populations are referred to as quasispecies.

Natural selection works like this: mutations occur randomly, and when a certain mutation creates an advantage for its owner, that individual (officially called a carrier) is set apart from the pack. If the genetic mutation fails to injure the function or reproductive success of its carrier, the imbued privilege can be passed to its progeny. Extending the example of the *HCV* epitope mutation described above, viruses carrying such mutations will become more abundant in the host as their fitness outstrips that of other viruses neutered by the immune response. We are, therefore, able to readily observe them. This phenomenon is called escape mutation and represents evolution on the mini scale. Freed from immune attack, viruses with escape mutations can thrive.

As I have implied, examples of escape mutation by HCV have already been observed[6, 7] and are popularly invoked as a principal means of HCV persistence. Indeed, so talented is this changeling virus that perhaps no HCV epitope can be guaranteed to remain permanently intact – a consideration that might confound vaccine development. It is important to emphasize, however, that the true extent by which mutation underlies HCV persistence remains uncertain. Because of the implications for vaccine design, some researchers are eager to measure the effect of HCV mutations on the overall efficiency of the immune response. The virus may, for example, experience more difficulty in surviving with some mutations than others. If a hierarchy of HCV mutations exists, discovery of epitopes that are problematic for the virus and therefore advantageous to the immune system could significantly enhance prospects for vaccine development.

HCV Mutation Has Resulted in Genotypes and Subtypes
The same genetic plasticity that results in HCV diversification has resulted in the evolution of even more divergent forms of HCV. The most profound HCV genetic divergence is observed between hepatitis C viruses from different human populations. Such comparisons reveal at least six major HCV genetic families, called *genotypes*, numbered 1 through 6 in their order of discovery (see Figure 3). Genetic sequence variability has resulted in each genotype being further divided into subtypes, which are denoted by lower case letters (a, b, c and so on). Hence, we routinely specify that someone is infected with HCV genotype 1a or genotype 2b, etc. In the North America, HCV genotype 1 infection is most common

with genotypes 1a and 1b occurring with approximately similar frequency, except in African Americans among whom genotype 1a is predominant. Next most common are infections with genotypes 2 and 3 viruses. The tree shown in Figure 3 depicts the relationship between the HCV genotypes and subtypes.

It is possible that the natural history of infection may differ between HCV genotypes in different ethnic groups, though little evidence in support of this possibility is yet available. However, differences in interferon-based treatment outcome according to HCV genotype and ethnicity are now well described.[8] For example, genotype 1 causes most HCV infections in the West, where it is also the most difficult type of HCV to successfully treat. Furthermore, genotype 1 is significantly more treatment resistant in African Americans. Overall, infections with genotypes 2 or 3 are the most treatment receptive, at least in western populations, with genotype 2 being most susceptible. While treatment responsiveness is discussed in more detail in a different chapter, these differences remain largely unexplained and imply interplay between host and viral factors. We suspect that genetically determined differences in the immune response play an important role, but a discussion of this is beyond the scope of this chapter.

Finally, it should be stressed that viral mechanisms other than mutation are likely to also play a role in immune subterfuge.[9-12] We suspect that HCV mutation may only be a factor in viral persistence, which requires further study. References 3,4, and 13 are thoughtful reviews that should at least partly satiate those detail-oriented readers with lingering hunger.[3, 4, 13] Other potential viral mechanisms involved in immune subterfuge will be discussed in the relevant immunology sections.

Figure 3. Genetic Diversification of the Hepatitis C Viruses

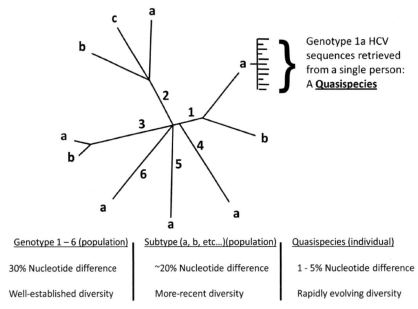

Genotype 1 – 6 (population)	Subtype (a, b, etc...)(population)	Quasispecies (individual)
30% Nucleotide difference	~20% Nucleotide difference	1 - 5% Nucleotide difference
Well-established diversity	More-recent diversity	Rapidly evolving diversity

Just as family trees depict the relatedness of human families, phylogenetic trees such as the one shown here, depict relatedness between different genetic sequences. A computer program has compared corresponding positions of many HCV genetic sequences and represented the degree of correspondence graphically. All members of each of the 6 major branches (the genotypes, numbered 1-6) are defined by shared genetic characteristics. Genetic variability exists at three levels. HCV genotypes (numbered 1-6) represent the highest level of divergence and probably the most ancient splits among HCV sequences. Each of the 6 major genetic groups contain a series of more closely related subtypes, typically different from each other by ~20% compared with >30% between genotypes. Genotypes 1a, 1b and 3a are now widely distributed due to unscreened blood transfusion and shared injection drug use, and now represent the vast majority of infections in Western countries. Each person is infected with a broad range of viral variants referred to as quasispecies, which exhibit up to 5% sequence differences.

The Immunology of HCV Infection

Like the body it protects, the human immune system has a physical and functional structure. Physically, it is made up of individual cells, receptors, and chemicals. The immune system deploys many types of cell and a considerably greater number of chemical substances.

Receptors are vitally important molecules embedded in the surface or the inside of a cell. Each receptor binds a specific chemical structure and then signals either activation (On) or inhibition (Off) of various cellular functions. In essence, receptors allow cells to detect and respond to certain things happening in their outside environment.

Functionally, the components of the immune system network to form a highly organized defense against invasion by abnormal cells and foreign organisms such as viruses. It is an integrated system with built-in control and failsafe mechanisms. If some components fail to work, others are in place to provide backup, an arrangement that inevitably generates complexity. That our ubiquitous species has survived every infection it has encountered in every niche of this planet attests to the sophistication and efficiency of the human immune system.

An approach that continues to serve students of immunology well is to categorize the immune system into two principal arms, called the innate and the adaptive systems. Typically, these are described as separate entities that defend in sequence (the innate system is first). As I will soon explain, in reality, these two systems are interactive and interdependent.

Innate Immunity

The innate immune system provides front-line defenses. It has a long list of chemical components, many of which are unstudied in the context of HCV infection and hence unnecessary to catalog here. Chemicals released inside infected cells that suppress viral replication may be the most ancient form of innate immunity. Interferons are in this category. Interferons can be effective inhibitors of viral replication and can suppress HCV in many people when used therapeutically. Why such innate immune mechanisms commonly fail to prevent HCV from establishing a foothold is deeply interesting but, as yet, relatively unstudied. Therefore, I will devote most attention here to the cellular arm of the innate immune system.

Cellular components of likely importance in influencing the outcome of HCV infection are:

- *antigen*-presenting cells (APCs)
- *natural killer cells* — the lymphocytes of innate immunity

Antigen Presenting Cells

Antigen presenting cells activate effector lymphocytes — natural killer and *T cells* — the immune system's front-line cells that attack foreign invaders. Antigen presenting cells include so-called dendritic cells and *macrophages*. A third type of cell, called a *B cell*, is also officially categorized as an APC, though the tenacious reader will later learn that B cells, like modern folk, multitask. B cells are also the cells that make *antibodies*. In summary, the three major categories of APC are dendritic cells, macrophages, and B cells.

Different APCs may serve to activate effector lymphocytes at different points in the immune response, and perhaps in different places. That is, there seems to be a subdivision of labor among APCs. The way in which APCs activate T cells (the effector lymphocytes of adaptive immunity) is relatively well worked out. But we have recently learned that dendritic cells (the most proficient APCs) also activate natural killer cells – the effector lymphocytes of the innate immune system.[14-17] However, the mechanism of natural killer cell activation by dendritic cells remains incompletely understood. An up-to-date review can be found in reference 18.

DENDRITIC CELLS INITIATE NEW IMMUNE RESPONSES

Dendritic cells were originally discovered in mice during the 1970s by Drs. Zanvil Cohn and Ralph Steinman at the

Rockefeller Institute, New York.[19] We now recognize a particular expertise of dendritic cells is their ability to kickstart a new immune response. Unlike macrophages and B cells, dendritic cells continuously express high levels of so called co-stimulatory molecules, which are inserted into their cell membranes. Co-stimulatory molecules are important because they are required for activating naïve T cells – rookies that have never previously interacted with a foreign invader.

Even dendritic cells come in different varieties. It now appears that there are distinct lineages of dendritic cells, each developing from a shared parental cell type in response to local microenvironmental conditions. In turn, each dendritic cell subset stimulates different lineages of T cells such as Th1, Th2, and Treg cells. (These T cell subsets will be discussed in the section on adaptive immunity, but please note here that we believe strong responses by the Th1 type of T cells are required for HCV clearance.)

Like military field commanders, dendritic cells can play a pivotal role in regulating an immune attack[20], by dictating the type of local forces deployed. Thus, dendritic cells may play an important role in determining the fate of HCV infection, a possibility that immunologists are beginning to consider.[21]

Because the local environment can influence the type of dendritic cells that develop, we are interested to learn more about dendritic cells in the human liver, the seat of HCV infection. As yet, information about dendritic cells in the liver remains relatively scant. Understanding the biology of the liver's dendritic cells and their likely role in governing immune responses against HCV should fill an important gap in current knowledge. In particular, unraveling the biology of the liver's version of a dendritic cell subset called plasmacytoid dendritic cells[22], which promote Th1 cells, might shed greatest light on the earliest determinants of HCV clearance. Readers wondering about the relevance of dendritic cell research for people with hepatitis C should recognize that dendritic cells are potential targets for vaccines aimed at eliminating HCV – and perhaps other persistent viral diseases.

DENDRITIC CELLS POSSESS ANTIQUE RECEPTORS FOR DETECTING VIRUSES

Like other APCs, dendritic cells take up foreign organisms, probably including HCV.[21, 23] Dendritic cells detect foreigners, take them into custody (uptake the organisms into the cell interior), then process them in a variety of ways. The following are two principal examples of how viruses are processed by dendritic cells and the immune response subsequently activated.

EXAMPLE 1: PATTERN RECOGNITION RECEPTORS

Dendritic cells possess pattern recognition receptors (PRR) that bind highly conserved structural motifs in the genetic material of different viruses and thereby distinguish the type of material (RNA or DNA) the virus is made from. Different PRRs recognize distinct motifs, and which PRR is bound determines what the response of the APC will be.

HCV and other single-stranded RNA viruses are bound by a brand of PRR named toll-like receptors (TLR)[24], perhaps especially TLR-7, 8, and 9 (humans have ten TLRs).[25] TLRs are themselves remarkably conserved molecules. Their close relatives, toll receptors, were originally discovered in flies. The common ancestor of humans and flies is estimated to have lived more than 1 billion years ago. When molecules are retained over long evolutionary time, it implies that they are so exceptionally useful that species cannot survive without them. As with PRRs in general, which TLR is bound determines the type of response.

TLR binding stimulates APCs to release chemicals called *cytokines*. Cytokines are small molecules that typically activate other immune cells. (A convenient description of individual cytokines can be found at www.copewithcytokines. de/cope.cgi).[26] APCs release cytokines to recruit the help of cells specialized in active combat (collectively called effectors). For students of trench warfare, cytokines are the immune system's runners, providing local and long distance communications. Therefore, using TLRs, dendritic cells identify the nature of the invading organism and turn on a response that is usually appropriate for repelling that type of invader.

Cytokines released following TLR binding by viral RNA include *interferon-alfa* (IFN-α) – the same chemical we use to treat hepatitis C – together with a variety of interleukins that stimulate activation of effector lymphocytes including natural killer and T cells. Notably, a variety of dendritic cells called pDC2 seem particularly important as major producers of IFN-α and other interferons, which we believe are essential for natural clearance of HCV.[27] Importantly, the profile of cytokines released during this earliest encounter with a virus (possibly even within the first hours) may set the stage for the type, strength, and eventual success of a person's immune response.

It is important to note that the amount and type of cytokine released by APCs during an *antiviral* immune response can differentially promote the function of natural killer cells, T cells, and B cells (in their mode as producers of antibodies). In the response against HCV, the lymphocytes that are recruited and the vigor of those responses almost certainly dictate whether HCV will be cleared or persist. I will develop this concept further later in the chapter. However, it is possible that HCV is already waging trickery during this earliest phase of infection by undertaking strategies for deviating the immune response away from a path that would otherwise lead to its removal from the host.[28]

Recent studies have suggested that by the time chronic infection is established, dendritic cell numbers are reduced and their ability to produce beneficial cytokines diminished.[29] Precisely how the virus pulls this off and at what stage of infection currently remains unclear. These central questions will be most accurately addressed by carefully studying dendritic cells during the course of acute HCV infection.

Example 2:
Antigen presenting cells not only detect the genetic material of internalized viruses, they also pay attention to the wrappings. Viral proteins are chopped into small fragments then transported back to the cell surface where they are firmly held and paraded by dedicated molecular scaffolds called antigen receptors. These bits of viral protein are closely inspected by lymphocytes, some of which will recognize their presence, become activated, and embark upon an attempt to rid the body of the virus.

For natural killer lymphocytes, the details of this recognition mechanism have not been fully worked out. But we know that interaction of natural killer cells with dendritic cells leads to activation, whereby the natural killer cell itself releases a variety of cytokines and small packets of lethal chemicals.[30] In the immunological squad dispatched to challenge HCV, natural killer cells are emerging as very probable players. This area of research is likely to mature quickly and I will therefore provide the reader with an essential guide to relevant aspects of natural killer cell function.

Natural Killer Cells
Natural killer cells are large lymphocytes that kill infected cells during the very early stages of viral infection.[31] Natural killer cells are always ready for action. Within minutes of activation they release an assortment of potent chemicals. Prepackaged combinations of perforin and granzymes, a cocktail of lethal proteins, are lobbed onto the outer membranes (the cell's equivalent of skin) of any virus-containing dendritic cells with which natural killer cells have forged specific contact. Perforin punches holes in the dendritic cell membrane that allow granzymes to enter and cause the cell to commit a form of ritual suicide called *apoptosis* (a programmed sequence leading to cell death).

Activated natural killer cells are not silent assassins. They stir things up like the most accomplished agitators. Already highly prepared, they quickly manufacture and release a set of cytokines, including interferons (IFN-α, IFN-γ), interleukin 12 (IL-12), and tumor necrosis factor alfa (TNF-α)[31, 32], which activate and attract other cells including cells of the adaptive immune system – the subject of the next section. As will be discussed, the cytokines released by activated natural killer cells closely resemble those produced by a type of T cell called a T helper 1 (Th1) cell, which promotes antiviral immunity by a far more selective virus-killing lymphocyte, called a *cytotoxic T cell*. Hence natural killer cells not only serve the innate immune system, they act to bridge innate and adaptive immunity. This is an important concept. It seems reasonable to assume that the efficiency of natural killer cell activation in response to a particular virus may be a critical factor determining whether the virus is eliminated or persists. And this may be especially pertinent in early HCV infection, when the balance between clearance and persistence could be finely suspended.

This emphasizes the value of natural killer cells in innate immune defense. However, at this point I would like the reader to reflect on a potential problem faced by nature in allowing natural killer cells to evolve. (Their presence in jawed cartilaginous fish suggests that natural killer cells first arose more than 350 million years ago.) The advantage of having cells capable of such potent ready-to-go effects in our organs and blood could result in catastrophe if they were to activate by mistake – a self-destructive condition referred to as horror autotoxicus by the 1908 Nobel Laureate, Dr. Paul Ehrlich.[33]

Since seminal experiments by Karre and colleagues in 1986[34], several teams of scientists have shown that nature's elegant solution involves regulation of natural killer cell activation using an intricate system of cell surface receptors. Natural killer cells integrate signals from arrays of activating and inhibitory receptors, but inhibitory receptors – which dampen cellular activation – play the dominant role. Nature has chosen safety. Therefore, as one would predict, every natural killer cell has at least one inhibitory receptor. Without one, by default, the natural killer cell will activate. By the same principle, if a natural killer cell's inhibitory receptor(s) is not engaged, the natural killer cell will activate.

A thorough discussion of natural killer cell receptor biology is beyond this chapter's scope, but diehard readers can seek additional information in a recent review by one of the field's pioneers in reference 31. Of relevance for HCV infection, a collaborative study led by Drs. Salim Khakoo and Mary Carrington recently provided the first evidence that certain natural killer cell inhibitory receptors significantly influence the chance of clearing acute hepatitis C.[35] This striking discovery holds potentially exciting prospects for future HCV therapies, and for readers craving more insight, I will next provide the necessary framework.

THE CONTROL OF NATURAL KILLER CELL ACTIVATION BY RECEPTORS FOR HLA CLASS I MOLECULES

Natural killer cells sample the health of body tissues by briefly touching cells – all of which are potential targets for natural killer cells if something goes awry, such as a virus infection. Each touch is carefully contrived and mediated by the natural killer cell receptor system. Readers have already learned that in the immune system, receptor is a general term encompassing many different types of signaling molecules. At this point it will be helpful to know that the molecular partners specifically bound by receptors are called ligands. Simply put, receptors bind ligands.

Binding to cells by the inhibitory natural killer cell receptors (iNKR) is accomplished by engaging ligands called HLA class I (one) molecules, which are embedded in the surface of virtually every normal cell in the body.

HLA molecules happen to be the things that create your tissue type, and therefore the things that transplant surgeons want to match as closely as possible before organ transplantation. The matching problem surrounding HLA class I molecules arises because the HLA genes and the proteins they encode are so remarkably variable that very few individuals are identical. Extreme variability at a population level is the hallmark of the three so-called classical HLA class I genes (HLA-A, HLA-B and HLA-C), which are nestled closely together on chromosome number 6. As of October 2004, 338 versions (called alleles) of HLA-A genes, 617 versions of HLA-B, and 179 versions of HLA-C have been found in people around the world (IMGT Database: www.ebi.ac.uk/imgt/). Please note that each genetically normal person can have a maximum of only two versions of each HLA gene.

Each cell in the body harbors two copies of chromosome 6, one inherited from each parent. Therefore, each person carries up to six different HLA class I genes (two HLA-A + two HLA-B + two HLA-C). Genes encode proteins, the entities that perform biological functions. Therefore, a person can express 3 to 6 HLA class I proteins. A major function of HLA class I proteins is to bind short pieces of processed viral proteins (pieces about 8 to 11 amino acids in length) and to display them at the cell surface where they can be detected and engaged by T lymphocytes.[36]

Figure 4A. Ribbon Diagram of the HLA-C Protein Structure Showing the Natural Killer Cell "Control Zone"

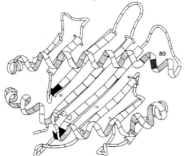

The ribbon diagram is based upon the known crystal structure of HLA class I molecules[36] and depicts part of an HLA-C molecule viewed from above. The part shown is held outside of the cell by the remainder of the structure which forms a subframe that traverses the cell membrane (not shown). Two spirals of amino acids form the respective lips of a mouth whose base is formed by parallel strands of amino acids[39]. Some amino acids are numbered to show their order in the protein sequence. Conspicuously, position 80 (shown in red) – either the amino acid asparagine or lysine in all HLA-C molecules – is located on the outer edge of the upper spiral, easily available for interaction with KIR2DL receptors on patrolling natural killer cells (see Figure 4B). Typically, self or viral peptides fill the groove (oriented horizontally across the page) and may influence, but not prevent, KIR2DL binding to position 80.

Figure 4B. Control of Natural Killer Cell Activation by KIR2DL

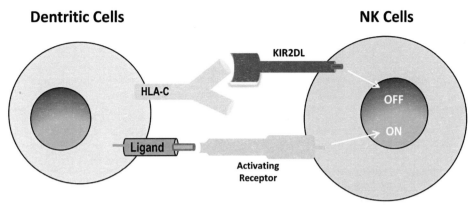

Triggering of an *NK cell* to kill and release cytokines is determined by the integration of activating and inhibitory signals delivered into the natural killer cell by various receptors. KIR2DL receptors (dark blue) deliver inhibitory (off) signals after engaging appropriate HLA-C molecules.

The most variable parts of HLA genes encode the regions of HLA proteins that physically contact viral protein pieces called *peptides*. Therefore, different HLA proteins have a strong tendency to bind different sets of viral peptides. We believe that the adaptive immune response benefits greatly from this HLA class I genetic and protein diversity, which imbues ability (particularly at a population level) to bind huge numbers of viral peptides. The work that spawned these discoveries started in the 1970's[37, 38], eventually earning Drs. Peter Doherty and Rolf Zinkernagel the 1996 Nobel Prize in Medicine. This occurred well before the discovery that HLA class I molecules possessed a second major function in innate immunity as mediators of natural killer cell inhibition.[34]

T cells are equipped to embrace HLA structural diversity by possessing a huge number of dedicated receptors (T cell receptors or TCR). On the other hand, HLA diversity poses a potential headache for natural killer cells, which possess only a limited number of inhibitory receptors. How could relatively few inhibitory receptors reliably detect so many different HLA structures? The solution, like many in nature, is extremely elegant and results from the simplicity of a natural killer cell's primary concern: are HLA class I molecules present? If not, then something is wrong with that cell and it should be destroyed. Many viruses and cancers prevent HLA class I molecules from appearing at the cell surface. If HLA class I molecules are not present, inhibitory receptors will not be engaged and natural killer cells will, by default, activate. Now clear is that over evolutionary time, inhibitory NKRs have rigorously frisked HLA class I molecules to identify discrete spots that do not change, or that change in only limited and predictable ways. Because Dr. Khakoo's recent paper in the journal Science indicated that joint possession of an inhibitory NKR, called KIR2DL3, with its HLA-C ligand increases the chance of clearing HCV, I will devote all remaining attention to this system.

According to inheritance, natural killer cells deploy up to three types of inhibitory receptors with the dedicated task of engaging self (your own) HLA-C molecules. All three inhibitory receptors are members of the same molecular family, given the tongue-twisting name killer-cell immunoglobulin-like receptors shortened to KIR. More specifically, the inhibitory KIR that engage HLA-C molecules are called KIR2DL, and, the three types are logically named KIR2DL1, KIR2DL2 and KIR2DL3. These three inhibitory receptors effectively collapse all known HLA-C molecules into two types. Of the 340-odd amino acids in most cell membrane-bound HLA-C molecules, all three KIR2DL receptors focus interest on amino acid number 80 in the HLA-C protein sequence (see Figures 4A and 4B).

In all known HLA-C molecules, position 80 is occupied by either the amino acid asparagine or lysine. There is a single letter code used to denote amino acids and by a befitting twist of fate, the single letter code for asparagine is "N" and for lysine it is "K". We refer to HLA-C molecules possessing asparagine (N) at position 80 as HLA-C1-type and those with lysine as HLA-C2-type.

Table 1. KIR2DL Receptors and HLA-C Ligands

INHIBITORY RECEPTOR	HLA-C Ligand	Position 80	Natural Killer Inhibitory Potency
KIR2DL1	C2	Lysine (K)	Strong
KIR2DL2	C1	Asparagine (N)	Intermediate
KIR2DL3	C1	Asparagine (N)	Weak

As shown in Table 1, KIR2DL1 is the receptor for HLA-C2 (K80) types and KIR2DL2 and KIR2DL3 each engage HLA-C1 (N80) molecules. Now for some apparently important subtlety: it seems that the strength of inhibitory signals delivered by each KIR2DL is not equal. The hierarchy of inhibitory potency is shown, also in Table 1.

KIR2DL1 most potently inhibits natural killer cells carrying this receptor and KIR2DL3 inhibits its carriers least. Clearly in this scheme, if people have two versions of an HLA-C2 type (one inherited from each parent – a state called homozygous) and their natural killer cells carry KIR2DL1, their natural killer cells will be most resistant to activation. On the other hand, in people who only inherit HLA-C1 types (HLA-C1 homozygotes) KIR2DL1 is functionally redundant – it is there but does nothing. People carrying only HLA-C1 types therefore rely on either KIR2DL2 or KIR2DL3 for HLA-C mediated natural killer cell inhibition. And because KIR2DL3 delivers the weakest inhibition, natural killer cells carrying only KIR2DL3 should activate most readily. In fact, it turns out that nature has made this latter situation possible and it seems that such individuals, who are homozygous for both KIR2DL3 and HLA-C1, are privileged in the battle against HCV infection. Among the 1,037 people studied by Khakoo et al, those homozygous for KIR2DL3 and HLA-C1 were significantly more likely to clear acute HCV infection.[35] In the natural killer world, these (KIR2DL3-HLA-C1 homozygotes) might be the type A personalities, genetically wired to be most highly resistant to viral infections.

DOES NATURAL KILLER CELL RECEPTOR BIOLOGY HOLD IMPLICATIONS FOR PEOPLE WITH HEPATITIS C?

We have suspected that vigorous early immune interaction is necessary for HCV clearance[1] but these recent findings suggest that vigor during even the very earliest interaction may influence the fate of HCV infection. Furthermore, that inhibitory signaling by KIR2DL-HLA-C has been so emphatically implicated offers some intriguing possibilities for new treatments. For example, if individuals with KIR2DL3-HLA-C1 are so gifted, could natural killer cells in people with the other KIR2DL-HLA-C combinations be manipulated to become more KIR2DL3-HLA-C1-like – that is, rendered more excitable?

The answer is: possibly. One strategy might be to administer agents (like monoclonal antibodies) that bind and block KIR2DL1 and KIR2DL2. The intent would be to diminish the inhibitory signals delivered by each receptor and convert these equivalents of couch-potato natural killer cells into gym flies. (The concept of inhibiting an inhibitor proves difficult for many; I hope readers will now understand that for a natural killer cell this means natural killer activation will occur more readily.)

Dr. Khakoo's study implied that sole possession of KIR2DL3 and HLA-C1 molecules wrought enhanced clearance of HCV during acute infection. However, receptor manipulations of the type discussed in the last paragraph could conceivably improve chances of HCV clearance in people undergoing treatment for chronic hepatitis C. Increased local release of the so-called Th1 cytokines (IFN-γ, TNF-α, IL-12) by liver natural killer cells seems likely to augment the type of T cell response that we now believe is important for treatment-induced clearance of chronic hepatitis C.

Another potentially positive twist arises from the fact that the HLA-C-specific KIR2DL inhibitory receptor system has also been found on some T cells, including some that have been shown to engage HCV. We suspect that, as on natural killer cells, KIR2DL will dampen activation of T cells and make them less vigorous.[40] Thus, the same therapeutic manipulations suggested for natural killer cells might make at least some HCV-targeting T cells also work more efficiently.

NATURAL KILLER CAVEAT EMPTOR

Before letting enthusiasm overwhelm caution, I should point out that the above study indicated advantage in carrying KIR2DL3 and HLA-C1 only in people presumed to have contracted HCV in relatively low dose, for example, by needle-sharing among injection drug users. This is now the typical acquisition route for new HCV infections in the West so the caveat certainly does not weaken the importance of the research team's observations. However, it suggests that other mechanisms for defeating host immunity are afoot when HCV is acquired in high dose, for example, following transfusion of HCV- infected blood products. Among the possibilities, natural killer cells may still be involved.

Many things other than HLA class I receptors litter the surface of natural killer cells. Among these is a common molecule called *CD81*, which has been shown by Dr. Sergio Abrignani's research team at Chiron Corporation to bind the HCV envelope (outer coat) proteins.[41] Recently, another group of Chiron researchers led by Dr. Nick Valiante made the interesting discovery that when HCV binds and sticks together adjacent CD81 molecules in the natural killer cell surface, all aspects of natural killer cell activation (killing and cytokine production) are prevented.[42] Therefore, we might anticipate that this HCV-triggered off switch for natural killer cells would be most firmly thrown in the presence of a large number of HCV particles. If this mechanism indeed plays a significant role, might advantage be swayed back in the host's favor if we blocked both the HCV envelope proteins and the natural killer cell KIR2DL inhibitory receptors as part of a therapeutic regimen? Such questions can keep immunologists awake at night.

The Intracellular Response to HCV Infection

As noted above, the reaction of a single cell to limit damage from viral infection probably represents one of the earliest types of (innate) immune response. Following pioneering studies by Dr. Markus Heim and colleagues in Basel, Switzerland[43], recent work suggests that HCV interferes with a principal signaling pathway used by IFN-α and IFN-β (the so-called type 1 interferons) to transmit messages into the nucleus of an infected cell. Type 1 interferons are among the most potent cytokines and are produced in most cell types, including liver cells.

Scientists who work on signal transmission inside cells (usually called transduction) have been as inventive with their shorthand as particle physicists. Hence the specific IFN signaling pathway inhibited by HCV is called JAK-STAT. In longhand, this respectively converts to Janus family of tyrosine kinases (JAK), and signal transducers and activators of transcription (STATs). JAKs add phosphate molecules (in chemical notation PO4) to STATs (there are two, STAT1 and STAT2) and thereby activate them. Adding phosphate groups is a biological trick for energizing molecules – somewhat akin to the double espressos imbibed by the scientists who study such systems. Enzymes that energize molecules by adding phosphate groups are generically called kinases – a name with two roots: a Greek word for moving (*kinetikos*) and, by convention, all enzymes end in -*ase*.

In general, an understanding of overarching principles is more indelible than attempts to memorize snippets of detail. Thus, cytokine receptors fall into two basic classes: those possessing their own kinase domain (like a couch potato with a firmly grasped TV remote – well equipped to make things happen at a distance), and those lacking a kinase domain (the remote always out of reach). For both types, however, kinase activity is essential for transmitting messages downstream. Cytokine receptors that lack their own kinase domain seem to often recruit JAK kinases for this purpose. This is the type of receptor bound by the cytokines IFN-α and IFN-β. Recruited JAKs link membrane receptors to nuclear genes.

Now some details that seem relevant to the immune subterfuge wrought by HCV. In the cellular fluid, JAKs activate both STAT molecules, which causes each STAT to combine with a third molecule called IRF-9. This huddle of three scurries across the nuclear membrane to bind and activate more than 30 target genes, collectively known as interferon α/β stimulated genes –ISGs. [With this surfeit of acronyms, the reader can be forgiven for believing that most immunologists have a military background.] Some ISGs have antiviral properties, among them OAS (oligoadenylate synthase) and PKR (protein kinase R) enzymes, which inhibit the generation of viral proteins. Many viruses have evolved strategies to down-regulate this system and HCV seems to be one of them.

Recently, de Lucas and colleagues showed that the HCV core protein disrupts IFN-α-induced induction of ISGs.[44] In these studies, the HCV core seems to decrease binding of a protein called ISGF3 to an important piece of DNA called the ISRE (interferon-stimulated response element), which controls expression of ISGs. In other studies using different experimental conditions, the HCV core protein appeared to prevent importation into the cell nucleus of STAT1 and the expression of another antiviral protein, MxA (myxovirus resistance A).[45] In summary, interference by HCV with IFN-α-induced signaling through the JAK-STAT pathway seems likely. It could contribute to the resistance to IFN-α therapy observed in many treated patients and may represent a basic strategy contributing to HCV persistence. More research is needed to determine the precise details and the extent to which such mechanisms of immune evasion operate during acute HCV infection. If a compelling case can be made, we can expect development of therapeutic agents designed to inhibit the viral protein inhibitors of JAK-STAT signaling.

In this section, I initially stressed that while innate immunity forms the immediate line of defense against viral infections, it seamlessly integrates with and triggers the adaptive immune response. I will now devote the remainder of this chapter to the adaptive immune system, particularly those components that have been shown to engage HCV with varying degrees of success.

Adaptive Immunity

CD4+ T Cells

When innate immune responses fail to dispatch viruses, CD4+ T cells emerge as the central controllers of viral immunity. CD4+ T cells are also called *T helper cells* because their activation helps other immune cells to combat viruses. Among the other cells are B cells that make antibodies and CD8+ T cells, which directly attack virus-infected cells. CD4+ T cells that promote antibody production by B cells are called T helper type 2 or Th2 cells. Those that stimulate CD8+ T cells are called Th1 cells. Although Th1 and Th2 responses can coexist, a very strong Th1 response suppresses Th2 responses and vice versa. Thus, a strong T cell response is often described as having a certain polarity, Th1 or Th2. A pivotal role for strong Th1-type CD4+ T cell activation in HCV clearance is now virtually certain.

It is important to understand that T cells only recognize tiny fragments of viral proteins not whole viruses. These tiny fragments (called peptides) are recognized only when they are presented at the infected cell surface by major histocompatibility complex (MHC) molecules. The reason for this is clever and subtle, but beyond the scope of this chapter.

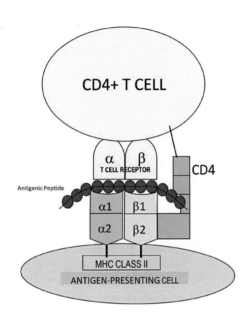

Figure 5. Recognition of MHC Class II-Viral Peptide Complexes by CD4+ T Cells

CD4+ T cells are activated when specific receptors (called T-cell receptors or TCR) engage molecular complexes of viral peptides embedded within MHC class II molecules (see Figure 5). The CD4 molecule is a co-receptor that binds and provides specificity for the MHC class II molecule.

Typically, CD4+ T cell responses are characterized by measuring the amount of proliferation (the extent to which the T cells divide) and/or cytokine secretion when they are incubated with viral versus negative control proteins. Using these techniques, involvement of CD4+ T cells in successful HCV immunity was first noted by Diepolder and colleagues after comparing T cell responses in the peripheral blood of people with self-limited versus chronic infection.[46] These studies suggested that prominent CD4+ T cell activation distinguished resolved infection.

A series of subsequent experiments have fairly consistently shown that vigorous CD4+ T cell responses, simultaneously targeting multiple HCV proteins, correlate with HCV clearance.[47-50] A characteristic of such CD4+ T cells is secretion of the Th1 cytokines, interferon gamma (IFN-γ), tumor necrosis factor alpha (TNF-α), and interleukin 2 (IL-2), which stimulate CD8+ cytotoxic T cells (CTL). In contrast, people whose HCV progresses to chronic infection appear to display less vigorous proliferation of CD4+ T cells, which secrete the Th2-type cytokines, IL-4, IL-5, and *IL-10*.

Although an HCV-specific CD4+ T cell response has been shown capable of persisting for 20 years after recovery[51], its robustness, duration, and potential for protecting the host from further infection are not yet clear.

CD4+CD25+ T cells (Treg)

Seminal studies in the 1990's by Sakaguchi[52, 53] and Shevach[54] showed that the tendency for experimentally manipulated newborn mice to develop *autoimmune* disease pivots around a subset of T cells that co-express the CD4 molecule (in common with T helper cells) together with the low affinity interleukin 2 receptor (IL-2R) α chain, called CD25. The presence of CD4+CD25+ regulatory T cells (abbreviated to Treg) prevents, whereas depletion portends, autoimmunity.

Although their precise mode of action remains uncertain, it has been shown that Treg suppress T-cell activation. Thus, Treg appear to dampen T cell responses and protect against the development of autoimmune diseases. This natural immunological braking system appears not only to protect against autoimmunity but also to benefit host immune responses to certain *pathogens* like Schistosomes[55] and Leishmania[56], where the immune response can cause tissue destruction. Thus, Treg are a prominent T cell population initially shown capable of mediating peripheral tolerance to self-antigens, but whose functions have now been extended to include regulation of T cell responses to viral antigens. There is, however, a potential downside of this natural dampening system. In some infectious diseases, like hepatitis C where the immunological balance between resolution and chronicity is finely poised[1], intervention by Treg could prematurely dampen the antiviral response and tip the balance in favor of persistence. Key in this regard may be the timing of Treg activation.

Clearly more needs to be known about involvement of Treg in HCV-specific immune responses. The potential for manipulating Treg and improving the outcome of hepatitis C makes this a fertile area of research. Intriguingly, one of the Treg on/off switches appears to be tilted by compounds naturally found in the brain. Dopamine has been shown to block the Treg-mediated suppression of T-effector cells, a finding with exciting potential for therapy.

CD8+ T Cells (Cytotoxic T Cells or CTL)

Like CD4+ T cells, these cells use a specific receptor (TCR) to detect viral peptides bound by MHC molecules expressed at the surface of infected cells. The principal difference is that CTL possess the CD8 co-receptor (instead of CD4), which binds MHC class I (instead of class II) molecules on the surface of infected cells. CTL are therefore activated by cell-surface complexes of viral peptides with MHC class I molecules (see Figure 6). Activation of CD8+ T cells by peptide/MHC complexes results in local release of chemicals that can kill and/or disinfect virus-infected cells and lead to viral eradication.[57] Because CTL can directly bring about viral clearance, they are often called effector cells.

Evidence that CD8+ T cells play a direct role in terminating hepatitis C was initially provided by prospective studies of acute infection in chimpanzees.[58] Chimpanzees are the only non-human species in which HCV replicates efficiently. Exceptionally for an animal model of human disease, chimpanzees and humans share MHC class I and II molecules, T cell receptors, and other immune response genes that are genetically indistinguishable.[59-62] The chimpanzee infection study revealed that a strong CTL response in the liver during acute infection correlated with HCV clearance.

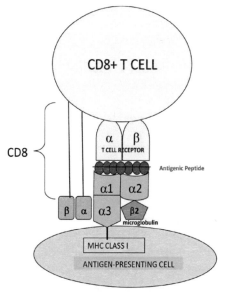

Figure 6. Recognition of MHC Class I-Viral Peptide Complexes by CD8+ T Cells

In six chimpanzees with acute hepatitis C, HCV was eradicated in the two who mounted the broadest CTL response. In contrast, both of these chimpanzee resolvers mounted extremely weak antibody responses, which quickly disappeared in one. The number and breadth of CTL that were synchronously operational in early infection seemed critical for HCV resolution. Rigorous dissection of the CTL repertoire in one chimpanzee resolver revealed at least nine distinct targets; one target defined as a specific viral peptide presented by an individual MHC class I molecule. In that individual, every class I molecule (like humans, chimpanzees can possess six) engaged CTL with peptides derived from most of the ten HCV proteins. The plasticity of this response was striking and suggested that plasticity might indeed be key in allowing the immune response to successfully confront the spectrum of viral variants.

In chronic infection, CTL seem to emerge sequentially but not in concert: a frugal property that seems unable to eradicate HCV, perhaps due, at least in part, to evolving quasispecies diversity. In chronic HCV infection, CTL select for viruses that have lost their target epitopes.[63] Because viruses possessing such mutated epitopes avoid immune responses, they emerge to detectable and perhaps dominant frequency, a phenomenon that can occur in weeks. CTL, however, endure as memory cells despite epitope loss.[58, 63] Therefore, the number of CTL identifiable at a given point in chronic infection might overestimate the number that are functional. Additionally, it is worth noting that when examined in bulk (not as individual clones), CTL responses tend to wane following HCV resolution but gradually expand in persistent infection.[6, 33] Therefore, examination of CTL beyond the acute phase could deceive the observer, revealing either no quantitative difference between chronics and resolvers or even an apparently broader CTL response in chronically infected individuals.

Subsequent studies in human resolvers similarly supported a role for multispecific CTL responses in HCV resolution.[6, 45, 46, 56, 57] For example, Grüner et al compared virus-specific CD8+ T cell responses in patients with self-limited versus chronic infection and found significant correlation between HCV clearance and the appearance of virus-specific CD8+ T cells in the first 6 months of infection.[47] Taken together, these chimpanzee and human studies suggest an inverse relationship between the extent of the CTL response in early infection (which may have qualitative and quantitative components) and the likelihood of viral persistence.

Factors underpinning differences in the strength and polarity of T cell responses during early HCV infection are under intense investigation. It appears that Th1-type cellular immune responses are essential for resolution of acute hepatitis C. Why so few hosts generate sufficiently potent Th1 responses is unknown and understanding this phenomenon is likely to be crucial for developing an effective *vaccine*.

T Cell Memory Following HCV Infection

Fundamentally, the effectiveness of a T cell vaccine will depend upon efficient induction and maintenance of an adequate repertoire of HCV-specific memory cells. Given that the principal site of HCV replication and probably antigen presentation is the liver cell, this may require (or at least benefit from) preferential memory cell induction and/or maintenance in the liver. This could be problematic because the liver is a site where T cells can be tolerized[64] or removed[65], properties that perhaps contribute to viral persistence.

Several studies have examined multiply HCV-exposed but seemingly uninfected individuals and found apparent HCV-specific CD4+ and CD8+ T cell responses following stimulation with HCV protein antigens.[60, 61] Although this suggested the possibility that HCV-specific T cells could endure following subclinical exposure, concern existed that such T cells may have been low affinity, cross-reactive cells rather than true HCV-specific memory cells that could respond to naturally processed antigens. CTL characterized from liver biopsies of chimpanzees studied during and after acute self-limited infection confirmed that HCV-specific memory cells could endure for at least 18 months.[33] The latter study hinted that memory CD8+ T cells might reside preferentially in liver tissue. More recently, HCV-specific memory CD8+ T cells have also been shown to endure in humans who clear the virus.[6, 75] Persistence of HCV-specific memory CD8+ T cells following self-limited infection suggests that virus-specific CD4+ T cells similarly persist.

Antibody-Mediated Immunity

In hepatitis B virus (HBV) infection, the capacity for antibodies to neutralize the virus is clear. But a role for antibodies in protection against HCV infection has been difficult to prove. The first detectable antibody responses against HCV antigens usually target the NS3 and core proteins (see Figure 1). Later, antibodies against NS4 and envelope proteins E1 and E2 develop. With continued presence of virus, antibody responses typically broaden further such that chronically infected hosts display antibodies against multiple viral epitopes.[30] In contrast, viral suppression or clearance is accompanied by reduction in (or even failure to generate) specific antibodies both in humans and chimpanzees.[31-33]

While antibodies appear to select HCV envelope protein variants,[19, 22, 23] clear evidence that antibodies protect against natural infection remains elusive. For example, a recent report of successful antibody responses during early infection described similar responses in a substantial proportion of patients who failed to clear virus.[35] And in HCV-challenged chimpanzees, Bassett et al showed that viral clearance was not associated with anti-E1 or anti-E2 antibodies[32]; indeed, antibody to E2 was observed only in viremic chimpanzees. Similar findings were reported in a group of Irish women who received HCV-contaminated anti-Rhesus D *immunoglobulin*.[36] In the latter study, anti-E2 antibody was found in all viremic women but in only about 60% of women who had cleared HCV RNA.

Another approach has been to study the influence of high titer HCV antibodies induced before or co-inoculated at the time of viral challenge. Using HCV *immune globulin*, Krawczynski et al showed hepatitis is delayed but not prevented.[37] On the other hand, Farci et al reported the ability to prevent hepatitis C in chimpanzees if the inoculum was first incubated with hyperimmune serum.[38] And at Chiron Corporation, Choo et al reported prevention of chronic infection in five out of seven chimpanzees when high titer anti-envelope antibodies were raised against homologous virus (i.e., the strain against which the antibodies were raised).[39]

These experiments suggested that high titer antibodies directed against certain structural antigens, especially envelope hypervariable regions (HVR), might at least modulate or even potentially protect against HCV infection. This was further supported by a retrospective study of 23 German women who had been infected, like their Irish counterparts, by HCV-contaminated anti-D globulin.[40] In the German study, Zibert et al found that antibodies against a 16 amino acid stretch of the second envelope protein were more frequent among 12 resolvers than among 11 women with chronic infection. The potential pitfalls of retrospective analysis notwithstanding, these data suggest that such antibodies may have played a role in resolution. Hence, finding the right recombinant HCV protein, and the best *adjuvant* for elicitation of protective antibodies, remains the Holy Grail for some vaccine researchers.

However, there are important caveats. Conclusive evidence that antibodies reliably afford protection is still lacking, particularly against different HCV strains, and putatively protective antibody titers may yet prove difficult to sustain. Of particular interest are studies of hepatitis C outcomes in antibody-deficient patients. Although numbers are limited, it is notable that spontaneous clearance has been reported in children who have congenital antibody deficiency[41-43], providing strong evidence that control of HCV can occur independently of antibodies. Indeed, it is notable that when data from these small studies are combined, disease termination occurred in approximately 15% of antibody-deficient children, a proportion tantalizingly similar to that anticipated in the general population. So while antibodies appear to exert selective pressure upon HCV, the ability to terminate infection remains uncertain, particularly against different strains and genotypes.

Cryoglobulins: Antibodies That Can Cause Harm

In up to 50% of people, HCV infection is associated with the presence of antibodies that bind to each other and precipitate out of solution when cooled below body temperature. These are called *cryoglobulins*. When these antibodies deposit in small blood vessels, inflammation and blockage can occur (a condition called *vasculitis*) and give rise to related damage and *clinical* syndromes. Vasculitic damage is most commonly apparent in the skin and kidney. However, many people (up to 2/3) who have these antibodies do not develop overt disease. The antibody precipitates usually contain *anti-HCV antibody*, HCV RNA, and IgM rheumatoid factor (an anti-IgG *autoantibody)*. In many cases successful treatment of HCV with pegylated interferon and ribavirin clears the cryoglobulins.

Summary

The human immune system is both elegantly efficient and sometimes maddeningly complex. The capacity of the small, single-stranded RNA virus that is the hepatitis C virus to evade the robust redundant abilities of immune system is the focus of much ongoing basic and applied laboratory research. The information presented in this chapter has been intellectually challenging, but it is hoped that it inspires excitement and hope.

References

1. Orland JR, Wright TL, Cooper SL. Acute hepatitis C. *Hepatology.* 2001;33:321.
2. Choo Q-L, Kuo G, Weiner AJ, Overby LR, Bradley DW, and Houghton M. Isolation of a cDNA clone derived from blood-borne non-A, non-B viral hepatitis genome. *Science.* 1989;244:359.
3. Bartenschlager R, Lohmann V. Replication of hepatitis C virus. *J Gen Virol.* 2000;81:1631.
4. Simmonds P. Genetic diversity and evolution of hepatitis C virus--15 years on. *J Gen Virol.* 2004;85:3173.
5. Martell M, Esteban JI, Quer J *et al.* Hepatitis C virus (HCV) circulates as a population of different but closely related genomes: quasispecies nature of HCV genome distribution. *J Virol.* 1992;66:3225.
6. Weiner A, Erickson A, Kansopon J *et al.* Persistent hepatitis C virus infection in a chimpanzee is associated with emergence of a cytotoxic T lymphocyte escape variant. *Proc Natl Acad Sci USA.* 1995;92:2755.
7. Erickson AL, Kimura Y, Igarashi S *et al.* The outcome of hepatitis C virus infection is predicted by escape mutations in epitopes targeted by cytotoxic T lymphocytes. *Immunity.* 2001;15:883.
8. Hepburn, MJ, Hepburn LM, Cantu NS, Lapeer MG, Lawitz EJ. Differences in treatment outcome for hepatitis C among ethnic groups. *Am J Med* 2004;117:163.
9. Large MK, Kittlesen DJ, Hahn YS. Suppression of host immune response by the core protein of hepatitis C virus: possible implications for hepatitis C virus persistence. *J Immunol* 1999;162:931.
10. Gale M, Kwieciszewski B.Jr, Dossett M, Nakao H, Katze MG. Antiapoptotic and oncogenic potentials of hepatitis C virus are linked to interferon resistance by viral repression of the PKR protein kinase. *J Virol* 1999;73:6506.
11. Chen CM, You LR, Hwang LH, Lee YH. Direct interaction of hepatitis C virus core protein with the cellular lymphotoxin-beta receptor modulates the signal pathway of the lymphotoxin-beta receptor. *Journal of Virology* 1997;71:9417.
12. Taylor DR, Shi ST, Romano PR, Barber GN, Lai MM. Inhibition of the interferon-inducible protein kinase PKR by HCV E2 protein. *Science* 1999;285:107.
13. Bartenschlager R, Frese M, Pietschmann T. Novel insights into hepatitis C virus replication and persistence. *Adv Virus Res* 2004;63:71.
14. Nishioka Y, Nishimura N, Suzuki Y, Sone S. Human monocyte-derived and CD83(+) blood dendritic cells enhance natural killer cell-mediated cytotoxicity. *Eur J Immunol* 2001;31:2633.
15. Gerosa F, Baldani-Guerra B, Nisii C, Marchesini V, Carra G, Trinchieri G. Reciprocal activating interaction between natural killer cells and dendritic cells. *J Exp Med* 2002;195:327.
16. Ferlazzo G, Tsang ML, Moretta L, Melioli G, Steinman RM, Munz C. Human dendritic cells activate resting natural killer (natural killer) cells and are recognized via the natural killerp30 receptor by activated natural killer cells. *J Exp Med* 2002;195:343.
17. Fernandez NC, Lozier A, Flament C, et al. Dendritic cells directly trigger natural killer cell functions: cross-talk relevant in innate anti-tumor immune responses in vivo. *Nat Med* 1999;5:405.
18. Andrews DM, Andoniou CE, Scalzo AA, et al. Cross-talk between dendritic cells and natural killer cells in viral infection. *Mol Immunol* 2005;42:547.
19. Steinman RM, Cohn ZA. Identification of a novel cell type in peripheral lymphoid organs of mice. I. Morphology, quantitation, tissue distribution. *J Exp Med* 1973;137:1142.
20. de Jong EC, Smits HH, Kapsenberg ML. Dendritic cell-mediated T cell polarization. *Springer Semin Immunopathol* 2005;26:289.
21. Barth H, Ulsenheimer A, Pape GR, et al. Uptake and presentation of hepatitis C virus-like particles by human dendritic cells. *Blood.* 2005
22. Colonna M, Trinchieri G, Liu YJ. Plasmacytoid dendritic cells in immunity. *Nat Immunol* 2004;5:1219.
23. Goutagny N, Fatmi A, De Ledinghen V, et al. Evidence of viral replication in circulating dendritic cells during hepatitis C virus infection. *J Infect Dis* 2003;187:1951.
24. Underhill DM, Ozinsky A. Toll-like receptors: key mediators of microbe detection. *Curr Opin Immunol* 2002;14:103.
25. Heil F, Hemmi H, Hochrein H, et al. Species-specific recognition of single-stranded RNA via toll-like receptor 7 and 8. *Science* 2004;303:1526.
26. Blalock JE. The immune system as the sixth sense. *J Intern Med* 2005;257:126.
27. Liu YJ. IPC: Professional Type 1 Interferon-Producing Cells and Plasmacytoid Dendritic Cell Precursors. *Annu Rev Immunol.* 2004
28. Siavoshian S, Abraham JD, Thumann C, Paule Kieny M, Schuster C. Hepatitis C virus core, NS3, NS5A, NS5B proteins induce apoptosis in mature dendritic cells. *J Med Virol* 2005;75:402.
29. Kanto T, Inoue M, Miyatake H, et al. Reduced numbers and impaired ability of myeloid and plasmacytoid dendritic cells to polarize T helper cells in chronic hepatitis C virus infection. *J Infect Dis* 2004;190:1919.
30. Moretta A. Natural killer cells and dendritic cells: rendezvous in abused tissues. *Nat Rev Immunol* 2002;2:957.
31. Lanier LL. Natural killer Cell Recognition. *Annu Rev Immunol.* 2004
32. Stetson DB, Mohrs M, Reinhardt RL, et al. Constitutive cytokine mRNAs mark natural killer (natural killer) and natural killer T cells poised for rapid effector function. *J Exp Med* 2003;198:1069.

33. Ehrlich P: On immunity with special reference to cell life, Croonian Lecture, 1900. In: F. Himmelweit, ed. *The Collected Papers of Paul Ehrlich*, Vol. 2, 1957. London, Pergamon Press, p. 178.

34. Karre K, Ljunggren HG, Piontek G, Kiessling R. Selective rejection of H-2-deficient lymphoma variants suggests alternative immune defence strategy. *Nature* 1986;319:675.

35. Khakoo SI, Thio CL, Martin MP, et al. HLA and natural killer cell inhibitory receptor genes in resolving hepatitis C virus infection. *Science* 2004;305:872.

36. Bjorkman PJ, Parham P. Structure, Function and Diversity of Class I Major Histocompatibility Complex Molecules. *Annu Rev Biochem* 1990;59:253.

37. Zinkernagel RM, Doherty PC. Immunological surveillance against altered self components by sensitized T lymphocytes in lymphocytic choriomeningitis. *Nature* 1974;251:547.

38. Zinkernagel RM, Doherty PC. MHC-restricted cytotoxic T cells: studies on the biological role of polymorphic major transplantation antigens determining T cell restriction-specificity, function and responsiveness. *Adv Immunol* 1979:27:51.

39. Parham P. Immunology. Deconstructing the MHC. *Nature* 1992;360:300.

40. Bakker AB, Phillips JH, Figdor CG, Lanier LL. Killer cell inhibitory receptors for MHC class I molecules regulate lysis of melanoma cells mediated by natural killer cells, gamma delta T cells, and antigen-specific CTL. *J Immunol 1998*;160:5239.

41. Pileri P, Uematsu Y, Campagnoli S, et al. Binding of hepatitis C virus to CD81. *Science* 1998;282:938.

42. Crotta S, Stilla A, Wack A, et al. Inhibition of natural killer cells through engagement of CD81 by the major hepatitis C virus envelope protein. *J Exp Med* 2002;195:35.

43. Heim MH, Moradpour D, Blum HE. Expression of hepatitis C virus proteins inhibits signal transduction through the Jak-STAT pathway. *J Virol* 1999;73:8469.

44. de Lucas S, Bartolome J, Carreno V. Hepatitis C virus core protein down-regulates transcription of interferon-induced antiviral genes. *J Infect Dis* 2005;191:93.

45. Melen K, Fagerlund R, Nyqvist M, Keskinen P, Julkunen I. Expression of hepatitis C virus core protein inhibits interferon-induced nuclear import of STATs. *J Med Virol* 2004;73:536.

46. Diepolder H, Zachoval R, Hoffmann R, et al. Possible mechanism involving T-lymphocyte response to non-structural protein 3 in viral clearance in acute hepatitis C virus infection. *Lancet* 1995;346:1006.

47. Cucchiarini M, Kammer AR, Grabscheid B, et al. Vigorous peripheral blood cytotoxic T cell response during the acute phase of hepatitis C virus infection. *Cell Immunol* 2000;203:111.

48. Gruner NH, Gerlach TJ, Jung MC, et al. Association of Hepatitis C Virus-Specific CD8+ T Cells with Viral Clearance in Acute Hepatitis C. *J Infect Dis* 2000;181:1528.

49. Missale G, Bertoni R, Lamonaca V, et al. Different clinical behaviors of acute hepatitis C infection are associated with different vigor of the anti-viral cell-mediated immune response. *J Clin Invest* 1996;98:706.

50. Tsai SL, Liaw YF, Chen MH, Huang CY, Kuo GC. Detection of type 2-like T-helper cells in hepatitis C virus infection: implications for hepatitis C virus chronicity. *Hepatology* 1997;25:449.

51. Diepolder HM, Scholz S, Pape GR. Influence of HLA alleles on outcome of hepatitis C virus infection [comment]. *Lancet* 1999;354:2094.

52. Sakaguchi S, Sakaguchi N, Asano M, Itoh M, Toda M. Immunologic self-tolerance maintained by activated T cells expressing IL-2 receptor alpha-chains (CD25). Breakdown of a single mechanism of self-tolerance causes various autoimmune diseases. *J Immunol* 1995;155:1151.

53. Asano M, Toda M, Sakaguchi N, Sakaguchi S. Autoimmune disease as a consequence of developmental abnormality of a T cell subpopulation. *J Exp Med* 1996;184:387.

54. Suri-Payer E, Amar AZ, Thornton AM, Shevach EM. CD4+CD25+ T cells inhibit both the induction and effector function of autoreactive T cells and represent a unique lineage of immunoregulatory cells. *J Immunol* 1998;160:1212.

55. Hesse M, Piccirillo CA, Belkaid Y, et al. The pathogenesis of schistosomiasis is controlled by cooperating IL-10-producing innate effector and regulatory T cells. *J Immunol* 2004;172:3157.

56. Belkaid Y, Piccirillo CA, Mendez S, Shevach EM, Sacks DL. CD4+CD25+ regulatory T cells control Leishmania major persistence and immunity. *Nature* 2002;420:502.

57. Guidotti LG, Rochford R, Chung J, Shapiro M, Purcell R, Chisari FV. Viral clearance without destruction of infected cells during acute HBV infection. *Science* 1999;284:825.

58. Cooper SL, Erickson AL, Adams EJ, et al. Analysis of a Successful Immune Response against Hepatitis C Virus. *Immunity* 1999;10:439.

59. Cooper SL, Adams EJ, Wells RS, Walker CM, Parham P. A Major Histocompatibility Complex Class I Allele Shared By Two Species Of Chimpanzee. *Immunogenetics* 1998;47:212.

60. Lawlor D A, Warren E, Ward FE, Parham P. Comparison of MHC Alleles in Humans and Apes. *Immunological Reviews* 1990;113:147.

61. Bontrop RE, Otting N, Slierendregt BL, Lanchbury JS. Evolution of Major Histocompatibility Complex Polymorphisms and T-Cell Receptor Diversity in Primates. *Immunological Reviews* 1995;143:33.

62. Jaeger EE, Bontrop RE, Lanchbury JS. Structure, diversity, and evolution of the T-cell receptor VB gene repertoire in primates. *Immunogenetics* 1994;40:184.

63. Houghton M, Choo Q-L, Kuo G, et al. Prospects for prophylactic and therapeutic hepatitis C virus vaccines. *Princess Takamatsu Symp* 1995;25:237.

64. Qian S, Lu L, Fu F, et al. Apoptosis Within Spontaneously Accepted Mouse Liver Allografts. *J Immunol* 1997;158:4654.

65. Nuti S, Rosa D, Valiante NM, et al. Dynamics of intra-hepatic lymphocytes in chronic hepatitis C: enrichment for Valpha24+ T cells and rapid elimination of effector cells by apoptosis. *Eur J Immunol* 1998;28:3448.

WESTERN (ALLOPATHIC) MEDICINE

Douglas R. LaBrecque, MD

SECTION

1

ALLOPATHIC HEPATITIS C TREATMENT OVERVIEW

Introduction

The majority of people in the United States receive most of their healthcare from medical doctors (MDs) or doctors of osteopathy (DOs). MDs practice "allopathic" medicine, the most common form of healthcare in the United States and the western world. Allopathic medicine is more commonly called western medicine. When selecting your own approach to maintaining health and treating disease, it is important to understand the basic concepts and philosophy that underlie the western medical approach to treating *hepatitis C*.

The Principles of Western Treatments for Hepatitis C

Three basic concepts guide the western medical approach to the treatment of hepatitis C.

- to understand and eliminate the cause of the disease (the virus)

- to treat the disease with medicines that have been shown to be effective against the virus in controlled, scientific studies and have been approved by the U.S. Food and Drug Administration (FDA)

- to improve the health and well-being of those with hepatitis C by relieving their *symptoms*, even if the virus is resistant to therapy

Understanding and Eliminating the Cause of Disease

Allopathic medicine is based on an understanding of the causes of disease and eliminating those causes. The hepatitis C virus (*HCV*) is understood to be the cause of *chronic hepatitis* C and the symptoms that result. Many studies have shown that eliminating HCV from the body prevents the disease from progressing further.[1-11] Both short- and long-term improvements in liver health and quality of life are associated with having undetectable levels of HCV in the blood.[1, 12-16] An undetectable level of virus is also associated with decreasing the rate of progression to *liver failure* and/or *liver cancer*.[15-25]

Hepatitis C can be cured. At least 95% of people in whom the virus has been eliminated continue to have undetectable virus, normal *liver function tests*, and improved health 5 to 15 years after treatment.[26–30] The primary goal in attempting to improve the health and well-being of those with hepatitis C is elimination of the virus.

Treating Hepatitis C with Effective, FDA-Approved Medicines

Western physicians make decisions about which treatment will be most helpful to their hepatitis C patients based on controlled, scientific studies. This approach is known as evidence-based medicine. The studies used to gather evidence about what is and is not effective are called *clinical trials*.

In clinical trials, a new drug or treatment is compared to a *placebo* (an inactive pill or treatment) or to the best currently available therapy. These trials are conducted to avoid the possibility of misinterpreting a patient's improvement as resulting from a particular treatment when it was actually due to the natural course of the disease, spontaneous improvement, or coincidence.

Most western doctors have had the experience of a new drug or therapy producing almost miraculous results in one person, only to find it to be a total disappointment in many other people. While it is possible that the treatment was the cause of the improvement in these cases, it is more likely that the improvement would have occurred without any therapy. The apparent benefit was a coincidence of timing, that is, the treatment was started just before the person was about to improve on his or her own. Even if the treatment did improve the health of one person, without scientific studies, we have no way to separate those people who might benefit from the treatment from the many others who will not benefit or may even be harmed by the treatment.

> **In western medicine, new treatments are tested in special studies called clinical trials to determine if there is scientific evidence showing treatment benefits for patients.**

Regardless of who recommends them, we strongly advise our patients to be wary of therapies for which fantastic claims are made if there is no scientific evidence to support the claims. If such treatments were clinically effective, many healthcare providers would gladly recommend them. There is a saying in western medicine that states, "The degree of enthusiasm for a treatment is inversely proportional to the degree to which it has been studied." In other words, once new treatments have been studied in a controlled, scientific way, many initially exciting new approaches prove to be ineffective or no better than safer, less expensive therapies. American consumers are being told of such situations with increasing frequency by the national media.

The Placebo Effect

The *placebo* effect (so-called "mind over matter") is well documented. A person who strongly believes that a particular treatment will make him or her feel better often does feel better, even if an inactive placebo is used.[31, 32] The placebo effect has many therapeutic implications. Researchers are actively exploring the complexes relationships between the mind and the body in illness and healing (see *Chapter 13, Mind-Body Medicine and Spiritual Healing*). The strength of placebo effect is one of the fundamental reasons western doctors insist on specifically measurable results and carefully controlled trials when evaluating a new therapy. In these clinical trials, neither the participants nor their doctors know who is taking placebo and who is taking active drug. This is done to eliminate even unintentional bias on the part of the participants or the healthcare providers.

Natural Versus Manufactured Drugs

Western doctors consider any compound that is ingested to improve health or fight disease to be a drug. The distinction between so-called natural compounds and those that are manufactured is often an artificial one.

Many manufactured drugs are derived from natural sources by taking extracts from plants, living organisms, or other naturally occurring materials. Other manufactured drugs are exact copies of naturally occurring compounds. For example, the drug alfa *interferon*, the basis of all current western therapies for HCV, is a copy of the alfa interferon the human body manufactures to combat viruses. The flu-like side effects of *interferon-based therapy* are not surprising when you realize that the same symptoms occur when the body releases its own interferons to combat a viral infection.

Any manufactured drug can have uncomfortable, even sometimes dangerous, side effects. The same holds true for natural drugs. Western doctors consider it wise to regard anything we take into our bodies as potentially dangerous. They look for evidence-based proof not only that a drug is effective, but also that it has been adequately studied to be certain that it is not harmful. The FDA requires documentation of both safety and usefulness for each newly approved drug. However, the FDA does not evaluate or regulate natural additives, herbal therapies, or dietary supplements. Therefore, you must read the advertisements for such products carefully. The phrase, "meets all FDA guidelines" does not mean a substance is FDA approved. In fact, the FDA has no guidelines for the use of natural additives, herbal therapies, or dietary supplements. Do not be fooled by slick advertising, whether it is for an FDA approved treatment, an herbal remedy, or any other product.

Goals of Western Treatment for Hepatitis C

The goal of western treatment for people infected with HCV is to eliminate the virus so that:

- progression of the disease to *cirrhosis*, liver failure, and/or liver cancer (*hepatocellular carcinoma*) are prevented

- symptoms of hepatitis C infection are reduced or eliminated

- quality of life is preserved and/or improved.

- Defining Successful Western Therapy

- Defining "success" in the western treatment of chronic hepatitis C is an outgrowth of the goals stated above. Treatment is considered successful if:

- ALT levels are below 30 IU/mL

- HCV *viral load* is undetectable using the most sensitive *PCR* test

- there is no progression of *inflammation* and/or *fibrosis* on *liver biopsy*

Approximately 50% to 60% of people treated with current western therapy (*pegylated interferon* plus *ribavirin*) achieve sustained hepatitis C *viral clearance*.[9-11, 33, 34] While interferon-based therapy is not always successful in ridding the body of HCV, several studies have shown that these therapies can still benefit most patients by slowing disease progression, reducing the risk of liver cancer, and reducing liver cell *necrosis*, inflammation, and fibrosis.[5, 26, 15-18, 35-38] Virtually none of the severe, life-threatening complications of hepatitis C occur until a person develops cirrhosis. Therefore, preventing progression to cirrhosis is critical, even if the virus cannot be eliminated.

Interferon has been shown to decrease the activation of *stellate cells* (the cells that produce fibrosis or scarring in the liver) in laboratory experiments[39, 40] and in human studies.[41] This effect occurs even when interferon fails to decrease the amount of circulating virus. Interferon also reduces liver cell necrosis and inflammation.

Summary

The two basic tenants of western medicine regarding the treatment of hepatitis C are:

- to determine the cause disease

- to eliminate that cause of disease

The goal of western medical doctors in treating people with hepatitis C is to eliminate the virus in order to stop disease progression, relieve the symptoms associated with the disease, prevent the spread of the infection outside the liver, and improve quality of life.

With recent advances in the treatment of chronic hepatitis C, many people are candidates for treatment. If you have elevated ALT levels, other conditions related to your HCV infection, a detectable viral load, and/or chronic inflammation on liver biopsy, you might be a candidate for therapy.

Hepatitis C is a curable disease. At least 95% of people in whom HCV has been eliminated using interferon-based therapy continue to have undetectable virus levels 5 to 15 years after the conclusion of treatment.

References

1. Bonkovsky HL, Woolley JM. Reduction of health-related quality of life in chronic hepatitis C and improvement with interferon therapy. The Consensus Interferon Study Group. *Hepatology*. 1999;29(1):264-270.
2. McHutchison JG, Gordon SC, Schiff ER, et al. Interferon alfa-2b alone or in combination with ribavirin as initial treatment for chronic hepatitis C. Hepatitis Interventional Therapy Group. *N Engl J Med*. 1998;339(21):1485-1492.
3. EASL: International Consensus Conference on Hepatitis C Consensus Statement. *J Hepatol*. 1999;30(5):956-961.

4.   Schalm SW, Weiland O, Hansen B, et al. Interferon-ribavirin for chronic hepatitis C with and without cirrhosis: analysis of individual patient data of six controlled trials. Eurohep Study Group for Viral Hepatitis. *Gastroenterology*. 1999;117(2):408-413.

5.   Zeuzem S, Feinman SV, Rasenack J, et al. Peginterferon alfa-2a in patients with chronic hepatitis C. *N Engl J Med*. 2000;343(23):1666-1672.

6.   Heathcote EJ, Shiffman ML, Cooksley WG, et al. Peginterferon alfa-2a in patients with chronic hepatitis C and cirrhosis. *N Engl J Med*. 2000;343(23):1673-1680.

7.   Serfaty L, Aumaitre H, Chazouilleres O, et al. Determinants of outcome of compensated hepatitis C virus-related cirrhosis. *Hepatology*. 1998;27(5):1435-1440.

8.   Giannini E, Fasoli A, Botta F, et al. Long-term follow up of chronic hepatitis C patients after alfa-interferon treatment: a functional study. *J Gastroenterol Hepatol*. 2001;16(4):399-405.

9.   Manns MP, McHutchison JG, Gordon SC, et al. Peginterferon alfa-2b plus ribavirin compared with interferon alfa-2b plus ribavirin for initial treatment of chronic hepatitis C: a randomised trial. *Lancet*. 2001;358(9286):958-65.

10.   Fried MW, Shiffman ML, Reddy KR, et al. Peginterferon alfa-2a plus ribavirin for chronic hepatitis C virus infection. *N Engl J Med*. 2002;347(13):975-82.

11.   Hadziyannis SJ, Sette H Jr, Morgan TR, et al. Peginterferon-alfa2a and ribavirin combination therapy in chronic hepatitis C: a randomized study of treatment duration and ribavirin dose. *Ann Intern Med*. 2004;140(5):346-55.

12.   Foster GR, Goldin RD, Thomas HC. Chronic hepatitis C virus infection causes a significant reduction in quality of life in the absence of cirrhosis. *Hepatology*. 1998;27(1):209-212.

13.   Rodger AJ, Jolley D, Thompson SC, et al. The impact of diagnosis of hepatitis C virus on quality of life. Hepatology. 1999;30(5):1299-1301.

14.   Ware JE, Jr., Bayliss MS, Mannocchia M, Davis GL. Health-related quality of life in chronic hepatitis C: impact of disease and treatment response. The Interventional Therapy Group. *Hepatology*. 1999;30(2):550-555.

15.   Yu ML, Lin SM, Chuang WL, et al. A sustained virological response to interferon or interferon/ribavirin reduces hepatocellular carcinoma and improves survival in chronic hepatitis C: a nationwide, multicentre study in Taiwan. *Antivir Ther*. 2006;11(8):985-94.

16.   Arase Y, Ikeda K, Suzuki F, et al. Long-term outcome after interferon therapy in elderly patients with chronic hepatitis C. *Intervirology*. 2007;50(1):16-23.

17.   Ikeda K, Kobayashi M, Saitoh S, et al. Recurrence rate and prognosis of patients with hepatocellular carcinoma that developed after elimination of hepatitis C virus RNA by interferon therapy. A closed cohort study including matched control patients. *Oncology*. 2003;65(3):204-10.

18.   Toccaceli F, Laghi V, Capurso L, et al. Long-term liver histology improvement in patients with chronic hepatitis C and sustained response to interferon. *J Viral Hepat*. 2003 Mar;10(2):126-33.

19.   Nishiguchi S, Kuroki T, Nakatani S, et al. Randomized trial of effects of interferon-alfa on incidence of hepatocellular carcinoma in chronic active hepatitis C with cirrhosis. *Lancet*. 1995;346(8982):1051-1055.

20.   Fattovich G, Giustina G, Degos F, et al. Effectiveness of interferon-alfa on incidence of hepatocellular carcinoma and decompensation in cirrhosis type C. European Concerted Action on Viral Hepatitis (EUROHEP). *J Hepatol*. 1997;27(1):201-205.

21.   Fattovich G, Giustina G, Degos F, et al. Morbidity and mortality in compensated cirrhosis type C: a retrospective follow-up study of 384 patients. *Gastroenterology*. 1997;112(2):463-472.

22.   Mazzella G, Accogli E, Sottili S, et al. Alfa-interferon treatment may prevent hepatocellular carcinoma in HCV- related liver cirrhosis. *J Hepatol*. 1996;24(2):141-147.

23.   Camma C, Giunta M, Andreone P, Craxi A. Interferon and prevention of hepatocellular carcinoma in viral cirrhosis: an evidence-based approach. *J Hepatol*. 2001;34(4):593-602.

24.   Baffis V, Shrier I, Sherker AH, Szilagyi A. Use of interferon for prevention of hepatocellular carcinoma in cirrhotic patients with hepatitis B or hepatitis C virus infection. *Ann Intern Med*. 1999;131(9):696-701.

25.   Ikeda K, Saitoh S, Kobayashi M, et al. Long-term interferon therapy for 1 year or longer reduces the hepatocellular carcinogenesis rate in patients with liver cirrhosis caused by hepatitis C virus: a pilot study. *J Gastroenterol Hepatol*. 2001;16(4):406-415.

26.   Marcellin P, Boyer N, Gervais A, et al. Long-term histologic improvement and loss of detectable intrahepatic HCV RNA in patients with chronic hepatitis C and sustained response to interferon-alfa therapy. *Ann Intern Med*. 1997;127(10):875-881.

27.   Lau DT, Kleiner DE, Ghany MG, Park Y, Schmid P, Hoofnagle JH. 10 year follow-up after interferon-alfa therapy for chronic hepatitis C. *Hepatology*. 1998 Oct;28(4):1121-1127.

28.   Veldt BJ, Heathcote EJ, Wedemeyer H, et al. Sustained virologic response and clinical outcomes in patients with chronic hepatitis C and advanced fibrosis. *Ann Intern Med*. 2007 Nov 20;147(10):677-84.

29.   Chavalitdhamrong D, Tanwandee T. World J Long-term outcomes of chronic hepatitis C patients with sustained virological response at 6 months after the end of treatment. *Gastroenterol*. 2006 Sep 14;12(34):5532-5.

30.   Swain,M. G. Lai, M. Shiffman, M. L. et al. Sustained Virologic Response (SVR) Resulting From Treatment with Peginterferon Alfa-2a (40KD) (PEGASYS®) Alone or in Combination with Ribavirin (COPEGUS®) is Durable and Constitutes a Cure: an Ongoing 5-year Follow-up Poster # 444 DDW May 2007.

31.   Bailar JC, III. The powerful placebo and the Wizard of Oz. *N Engl J Med*. 2001;344(21):1630-1632.

32.   Hrobjartsson A, Gotzsche PC. Is the placebo powerless? An analysis of clinical trials comparing placebo with no treatment. *N Engl J Med*. 2001;344(21):1594-1602.

33.   Mangia A, Minerva N, Bacca D, et al. Individualized treatment duration for hepatitis C genotype 1 patients: A randomized controlled trial. *Hepatology*. 2008 Jan;47(1):43-50.

34.   Shepherd J, Brodin H, Cave C, et al. Pegylated interferon alfa-2a and -2b in combination with ribavirin in the treatment of chronic hepatitis C: a systematic review and economic evaluation. *Health Technol Assess*. 2004 Oct;8(39):iii-iv, 1-125.

35.   Shiffman ML, Hofmann CM, Contos MJ, et al. A randomized, controlled trial of maintenance interferon therapy for patients with chronic hepatitis C virus and persistent viremia. *Gastroenterology*. 1999;117(5):1164-1172.

36.   Balart L, Lee S, Schiffman M, et al. Histologic improvement following treatment with once weekly pegylated interferon alfa-2a (Pegasys) and thrice weekly interferon alfa-2a (Roferon) in patients with chronic hepatitis C and compensated cirrhosis. *Gastroenterology*.

2000;118:A961 (abstract). [Note: This abstract is not available on the National Library of Medicine database PubMed.]

37. Poynard T, McHutchison J, Davis GL, et al. Impact of interferon alfa-2b and ribavirin on progression of liver fibrosis in patients with chronic hepatitis C. *Hepatology*. 2000;32(5):1131-1137.

38. Poynard T, Ratziu V, Benmanov Y, et al.. Fibrosis in patients with chronic hepatitis C: detection and significance. *Semin Liver Dis*. 2000;20(1):47-55.

39. Muriel P. Alfa-interferon prevents liver collagen deposition and damage induced by prolonged bile duct obstruction in the rat. *J Hepatol*. 1996;24(5):614-621.

40. Fort J, Pilette C, Veal N, et al. Effects of long-term administration of interferon alfa in two models of liver fibrosis in rats. *J Hepatol*. 1998;29(2):263-270.

41. Reeves HL, Dack CL, Peak M, Burt AD, Day CP. Stress-activated protein kinases in the activation of rat hepatic stellate cells in culture. *J Hepatol*. 2000 Mar;32(3):465-72.

WESTERN (ALLOPATHIC) MEDICINE

Douglas R. LaBrecque, MD

INITIAL TREATMENT OPTIONS

Introduction

It has only been possible to diagnose *hepatitis C* since 1990. However, great progress has been made in the treatment of hepatitis C in this short period. Currently, all western therapy for hepatitis C is based on the use of alfa *interferons*. However, alfa interferons alone (*monotherapy*) provided only limited success. The allopathic standard of care as of this writing (April 2008) is *combination therapy* with *pegylated interferon* plus *ribavirin*. *Hepatologists* (liver doctors) generally agree that it is no longer advisable to treat hepatitis C with interferon alone unless the use of ribavirin is *contraindicated*.

Western Treatment: Who and Why

The discussion in this chapter is focused primarily on western treatment for *chronic hepatitis* C. A person is said to have chronic hepatitis C if he/she continues to have the virus for six or more months after the time of initial infection. (Note: A brief discussion on the treatment of *acute hepatitis* C appears later in this chapter section.)

This section discusses the treatment options available to those with chronic hepatitis C who have not previously received interferon-based therapy. The term used to describe this group of patients in western medicine is "treatment naïve." Although each person <u>must</u> be evaluated on a case-by-case basis, there are some generally accepted characteristics of persons for whom *interferon-based therapy* is widely accepted.[1] These characteristics include:

- abnormal ALT
- chronic hepatitis with significant *fibrosis* on *liver biopsy*
- no evidence of liver *decompensation*
- no absolute contraindications to treatment
- willingness to undergo and commit to the requirements of treatment

The only way to know if you are a candidate for interferon-based therapy is to talk with your doctor. The criteria listed above only give a broad view. Each person with hepatitis C is different, and only you and your doctor can determine whether interferon-based therapy is appropriate for you, taking into consideration all the unique characteristics of your personal situation.

The five major goals of western treatment for chronic hepatitis C are:

- eliminate the virus from the body
- restore normal liver function (as shown by liver-specific blood tests)
- prevent further liver damage (shown by improvement or stabilization on the liver biopsy)
- improve overall health and well-being
- produce a response to therapy (a durable or *sustained response*) that will last for the rest of the patient's life

A *sustained response* is defined as continued undetectable *HCV* in the blood 6 months after the completion of treatment. At this point, a person is considered *cured* of chronic hepatitis C.[2]

Interferon-Based Therapies

From Past to Present

Interferon *monotherapy* refers to hepatitis C treatment with interferon alone (that is, without *ribavirin*). Standard interferon was the first therapy approved by the U.S. Food and Drug Administration (FDA) for chronic hepatitis C in 1991. With overall durable response rates of 20% to 25%[3-8], *hepatologists* and patients were encouraged, but also determined to find other options that would lead to successful outcomes for a much greater proportion of those undergoing treatment. The addition of ribavirin to interferon was a big breakthrough in the western treatment of hepatitis C improving overall durable response rates to approximately 40%.[9-16] The improvement was encouraging, but insufficient.

Standard interferon is cleared from the body very quickly, within 6 to 7 hours. With thrice weekly dosing, there were long periods with no interferon circulating in the blood. This gives the virus time to recover from the effects of the interferon. The development of pegylated interferons came about from an effort to solve these problems and to keep interferon continuously circulating in the blood.[17, 18] It was hoped that a longer-acting form of interferon would provide a great improvement in the treatment success rate, and this has proven to be the case.

The attachment of polyethylene glycol (a long-chain sugar molecule known as "peg") to a protein such as interferon slows its absorption, and decreases its breakdown and *clearance* from the body. Based on this knowledge, pegylated interferons were developed and tested.[19-31] Treatment with pegylated interferon provides a relatively constant level of interferon in the blood when given only once a week. This makes it more convenient (one injection each week rather than three) and produces a continuous interferon level to combat the virus.

Landmark studies have shown that approximately 80% of people with genotypes 2 and 3 who receive pegylated interferon plus ribavirin achieve a durable response. Just under 50% of people with genotype 1 achieve a durable response with this treatment protocol.[23, 32-34] Side effects are similar to those seen with standard *combination therapy*.[22, 23, 32, 35-38]

> Pegylated interferon plus ribavirin is standard of care for chronic hepatitis C in western medicine

Combination Therapy: Pegylated Interferon Plus Ribavirin

The current treatment of choice for chronic hepatitis C among western doctors is pegylated interferon plus ribavirin. The hepatitis C treatment guidelines from the American Association for the Study of Liver Diseases include the following recommendations regarding the dose and duration of therapy (see Table 1).

Table 1. AASLD Guidelines on Pegylated Interferon Plus Ribavirin Therapy[1]

	Genotype 1	Genotype 2 or 3
Duration of Therapy	48 weeks	24 weeks
Ribavirin Dose	1000 mg for those ≤ 75 kg 1200 mg for those > 75 kg	800 mg
Early Viral Response Check	Week 12	
Sustained Viral Response Check	24 weeks after completion of therapy	

Important: Research on dosing, when to test for response to therapy, and duration of therapy is ongoing, and new studies are reported each week. Your doctor will customize your treatment protocol based on not only standard guidelines, but also the unique circumstances of your situation, and the latest medical research data.

Response to Interferon-Based Therapy

Western medicine's key measurement of successful treatment of hepatitis C is undetectable virus in the blood. Among those for whom therapy is successful, this usually occurs very early during the treatment course. If therapy fails to produce an undetectable or very low *viral load* test after 12 weeks of treatment, it is highly unlikely that the therapy will be successful.[23, 32]

Most doctors discontinue treatment if HCV is not undetectable by week 12 after the initiation of interferon-based therapy. However, the decision to continue therapy for another 12 weeks is sometimes made if the viral load has dropped by at 100-fold (for example from 1,000,000 to 10,000). It is a rare and unusual occurrence for a doctor to continue therapy for an additional 12 weeks if there is no viral response to treatment within the first 12 weeks.

If a durable response is to occur, HCV should be undetectable after 24 weeks of therapy. It is important to recognize that measurement of viral levels can vary greatly from one laboratory to another. Therefore, you should try to have the same laboratory perform your HCV viral load tests before and during your treatment.

Also, be aware that small changes in viral load are not significant. Recall that viral levels must fall at least 100-fold to be considered significant. For example, even a seemingly large drop from 800,000 to 200,000 would not be considered significant because it is not a 100-fold decrease and would not be an indication of successful therapy.

There are several different phrases your doctor may use when talking about your response to treatment. Table 2 below summarizes some of the most common of these terms.

Table 2. Terms Used to Describe Response to Therapy

Term	Definition
Rapid Viral Response (RVR)	100-fold or greater drop in HCV viral load by week 4 of treatment
Early Viral Response (EVR)	100-fold or greater drop in HCV viral load by week 12 of treatment
End of Treatment Response (ETR)	Undetectable HCV (by molecular testing) at the end of the treatment period
Sustained Viral Response (SVR)	Undetectable HCV (by molecular testing) 24 weeks after the completion of treatment
Relapse	Return of detectable HCV (by molecular testing) after a documented end of treatment response
Non-Response	Treatment fails to produce a 100-fold or greater drop in HCV viral load by week 12 of treatment

A *relapse* is defined as having no detectable virus during treatment, but the return of detectable virus after treatment ends. If the virus becomes detectable after treatment, there are usually no *symptoms* but ALT levels often rises. A relapse typically occurs within 4 to 24 weeks after completing therapy. Developing detectable virus more than 12 to 24 weeks after completing treatment is rare and occurs in less than 5% of those treated.[5, 39, 40] Relapse beyond two years after completing therapy is exceedingly rare. Retreatment for people who have a relapse is discussed in *Section 3* of this chapter.

It is notable that a recent report from a study that followed *sustained responders* for up to seven years after the successful completion of interferon-based therapy found that 99% remained free of detectable hepatitis C virus. This study, conducted at nearly 40 sites worldwide, has given both doctors and patients the news they have long awaited: **hepatitis C is a curable disease**.

The best measure of treatment success is improvement on liver biopsy. However, a follow-up liver biopsy after successful treatment is rarely performed outside of research studies. Liver biopsy is an invasive procedure with potential complications such as bleeding and infection. It is also much more costly and time-consuming to do than simple blood tests for liver enzyme levels and viral load. If the virus is undetectable and ALT levels have returned to normal, it is assumed that the biopsy will show improvement based on a large amount of information obtained from carefully controlled research studies.[41] In addition to improved liver *histology*, there is evidence that *antiviral* therapy may reduce the risk of developing hepatocellular carcinoma (*liver cancer*).[42-51]

Special Situations

Treatment of Acute HCV Infection

The initial phase of hepatitis C infection is called acute hepatitis C. This acute phase describes the first 6 months after HCV enters the body. Acute hepatitis C is rarely diagnosed because there are either no symptoms, or they are so mild that no medical care is sought.

The acute phase of hepatitis C infection is when most cases of *spontaneous clearance* occur. Spontaneous clearance refers to the *immune system* successfully getting rid of the virus without medical intervention. We do not know the true rate of spontaneous clearance of HCV. Many experts think it is in the range of 15% to 30%, but it may vary by age, gender, genotype, immune status, and other factors yet to be identified.

Because acute hepatitis C is so rarely encountered, large scale controlled trials to study its treatment have not been feasible. As a result, there is no currently approved therapy for acute hepatitis C. Nonetheless, both standard interferon monotherapy and pegylated interferon monotherapy have been reported to produced durable *viral clearance* in more than 85% of patients treated for 24 weeks.[52-54] Most experts believe that if interferon treatment is a consideration, it is advisable to wait until 8 to 12 weeks after the exposure to allow time for possible spontaneous clearance.

The role of combination therapy for the treatment of acute hepatitis C is presently unknown. *Clinical trials* must be conducted to determine if combination therapy is a valuable option to reduce the frequency of chronic hepatitis C.

Treatment of Chronic Hepatitis C with Normal Liver Enzymes

The treatment of people with chronic hepatitis C who have persistently normal liver enzyme levels is controversial. The question is one of risk versus benefit. If one believes that the majority of people with normal *liver enzymes* are (overall) not at significant risk for the development of debilitating liver disease in their lifetime, the scale tips in favor of not treating. This is because the inherent medical risks, cost, and personal toll of treatment seem unjustified in the face of a treatment that seems unlikely to benefit the patient in any substantive way. On the other hand, studies have shown that up to 10% of people with persistently normal liver enzymes have significant fibrosis on liver biopsy.[55-58] This calls into the doubt the assumption of little risk of harm just because the liver enzyme levels are normal, and begins to tip the scale back in favor of treatment.

As one might expect, this leads one back to the gold standard of liver evaluation in people living the hepatitis C: the liver biopsy. AASLD hepatitis C treatment guidelines state that, "Regardless of the *serum aminotransferase* levels, the decision to initiate therapy with interferon and ribavirin should be individualized based on the severity of liver disease by liver biopsy, the potential of serious side effects, the likelihood of response, and the presence of comorbid conditions."[1]

Research must be conducted to look at the natural course of hepatitis C disease when ALT levels remain normal. Clinical trials are also needed to determine whether combination therapy or alternative therapeutic approaches are helpful in this situation. It is hoped that a more standardized approach will be developed for defining what normal liver enzyme levels are. This should include correction for body weight or body mass, and gender.

Treatment of Chronic Hepatitis C in Patients with Cirrhosis

Overall, there is an inverse trend between the degree of fibrosis and the probability of response to interferon-based therapy. In other words, the greater the degree of fibrosis, the lower the chance for sustained viral response. Thus, it is known that people who have developed *cirrhosis* are somewhat less likely to respond to pegylated interferon plus ribavirin than those who have not. However, <u>many</u> people with cirrhosis are successfully treated even with cirrhosis.

In two studies using combined pegylated interferon plus ribavirin, 43% and 44% of patients with cirrhosis achieved a durable response. These study data demonstrate that patients with cirrhosis can and do benefit from state-of-the-art interferon-based therapy.[23, 32, 33] This holds true even for patients who have had previous unsuccessful treatment.[59]

POTENTIAL THERAPY-RELATED COMPLICATIONS FOR PATIENTS WITH CIRRHOSIS

Patients with cirrhosis require somewhat more intensive medical supervision during treatment than those without cirrhosis. People with cirrhosis have an increased risk during treatment of developing serious bacterial infections and other liver disease complications because the liver has been damaged and may not be functioning properly. People with cirrhosis also more likely to develop low *neutrophil, platelet*, or *hemoglobin* levels than someone without cirrhosis. Neutrophils are a type of white blood cell, and a low level makes you more susceptible to bacterial infections. A low platelet count makes it more difficult for your blood to clot normally, and may cause you to bleed and/or bruise easily. *Anemia* is present when the hemoglobin gets low, which can cause *fatigue*.

If you have cirrhosis and are undergoing treatment, it is very important that you tell your healthcare provider about any problems you experience. Your healthcare provider should check your blood counts frequently to identify potential problems and treat them early.

Treatment of Patients with HCV-Related Diseases Outside the Liver

HCV has been associated with a wide variety of diseases outside the liver including *cryoglobulinemia*, *lichen planus*, and *porphyria cutanea tarda*.[60, 61] All of these cause disfiguring skin problems. Cryoglobulinemia can also cause kidney, nerve, blood vessel, and other tissue damage that, in the most severe cases, may be life threatening.

If you have an *immune* complex disease, you may still be a candidate for interferon-based therapy. Successful treatment often results in not only HCV clearance, but also the resolution of HCV-related immune complex syndromes.

Treatment of Coinfection (Hepatitis B Virus or Human Immunodeficiency Virus)

HEPATITIS B VIRUS

Coinfection with HCV and the *hepatitis B* virus (*HBV*) increases your risk of developing cirrhosis and other liver complications compared to infection with either virus alone. There is no standard of care treatment recommendation for patients coinfection with both hepatitis B and hepatitis C. Treatment is individualized and is based on many factors, including which virus appears to be "dominant" in the liver disease process. A number of different therapies have been tried in clinical trials including standard interferon (with and without ribavirin), pegylated interferon (with and without ribavirin). Flares have been reported while on treatment, so close medical supervision is a must. Working with a hepatologist who has experience in the management and treatment of HBV/HCV is encouraged. In the end, you and your doctor will need to make decisions about what is best in your specific circumstance.

HUMAN IMMUNODEFICIENCY VIRUS

People infected with both HCV and the *human immunodeficiency virus* (*HIV*) have more rapidly progressive liver disease compared to people infected with HCV alone.[62-65] End-*stage* liver disease is now a leading cause of death in the HIV-positive population.[66]

As in monoinfected patients, the standard treatment choice of hepatitis C in HCV/HIV coinfected patients is combination therapy with pegylated interferon plus ribavirin. Overall, the response rate among coinfected patients are lower than among HCV-monoinfected patients.[67-69] A low *CD4 count* (less than 200), high *alcohol* consumption (more than 1.75

ounces per day), and older age at the time of HCV infection are associated with an increased rate of progression to liver fibrosis.[63, 66, 70]

If you are living with HIV and HCV, discuss your treatment options with both a liver specialist and your HIV healthcare provider. While treatment is more complex and requires more intensive medical monitoring than in HCV monoinfected individuals, successful treatment has been shown to lead to significant stabilization or regression of fibrosis.[71]
There is also evidence that even in the absence of a sustain viral response, interferon-based treatment may lead to improvements in liver histology (fibrosis).[72] See *Chapter 21, Sections 1 and 2* for additional information about western treatment of HCV/HIV coinfection.

Possible Side Effects of Combination Therapy and Successful Management

Strong medicines such as interferon and ribavirin carry with them the possibility of some side effects. Not everyone experiences side effects. In those that do, they range from barely noticeable to severe. Many of these side effects can be managed, especially if caught early. Nonetheless, side effects are unpredictable and quite variable. With severe side effects, your doctor may need to reduce the dose of your medications. In rare cases, therapy is discontinued, but this is quite uncommon.

A few thoughts to keep in mind before you read the rest of this section:

- Because "bad news travels fast" and "no news" travels nowhere, you are much more likely to hear about the worst case scenarios than you are the experiences of those who underwent treatment without any significant difficulty.

- "Attending" is a psychological term that refers to how much attention or focus we devote to something. How much we "attend" to something affects how we experience it. We attend to or don't attend to literally hundreds of different thoughts, feelings, and experiences every day. For example, if you are watching an engrossing television program at the same time you are eating your dinner, you may well find that you finish your meal without even tasting it much. That is because you were attending to the television program, and not attending to the taste of your food. The same holds true for other physical experiences. If we've heard that a certain food is likely to make people feel ill, we attend to any feelings that may arise in our gut after having eaten the food with much more attention and vigor than we normally give our gut after a meal. Similarly, if we have heard horror stories about certain medications, we are more likely to experience anything remotely related to what we've heard about with greater intensity. This is not a weakness, it's just part of being human. But we are not helpless in these situations. If we are aware of how attending affects our experiences, we can often willfully damp down the attending response. This is not to say that we should not "listen" to our bodies – of course we should! But we can listen to our bodies and also be aware of the power of our attentions on our experiences.

- Thousands of people have successfully made it through interferon-based therapy.

- The decision to undergo treatment is highly personal, and the experiences you have will be as well. A good rule of thumb is to be aware of the possibilities so that you're prepared, but to take each day as it comes.

Interferon Side Effects
Interferons all have similar side effects. The most common side effects are fever and flu-like symptoms. Other potential side effects include injection site reactions, decreased blood cell counts, hair loss, depression, and *thyroid* abnormalities. One of the most serious side effects of interferon is depression or the worsening of other psychiatric disorders. With the exception of hypothyroidism, virtually all of these side effects go away after treatment has ended. Following are brief discussions of these potential side effects of interferon therapy.

FEVER AND FLU-LIKE SYMPTOMS

Up to 66% of people taking interferon experience some form of flu-like symptoms including fever, chills, fatigue, myalgia (muscle pains), *arthralgia* (joint pains), and weight loss. These symptoms wax and wane and usually decrease after the first two or three treatments. Taking *acetaminophen* or a *nonsteroidal analgesic* (pain medicine) such as ibuprofen or naproxen 30 to 60 minutes before your dose can further reduce these symptoms. However, you should discuss using these or any other medicines with your doctor before taking them.

Most patients prefer taking their interferon in the late afternoon or early evening so that the worst side effects occur while they are asleep. However, this must be individualized as some patients feel better taking their injections early in the morning. People have also reported that drinking at least eight eight-ounce glasses of non-caffeinated or decaffeinated beverages per day markedly reduces their flu-like symptoms. Those who have tried this approach swear by the value of increasing their fluid intake. A good rule of thumb to determine how much water you should be drinking each day is to divide your weight in pounds in half, and drink that many ounces of fluid per day. For example, a 120 pound female should drink at least 60 ounces of fluid, preferably water, per day. Good indicators that you are drinking enough fluids are clear to very pale yellow urine, and having to get up at least once during the night to urinate.

DECREASED BLOOD CELL COUNTS

Mild *bone marrow suppression*, especially leukopenia (a low white cell count) and thrombocytopenia (a low platelet count) can occur with interferon-based treatment. This can be easily monitored and managed.

THYROID ABNORMALITIES

Hypothyroidism among people taking interferon is usually due to stimulation of an unsuspected *autoimmune* thyroid disorder. This side effect of treatment can occur in 3% to 5% of patients. Hypothyroidism is managed with thyroid *hormone* replacement therapy. Patients may require continued thyroid hormone replacement after treatment has ended.

INJECTION SITE REACTIONS

The development of redness and warmth with or without itchiness at the injection site is a common side effect of interferon treatment. This often does not occur until 24 to 48 hours after the injection. This is a common and does not lead to complications. However, it is important to rotate injection sites in order to avoid injecting the same spot over and over again. This is particularly true with the pegylated interferons, which are absorbed more slowly and may stay in the skin for a prolonged period. Injection site reactions can take 2 to 3 weeks to clear. It is important not to inject interferon into an area that is still red from a prior injection. Repeated injections into the same area can lead to severe skin reactions including deep skin ulcers that take many weeks or months to heal.

HAIR LOSS

Limited hair loss occurs in about 20% of patients taking interferon. When it occurs, this side effect last only during treatment.

DEPRESSION AND PSYCHIATRIC DISORDERS

Interferon can worsen existing depression (and possibly other psychiatric disorders), and can lead to new depression among people who have not previously suffered from this condition. Studies show that about 1/3 of those on interferon therapy experience depression. Suicidal thoughts or attempts occur in less than 1% of those taking interferon. It is very important to tell your healthcare provider if you have had any psychiatric counseling or have been dealing with depression before you consider treatment. If you have ever attempted or seriously considered suicide, you must tell your doctor. You should not be treated with interferon if you have recently struggled with thoughts of or have attempted suicide because interferon could intensify these thoughts and feelings. Once you and your healthcare provider are confident your depression and it is under control, you may reconsider therapy. Depression can usually be managed with counseling and/or antidepressant medications.

ANECDOTAL STORY OF SUCCESS WITH INTERFERON THERAPY DESPITE PSYCHIATRIC COMPLICATIONS

A 44-year-old female was found to have elevated liver enzymes when she donated blood in 1990. She tested positive for hepatitis C (genotype 1b) in 1992. Enzyme levels remained 1to 2 times normal until 1998 when they were noted to be 4 to 6 times above normal. The patient had abused alcohol and used multiple oral and IV drugs until 1994. She was *asymptomatic*, and her physical exam was unremarkable. She had a history of depression while actively using drugs, but no suicide attempts. A liver biopsy showed moderate activity and moderate fibrosis.

The patient was treated with pegylated interferon alfa 2b plus ribavirin for 48 weeks. Fever, decreased appetite, "weird dreams," and increased moodiness complicated the patient's therapy during the first few weeks. These symptoms resolved except for worsening mood swings. Three months into therapy, the patient was referred for psychiatric help due to decreased ability to concentrate, insomnia, excessive crying, anxiety, feelings of loss of control, and hopelessness. She was diagnosed with a mood disturbance related to interferon and started taking Xanax® and Effexor.® Because of intolerance to Effexor®, she was switched to Prozac® with occasional Xanax®. Xanax® was changed to Klonopin® to manage residual anxiety. This was later switched to Ativan® due to oversedation with the Klonopin®. The patient was also started on intensive psychotherapy to address her personal problems. She remained on Prozac® and a variety of anti-anxiety drugs throughout therapy with no more active depression. She has continued with psychotherapy since completing her hepatitis C treatment

The patient remains virus-free with normal liver enzymes for more than one year after completing therapy. Follow-up liver biopsy showed a definite decrease in activity and fibrosis.

This patient's experience demonstrates the importance of close follow-up for early recognition of the development of psychological problems. It also shows that the majority of such problems can be successfully overcome and therapy completed with the cooperation of a psychiatrist experienced in the management of interferon-related depression. This patient's experience stresses the concept that there is no simple "one drug fits all" approach to interferon-related psychiatric problems. Therapy must be individualized.

Ribavirin Side Effects

Ribavirin can lead to side effects such as cough, dyspnea (difficulty breathing), insomnia, *pruritus* (itching), rash, and reduced appetite (anorexia). These side effects are generally mild and usually do not require discontinuation of therapy or dose reduction. Most side effects go away over several weeks to months after stopping therapy.

Ribavirin can cause two serious side effects, *hemolytic anemia* and birth defects, which are discussed below.

HEMOLYTIC ANEMIA

The most serious side effect of ribavirin is hemolytic anemia, which occurs in up to 54% of patients on the medication.[33] The severity of this type of anemia depends on the amount of ribavirin you are taking. Hemolytic anemia means your *red blood cells* are breaking down at an abnormally high rate. Red blood cells are necessary to carry oxygen from your lungs to all the tissues of the body. Anemia causes a generalized feeling of tiredness as the number of red blood cells decreases. Your blood will be checked frequently during the first few months of therapy with ribavirin to test for hemolytic anemia. Your hemoglobin should be checked at 2, 4, 8, and 12 weeks after starting therapy (at a minimum). After 12 weeks of treatment, your hemoglobin should be checked every 4 to 8 weeks. This is especially important if you have coronary artery disease, or have suffered a stroke or transient ischemic attacks (TIAs) in the past.

Hemoglobin levels typically decrease by 2 to 3 grams/dL during the first 4to 8 weeks of therapy. If your hemoglobin falls below 10 grams/dL, your healthcare provider will probably reduce your ribavirin dosage. Hemolytic anemia is the most common reason for reducing the dose of ribavirin, however, it rarely causes therapy to be stopped. Hemoglobin levels usually increase within 4 to 8 weeks of completing therapy.

If you already have severe anemia, active coronary artery disease, peripheral *vascular* disease, or if you cannot tolerate anemia for any other reason, you are not a suitable candidate for combination therapy. Your healthcare provider may suggest treatment with pegylated interferon monotherapy or may advise no treatment. An injectable form of erythropoietin, a hormone produced by the body to stimulate red blood cell production, is sometimes used to counteract the effects of hemolytic anemia and enable you to complete therapy.[73-77]

ANECDOTAL STORY OF PEGYLATED INTERFERON AND USE OF ERYTHROPOIETIN TO MANAGE ANEMIA DUE TO RIBAVIRIN

A 49 year old nurse was diagnosed with hepatitis C in 1993, two years after an accidental needle stick from a known hepatitis C patient. She also had a remote history of IV drug use in 1969. She was asymptomatic and had a normal physical exam. A liver biopsy revealed minimal *nonspecific* changes with no fibrosis. She had healthcare 2b virus. The patient's ALT remained mildly elevated over the next six years. A repeat liver biopsy in 1999 showed the development of mild activity and moderate fibrosis.

The patient was treated with pegylated interferon alfa 2b plus ribavirin, and her hemoglobin dropped to 8.7 grams/dL. She had severe fatigue and was unable to carry out her normal work. Ribavirin was initially stopped, allowing her hemoglobin to recover to 10.4 grams/dL. Ribavirin was restarted at half dose, but her hemoglobin again fell to 8.7 grams/dL. Erythropoietin therapy was added to stimulate red blood cell production. This allowed the patient to continue ribavirin therapy and to return to work with a hemoglobin of 11.0 to 12.1 grams/dL. Three years after completion of therapy, the patient has undetectable virus and her liver enzymes remain normal.

This patient's experience demonstrates the value of working through side effects to complete treatment if early viral tests indicate that therapy is likely to be successful. It also demonstrates the usefulness of the red blood cell growth factor, erythropoietin, in increasing the hemoglobin level so that the patient was able to complete therapy.

BIRTH DEFECTS

A major concern with ribavirin therapy is its ability to cause birth defects or miscarriage. If you are a woman of childbearing age and have not had a hysterectomy, you must have a pregnancy test prior to starting therapy, and periodically thereafter. Reliable birth control is essential during therapy with ribavirin. Neither the male nor the female in a partnership can take ribavirin if the female is pregnant or could become pregnant. Ribavirin <u>cannot</u> be given to pregnant women, or to men or women who cannot comply with the requirement for adequate birth control for the duration of treatment and six months following the conclusion of treatment. If you are planning to have children, it is important to discuss this with your healthcare provider.

Making Therapy Work

As discussed elsewhere in Hepatitis C Choices, the most important risk factors contributing to rapid progression of hepatitis C are being over age 40 years, being male, and drinking alcohol. Of course, you cannot change your age or sex. Therefore, the single most important thing you <u>can</u> do to slow the progression of hepatitis C is to eliminate <u>all</u> alcohol. This includes hard liquor, beer, and wine, and any products that may contain alcohol such as certain over-the-counter cough remedies, mouthwashes, and other products. Remember, even so-called nonalcoholic beer contains some alcohol.

Your liver is damaged by infection with the hepatitis C virus. It has to both fight the virus and repair itself. As discussed in other chapters in this book, a well-balanced diet will give your liver the building blocks and energy it needs to repair itself. Adequate exercise and sleep can also help the repair process and improve your immune function.

Alternative approaches to managing the symptoms of hepatitis C and the side effects associated with interferon and ribavirin treatment are discussed elsewhere in this book. It is critical to make sure your western doctor is aware of everything you are taking so that he or she can coordinate all of your medicines, including both prescription and over-the-counter medicines. This includes supplements you may be taking such as Chinese and Ayurvedic herbs, *amino acids*, *nutritional supplements*, minerals, and any other substances you are taking. In other words, you should tell your doctor about <u>anything</u> you ingest, put on your skin, inject, or in any other way introduce into your body. Your doctor must have the full picture in order to best advise you and evaluate the results of your treatment.

The 80-80-80 Goal

Combination therapy with interferon plus ribavirin can be challenging. Hepatitis C treatment requires serious commitments from both you and your healthcare provider. Studies have shown that if you do not take at least 80% of the prescribed interferon and ribavirin doses at least 80% of the time, your chances of long-term success are dramatically reduced.[78] Thus, the phrase "the 80-80-80 goal" was coined. Achieving the 80-80-80 goal increases the likelihood of a durable response rate. Careful attention from you and your healthcare provider to prevent and treat side effects, anticipate complications, and support one another's efforts will produce a high likelihood of success. Failure to make every effort to achieve at least the 80-80-80 goal described above is likely to be a fruitless exercise, wasting your effort and causing discomfort.

While this goal may sound formidable, remember, you are initially committing to only a 12-week trial of therapy. At the end of that period, it should be clear if therapy is not working and should be stopped.[23, 32, 33, 79] However, if you are responding at week 12, it is critical that you make every effort to complete a full course of therapy.

Studies suggest that taking full dose therapy, especially of ribavirin, during the first 12 weeks of treatment is the single most important factor in achieving a durable response.[33, 79-82] The use of substances called growth factors to stimulate the body's production of red and *white blood cells* is sometimes necessary to enable a person to complete a full course of adequate dose therapy.[73-76]

Reasons for Using the Allopathic Treatment Approach and Who Might Benefit

Chronic hepatitis C is often a silent in the early years of infection, but eventually progresses to liver *cirrhosis, liver failure*, and/or liver cancer in 20% to 30% of those infected. Now that successful therapy is available, these serious consequences can be avoided in over 50% of patients. Most people infected with HCV remain asymptomatic until the disease is quite advanced. However during this time, infected people can pass HCV on to others.

You are urged to consider combination therapy if one or more of the following circumstances applies to you.

- If you have HCV genotype 2 or 3, combination therapy should be considered because the durable response rate is greater than 70-80%[83] with 24 weeks of therapy with pegylated interferon plus ribavirin.

- If your liver biopsy shows stage 2 to 3 fibrosis and/or grade 2 to 4 *necrosis/inflammation* (see *Chapter 4.1, Liver Disease Progression*), you should consider therapy regardless of your genotype. Without treatment, you will eventually progress to cirrhosis. Almost all serious complications and deaths due to hepatitis C are related to the development of cirrhosis.

- If you have active disease, stage 4 fibrosis (cirrhosis), and your liver disease is compensated, you should consider combination therapy because if your disease cannot be stabilized, the next step is liver transplantation.

Reasons for Not Using the Allopathic Treatment Approach

You may wish to delay therapy if you are asymptomatic, have minimal disease on liver biopsy (stage 0-1, grade 0-1), and have no manifestations of hepatitis C outside the liver. This is particularly true if you have had the disease for over 20 years, are over 60 years of age, and/or have HCV genotype 1 or 6 (the most difficult genotypes to treat). However, even if you decide not to pursue treatment at this time, you still need regular medical follow-up and a repeat liver biopsy in 3 to 5 years to look for evidence of disease progression.

You cannot safely take interferon if you:

- have an uncontrolled psychiatric condition

- are actively using drugs or alcohol

- have severe heart disease, very low white blood cell or platelet counts, organ transplantation (except liver), and/or uncontrolled seizures

If you have decompensated cirrhosis (liver failure), you should be evaluated at a transplant center promptly to determine whether you are a candidate for liver transplantation. You may be put on carefully monitored therapy in an attempt to reduce HCV viral load prior to transplant.

Other conditions such as uncontrolled diabetes or *hypertension*, moderately decreased white blood cells or platelets, uncontrolled autoimmune disease, *psoriasis*, and *rheumatoid* arthritis may make interferon treatment unsafe. Your doctor will advise you of the relative safety of interferon treatment if you have one or more of these conditions.

Pregnant women and women of childbearing age who do not use a reliable form of birth control cannot take ribavirin due to the risk of birth defects. Because ribavirin is cleared from the blood by the kidneys, patients on hemodialysis or with end-stage renal failure cannot take ribavirin. Severe anemia (hemoglobin less than 11gm/dL), *hemoglobinopathies*, or other conditions in which anemia can be dangerous may make it unsafe to take ribavirin.

What You Need to Know Regarding Therapy

There are a number of things you and your doctor need to know about your situation before you decide to begin interferon-based therapy and at various stages of treatment once it has begun. Most of this information can only be gained through testing.

Before Starting Therapy

Before therapy begins, you will need to have the following tests, and discuss these aspects of your medical history.

- HCV genotype and viral load

- liver biopsy grade (inflammation/necrosis) and stage (fibrosis)

- hemoglobin level

- white blood cell count with neutrophil count

- platelet count

- cryoglobulin level

- *thyroid stimulating hormone* (*TSH*) level to check thyroid status

- electrocardiogram (EKG) if you are over 50 years of age

- presence or absence of other liver diseases (for example, hepatitis B, *alcoholic liver disease*, etc.), autoimmune diseases, heart or kidney disease, seizure disorder, diabetes, and/or severe lung disease

- presence or history of any psychiatric disorder, especially depression or suicidal thoughts; psychiatric consultation may be required if one of these is present

- pregnancy or ability to become pregnant and the use of appropriate means to prevent pregnancy

During Therapy

During therapy, the following tests need to be done.

- *complete blood count* (*CBC*) and differential cell count (neutrophils) at 2, 4, 8, and 12 weeks, and then every 4 to 8 weeks until therapy is completed
- ALT levels are usually checked at the same time points as your CBC
- HCV viral load at week 12
- TSH (thyroid stimulating hormone) at 12, 24, and 48 weeks
- a standardized test for depression (for example, Beck's Inventory or the Hospital Anxiety/Depression Index) as well as a clinical evaluation for depression at the time of each visit to screen for the development of psychological problems

You must eliminate <u>all</u> alcohol and strive to take more than 80% of your prescribed interferon and ribavirin doses more than 80% of the time in order to have the best chance of achieving a durable response.

After Therapy

If your HCV viral load is negative at the end of treatment, the following tests need be done after therapy is completed.

- ALT at 4, 12, 24, and 48 weeks
- HCV viral load at 12, 24, and 48 weeks, or at any time your ALT becomes elevated
- yearly tests after these time points

If you have detectable virus the end of treatment, or if the virus becomes detectable again after the completion of treatment, see *Section 3* of this chapter for additional treatment options.

Summary

Many people are candidates for interferon-based treatment of chronic hepatitis C. You may be a candidate for therapy if you have an elevated ALT, other conditions related to your HCV infection, a detectable HCV viral load, and/or chronic inflammation or fibrosis on liver biopsy. Currently, the best initial treatment for chronic hepatitis C is pegylated interferon plus ribavirin. This combination has resulted in a sustained response in 54% to 56% of patients studied in clinical trials. If you are not a candidate for combination therapy, you may be a candidate for pegylated interferon monotherapy.

Therapy for hepatitis C is rapidly changing with the primary goals of eliminating the virus, improving quality of life, and alleviating the effects of HCV infection on the liver and other organs. In this rapidly changing environment, the recommendations for therapy will probably change every few years. It is hoped that new approaches will provide more effective therapy for the majority of people infected with hepatitis C.

References

1. Strader DB, Wright T, Thomas DL, Seeff LB; American Association for the Study of Liver Diseases. Diagnosis, management, and treatment of hepatitis C. *Hepatology*. 2004;39(4):1147-71.
2. Swain MG, Lai M, Shiffman ML, et al. Sustained Virologic Response (SVR) Resulting From Treatment with Peginterferon Alfa-2a (40KD) (Pegasys®) Alone or in Combination with Ribavirin (Copegus®) is Durable and Constitutes a Cure: an Ongoing 5-year Follow-up. DDW 2007. May 19-24, 2007. Abstract 444.
3. Poynard T, Leroy V, Cohard M, et al. Meta-analysis of interferon randomized trials in the treatment of viral hepatitis C: effects of dose and duration. *Hepatology*. 1996;24(4):778-789.
4. Lin R, Roach E, Zimmerman M, et al. Interferon alfa-2b for chronic hepatitis C: effects of dose increment and duration of treatment on response rates. Results of the first multicentre Australian trial. Australia Hepatitis C Study Group. *J Hepatol*. 1995;23(5):487-496.
5. Manesis EK, Papaioannou C, Gioustozi A, et al. Biochemical and virological outcome of patients with chronic hepatitis C treated with

interferon alfa-2b for 6 or 12 months: a 4-year follow- up of 211 patients. *Hepatology*. 1997;26(3):734-739.

6. Poynard T, Bedossa P, Chevallier M, et al. A comparison of three interferon alfa-2b regimens for the long-term treatment of chronic non-A, non-B hepatitis. Multicenter Study Group. *N Engl J Med*. 1995;332(22):1457-1462.

7. Reichard O, Foberg U, Fryden A, et al. High sustained response rate and clearance of viremia in chronic hepatitis C after treatment with interferon-alfa 2b for 60 weeks. *Hepatology*. 1994;19(2):280-285.

8. Carithers RL, Jr, Emerson SS. Therapy of hepatitis C: meta-analysis of interferon alfa-2b trials. Hepatology. 1997;26(3 Suppl 1):83-88S.

9. Tong MJ, Reddy KR, Lee WM, et al. Treatment of chronic hepatitis C with consensus interferon: a multicenter, randomized, controlled trial. Consensus Interferon Study Group. *Hepatology*. 1997;26(3):747-754.

10. EASL: International Consensus Conference on Hepatitis C Consensus Statement. *J Hepatol*. 1999;30(5):956-961.

11. Schalm SW, Weiland O, Hansen BE, et al. Interferon-ribavirin for chronic hepatitis C with and without cirrhosis: analysis of individual patient data of six controlled trials. Eurohep Study Group for Viral Hepatitis. *Gastroenterology*. 1999;117(2):408-413.

12. Recommendations for prevention and control of hepatitis C virus (HCV) infection and HCV-related chronic disease. MMWR. 1998;47(No. RR-19):1-39.

13. Poynard T, Marcellin P, Lee SS, et al. Randomised trial of interferon alfa2b plus ribavirin for 48 weeks or for 24 weeks versus interferon alfa2b plus placebo for 48 weeks for treatment of chronic infection with hepatitis C virus. International Hepatitis Interventional Therapy Group (IHIT). *Lancet*. 1998;352(9138):1426-1432.

14. McHutchison JG, Gordon SC, Schiff ER, et al. Interferon alfa-2b alone or in combination with ribavirin as initial treatment for chronic hepatitis C. Hepatitis Interventional Therapy Group. *N Engl J Med*. 1998;339(21):1485-1492.

15. Poynard T, McHutchison J, Goodman Z, et al. Is an "a la carte" combination interferon alfa-2b plus ribavirin regimen possible for the first line treatment in patients with chronic hepatitis C? The ALGOVIRC Project Group. *Hepatology*. 2000;31(1):211-218.

16. Schalm SW, Hansen BE, Chemello L, et al. Ribavirin enhances the efficacy but not the adverse effects of interferon in chronic hepatitis C. Meta-analysis of individual patient data from European centers. *J Hepatol*. 1997;26(5):961-966.

17. Reddy KR. Controlled-release, pegylation, liposomal formulations: new mechanisms in the delivery of injectable drugs. *Ann Pharmacother*. 2000;34(7-8):915-923.

18. Kozlowski A, Harris JM. Improvements in protein PEGylation: pegylated interferons for treatment of hepatitis C. *J Control Release*. 2001;72(1-3):217-224.

19. Zeuzem S, Feinman SV, Rasenack J, et al. Peginterferon alfa-2a in patients with chronic hepatitis C. *N Engl J Med*. 2000;343(23):1666-1672.

20. Heathcote EJ, Shiffman ML, Cooksley W, et al. Peginterferon alfa-2a in patients with chronic hepatitis C and cirrhosis. *N Engl J Med*. 2000;343(23):1673-1680.

21. Glue P, Rouzier-Panis R, Raffanel C, et al. A dose-ranging study of pegylated interferon alfa-2b and ribavirin in chronic hepatitis C. The Hepatitis C Intervention Therapy Group. *Hepatology*. 2000;32(3):647-653.

22. Fried M, Shiffman M, Reddy R, et al. Pegylated (40 kDa) interferon alfa-2a (PEGASYS) in combination with ribavirin: efficacy and safety results from a phase III, randomized, actively-controlled, multicenter study. *Gastroenterology*. 120 (Suppl), A55. 2001. (Abstract).

23. Manns M, McHutchison J, Gordon S, et al. Peginterferon alfa-2b plus ribavirin compared with interferon alfa-2b plus ribavirin for initial treatmentof chronic hepatitis C: a randomized trial. *Lancet*. 2001;358(9286):958-965.

24. Trepo C, Lindsey K, Niederau C, et al. Pegylated interferon alfa-2b (PEG-INTRON) monotherapy is superior to interferon alfa-2b (INTRON A) for the treatment of chronic hepatitis C. *J Hepatol*. 2000;32(S2):29.

25. Sulkowski M, Reindollar R, Yu J. Pegylated interferon alfa-2a (PEGASYS) and ribavirin combination therapy for chronic hepatitis C: a phase II open-label study. *Gastroenterology*. 188(S2), A950. 2000. (Abstract).

26. Jacobson IM, Russo M, Brown R, et al. Pegylated interferon alfa-2b plus ribavirin in patients with chronic hepatitis C: a trial in prior nonresponders to interferon monotherapy or combination therapy, and in combination therapy relapsers. *Gastroenterology*. 120(S1). 2001. (Abstract).

27. Craxi A, Licata A. Clinical trial results of peginterferons in combination with ribavirin. *Semin Liver Dis*. 2003;23 Suppl 1:35-46.

28. Zeuzem S, Welsch C, Herrmann E. Pharmacokinetics of peginterferons. *Semin Liver Dis*. 2003;23 Suppl 1:23-8.

29. Pedder SC. Pegylation of interferon alfa: structural and pharmacokinetic properties. *Semin Liver Dis*. 2003;23 Suppl 1:19-22.

30. Powers KA, Dixit NM, Ribeiro RM, Golia P, Talal AH, Perelson AS. Modeling viral and drug kinetics: hepatitis C virus treatment with pegylated interferon alfa-2b. *Semin Liver Dis*. 2003;23 Suppl 1:13-8.

31. Sherman KE. Implications of peginterferon use in special populations infected with HCV. *Semin Liver Dis*. 2003;23 Suppl 1:47-52.

32. Fried MW, Shiffman ML, Reddy KR, et al. Peginterferon alfa-2a plus ribavirin for chronic hepatitis C virus infection. *N Engl J Med*. 2002;347(13):975-982.

33. Hadziyannis SJ, Sette H Jr, Morgan TR, et al. Peginterferon-alfa2a and ribavirin combination therapy in chronic hepatitis C: a randomized study of treatment duration and ribavirin dose. *Ann Intern Med*. 2004;140(5):346-55.

34. Borroni G, Andreoletti M, Casiraghi MA, et al. Effectiveness of pegylated interferon/ribavirin combination in 'real world' patients with chronic hepatitis C virus infection. *Ailment Pharmacol Ther*. 2008 May;27(9):790-7. Epub 2008 Feb 21.

35. Reddy KR, Wright TL, Pockros PJ, et al. Efficacy and safety of pegylated (40-kd) interferon alfa-2a compared with interferon alfa-2a in noncirrhotic patients with chronic hepatitis C. *Hepatology*. 2001;33(2):433-438.

36. Liu CH, Liang CC, Lin JW, et al. Pegylated interferon alfa-2a versus standard interferon alfa-2a for treatment-naive dialysis patients with chronic hepatitis C: a randomized study. *Gut*. 2008 Apr;57(4):525-30. Epub 2007 Sep 19.

37. Quarantini LC, Bressan RA, Galvão A, et al.Incidence of psychiatric side effects during pegylated interferon- alfa retreatment in nonresponder hepatitis C virus-infected patients. *Liver Int*. 2007 Oct;27(8):1098-102.

38. C.Fontana RJ, Bieliauskas LA, Lindsay KL, et al. Cognitive function does not worsen during pegylated interferon and ribavirin retreatment of chronic hepatitis C. *Hepatology*. 2007 May;45(5):1154-63.

39. Lau DT, Kleiner DE, Ghany MG, Park Y, Schmid P, Hoofnagle JH. 10 year follow-up after interferon-alfa therapy for chronic hepatitis C. *Hepatology*. 1998 Oct;28(4):1121-1127.

40. Chavalitdhamrong D, Tanwandee T.Long-term outcomes of chronic hepatitis C patients with sustained virological response at 6 months

after the end of treatment. *World J Gastroenterol*. 2006 Sep 14;12(34):5532-5.

41. Marcellin P, Boyer N, Gervais A, et al. Long-term histologic improvement and loss of detectable intrahepatic HCV RNA in patients with chronic hepatitis C and sustained response to interferon-alfa therapy. *Ann Intern Med*. 1997 Nov 15;127(10):875-81.

42. Tanaka H, Tsukuma H, Kasahara A, et al. Effect of interferon therapy on the incidence of hepatocellular carcinoma and mortality of patients with chronic hepatitis C: a retrospective cohort study of 738 patients. *Int J Cancer*. 2000 Sep 1;87(5):741-9.

43. Nishiguchi S, Kuroki T, Nakatani S, et al. Randomised trial of effects of interferon-alfa on incidence of hepatocellular carcinoma in chronic active hepatitis C with cirrhosis. Lancet. 1995;346(8982):1051-1055.

44. Fattovich G, Giustina G, Degos F, et al. Effectiveness of interferon alfa on incidence of hepatocellular carcinoma and decompensation in cirrhosis type C. European Concerted Action on Viral Hepatitis (EUROHEP). *J Hepatol*. 1997;27(1):201-205.

45. Fattovich G, Giustina G, Degos F, et al. Morbidity and mortality in compensated cirrhosis type C: a retrospective follow-up study of 384 patients. *Gastroenterology*. 1997;112(2):463-472.

46. Mazzella G, Accogli E, Sottili S, et al. Alfa interferon treatment may prevent hepatocellular carcinoma in HCV-related liver cirrhosis. *J Hepatol*. 1996;24(2):141-147.

47. Camma C, Giunta M, Andreone P, Craxi A. Interferon and prevention of hepatocellular carcinoma in viral cirrhosis: an evidence-based approach. *J Hepatol*. 2001;34(4):593-602.

48. Baffis V, Shrier I, Sherker AH, Szilagyi A. Use of interferon for prevention of hepatocellular carcinoma in cirrhotic patients with hepatitis B or hepatitis C virus infection. *Ann Intern Med*. 1999;131(9):696-701.

49. Ikeda K, Saitoh S, Kobayashi M, et al. Long-term interferon therapy for 1 year or longer reduces the hepatocellular carcinogenesis rate in patients with liver cirrhosis caused by hepatitis C virus: a pilot study. *J Gastroenterol Hepatol*. 2001;16(4):406-415.

50. Yu ML, et al. A sustained virological response to interferon or interferon/ribavirin reduces hepatocellular carcinoma and improves survival in chronic hepatitis C: a nationwide, multicentre study in Taiwan. *Antivir Ther*. 2006;11(8):985-94.

51. Everson GT, et al. Histological benefits of virological response to peginterferon alfa-2a monotherapy in patients with hepatitis C and advanced fibrosis or compensated cirrhosis. *Aliment Pharmacol Ther*. 2008 Apr 1;27(7):542-51.

52. Jaeckel E, Cornberg M, Wedemeyer H, et al. Treatment of acute hepatitis C with interferon alfa-2b. N Engl J Med. 2001;345(20):1452-7.

53. Kamal SM, Moustafa KN, Chen J, et al. Duration of peginterferon therapy in acute hepatitis C: a randomized trial. *Hepatology*. 2006;43:923-931.

54. Kamal SM, Fouly AE, Kamel RR, et al. Peginterferon alfa-2b therapy in acute hepatitis C: impact of onset of therapy on sustained virologic response. *Gastroenterology*. 2006;130:632-638.

55. Marcellin P, Asselah T, Boyer N. Fibrosis and disease progression in hepatitis C. *Hepatology*. 2002;36(suppl 1):S-47-S56.

56. Pradar P, Alberti A, Poynard T, et al. Predictive value of ALT levels for histologic findings in chronic hepatitis C: a European collaborative study. *Hepatology*. 2002;36(pt 1):973-977.

57. Hui CK, Belaye T, Montegrande , Wright TL. A comparison in the progression of liver fibrosis in chronic hepatitis C between persistently normal and elevated transaminases. *J Hepatol*. 2003;38:511-517.

58. Alberti A, Morsica G, Chemello L, et al. Hepatitis C viraemia and liver disease in symptom-free individuals with anti-HCV. *Lancet*. 1992;340:697-698.

59. Everson GT, Hoefs JC, Seeff LB, et al. Impact of disease severity on outcome of antiviral therapy for chronic hepatitis C: Lessons from the HALT-C trial. *Hepatology*. 2006;44(6):1675-84.

60. Gumber SC, Chopra S. Hepatitis C: a multifaceted disease. Review of extrahepatic manifestations. *Ann Intern Med*. 1995;123(8):615-620.

61. Cacoub P, Poynard T, Ghillani P, et al. Extrahepatic manifestations of chronic hepatitis C. MULTIVIRC Group. Multidepartment Virus C. Arthritis Rheum. 1999;42(10):2204-2212.

62. Darby SC, Ewart DW, Giangrande PL, et al. Mortality from liver cancer and liver disease in haemophilic men and boys in UK given blood products contaminated with hepatitis C. UK Haemophilia Centre Directors' Organisation. *Lancet*. 1997;350(9089):1425-1431.

63. Benhamou Y, Bochet M, Di Martino V, et al. Liver fibrosis progression in human immunodeficiency virus and hepatitis C virus coinfected patients. The Multivirc Group. *Hepatology*. 1999;30(4):1054-1058.

64. Daar ES, Lynn H, Donfield S, et al. Relation between HIV-1 and hepatitis C viral load in patients with hemophilia. *J Acquir Immune Defic Syndr*. 2001;26(5):466-472.

65. Pineda JA, García-García JA, Aguilar-Guisado M, et al. Clinical progression of hepatitis C virus-related chronic liver disease in human immunodeficiency virus-infected patients undergoing highly active antiretroviral therapy. *Hepatology*. 2007;46(3):622-30.

66. Salmon-Ceron D, Lewden C, Morlat P, et al. Liver disease as a major cause of death among HIV infected patients: role of hepatitis C and B viruses and alcohol. *J Hepatol*. 2005;42(6):799-805.

67. Chung RT, Andersen J, Volberding P, et al. Peginterferon Alfa-2a plus ribavirin versus interferon alfa-2a plus ribavirin for chronic hepatitis C in HIV-coinfected persons. N Engl J Med 2004; 351(5): 451-459.

68. Torriani FJ, Rodriguez-Torres M, Rockstroh JK, et al. Peginterferon alfa-2a plus ribavirin for chronic hepatitis C virus infection in HIV-infected patients. N Engl J Med 2004; 351(5): 438-450.

69. Carrat F, Bani-Sadr F, Pol S, et al. Pegylated interferon alfa-2b vs standard interferon alfa-2b, plus ribavirin, for chronic hepatitis C in HIV-infected patients: a randomized controlled trial. *JAMA* 2004; 292(23): 2839-2848.

70. Opravil M, Sasadeusz J, Cooper DA, et al. Effect of baseline CD4 cell count on the efficacy and safety of peginterferon Alfa-2a (40KD) plus ribavirin in patients with HIV/hepatitis C virus coinfection. *J Acquir Immune Defic Syndr*. 2008;47(1):36-49.

71. Rodríguez-Torres M, Rodríguez-Orengo JF, Ríos-Bedoya CF, et al. Effect of hepatitis C virus treatment in fibrosis progression rate (FPR) and time to cirrhosis (TTC) in patients co-infected with human immunodeficiency virus: a paired liver biopsy study. *J Hepatol*. 2007;46(4):613-9.

72. Rodríguez-Torres M, Rodríguez-Orengo JF, Ríos-Bedoya CF, et al. Efficacy and safety of peg-IFN alfa-2a with ribavirin for the treatment of HCV/HIV coinfected patients who failed previous IFN based therapy. *J Clin Virol*. 2007;38(1):32-8.

73. Afdhal NH, Dieterich DT, Pockros PJ, et al. Epoetin alfa maintains ribavirin dose in HCV-infected patients: a prospective, double-blind, randomized controlled study. *Gastroenterology*. 2004;126(5):1302-11.

74. Dieterich DT, Wasserman R, Brau N, et al. Once-weekly epoetin alfa improves anemia and facilitates maintenance of ribavirin dosing in

hepatitis C virus-infected patients receiving ribavirin plus interferon alfa. *Am J Gastroenterol.* 2003;98(11):2491-9.

75. Soza A, Everhart JE, Ghany MG, et al. Neutropenia during combination therapy of interferon alfa and ribavirin for chronic hepatitis C. *Hepatology.* 2002;36(5):1273-9.

76. Van Thiel DH, Faruki H, Friedlander L, et al. Combination treatment of advanced HCV associated liver disease with interferon and G-CSF. *Hepatogastroenterology.* 1995;42(6):907-12.

77. Sharvadze L, Tsertsvadze T, Gochitashvili N, et al.Ifn/Rbv treatment induced anemia and its correction with epoetin alfa in patients with hepatitis C. *Georgian Med News.* 2006 Aug;(137):62-5.

78. McHutchison JG, Manns M, Patel K, et al. Adherence to combination therapy enhances sustained response in genotype-1-infected patients with chronic hepatitis C. *Gastroenterology.* 2002;123(4):1061-9.

79. Yu JW, Wang GQ, Sun LJ, et al. Predictive value of rapid virological response and early virological response on sustained virological response in HCV patients treated with pegylated interferon alfa-2a and ribavirin. *J Gastroenterol Hepatol.* 2007 Jun;22(6):832-6.

80. Davis GL, Wong JB, McHutchison JG, Manns MP, Harvey J, Albrecht J. Early virologic response to treatment with peginterferon alfa-2b plus ribavirin in patients with chronic hepatitis C. *Hepatology.* 2003;38(3):645-52.

81. Shiffman ML, Di Bisceglie AM, Lindsay KL, et al. Peginterferon alfa-2a and ribavirin in patients with chronic hepatitis C who have failed prior treatment. *Gastroenterology.* 2004;126(4):1015-23; discussion 947.

82. Furusyo N, Kajiwara E, Takahashi K, et al. Association between the treatment length and cumulative dose of pegylated interferon alfa-2b plus ribavirin and their effectiveness as a combination treatment for Japanese chronic hepatitis C patients: Project of the Kyushu University Liver Disease Study Group. *J Gastroenterol Hepatol.* 2008 Feb 1 [Epub ahead of print]

83. Shepherd J, Brodin H, Cave C, et al. Pegylated interferon alfa-2a and -2b in combination with ribavirin in the treatment of chronic hepatitis C: a systematic review and economic evaluation. *Health Technol Assess.* 2004 Oct;8(39):iii-iv, 1-125.

WESTERN (ALLOPATHIC) MEDICINE

Gregory T. Everson, MD

OPTIONS WHEN INITIAL TREATMENT FAILS TO CLEAR HCV

Introduction

The current standard for initial treatment of *chronic hepatitis C* is the combination of *pegylated interferon* plus *ribavirin*.[1-3] This combination is superior to previous treatments including *interferon* monotherapy, pegylated interferon monotherapy, or interferon plus ribavirin.

Despite the success of current treatment, approximately 20% of patients infected with hepatitis C *genotypes* 2 or 3 and over 50% of patients infected with genotype 1 fail to clear the hepatitis C virus (HCV). Since *sustained viral response* (*SVR*) after pegylated interferon plus ribavirin is much lower in patients with genotype 1 compared to genotypes 2 and 3, most patients remaining infected after an initial course of pegylated interferon plus ribavirin are infected with genotype 1. Options for treatment and management of patients who fail to clear HCV with an initial course of pegylated interferon/ribavirin are the key issues addressed in this chapter.

I will focus solely on retreatment of patients in whom the initial course of treatment was pegylated interferon plus ribavirin. Other patients who were initially treated with inferior regimens (interferon monotherapy, pegylated interferon monotherapy, or interferon plus ribavirin) should be retreated with pegylated interferon plus ribavirin.

As already stated, more than 50% of people with genotype 1 who were treated with pegylated interferon plus ribavirin do not clear HCV from their bodies.[3] These patients have either *relapsed* despite on-treatment clearance of *HCV RNA* from their blood or never cleared HCV RNA during or after treatment (called *nonresponse*). For these patients, the key questions are, "Should I be retreated? If I should be retreated, with what?"

In addressing these questions, this chapter covers the following topics:

- What are the goals of retreatment?
- Who should consider retreatment?
- Should I be retreated with pegylated interferon or another interferon, plus ribavirin?
- What are the chances that retreatment will clear HCV?
- Should I consider maintenance therapy with low-dose pegylated interferon?
- What is the evidence that treatment slows disease progression?
- What is the evidence that treatment reduces the risk of *liver cancer*?
- Who should be screened for liver cancer? What tests should be done?

What are the Goals of Retreatment?

The main goal of retreatment is achievement of SVR. Clearing HCV from your body is the one sure way to reduce progression of liver disease and decrease your risk of complications including *hepatocellular carcinoma* (liver cancer). Options for retreatment include:

- second course of pegylated interferon plus ribavirin
- consensus interferon plus ribavirin
- *clinical trial* of new therapies
- interferon maintenance therapy

Successful retreatment with SVR will:

- clear HCV from your body
- slow disease progression
- reduce the risk of liver cancer (also known as *hepatoma*, hepatocellular carcinoma, and *HCC*)

The goals of retreatment vary from person to person. Table 1 summarizes the issues doctors take into account when recommending retreatment to people with hepatitis C. Each of these issues is important. We must determine which therapy gives a particular patient the best chance to clear the virus. We must also determine if there are supportive care measures needed to slow the rate of liver injury. These measures could include reducing the amount of *iron* in the body, *antioxidant* therapy, and/or long-term treatment with low-dose, pegylated interferon (maintenance therapy).

Table 1. Management Issues in Retreatment of Non-Responders to Previous Interferon-Based Therapy

Attempt to clear HCV with pegylated interferon plus ribavirin

Prevent disease progression (hypothetical)
   • antioxidants (vitamin E, silymarin, vitamin C, SAMe, and others) - unproven
   • iron unloading in patients with increased iron in the liver - unproven
   • maintenance interferon - unproven
   • anti-fibrotic agents - unproven
   • others

Detect liver cancer in patients with advanced fibrosis and/or cirrhosis
   • alfa-fetoprotein testing every six months
   • radiologic imaging (such as ultrasound) every six months

Monitor for liver decompensation with biochemical tests and for possible referral to a liver transplant center

Clearing the Hepatitis C Virus

Viral clearance is the elimination of HCV from the blood and the liver. Clearing HCV is the only sure way to slow or halt disease progression in patients with chronic hepatitis C.

The most common test used to measure *viral load* is the *polymerase chain reaction* (*PCR*) assay. Sustained viral clearance means HCV is undetectable in the blood for six months or more after completing a course of *antiviral* therapy. Clearance of HCV from the blood is usually accompanied by clearance of the virus from the liver. This is known as a *virologic cure*. A virologic cure is assumed to occur when a person maintains a sustained response for at least six months following completion of therapy. A small percentage of people (less than 1%) who have a sustained response may relapse, meaning the virus becomes detectable again. This usually occurs within a year of completion of therapy.[4]

Certain characteristics predict the likelihood of clearing HCV with retreatment using pegylated interferon plus ribavirin.

- <u>relative effectiveness of prior treatment</u> - Patients who received the least effective initial therapy (for example, interferon monotherapy) are most likely to respond to retreatment with pegylated interferon plus ribavirin.

- <u>features of the infected person</u> - Young individuals, women, and people without *cirrhosis* are more likely to respond than others are.

- <u>viral status</u> - Patients with non-1 genotype and relatively low levels of virus are more likely to respond than others are.

Slowing Disease Progression

If viral clearance cannot be achieved, the secondary goals of treatment are to reduce the extent of *liver damage*, slow disease progression, and reduce the risk of complications.

A *nonresponder* is at risk for disease progression and should be monitored for signs of *liver failure*. If you are a nonresponder, any sign of liver function deterioration should prompt your healthcare provider to refer you to a treatment center experienced in liver transplantation for evaluation.

Clinical information, laboratory tests, and/or *liver biopsy* results define the progression of liver disease. See *Chapter 5, Signs & Symptoms that May be Associated with Hepatitis C* and *Chapter 6, Laboratory Tests and Procedures* for further explanation of the following criteria that point toward disease progression.

<u>Clinical Criteria</u>
- ankle *edema*
- *ascites*
- *encephalopathy*
- *gastrointestinal* bleeding from *varices*
- skin manifestations (spider telangiectasia, palmar erythema)
- varices

<u>Blood Tests</u>
- increased *bilirubin*
- increased *prothrombin time*
- reduced *albumin*
- reduced *platelet* and/or *neutrophil* count

<u>Liver Biopsy Findings</u>
- increased *fibrosis*
- development of cirrhosis

Despite increased awareness of the potentially serious consequences of hepatitis C, many people ignore early warning signs and see their healthcare provider only when they already have late *stage* disease. Unfortunately, it is more difficult to treat people with late stage disease using *interferon-based therapy*. Many of these patients progress to liver failure and may ultimately need a liver transplant.

Reducing the Risk of Liver Cancer

The third goal of retreatment is to reduce or eliminate the risk of developing liver cancer. Among people with chronic hepatitis C, the risk of liver cancer is mainly limited to those with cirrhosis.[5] Screening tests for liver cancer often include twice-yearly blood tests for *alfa-fetoprotein* and radiologic imaging of the liver (usually *ultrasonography* or ultrasonography alternating with CT scans).

Despite aggressive screening efforts, at least one-third of liver cancers are not detected in the early stages of the disease. Later stage *tumors* may not be curable with surgery and cannot be cured with liver transplantation. Existing studies strongly suggest that achievement of SVR reduces, but does not eliminate, the risk of developing liver cancer.[6] In contrast, it is not clear that interferon-based treatment reduces the risk of liver cancer in patients who fail to clear HCV. Cancer risk in patients who remain infected with HCV is primarily related to the stage of liver fibrosis. The lowest risk is in patients with minimal or no fibrosis; the highest risk is in patients with cirrhosis.

Other studies have suggested, but not proven, that interferon may slow the growth or spread of existing liver cancer. Detection of slow-growing liver cancer at an early stage can allow for effective and possibly curative therapy such as liver transplantation. Since urgent transplantation may be required for cure, living donor transplantation may be of particular benefit for people with liver cancer. This type of liver transplantation can be performed relatively quickly once the cancer has been diagnosed.[7]

Who Should Consider Retreatment?

Assuming you did not respond or clear HCV with the initial course of therapy, you may want to consider retreatment with pegylated interferon plus ribavirin therapy if:

- you did not receive full doses of pegylated interferon plus ribavirin during the initial therapy, or
- you had *side effects* that led to discontinuation, which might now be better tolerated or manageable with supportive care and treatments, or
- you had decreases in *blood counts* that lead to decreases in pegylated interferon, ribavirin, or both.

If your prior therapy was pegylated interferon plus ribavirin and you took full doses of both drugs, retreatment with the same or another pegylated interferon plus ribavirin is unlikely to achieve SVR.

Nonresponse

Nonresponse is the inability of a treatment to clear HCV both during and after a course of antiviral therapy. There are five main reasons for nonresponsive treatment failures.

- The type of hepatitis C infection was resistant to interferon-based treatment.
- The therapy used was inferior to the best current therapy.
- The patient did not adhere to the prescribed treatment regimen.
- Treatment doses had to be reduced because of low levels of *white blood cells*, *red blood cells*, and/or *platelets*.
- The length of treatment was reduced due to side effects and/or poor quality of life.

Relapse

Relapse is not the same as nonresponse. In people who relapse, the virus is undetectable during treatment, but becomes detectable again after treatment ends. Relapse is a common occurrence with interferon monotherapy (interferon used as single agent therapy). It is less common with the combination of interferon plus ribavirin, especially when pegylated interferon is used.

What is the Evidence that Retreatment Can Clear HCV?

The probability that retreatment will clear HCV is affected by the type of prior treatment, your personal characteristics, and viral characteristics.

For example, there is a good chance retreatment will provide virologic cure in a person without cirrhosis who did not respond to six months of interferon monotherapy, and who has less than a million copies of genotype 2b HCV per milliliter of blood.

In contrast, retreatment is unlikely to clear virus in people with cirrhosis whose initial treatment was interferon alfa-2b plus ribavirin and who have high levels of genotype 1b HCV. Virus levels greater than 2 million copies of virus per milliliter of blood are considered high. The treatment goals for a person in this situation are to slow disease progression and reduce the risk of liver cancer. The results of a large clinical trial, HALT C, are discussed below and provide confirmation of these trends.

Results from Lead-In Phase of HALT C

The results of the lead-in phase of the National Institutes of Health (NIH) sponsored trial known as HALT C have recently become available.[8] All HALT C participants experienced prior treatment failure with interferon-based therapy and biopsy proven liver fibrosis. The study incorporated a lead-in phase where all patients, previously treated with either interferon monotherapy or a combination of non-pegylated interferon plus ribavirin, were retreated with pegylated interferon alfa-2a plus ribavirin. Responders who were HCV RNA negative after 20 weeks of treatment continued treatment for a total of 48 weeks.

Virologic cure (sustained viral response or SVR) was observed as follows, based on prior interferon-based treatment:[8]

- 27% of patients previously treated with interferon monotherapy

- 34% of patients previously treated with pegylated interferon monotherapy

- 13% of patients previously treated with standard interferon plus ribavirin

- 11% of patients previously treated with pegylated interferon plus ribavirin

Genotype, race and the presence or absence of cirrhosis were also found to affect the observed rates of SVR.[9]

- SVR was 14% for genotype 1, 65% for genotype 2, and 54% for genotype 3.

- SVR was more likely in Caucasians (20%) and Hispanics (18%) compared to African Americans (6%).

- SVR was 23% among people without cirrhosis and 11% in people with cirrhosis.

Further, ribavirin dose reductions during the first 24 weeks from greater than 80% of the prescribed dose to less than 60% of prescribed dose reduced SVR from 21% to 11%. Viral clearance or a 100-fold reduction in HCV viral load by week 12 (early viral response or EVR) correlated strongly with treatment response (34% for those with EVR versus 1% for those without EVR). These results will help doctors group people into high and low responder categories for selection of retreatment.

**Table 2. Actual Sustained Response Rates
After Retreatment with Pegylated Interferon Plus Ribavirin in the HALT C Trial[8,9]**

Independent Variable	Sustained Response (%)	
	After Retreatment with Pegylayed interferon alfa-2a Plus Ribavirin	
Interferon Monotherapy vs. Combination	28%	12%
Genotype 1 vs. 2 & 3	14%	65% and 54%
Caucasians & Hispanic vs. African American	20%, 18%	6%
Adherence vs. Dose Reductions	21%	11%
No Cirrhosis vs. Cirrhosis	23%	11%
EVR vs. No EVR	34%	1%

Abbreviations
HALT C: Hepatitis C Antiviral Long-Term Treatment to Prevent Cirrhosis trial
EVR: early virologic response defined by greater than a 100-fold drop in HCV RNA after 20 weeks of treatment
Pegylated interferon alfa-2a is marketed as Pegasys® and the ribavirin used in this trial was Copegus®.
Adherence was defined as taking 80% or more of the prescribed dose of both pegylated interferon alfa-2a and ribavirin.
Dose reduction was defined as taking 60% or less of the prescribed dose of either medication.

Your doctor may not recommend pegylated interferon plus ribavirin for clinical reasons. In this situation, options include retreatment with either interferon alfa-2b plus ribavirin or pegylated interferon monotherapy. The chance for a virologic cure with these regimens is less than that for pegylated interferon plus ribavirin. Pegylated interferon monotherapy might be preferred over interferon plus ribavirin for patients with *renal* failure, cardiac conditions, anemia, or for women of childbearing age.

What is the Evidence that Treatment Slows Disease Progression?

Pegylated interferon reduces *inflammation* and may slow fibrosis progression in patients with chronic hepatitis C. Thus, one strategy is to use low-dose or "maintenance" pegylated interferon in patients who fail to clear HCV with pegylated interferon plus ribavirin. The goal of maintenance therapy is to slow or halt disease progression. Potential benefits include reducing liver inflammation and the rate of fibrosis, slowing the rate of progression to cirrhosis, and reducing the rate of liver failure.

One published trial evaluated the effectiveness of long-term interferon therapy in preventing progressive fibrosis in patients who had not responded to therapy.[10] Patients had a pre-treatment liver biopsy and a second biopsy following a six-month course of interferon therapy. Those patients whose liver biopsies showed improvement were randomly assigned to stop interferon therapy or to continue on interferon treatment for a two-year follow-up period. Those who continued interferon therapy had a reduction in liver inflammation and a decline in liver fibrosis. Those who did not continue therapy had increases in liver inflammation and fibrosis.

In another study, 499 patients with chronic hepatitis C who experienced virologic response during treatment with standard interferon monotherapy were given long-term interferon treatment.[11] The results suggested that long-term treatment was associated with reduction in both *hepatic* inflammation and hepatic fibrosis. The key point regarding criteria for treatment was that patients selected for this trial had to demonstrated both virologic response and biochemical improvement with the initial course of treatment.

The HALT C Trial: Pegylated Interferon as Maintenance Therapy
The primary goal of the NIH-sponsored HALT C trial was to determine if maintenance therapy with pegylated interferon alfa-2a could halt disease progression in people with chronic hepatitis C.[12] Recall that all HALT C participants

(1,050 patients) experienced prior treatment failure with interferon-based therapy and biopsy proven liver fibrosis. Approximately 60% had bridging fibrosis and 40% had cirrhosis. Ninety-four percent had genotype 1 HCV.

Patients were randomized (selected by chance) to receive either pegylated interferon-alfa-2a monotherapy (90 ug/wk) or no treatment for 3 ½ years. Prior to randomization, all patients were treated with full dose pegylated interferon/ribavirin in the lead-in phase of HALT-C for ½ year. Thus, patients allocated to maintenance therapy received 4 years of pegylated interferon, whereas those randomized to the control group received only 1/2 year of pegylated interferon.

Clinical evaluations, laboratory tests, *radiologic* imaging, endoscopy, and liver biopsy were performed throughout the trial.

Unfortunately, pegylated interferon monotherapy had no effect on clinical outcome in the HALT C trial. In other words, there was no significant different in the rate of death, liver transplantation, liver cancer, or liver failure between the maintenance therapy group and the control group. The result was the same for both fibrosis and cirrhosis groups. Although there was a trend toward reduced adverse clinical outcomes in patients with marked reduction in HCV RNA during the lead-in phase, overall, there was no significant relationship between viral reduction and clinical outcome.

Thus, the results from HALT C do not support a recommendation for maintenance therapy for nonresponders or relapsers to prior therapy with pegylated interferon plus ribavirin.[13]

What is the Evidence that Treatment Reduces the Risk of Liver Cancer?

Several studies have suggested that SVR after interferon-based therapy reduces the risk of developing liver cancer.[14, 15] A study involving patients with cirrhosis showed that only 4% of those previously treated with interferon developed liver cancer, while 38% of those not treated with interferon went on to develop liver cancer.[16] The patients in this study were followed for an average of 4.4 years after treatment. There were two surprising aspects of this study. The first was that the reduction in cancer risk was achieved with a limited, six-month course of interferon therapy. The second was that the beneficial effect occurred in both those who cleared the virus and in those who did not.

A review article reported the results of three studies addressing the effect of interferon therapy on the development of liver cancer in hepatitis C patients with cirrhosis.[6] The studies involved a total of 272 patients who received no treatment, 371 patients who received but did not respond to interferon treatment, and 60 patients who had a sustained response to interferon treatment. The incidence of liver cancer was 15% among those who received no treatment, 4% among those who did not respond to treatment, and 0% among those who had a sustained response. The greatest reduction in the incidence of liver cancer was among those who had sustained viral clearance.

However, it is important to conduct properly *controlled trials* to determine if antiviral therapy can slow the progression of fibrosis to cirrhosis, and reduce the risk of cancer. These trials must involve large populations of hepatitis C patients who have significant fibrosis or cirrhosis and are willing to be treated with antiviral therapy for an extended period of time. The HALT C trial meets these criteria and examined the role of antiviral therapy in preventing liver cancer and slowing disease progression.

Data indicate that interferon therapy has anti-inflammatory, *antifibrotic*, and anti-proliferative effects.[17] These effects may slow disease progression and prevent liver cancer. The HALT C trial examined the ability of maintenance therapy with low-dose pegylated interferon alfa-2a to prevent liver cancer. Unfortunately the therapy was ineffective. Rates of development of liver cancer were identical between treatment and control arms.[18] Maintenance therapy using low-dose pegylated interferon monotherapy has not been shown to reduce risk of liver cancer.

Who Should Be Screened for Liver Cancer?
What Tests Should Be Done?

Because chronic hepatitis C increases your risk for liver cancer, screening is recommended for people with advanced fibrosis or cirrhosis. However, there are no screening guidelines with which everyone agrees.

Liver cancer can be effectively treated if detected early. For this reason, I recommend that people with bridging fibrosis or cirrhosis have ultrasonography (or ultrasonography alternating with CT scans) of the liver and an alfa-fetoprotein blood test every six months. A persistent, progressive rise in alfa-fetoprotein levels or the development of a new liver mass indicates the need for additional tests. These tests might include special radiologic studies or a biopsy of the mass. If liver cancer is diagnosed, it may be treated with surgery, liver transplantation, and/or other non-surgical approaches.

Options for People Who Are Not Candidates for Retreatment or Who Choose Not To Be Retreated

Despite many advances in antiviral treatment for HCV, some people decide against retreatment with currently available combination therapies. They may choose different therapies or decide not to have any therapy.

Alternatives to interferon-based retreatment *protocols* include:

- clinical trials
  - *protease*, helicase, or *polymerase* inhibitors
  - new interferons (Albuferon®, continuous infusion pumps, others)
  - therapeutic vaccines
  - *complementary and alternative therapies* (CAM)
- no treatment

Factors such as religious beliefs, lifestyle, lack of financial resources or health insurance coverage, and/or health conditions that might make undergoing existing interferon-based treatment difficult can affect the decision each person makes.

Clinical Trials

If you are being treated at a major teaching hospital and/or by a hepatitis C specialist, you may have access to any of a number of clinical trials. Some of these trials will study new formulations of standard interferon and other antiviral agents. Others will be looking at completely new drugs or approaches to the treatment of hepatitis C. Talk with your doctor about which of these trials might be available and appropriate for you. The Internet is a good source of information about clinical trials. Check the *Resource Directory* at the back of this book for Internet addresses.

Many new drugs are under development and preliminary evaluation of them may have a therapeutic role in the management of those who do not respond to conventional, interferon-based therapy. These options may include new interferons, new methods for administering interferons, protease inhibitors, polymerase inhibitors, additional agents targeting other molecular sites of HCV, therapeutic *vaccines*, and others. See *Chapter 8.4, Western (Allopathic) Medicine: The Future of Allopathic Treatment for Hepatitis C* for additional information about emerging therapies. To date, none of these agents has been completely evaluated, nor have they been shown to slow disease progression or reduce the risk of liver cancer. Early results with a combination of pegylated interferon plus ribavirin and telaprevir (a protease inhibitor) suggest that this treatment may be effective in a sizeable proportion of nonresponders and relapsers.[19]

Complementary and Alternative Medicine (CAM)

If your treatment with western medicine failed to clear HCV and there is little hope that retreatment will be successful, you may choose a CAM treatment approach. Treatment strategies for most CAM approaches are generally focused on reducing the amount and rate of liver damage caused by the virus and slowing the progression of liver fibrosis.

CAM approaches to chronic hepatitis C include antioxidant therapy, Chinese herbal remedies, Ayurvedic practices, and others. The rationale, goals, and objectives of these treatment approaches are described in other chapters of this book.

People exploring CAM options should be advised that these therapies have not been fully evaluated for proof of effectiveness in controlled clinical trials. Specifically, you must understand there is no evidence that CAM clears HCV, slows disease progression, or reduces the risk of liver cancer.

No Treatment

You may decide against retreatment with any of the options discussed. This is a personal decision, but it must be made after you have carefully weighed the information concerning the natural progression of hepatitis C and your treatment options. The reasons people choose not to be treated vary. Often, these decisions are related to cost, inconvenience, and fears of the severity of side effects of treatment.

There are major health issues that are important for you to understand even if you elect not to be retreated. You need to understand the natural history of hepatitis C and the long-term consequences of infection. You need to know how the virus affects other parts of the body in addition to the liver. This is particularly crucial if you have advanced fibrosis or cirrhosis. If you have advanced fibrosis or cirrhosis, you are at risk for liver deterioration, liver failure, and the development of liver cancer. You may eventually need a liver transplant. Your doctor must examine you regularly for signs of advancing disease. He or she may order tests to screen for the development of liver cancer.

Summary

This chapter addresses several important clinical issues for an increasingly large population of patients with chronic hepatitis C — those in whom treatment failed to clear HCV. You have been provided with information to help you determine if you should consider retreatment with pegylated interferon plus ribavirin. You have also learned about some of the issues surrounding maintenance interferon.

The goals of retreatment are to clear virus, slow disease progression, and reduce the risk of liver cancer. This chapter identifies criteria for selection of patients for retreatment and provides definitions for response. Studies are summarized that provide information on expected response rates should you elect to undergo retreatment with interferon-based therapy.

Results from past and current clinical trials suggest retreatment clears virus in a small but significant subset of nonresponders. They also show that viral clearance is especially dependent upon viral genotype. New drugs, such as protease- or polymerase-inhibitors, may improve the chance for nonresponders and relapsers to clear HCV. *Phase III clinical trials* of at least two new drugs are ongoing at the time of this writing.

Even if HCV is not cleared by retreatment, you may still benefit from treatments that slow disease progression and reduce your risk of liver cancer. However, results from the largest trial of maintenance therapy, HALT C, were disappointing as treatment with low-dose pegylated interferon monotherapy failed to positively influence any clinical outcome.

Regardless of whether you decide to pursue retreatment, if you have advanced fibrosis or cirrhosis, you must have regular clinical follow-up to monitor for liver decompensation, liver failure, and the development of liver cancer.

References

1. Fried MW, Shiffman ML, Reddy RK, et al. Peginterferon alfa-2a plus ribavirin for chronic hepatitis C virus infection. *N Engl J Med.* 2002;347:975-982.
2. Deutsch M, Hadziyannis SJ. Old and emerging therapies in chronic hepatitis C: an update. *J Viral Hepat.* 2008 Jan;15(1):2-11.
3. Manns MP, McHutchison JG, Gordon SC,et al and the International Hepatitis Interventional Therapy Group. Peginterferon alfa-2b plus ribavirin compared with interferon alfa-2b plus ribavirin for initial treatment of chronic hepatitis C: A randomized trial. *Lancet.* 2001;358(9286):958-965.
4. Lau DT, Kleiner DE, Ghany MG, et al. 10 years follow-up after interferon alfa therapy for chronic hepatitis C. *Hepatology.* 1998;28(4):1121-1127.
5. Imai Y, Kawata S, Tamura S, et al. Relation of interferon therapy and hepatocellular carcinoma in patients with chronic hepatitis C. Osaka Hepatocellular Carcinoma Prevention Study Group. *Ann Intern Med.* 1998;129(2):94-99.
6. Schalm SW, Fattovich G, Brouwer JT. Therapy of hepatitis C: Patients with cirrhosis. *Hepatology.* 1997;26 (Suppl 1):128-132S.
7. Trotter JF, Wachs M, Everson GT, Kam I. Adult-to-adult transplantation of the right hepatic lobe from a living donor. *N Engl J Med.* 2002;346(14):1074-1082.
8. Shiffman ML, Di Bisceglie AM, Lindsay KL, et al. Peginterferon alfa-2a and ribavirin in patients with chronic hepatitis C who have failed prior treatment. *Gastroenterology.* 2004;126(4):1015-23.
9. Everson GT, et al. Impact of Disease Severity on Outcome of Antiviral Therapy for Chronic Hepatitis C: Lessons from the HALT-C Trial. *Hepatology.* 2006; 44:1675-1684.
10. Shiffman ML, Hofmann CM, Contos MJ, Luketic VA, Sanyal AJ, Sterling RK, Ferreira-Gonzalez A, et al. A randomized, controlled trial of maintenance interferon therapy for patients with chronic hepatitis C virus and persistent viremia. *Gastroenterology.* 1999;117:1164-1172.
11. McHutchison JG, Patel K, Schiff ER, et al. Clinical Trial: interferon alfa-2b continuous long-term therapy versus repeated 24 week cycles for re-treating chronic hepatitis C. *Aliment Pharmacol Ther.* 2008;27:422-432.
12. Lee WM, Dienstag JL, Lindsay KL, Lok AS, Bonkovsky HL, Shiffman ML, Everson GT, et al. Evolution of the HALT-C Trial: pegylated interferon as maintenance therapy for chronic hepatitis C in previous interferon nonresponders. *Controlled Clinical Trials.* 2004;25:472-492.
13. Di Bisceglie AM, et al. Prolonged Therapy of Advance Chronic Hepatitis C with low dose peginterferon. *N Engl J Med* 2008;in press.
14. Imai Y, Kawata S, Tamura S, Yabuuchi I, Noda S, Inada M, Maeda Y, et al. Relation of interferon therapy and hepatocellular carcinoma in patients with chronic hepatitis C. Osaka Hepatocellular Carcinoma Prevention Study Group. *Annals of Internal Medicine* 1998;129:94-99.
15. Yoshida H, Shiratori Y, Moriyama M, Arakawa Y, Ide T, Sata M, Inoue O, et al. Interferon therapy reduces the risk for hepatocellular carcinoma: national surveillance program of cirrhotic and noncirrhotic patients with chronic hepatitis C in Japan. *IHIT Study Group.* Inhibition of Hepatocarcinogenesis by Interferon Therapy. *Annals of Internal Medicine* 1999;131:174-181.
16. Fattovich G, Giustina G, Degos F, et al. Effectiveness of interferon alfa on incidence of hepatocellular carcinoma and decompensation in cirrhosis type C. *J Hepatol.* 1997;27(1):201-205.
17. Pestka SS. Langer JA, Zoon KC, Samual KC. Interferons and their actions. *Annu Rev Biochem.* 1987;56:727-777.
18. Fartoux L, Degos F, Trépo C, et al. Effect of prolonged interferon therapy on the outcome of hepatitis C virus related cirrhosis: a randomized trial. *Clin Gastroenterol Hepatol.* 2007 Apr;5(4):502-7.
19. Vertex Pharmaceuticals Press Release, June 9, 2008. Accessed online August 20, 2008 at investors.vrtx.com/releasedetail.cfm?ReleaseID=314874.

WESTERN (ALLOPATHIC) MEDICINE

Robert G. Gish, MD

FUTURE OF ALLOPATHIC HEPATITIS C TREATMENT

Introduction

Despite ongoing advances in treatments for *chronic hepatitis* C, more effective and safer treatments are still needed. About one-half of people infected with the hepatitis C virus (*HCV*) worldwide will not have a long-term response to the best current western therapy or to any treatments on the immediate horizon.

Progress has been made determining how HCV infects human cells. Cell culture models are now available to determine what medications work to stop HCV *replication*. These models have also advanced our understanding of how receptor sites allow HCV to enter cells and the processes in liver cells that allow HCV to thrive.

Despite these advances, we need to learn more about the hepatitis C virus itself. We need to know more about the virus *proteins* and how they help the virus multiply and infect other cells. We need a better understanding of how the *immune system* responds to the virus. Finally, we need a better understanding of disease progression. What causes hepatitis C to progress in some people but not in others? All this information will lead to the development of new *antiviral* agents. New therapies may be used as single agents. However, it is more likely they will be used in combination with current agents such as *interferon* and *ribavirin*.

This section discusses western therapies currently being studied as potential treatments for hepatitis C. Although some of the concepts are technical and may be challenging to understand, try not to let that keep you from seeing what the future might hold for hepatitis C treatment. Many of the medical and technical terms are defined in the *Glossary*. These definitions should make it easier to understand the concepts presented in this section.

There are many references in this section to *clinical trials*. If you are unfamiliar with the clinical trial process, it may be helpful to review the definitions of the different phases of clinical trials in the *Glossary*. As you read about potential therapies currently in development, keep in mind that many new drugs or treatments that appear promising in the laboratory, or in clinical trials are withdrawn from development because of unexpected side effects and/or lack of effectiveness. At the time this book was published (August 2008), there were more than 40 drugs in clinical development for HCV. However, in general, for every 100 drugs taken through *phase I* testing, only one will eventually be approved by the Food and Drug Administration (FDA).

Interferons

Pegylated Interferon

Interferon is an important, naturally occurring chemical produced in small quantities by many different cells of the body. Interferon helps regulate the body's *immune system*. Man-made versions of naturally occurring interferons are the mainstay of current treatment for hepatitis C. The first man-made interferons (standard interferons) were rapidly processed and eliminated from the body, making frequent dosing a necessity. These interferons were improved upon by attaching a molecule called polyethylene glycol (peg) to different sites on the interferon. The result is *pegylated interferon* or *peginterferon*. The kidneys do not clear pegylated interferon as quickly as standard interferon. Thus, pegylated interferon remains active in the body much longer than standard interferon does.[1-9] In theory, long-acting pegylated interferons deliver a more constant interferon dose than standard interferons. Because the drug is cleared from the body slowly, pegylated interferon can be given once a week. Although the activity of interferon is decreased by the attachment of peg molecules to it, the longer duration of action counteracts the reduction in immune activity. The effects of weekly pegylated interferon on the immune system and HCV are an enhanced version of those produced by standard interferon.

The FDA approved PegIntron® (pegylated interferon alfa-2b) as stand-alone for treatment of chronic hepatitis C in January 2001. It was approved for use in combination with ribavirin (Rebetol®) in August 2001. Pegasys® (pegylated interferon alfa-2a) has also been FDA-approved for use as stand-alone therapy or in combination with ribavirin. The overall *sustained response* rates with these two pegylated interferons in combination with ribavirin are approximately 53% to 55%.[10, 11] Emerging data show overall response rates with pegylated interferon plus ribavirin in the 60% range if patients are adherent with optimal dosing of both medications. Among people with HCV *genotype* 1, response rates of approximately 50% have been observed in patients taking weight-based doses of PegIntron® plus ribavirin (at full dose) or Pegasys® with weight-based doses of ribavirin.[12, 13]

The response rates to pegylated interferon plus ribavirin specifically among patients with *cirrhosis* or compensated *liver failure* are more modest than the overall response rates. One trial conducted exclusively among patients with cirrhosis reported a 29% sustained response rate with pegylated interferon alfa-2a compared to a 6% response rate with non-pegylated interferon alfa-2a. Another international, multi-center trial wherein 28% of the patients had cirrhosis reported that this group of patients had a overall sustained response rate of 39% with pegylated interferon alfa-2a compared to a 19% sustained response rate for non-pegylated interferon alfa-2a.[14, 15] In a large, multicenter randomized trial known as HALT-C, among patients who had not responded to previous therapy and had either cirrhosis or advanced fibrosis, the overall sustained response rate to pegylated interferon plus ribavirin was 18%.[16] Among these populations of so-called difficult to treat patients, which include patients who have undergone liver transplantation, there is clearly a need for safe treatments that will be effective in greater numbers of patients.

Other Interferons

Albinterferon alfa-2b (Albuferon™) is a long-acting interferon that has the potential for every 2 week or every 4 week dosing. The attachment of interferon alfa to the naturally occurring *protein albumin* keeps active interferon molecules circulating in the body for an extended period of time (a prolonged half-life). *Phase I/II clinical trial* data demonstrated albinterferon alfa-2b is well tolerated, has a prolonged half-life, and is biologically active in adults with chronic hepatitis C.[17] Albinterferon alfa-2b is in final, *phase III* development. Two large studies with this drug include treatment naïve patients with genotypes 1 and genotypes 2/3 using an every two week dosing schedule for albinterferon alfa-2b. Results are expected in early 2009.

Controlled-release recombinant interferon alfa-2b (Locteron™), omega interferon (being developed to be delivered by a continuous release device), and peginterferon lambda (interleukin 29) are in phase I-II clinical trials.

Possible treatment advances that may be possible with the successful development of longer acting interferons include:

- longer intervals between interferon dosing
- improved sustained viral response rates
- fewer treatment side effects

New delivery systems for interferons are also being explored including continuous release preparations, pumps, and depo preparations.

Therapies That Modulate the Immune Response

Vaccines

Vaccine research has historically focused on preventing infection. More recently, vaccine research has taken a new direction. Scientists are now attempting to develop vaccines to either protect people from developing chronic infection or to modify the course of chronic infection. A preliminary study conducted in chimpanzees found an experimental HCV vaccine led to the production of antibodies and inflammatory *T cells* (immune cells) against the virus. The experimental vaccine contained recombinant HCV envelope proteins (proteins found on the outside of the virus). The antibody and T cell responses observed in the chimpanzees prevented chronic HCV infection in the majority of the animals tested in this very small study.[18] A study reported in 2008 among hepatitis C patients who had not responded to prior therapy found that experiment vaccine IC41 resulted in T-cell proliferation in up to 67% who received the vaccine. However, significant reduction in *HCV RNA* was observed in only 3 of the 60 patients in the study.[19]

Recent advances in recombinant protein technology, novel vaccine *adjuvants*, and *DNA*-based vaccines are providing essential tools for the development of HCV vaccines. While several companies are working on developing therapeutic HCV vaccines, there has been no proven benefit to date. Although the preliminary research is encouraging, it will probably take many years to develop an effective HCV vaccine. Some of the many challenges of HCV vaccine research are described below.[20-24]

- HCV is difficult to grow in a laboratory setting.

  Vaccine development begins in the research laboratory where potential vaccine components are studied in animals and living cells. In the past, HCV was found only in humans and chimpanzees. A breakthrough was realized when scientists at the University of Alberta, Canada developed a mouse model that supports HCV replication.[25] An additional animal model called the Trimera mouse has been developed by XTL Pharmaceuticals. Cell culture models have also been reported. The discovery of these culture systems and animal models is an important step in HCV vaccine research. In addition, they will aid in drug discovery and our understanding of how HCV behaves in humans.

- HCV is highly susceptible to *mutation*. This characteristic of the virus makes it difficult to provide long-term, antibody-based *immunity*. Thus, an effective vaccine must stimulate T cells, immune system partners to the antibody-producing *B cells*. T cells interact directly and indirectly with HCV-infected cells and other immune cells.

  The underlying concept behind *vaccination* is that a vaccine will stimulate the immune system to respond to a specific infectious agent leading to elimination of the agent or limitation of its harmful activities. Immune system responses are highly specific. A specific antibody will react only with the agent that stimulated its production. This highly specific interaction is often described as being similar to a lock and key. HCV is known to mutate frequently, meaning the virus frequently makes small changes in its structure. These small changes may make the virus unrecognizable to specific antibodies against the virus. Therefore, developing a vaccine to stimulate the production of antibodies that will continue to recognize the virus long-term and provide protection is challenging.

- HCV can avoid detection by the human immune system.

  The immune system has a highly developed surveillance system to detect the presence of any substance foreign to the body (such as viruses and bacteria). The detection of an "invader" leads to a complex series of immune response that are intended to eliminate the invader. Thus, the detection of a foreign substance is the first step in the immune response. HCV appears to have the ability to escape detection by the immune system allowing the virus to flourish with little disruption.

- HCV-neutralizing immune cells (specific *CD4* and *CD8 T cells)* are not efficiently produced in all persons.

  As noted above, immune reactions are highly specific. Researchers have found that the cellular immune response to HCV varies from person to person. This may be partially responsible for the fact that some people clear HCV on their own while others do not. This variability could also be a factor in potential treatments and vaccines.

- HCV can become resistant to drug treatments.

As noted earlier, HCV is prone to mutations. These mutations can result in the emergence of resistance to specific treatments for HCV. Resistance to drug therapy refers to the ability of the virus to "escape" the effects of a drug and continue to multiply after an initial period of response. Drug resistance is caused by mutations in the genes of the virus. The evolution of HCV strains that are resistant to certain treatments is problematic for both vaccine and new drug development. The ability of HCV to develop resistance to drug therapy has been documented for a number of *protease* inhibitors.[26, 27] Studies with telaprevir and boceprevir have shown that resistant strains have poor replication efficiency and gradually fall to undectable levels after the therapy is stopped.[28-32]

To date, there has been no documented evidence of the development of resistance to ribavirin or interferon in persons undergoing HCV treatment. However, the emergence of treatment resistance remains a serious concern as more therapies are developed.

Immune Globulin Preparations

Approximately 22% to 29% of adults infected with HCV clear the virus through a naturally occurring immune process,[33] but approximately 70% to 80% do not. Studies suggest that children spontaneously clear HCV more often than adults do, especially those infected at a young age.[34]

While we do not yet know exactly how the immune system spontaneously clears HCV, we have discovered some of the mechanisms that allow HCV to persist in the body. HCV has the ability to rapidly change its structure (that is, to mutate). This helps the virus survive by allowing it to escape detection and recognition by the immune system's B cells and T cells. B cells produce antibodies (also called globulins). T cells are immune cells that interact directly with infectious agents and infected cells. For additional information on this topic, see *Chapter 7.2 The Immune System and Hepatitis C*.

Researchers are exploring the possible uses of antibody preparations (*immune globulin*) to treat HCV. Current development is focused on liver transplantation. Investigators theorize that immune globulins may prevent transplanted livers from becoming infected with HCV when they are placed in HCV-positive persons. If the use of immune globulin preparations is successful in this setting, they may be tested for prevention of HCV infection after accidental exposure to blood or body secretions.

Civacir™ is an antibody preparation targeted specifically to HCV. The initial clinical trials for the prevention of hepatitis C infection of transplanted livers among HCV-infected transplant patients did not show any clinical benefit.[35] HCV-AB[XTL]-68 has also been studied for the prevention of reinfection in HCV-positive people undergoing liver transplantation. The study concluded HCV-AB[XTL]-68 may decrease viral load after transplantation, but further studies are needed.[36]

Products Derived from Thymus Extracts

The *thymus gland* is a small structure located in the chest under the breastbone. It is an important part of the immune system. Immune cells called *lymphocytes* are formed in the bone marrow. Lymphocytes that travel to the thymus gland to mature become *T lymphocytes* or T cells. T cells are the primary actors involved in the cellular immune response, which is particularly important in battling viral infections.

Thymosin fraction 5 and thymalfasin (Zadaxin®, also known as thymosin alfa-1) are two special types of proteins called *cytokines* derived from the thymus gland. Cytokines are produced by many cell types in the body. They cause specific reactions, many of which are important for immune function. Thymosin fraction 5 and thymalfasin may be able to change a person's response to HCV infection.[37] These compounds are being studied to determine if they are capable of preventing chronic HCV infection, or of slowing or halting disease progression.

Thymalfasin stimulates the immune system. Abnormally low levels of thymalfasin have been found in people chronically infected with the *hepatitis B* virus (HBV).[38] Initial studies in HBV-infected animals and humans suggested that thymalfasin and thymosin factor 5 increase the rate of *clearance* of HBV DNA (the genetic material of the virus).[39-41] However, another study showed no difference in HBV clearance when thymalfasin was compared to a *placebo* (an inactive substance). Therefore, the results from these studies were inconclusive. Small, preliminary studies suggested that the addition of thymalfasin to interferon-based therapy for HCV may enhance treatment response.[42, 43] However, two large phase III studies of thymalfasin in combination with Pegasys® (without ribavirin) were recently completed and showed no efficacy for the treatment of HCV-infected people who were non-responders to previous interferon plus ribavirin therapy. A phase III trial of thymalfasin in combination with pegylated interferon alfa and ribavirin is currently being conducted in Europe.

Other Therapies That Modulate the Immune System

Interferon works by stimulating the immune system. Currently, noninterferon substances that also stimulate the immune system are being explored as possible HCV treatments.

Toll-like receptor (TLR) agonists are a class of small molecules that specifically stimulate the innate immune system. Research has shown that these molecules have antiviral activity, but none have yet proven both safe and effective. For more information on how this class of drugs works, see *Chapter 7.2 The Immune System and Hepatitis C.*

GI-5005 is another substance that is being evaluated for its potential to enhance the body's cellular immune response to HCV. A phase II study of combination therapy with GI-5005 in combination with pegylated interferon plus ribavirin in genotype 1 *nonresponders* is underway.

STAT-C: Specifically Targeted Antiviral Therapy for HCV

Interferon-based therapy for hepatitis C is based on that notion that by enhancing the body's immune response to hepatitis C, it will be able to effectively clear the virus. In other words, interferon-based therapy boosts the immune system to that it can kill the virus.

Emerging therapies take a different, more direct approach. These agents are designed to interfere with the virus directly by targeting molecules essential to the lifecycle and replication of the hepatitis C virus. These agents are collectively referred to as STAT-C (specifically targeted antiviral therapy for HCV).

The total genetic blueprint of any living organism is called its genome. The genome contains the specific information that makes a tree a tree, a virus a virus, and a human a human. The genome is made up of individual genes. Each gene has the blueprint or code for a specific protein. The types of proteins made by an organism determine how it lives, functions, and survives.

The HCV genome contains the code for ten building blocks that make up the "house" the virus lives in and the machinery needed for the virus to make more copies of itself (replication). New virus particles infect other liver cells and can infect other people.[44] The machinery proteins of HCV act primarily as enzymes, which are needed for viral replication (reproduction) and processing other proteins. Enzymes are specialized proteins that are necessary for various chemical reactions.

Several HCV enzymes (called *proteases*, *helicases*, and *polymerases*) are the targets of STAT-C therapies currently in development. Researchers theorize that if the function of one or more of these enzymes can be interrupted, the replication and damage caused by HCV may also be interrupted. Several pharmaceutical companies are currently developing molecules that act as HCV enzyme inhibitors.

It is important to recognize there are many barriers to overcome in the development of effective HCV enzyme inhibitors. Such barriers include the need for inhibitors to have activity against a broad range of virus genotypes and *quasispecies*, and the potential development of resistance to the drugs. Due to the development of resistance with this class of drugs, it is unlikely in the near future that they will be considered for *monotherapy*.

Protease Inhibitors

NS3 is a non-structural (NS) protein encoded by the HCV genome. The protein is a specific type of enzyme called a serine protease. This protein is one of the potential targets for HCV inhibitor research.

Two promising protease inhibitors are currently going into *phase III clinical trials*, telaprevir and boceprevir. These agents are taken by mouth, and are intended to be used in conjunction with interferon-based therapy.

The results of the first phase I clinical trial of telaprevir (VX-950) were presented in late 2005. Three phase II clinical trials, PROVE 1, 2, and 3, were subsequently launched. PROVE 1 (conducted in the U.S.) evaluated short-duration therapy with telaprevir (VX-950) in combination with pegylated interferon and ribavirin in treatment-naive, genotype 1-infected patients. Sustained viral response was reported for 61% of those that received 24 weeks of treatment, and 67% for those receiving 48 weeks of treatment.[45]

PROVE 2 (conducted in Europe with a trial design like PROVE 1) researchers reported sustained viral response in 62% of those treated for 24 weeks and 68% in those that received 36 weeks of treatment. There was a greater incidence of rash in the telaprevir arms of these trials than in the control groups that were given pegylated interferon and ribavirin alone.[46]

PROVE 3 is an ongoing phase IIb study evaluating telaprevir-based treatment in patients with genotype 1 chronic hepatitis C virus (HCV) infection who did not achieve sustained virologic response (SVR) with at least one prior pegylated interferon (peg-*IFN)* and ribavirin (RBV) regimen. Interim results were reported in June 2008. Fifty-two percent of patients randomized to receive treatment with a 24-week telaprevir-based regimen (12 weeks of telaprevir in combination with peg-IFN and RBV, followed by 12 weeks of peg-IFN and RBV alone) maintained undetectable HCV RNA 12 weeks post-treatment. PROVE 3 is ongoing, and an additional phase III trial to be conducted among prior nonresponders is planned.[47]

Telaprevir resistance has been observed, but the rate of resistance to the drug is substantially reduced when used together with pegylated interferon.[48-51]

Boceprevir (SCH 503034) is another oral NS3 protease inhibitor currently in development. A phase I study found the drug to be well-tolerated and reduced HCV viral loads were observed.[52-54] In August 2008, preliminary data from a phase II study were reported. The group treated with a lead-in phase of Peg-Intron® plus ribavirin (standard doses) for 4 weeks followed with triple therapy (boceprevir/ Peg-Intron®/ribavirin) for another 44 weeks achieved 74% SVR12 (continued undetectable viral load 12 weeks after treatment ends). Patients who received 48-weeks of triple therapy (boceprevir/ Peg-Intron®/ribavirin) but who did not have a lead-in phase achieved a 66% SVR 12 weeks after the end of treatment.[55]

As with telaprevir, boceprevir resistance has been reported but is reduced when the drug is used in combination with pegylated interferon.[30, 56]

The clinical trial data for these protease inhibitors are promising. However, the upcoming phase III trial data will be important in determining how more diverse groups of patients respond to interferon and ribavirin therapy plus telaprevir or boceprevir.

TMC435350 is third oral NS3 protease inhibitor that will be evaluated in a phase II trial, genotype 1 known as OPERA 1. Whereas both telaprevir and boceprevir are taken three times daily, the developers of TMC435350 will be exploring a once daily dosing schedule in the OPERA 1 study. Phase I trial data indicate that TMC435350 is well-tolerated.[57]

Polymerase Inhibitors

The HCV RNA-dependent RNA polymerase is a key viral enzyme responsible for HCV replication. Potential target sites in this protein for polymerase inhibition include the polymerase active site, the GTP-binding site, nucleotide binding sites, and the template RNA binding groove.[58] Several companies are also developing drugs to target other key sites of the HCV RNA-dependent RNA polymerase cascade. Nine companies currently have drugs in phase I or II clinical trials.[59]

The polymerase inhibitor furthest along in clinical development at the time of this writing (August 2008) is oral drug R1626. The drug has been shown to be effective in significantly reducing HCV viral load both alone[60] and in combination with pegylated interferon plus ribavirin. Interim results from an ongoing phase II clinical trial indicated that 81% of patients receiving triple therapy (R1626/pegylated interferon/ribavirin) had undetectable HCV RNA at 4 weeks after the start of therapy[61] and 84% were virus-negative at the end of treatment.[62] No evidence of resistance to R1626 has been detected to date.[63] However, R1626 has been associated with high rates of significant leukopenia (a low white blood cell count), which could limit dosing and influence rates of effectiveness. Further study is needed into the appropriate balance between safety and effectiveness with this drug.

Anti-sense Oligonucleotides

The genome of a living organism exists in the form of either RNA (*ribonucleic acid*) or DNA (*deoxyribonucleic acid*), depending upon the type of organism. The HCV genome is made of RNA; the human genome is made of DNA. Because HCV "borrows" the protein-making machinery of human cells during replication, the blueprint for HCV's specific proteins must be "read" or translated into DNA before HCV proteins can be produced. Anti-sense oligonucleotides are small pieces of DNA or RNA molecules that are designed to block the "reading" (translation) of viral RNA.[64] ISIS 14803 (Isis Pharmaceuticals) is an antisense medication that inhibits HCV replication and protein production and release in cell cultures and animals. However, ISIS 14803 reduced HCV viral load only moderately in a small number of patients recently who experienced a high level of liver enzymes. This medication may possess direct antiviral effects or works through general immune stimulation. Development was discontinued, but it is unclear if other anti-sense oligonucleotides may have a role in HCV therapies of the future.

Ribozymes

At one time, scientists believed all enzymes were proteins. However approximately 20 years ago, researchers discovered that certain RNA molecules can act as enzymes. These specialized RNA molecules are called *ribozymes*. They act by binding to and cutting (cleaving) specific sites of larger RNA molecules.[65] *Anti-HCV* ribozymes have been developed in the laboratory. However, there were serious side effects when these molecules were administered to animals. Because of the toxicity of the anti-HCV ribozymes developed to date, further development has been halted for the time being. It is unclear whether ribozymes may have a role in therapy for chronic hepatitis C at some time in the future.

Ribozymes are RNA molecules that bind to and break specific RNA messages. Hepatzyme is an IRES-specific ribozyme that has also been investigated in phase II trials. However, development of this agent was halted because of heart problems in monkey. Whether other ribozymes may be developed as potential HCV therapies is yet to be determined.

Short Interfering RNAs

During the replication process of many viruses, including HCV, two strands of RNA come together to form a double-stranded RNA molecule (dsRNA). An enzyme called DICER binds to and cuts (cleaves) dsRNA. *0* (siRNA) molecules are small pieces of dsRNA produced when larger lengths of dsRNA are cleaved (see Figure 1).

Figure 1. Formation of siRNA

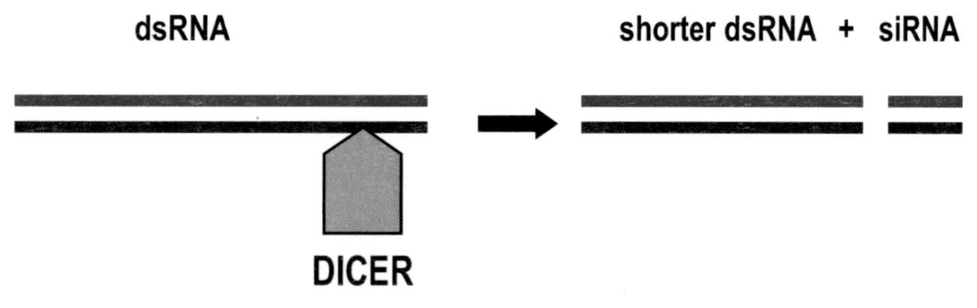

dsRNA → shorter dsRNA + siRNA

DICER

siRNA molecules bind with proteins to form a unit called the RNA-induced silencing complex (RISC). Through a series of complex interactions, RISC suppresses the expression of the gene it corresponds to in the viral genome. In other words, the gene from which the siRNA is derived is silenced. In theory, the ability to silence specific genes in the HCV viral genome could prevent viral replication. Recent studies have confirmed this theory. HCV-specific siRNAs have been shown to block HCV replication and protein expression.[66] These early findings suggest that RNA interference may have a role in treating people with chronic hepatitis C. It is yet to be determined whether siRNA molecules, which are relatively large compared to other molecules used to treat HCV, can be delivered in such a way that they are able to reach the site of viral replication inside infected cells.

Companies are currently conducting research to determine if products that work by this mechanism may be useful in the treatment of hepatitis C.

Therapies Targeting Host Factors

Another tack being taken in developing new therapies for HCV is to target molecular sites in the host (the patient) that may help in viral clearance.

Cyclophilin B Inhibitors

Cyclophilin B is a naturally occurring substance in the body that acts as a regulator of not only the immune system but also the HCV RNA-dependent RNA polymerase. In theory, inhibitors of cyclophilin B may well inhibit the activity of the HCV viral polymerase thereby halting viral replication.

DEBIO-025 has been evaluated in a phase Ib study of HIV/HCV coinfected patients. In this study, DEBIO-025 was found to be associated with significant reductions in both cyclophilin B and HCV viral load.[67, 68] Interim results from a phase II study of DEBIO-025 conducted in HCV monoinfected patients have been reported indicating that 66% of genotype 1/4 patients treated with 1,000 mg of DEBIO-025 daily plus pegylated interferon were virus negative at day 29.[69] Another phase II trial with DEBIO-025 is underway in interferon nonresponders.

Another cyclophilin B inhibitor in early clinical development is NIM811, which has shown antiviral activity against HCV that is enhanced in the presence of pegylated interferon.[70, 71]

Nitazoxanide

Nitazoxanide is a drug that is already on the market to treat protozoal infections such as giardiasis and cryptosporidiosis. Recently, researchers have found that nitazoxanide inhibits HCV replication, which has led to clinical studies to examine the use of this drug to treat hepatitis C.[72] In a study of Egyptian patients with genotype 4 infection, 79% of patients who received triple drug therapy (nitazoxanide/pegylated interferon/ribavirin) had a sustained viral response compared to 50% in those receiving only pegylated interferon plus ribavirin.[73] A phase II U.S. study among genotype 1 nonresponders is underway, and a phase II trial among genotype 1 patients who have not previously been treated is planned.[74]

Anti-Fibrotic Therapy

The liver damage caused by HCV is largely the result of an inflammatory response that leads to fibrosis. For people who do not respond to therapy it is important to find another way to mitigate the damage caused by HCV in the liver. To this end, companies are currently investigating therapies to slow down or prevent liver damage caused by the hepatitis C virus.

Ribavarin Analogues

Ribavirin is one component of current standard therapy. It is described as a nucleoside-like antiviral drug. Its structure resembles that of nucleosides, the building blocks of the gene-carrying molecules DNA and RNA. Ribavirin is minimally effective against HCV when used as monotherapy and has a troublesome side-effect profile. Several pharmaceutical companies are currently involved in developing improved versions of ribavirin. The new compounds are chemically altered versions of ribavirin and are known collectively as ribavirin analogues.

Taribavirin (also known as Viramidine)

Taribavirin is a liver-targeting prodrug of ribavirin. Taribavirin is converted to ribavirin by an enzyme called adenosine deaminase (ADA). The liver is rich in ADA, which leads to a higher concentration of ribavirin in the liver compared to other tissues when taribavirin is taken by mouth.

Two phase III clinical trials of taribavirin in combination with pegylated interferon alfa-2b (VISER1 and VISER2) lower rates of anemia but also lower SVRs compared to pegylated interferon alfa-2b plus ribavirin.[75, 76] A subsequent phase IIb study using pegylated interferon alfa-2b plus weight-base dosing of either taribavirin or ribavirin revealed equivalent rates of HCV RNA clearance with the two drugs but significantly less anemia associated with taribavirin.[77] The study is expected to continue through to end of treatment (48 weeks) and posttreatment (72 weeks) endpoints.

Future of Non-Western Treatments

One goal of researchers and practitioners of *complementary and alternative medicine* (CAM) is to determine the role of CAM therapies in the management of hepatitis C. This is important for both people living with HCV and their healthcare providers.

The role of herbal and other therapies in controlling *arthralgia*, *myalgia*, mental fogginess, and *fatigue* is clear to individual patients. However, research data are needed to support broad usage of these agents in symptom management across diverse populations. The possible anti-inflammatory role of herbal therapies to prevent or slow disease progression must also be explored. Carefully designed clinical trials may determine which therapies are most beneficial to specific subgroups of people with HCV. For instance, herbal therapy and acupuncture may benefit people with joint pain. Large-scale clinical studies are needed to obtain conclusive information about the efficacy of CAM therapies for these and other signs and symptoms of HCV. A series of anecdotes is not sufficient. NCCAM is currently sponsoring clinical trials using milk thistle in people with chronic liver disease.

Clinical research may clarify whether the use of CAM approaches is safe and beneficial in combination with western therapies. Such studies may also determine if CAM therapies are useful to control side effects of western therapies. Safety is an important issue since many CAM therapies have been anecdotally reported to cause side effects that may be serious. We need to determine the actual incidence of these reported side effects and document their severity with carefully designed clinical studies.

Proving the presence or absence of antiviral effects of nonwestern therapy is important. Some CAM practitioners claim to be able to cure HCV with a variety of therapies. But these claims are poorly documented. Scientifically sound studies are needed to discover which, if any, CAM agents have clinical benefit. Herbal remedies may actually decrease liver inflammation, the early component of liver disease that can lead to fibrosis and cirrhosis. Prevention of the development of cirrhosis would be of great benefit to people with chronic HCV who cannot be cured with interferon-based therapy. Integrative medicine utilizes both western and CAM therapies. For information on the integrative medicine approach to hepatitis C management, see *Chapter 9*.

References

1. Xu ZX, Hoffman J, Patel I, Joubert P. Single-dose safety/tolerability and pharmacokinetics/ pharmacodynamics (PK/PD) following administration of ascending subcutaneous doses of pegylated-interferon (PEG-IFN) and interferon alfa-2a (IFN alfa-2a) to healthy subjects. *Hepatology.* 1998;28:A702.
2. Heathcote EJ, Fried MW, Bain MA, DePamphilis J, Modi M. The pharmacokinetics of pegylated-40K interferon alfa-2A (PEG-IFN) in chronic hepatitis C (CHC) patients with cirrhosis. *Gastroenterology* 1999;116:A735.
3. Reddy KR. Controlled-release, pegylation, liposomal formulations: new mechanisms in the delivery of injectable drugs. *Ann Pharmacother.* 2000; 34(7-8):915-923.
4. Healthcote EJ, Shiffman ML, Cooksley WG, et al. Peginterferon alfa-2a in patients with chronic hepatitis C and cirrhosis. *N Engl J Med.* 2000;343(23):1673-1680.
5. Kozlowski A, Harris JM. Improvements in protein PEGylation: pegylated interferons for treatment of hepatitis C. *J Control Release.* 2001; 72(1-3):217-224.
6. Jen JF, Glue P, Ezzet F, Chung C, Gupta SK, Jacobs S et al. Population pharmacokinetic analysis of pegylated interferon alfa-2b and interferon alfa-2b in patients with chronic hepatitis C. *Clin Pharmacol Ther.* 2001; 69(6):407-421.
7. Lindsay KL, Trepo C, Heintges T, et al. A randomized, double-blind trial comparing pegylated interferon alfa-2b to interferon alfa-2b as initial treatment for chronic hepatitis C. *Hepatology.* 2001;34(2):395-403.
8. Bailon P, Palleroni A, Schaffer CA, Spence CL, Fung WJ, Porter JE et al. Rational design of a potent, long-lasting form of interferon: a 40 kDa branched polyethylene glycol-conjugated interferon alfa-2a for the treatment of hepatitis C. *Bioconjug Chem.* 2001; 12(2):195-202.
9. Glue P, Fang JW, Rouzier-Panis R, Raffanel C, Sabo R, Gupta SK et al. Pegylated interferon-alfa2b: pharmacokinetics, pharmacodynamics, safety, and preliminary efficacy data. Hepatitis C Intervention Therapy Group. *Clin Pharmacol Ther.* 2000; 68(5):556-567
10. Fried MW, Shiffman ML, Reddy KR, Smith C, Marinos G, Goncales FL, Jr. et al. Peginterferon alfa-2a plus ribavirin for chronic hepatitis C virus infection. *N Engl J Med.* 2002; 347(13):975-982.
11. Manns MP, McHutchison JG, Gordon SC, Rustgi VK, Shiffman M, Reindollar R et al. Peginterferon alfa-2b plus ribavirin compared with interferon alfa-2b plus ribavirin for initial treatment of chronic hepatitis C: a randomised trial. *Lancet.* 2001; 358(9286):958-965.
12. McHutchison JG, Manns M, Patel K, Poynard T, Lindsay KL, Trepo C et al. Adherence to combination therapy enhances sustained response in genotype-1-infected patients with chronic hepatitis C. *Gastroenterology.* 2002; 123(4):1061-1069.
13. Fried MW, Hadziyannis SJ. Treatment of chronic hepatitis C infection with peginterferons plus ribavirin. *Semin Liver Dis.* 2004;24 Suppl 2:47-54.
14. Zeuzem S. Treatment of chronic hepatitis C virus infection in patients with cirrhosis. *J Viral Hepat.* 2000; 7(5):327-334.
15. Zeuzem S, Herrmann E, Lee JH, et al. Viral kinetics in patients with chronic hepatitis C treated with standard or peginterferon alfa-2a. *Gastroenterology.* 2001;120(6):1438-1447.
16. Shiffman ML, Di Bisceglie AM, Lindsay KL, et al. Peginterferon alfa-2a and ribavirin in patients with chronic hepatitis C who have failed prior treatment. *Gastroenterology.* 2004 Apr;126(4):1015-23.
17. Davis GL, et al. A phase I study to evaluate the pharmacokinetics, safety, and tolerability of escalating doses of a novel recombinant human albumin-interferon-α fusion protein (Albuferon™) in subjects with chronic hepatitis C. Abstract 490. 53rd Annual Meeting of the American Association for the Study of Liver Diseases. November 2002. Boston, Massachusetts.
18. Abrignani S, Houghton M, Hsu HH. Perspectives for a vaccine against hepatitis C virus. *J Hepatology* 1999;31(Suppl 1):259-263.
19. Klade CS, Wedemeyer H, Berg T, et al, Therapeutic vaccination of chronic hepatitis C nonresponder patients with the peptide vaccine IC41. *Gastroenterology.* 2008 May;134(5):1385-95.
20. Hsu HH, Abrignani S, Houghton M. Prospects for a hepatitis C virus vaccine. *Clin Liver Dis.* 1999; 3(4):901-915.
21. Lechmann M, Liang TJ. Vaccine development for hepatitis C. *Semin Liver Dis.* 2000; 20(2):211-226.
22. Rosenberg S. Recent advances in the molecular biology of hepatitis C virus. *J Mol Biol.* 2001; 313(3):451-464.
23. Beyene A, Basu A, Meyer K, Ray R. Hepatitis C virus envelope glycoproteins and potential for vaccine development. *Vox Sang.* 2002; 83 Suppl 1:27-32.
24. Inchauspe G, Feinstone S. Development of a hepatitis C virus vaccine. *Clin Liver Dis.* 2003; 7(1):243-59
25. Tyrell DL, et al. Development of a mouse model to support hepatitis C viral replication. Frontiers for Drug Development. Abstract 024. HepDART 2001. Maui, Hawaii. 2001.
26. Yi M, Tong X, Skelton A, et al. Mutations conferring resistance to SCH6, a novel hepatitis C virus NS3/4A protease inhibitor. Reduced RNA replication fitness and partial rescue by second-site mutations. *J Biol Chem.* 2006;281(12):8205-15.
27. Mo H, Lu L, Pilot-Matias T, et al. Mutations conferring resistance to a hepatitis C virus (HCV) RNA-dependent RNA polymerase inhibitor alone or in combination with an HCV serine protease inhibitor in vitro. *Antimicrob Agents Chemother.* 2005;49(10):4305-14.
28. Lawitz EJ, et al. 28 days of the hepatitis C protease inhibitor VX-950 in combination with peg-interferon alfa-2a and ribavirin is well-tolorated and demonstrates robust antiviral effects (abstract). *Gastroenterology.* 2006; 130:686.
29. Courcambeck J, Bouzidi M, Perbost R, et al. Resistance of hepatitis C virus to NS3-4A protease inhibitors: mechanisms of drug resistance induced by R155Q, A156T, D168A and D168V mutations. *Antivir Ther.* 2006;11:847-855.
30. Tong X, et al. Identification and analysis of fitness of resistance mutations against the HCV protease inhibitor SCH 503034. *Antiviral Res.* 2006;70:28-38.
31. Kieffer T, et al. Combination of Telaprevir (VX-950) and peg-IFN-alfa suppresses both wild-type virus and resistance variants in HCV genotype 1 infected patients in a 14-day phase 1b study. Program and abstracts of the 57th Annual Meeting of the American Association for the Study of Liver Diseases. October 27-31, 2006. Boston, Massachusetts.
32. Forestier N, et al. Current status of subjects receiving peginterferon alfa-2a and ribavirin after a 14-day study of the hepatitis C protease inhibitor Telaprevir (VX-950), with peginterferon alfa-2a. Program and abstracts of the 57th Annual Meeting of the American Association for the Study of Liver Diseases. October 27-31, 2006. Boston, Massachusetts

33. Micallef JM, Kaldor JM, Dore GJ. Spontaneous viral clearance following acute hepatitis C infection: a systematic review of longitudinal studies. *J Viral Hepat.* 2006;13(1):34-41.

34. Zhang M, Rosenberg PS, Brown DL, et al. Correlates of spontaneous clearance of hepatitis C virus among people with hemophilia. *Blood.* 2006;107(3):892-7.

35. Davis GL, Nelson DR, Terrault N, et al. A randomized, open-label study to evaluate the safety and pharmacokinetics of human hepatitis C immune globulin (Civacir) in liver transplant recipients. *Liver Transpl.* 2005;11(8):941-9.

36. Schiano TD, Charlton M, Younossi Z, et al. Monoclonal antibody HCV-AbXTL68 in patients undergoing liver transplantation for HCV: results of a phase 2 randomized study. *Liver Transpl.* 2006 Sep;12(9):1381-9.

37. Fattovich G, Giustina G, Alberti A, et al. A randomized controlled trial of thymopentin therapy in patients with chronic hepatitis B. *J Hepatol.* 1994;21:361-366.

38. Eichberg JW, Seeff LB, Lawlor DL, et al. Effect of thymosin immunostimulation with and without corticosteroid immunosuppression on chimpanzee hepatitis B carriers. *J Med Virol.* 1987;21(1):25-37.

39. Davis GL. Treatment of chronic hepatitis B. *Hepatology.* 1991;14(3):567-569.

40. Mutchnick MG, Lindsay KL, Schiff ER, et al. Thymosin a-1 treatment of chronic hepatitis B: a multicenter randomized, placebo-controlled double blind study. *Gastroenterology.* 1995;108:A1127.

41. Saruc M, Ozden N, Turkel N, Ayhan S, Hock LM, Tuzcuoglu I, Yuceyar H. Long-term outcomes of thymosin-alfa 1 and interferon alfa-2b combination therapy in patients with hepatitis B e antigen (HBeAg) negative chronic hepatitis B. *J Pharm Sci.* 2003;92(7):1386-95.

42. Rasi G, DiVirgilio D, Mutchnick MG, et al. Combination thymosin alfa 1 and lymphoblastoid interferon treatment in chronic hepatitis C. *Gut.* 1996;39(5):679-683.

43. Andreone P, Gramenzi A, Cursaro C, et al. Thymosin-alfa 1 plus interferon-alfa for naïve patients with chronic hepatitis C: results of a randomized controlled pilot trial. *J Viral Hepat.* 2004;11(1):69-73.

44. Penin F, Dubuisson J, Rey FA, Moradpour D, Pawlotsky JM. Structural biology of hepatitis C virus. *Hepatology.* 2004;39(1):5-19.

45. McHutchison G, Everson GT, Gordon SC, et al. PROVE1: results from a phase 2 study of telaprevir with peginterferon alfa-2a and ribavirin in treatment-naive subjects with hepatitis C. Program and abstracts of the 43rd Annual Meeting of the European Association for the Study of the Liver; April 23-27, 2008; Milan, Italy. Abstract 4.

46. Dusheiko GM, Hézode C, Pol S, et al. Treatment of chronic hepatitis C with telaprevir (TVR) in combination with peginterferon alfa-2a with or without ribavirin: Further interim analysis results of the PROVE2 study. Program and abstracts of the 43rd Annual Meeting of the European Association for the Study of the Liver; April 23-27, 2008; Milan, Italy. Abstract 58.

47. Vertex Pharmaceuticals Press Release, June 9, 2008. Available at: http://investors.vrtx.com/releasedetail.cfm?ReleaseID=314874. Accessed August 20, 2008

48. Keiffer TL, Sarrazin C, Miller JS, et al. Telaprevir and pegylated interferon-alfa-2a inhibit wild-type and resistant genotype 1 hepatitis C virus replication in patients. *Hepatology.* 2007;46:631-639.

49. Kieffer T, Sarrazin C, Miller J, et al. Combination of telaprevir (VX-950) and peg-IFN-alfa suppresses both wild-type virus and resistance variants in HCV genotype 1-infected patients in a 14-day phase 1b study. Program and abstracts of the 57th Annual Meeting of the American Association for the Study of Liver Diseases; October 27-31, 2006; Boston, Massachusetts. Abstract 92.

50. McCown M, Rajyaguru S, Symons J, Cammack N, Najera I. In vitro resistance selection to the HCV nucleoside polymerase inhibitor R1479 and to the protease inhibitor VX-950. Program and abstracts of the 42nd Annual Meeting of the European Association for the Study of the Liver; April 11-15, 2007; Barcelona, Spain. Abstract 790.

51. Kieffer T, Zhou Y, Zhang E, et al. Evaluation of viral variants during a phase 2 study (PROVE2) of telaprevir with peginterferon alfa-2a and ribavirin in treatment-naive HCV genotype 1-infected patients. Program and abstracts of the 58th Annual Meeting of the American Association for the Study of Liver Diseases; November 2-6, 2007; Boston, Massachusetts. Abstract LB8.

52. Zhang J, Gupta S, Rouzier R, et al. Single dose pharmacokinetics of a novel hepatitis C protease inhibitor, SCH 503034, in an oral capsule formulation. Abstract 862. *Hepatology.* 2005;42(4) Suppl. 1: 535A.

53. Zeuzem S, Sarrazin C, Rouzier R, et al. Antiviral activity of SCH 503034, a HCV protease inhibitor, administered as monotherapy in hepatitis C genotype-1 (HCV-1) patients refractory to pegylated interferon (Peg-IFN-a). Abstract 94. *Hepatology.* 2005;42(4) Suppl. 1: 233A.

54. Zeuzem S et al. Combination therapy with the HCV protease inhibitor, SCH 503034, plus PEG-INTRON in hepatitis C genotype-1 PEG-INTRON nonresponders: phase Ib results. Abstract 201. *Hepatology.* 2005;42(4) Suppl. 1: 276A.

55. Schering-Plough Corporation Press Release, August 4, 2008. Available at: http://www.prnewswire.com/cgi-bin/stories.pl?ACCT=104&STORY=/www/story/08-04-2008/0004860889&EDATE. Accessed online August 25, 2008

56. Susser S, Welker MW, Zettler M, et al. Genotypic and phenotypic characterisation of mutations within the HCV NS3 protease in HCV genotype 1 infected patients treated with the protease inhibitor boceprevir (SCH503034). Program and abstracts of the Conference Hepatitis B and C Virus Resistance to Antiviral Therapies; February 14-16, 2008; Paris, France. Poster 54.

57. Verloes R, Farha KA, van Vliet A, et al. Results of a phase I placebo-controlled trial in healthy volunteers to examine the safety, tolerability, and pharmacokinetics of the HCV protease inhibitor TMC435350 after single and repeated dosing. Program and abstracts of the 58th Annual Meeting of the American Association for the Study of Liver Diseases; November 2-6, 2007; Boston, Massachusetts. Abstract 1318.

58. Pawlotsky JM & McHutchison JG. Hepatitis C. Development of new drugs and clinical trials: promises and pitfalls. Summary of an AASLD hepatitis single topic conference, Chicago, IL, February 27-March 1, 2003. *Hepatology* 2004; 39:554-567.

59. Franciscus A, Hepatitis C Treatments in Current Clinical Development. Available at: http://www.hcvadvocate.org/hepatitis/hepC/HCVDrugs.html. Accessed on August 8, 2008

60. Roberts S, Cooksley G, Dore G, et al. Results of a phase 1B, multiple dose study of R1626, a novel nucleoside analog targeting HCV polymerase in chronic HCV genotype 1 patients. Program and abstracts of the 57th Annual Meeting of the American Association for the Study of Liver Diseases; October 27-31, 2006; Boston, Massachusetts. Abstract LB2.

61. Pockros PJ, Nelson D, Godofsky E, et al. Robust synergistic antiviral effect of R1626 in combination with peginterferon alfa-2a (40KD), with or without ribavirin: interim analysis results of phase 2a study. Program and abstracts of the 58th Annual Meeting of the American Association for the Study of Liver Diseases; November 2-6, 2007; Boston, Massachusetts. Abstract 167.

62. Nelson D, Pockros PJ, Godofsky E, et al. High end-of-treatment response (84%) after 4 weeks of R1626, peginterferon alfa-2a (40kd) and ribavirin followed by a further 44 weeks of peginterferon alfa-2a and ribavirin. Program and abstracts of the 43rd Annual Meeting of the European Association for the Study of the Liver; April 23-27, 2008; Milan, Italy. Abstract 993.

63. Le Pogam S, Seshaadri A, Kosaka A, et al. A high barrier to resistance may contribute to the robust antiviral effect demonstrated by R1626 in HCV genotype 1-infected treatment-naive patients. Program and abstracts of the 58th Annual Meeting of the American Association for the Study of Liver Diseases; November 2-6, 2007; Boston, Massachusetts. Abstract 1298.

64. Dias N, Stein CA. Antisense oligonucleotides: basic concepts and mechanisms. *Mol.Cancer Ther.* 2002;1:347-355.

65. Lee PA, Blatt LM, Blanchard KS, et al. Pharmacokinetics and tissue distribution of a ribozyme directed against hepatitis C virus RNA following subcutaneous or intravenous administration in mice. *Hepatology.* 2000;32:640-646.

66. Kapadia SB, Brideau-Andersen A, Chisari FV. Interference of hepatitis C virus RNA replication by short interfering RNAs. *Proc Natl Acad Sci U S A.* 2003;100(4):2014-2018.

67. Flisiak R, Horban A, Kierkus J, et al. The cyclophilin inhibitor DEBIO-025 has a potent dual anti-HIV and anti-HCV activity in treatment-naive HIV/HCV co-infected subjects. Program and abstracts of the 57th Annual Meeting of the American Association for the Study of Liver Diseases; October 27-31, 2006; Boston, Massachusetts. Abstract 1130.

68. Flisiak R, Horban A, Gallay P, et al. The cyclophilin inhibitor Debio-025 shows potent anti-hepatitis C effect in patients coinfected with hepatitis C and human immunodeficiency virus. *Hepatology.* 2008;47:817-826.

69. Schiff ER, Everson GT, Tsai N, et al. HCV-specific cellular immunity, RNA reductions, and normalization of ALT in chronic HCV subjects after treatment with GI-5005, a yeast-based immunotherapy targeting NS3 and core: a randomized, double-blind, placebo-controlled phase 1b study. Program and abstracts of the 58th Annual Meeting of the American Association for the Study of Liver Diseases; November 2-6, 2007; Boston, Massachusetts. Abstract 1304.

70. Goto K, Watashi K, Murata T, Hishiki T, Hijikata M, Shimotohno K. Evaluation of the anti-hepatitis C virus effects of cyclophilin inhibitors, cyclosporin A, and NIM811. *Biochem Biophys Res Commun.* 2006;343:879-884.

71. Lin K, Boerner J, Ma S, Compton T. NIM811, a cyclophilin inhibitor, and NM107, an HCV polymerase inhibitor, synergistically inhibit HCV replication and suppress the emergence of resistance in vitro. Program and abstracts of the 42nd Annual Meeting of the European Association for the Study of the Liver; April 11-15, 2007; Barcelona, Spain. Abstract 608.

72. Korba BE, Montero AB, Farrar K, et al. Nitazoxanide, tizoxanide and other thiazolidesare potent inhibitors of hepatitis B virus and hepatitis C virus replication. *Antiviral Res.* 2008;77:56-63.

73. Rossignol JF, Elfert A, El-Gohary Y, Keeffe EB. Randomized controlled trial of nitazoxanide-peginterferon-ribavirin, nitazoxanide-peginterferon and peginterferon-ribavirin in the treatment of patients with chronic hepatitis C genotype 4. Program and abstracts of the 43rd Annual Meeting of the European Association for the Study of the Liver; April 23-27, 2008; Milan, Italy. Abstract 68.

74. Swan T. Hepatitis C: New Treatments in the Pipeline. Treatment Action Group 2008.

75. Jacobson I, Pockros P, Benhamou Y, et al. Impact of taribavirin and ribavirin exposure on efficacy and anemia rates when combined with pegylated interferon alfa-2b in the treatment of chronic HCV. Program and abstracts of the 57th Annual Meeting of the American Association for the Study of Liver Diseases; October 27-31, 2006; Boston, Massachusetts. Abstract 1133.

76. Marcellin P, Lurie Y, Rodrigues Torres M, Chasen R, Xu Y, Murphy B. The safety and efficacy of taribavirin plus pegylated interferon alfa 2a versus ribavirin plus pegylated interferon alfa 2a in therapy naive patients infected with HCV: phase 3 results. Program and abstracts of the 42nd Annual Meeting of the European Association for the Study of the Liver; April 11-15, 2007; Barcelona, Spain. Abstract 10.

77. Poordad F, Lawitz E, Chun E, Hammond J. Treatment week 12 results of weight-based taribavirin versus weight-based ribavirin, both with peginterferon alfa-2, in naive chronic hepatitis C, genotype 1 patients. Program and abstracts of the 43rd annual meeting of the European Association for the Study of the Liver; April 23-27, 2008; Milan, Italy. Abstract 996.

INTEGRATIVE MEDICINE

Randy J. Horwitz, MD, PhD and Julia Jernberg, MD

Introduction

Integrative medicine is far more than simply the combination of mainstream (western) medicine with *complementary and alternative medicine* (*CAM*). The concept of integrative medicine embraces the philosophies and practices of different healing disciplines and functions as a bridge between them. As it is currently practiced in the United States, integrative medicine is spearheaded by western doctors who have come to appreciate the benefits and the limitations of both conventional (western) medicine and alternative healing practices and philosophies. An integrative medicine doctor practices western medicine and also utilizes other healing techniques either in combination with or, in some cases, as an alternative to conventional healing practices.

Integrative medicine was borne of a desire to expand the conventional practice of medicine beyond the traditional boundaries of modern western medicine. Conventional medicine, as it is currently practiced in the west, is one of the youngest of the medical sciences. Yet it has a well-earned reputation for achievement in certain areas such as the introduction of antibiotic therapies, *vaccine* therapies, and organ transplantation, to name just a few.

Sophisticated diagnostic procedures such as magnetic resonance imaging (MRI) and computed tomography (CT) scans reveal the inner structures of the body in minute detail. *Ultrasound* technology enables us to see blood flow through the body and the tiny beating hearts of babies in the womb. A small amount of blood can be sent to the laboratory to determine a seemingly endless number of details about the body's chemistry. The wonders of modern medicine marvel and amaze us. Advances in western medicine have saved countless lives over the years. Yet despite these advances, many patients and doctors alike believe that some of the humanistic features of *clinical* medicine have been neglected in the whirlwind of technology. Integrative medicine seeks to restore these attributes to the field of medicine, and to utilize both the newest medical technologies and time-honored healing practices to optimize patients' health and wellness.

In a quest to expand upon the therapeutic choices available to patients, several visionaries from the conventional healthcare system looked to more traditional healing practices for insights that might aid the sick and suffering. Integrative medicine practitioners utilize a wide variety of healing techniques in addition to conventional treatments.

Healing Techniques Commonly Utilized in Integrative Medicine	
acupuncture	allopathic medicine and treatments
herbal medicine	homeopathy
nutrition	energy medicine
exercise	vitamins and nutritional supplements
spirituality	

Supporting the self-healing nature of the human body and affecting a positive influence over interactions between the mind and body are two fundamental principles of most integrative medicine practices. Scientific research conducted in recent years has shown the powerful influence of the mind on wellness and disease. Robert Ader's landmark experiments in the 1970's demonstrated the power a mental stimulus can have on the *immune system*. His work showed that psychological conditioning could destroy a mouse's immune function almost as effectively as a powerful *chemotherapy* drug.[1] Another study found that writing about one's emotions and thoughts can significantly reduce the level of illness experienced by people with chronic diseases such as asthma and *rheumatoid arthritis*.[2]

Definition and Principles of Integrative Medicine

There are many formal definitions of integrative medicine. The definition used by the University of Arizona, which established the first university program for fellowship training in integrative medicine, is as follows.

> Integrative medicine is healing-oriented medicine that takes account of the whole person (body, mind, and spirit), including all aspects of lifestyle. It emphasizes the therapeutic relationship and makes use of all appropriate therapies, both conventional and alternative.

In addition to this definition, the University of Arizona program has defined several principles that encompass the basic goals of integrative medicine.

- Establish a partnership between patient and practitioner.
- Facilitate the body's innate healing abilities.
- Neither reject conventional medicine nor embrace alternative medical practices uncritically.
- Realize that good medicine is grounded in good science and open to new paradigms.
- Focus on promoting health and preventing illness, as well as treating disease.

It is hoped that these principles will be integrated into the philosophy of medical care practiced by all doctors, obviating the need for a separate field of medicine.

How to Choose an Integrative Medicine Practitioner

An ideal integrative medicine practitioner must above all be a well-trained practitioner of conventional medicine. He or she must be able to diagnose ailments based on the medical history, physical examination, laboratory tests, x-ray exams, and other diagnostic tests. He or she is able to successfully treat acute ailments that lend themselves to conventional remedies such as antibiotics or surgery that are curative and potentially life-saving. In addition, an integrative medicine practitioner utilizes non-conventional (CAM) diagnostic and treatment techniques if they will benefit the patient. CAM healing techniques are often used when no conventional therapies are available or when they produce side effects that are unacceptable to the patient.

It can be challenging to find a qualified integrative medicine practitioner since this approach is relatively new in the United States, and there is no formal accreditation or certifying board. However, the following guidelines may be helpful. Be sure your integrative medicine doctor is a qualified conventional medical practitioner. He or she should have an M.D. (medical doctor) or D.O. (doctor of osteopathy) degree from a recognized medical school.

Board certification is another indicator of a doctor's qualifications. It means the doctor has completed several years of training after medical school in a particular specialty area and has passed a rigorous examination in that field. While this does not ensure that you have located a "good" doctor, it certainly reflects his or her level of training. Several national organizations certify doctors in the fields of internal medicine and family practice. The certification status of a doctor can be verified on the Internet at www.abim.org or www.abfp.org. Within certain medical specialties, there are also subspecialties. Subspecialty board certification (such as gastroenterology, a subspecialty of internal medicine) can also be verified at www.abms.org.

In recent years, several university medical schools have established fellowship programs in integrative medicine. While there is no board certification for integrative medicine, university-affiliated training programs must meet the university's quality standards. The University of Arizona, the University of California, San Diego with Scripps Institute, Beth Israel Medical Center in New York, and Harvard University (research only) have integrative medicine fellowship programs. A practitioner's participation in an integrative medicine fellowship program is one gauge of his or her qualifications.

However, many highly qualified and experienced doctors began practicing integrative medicine before formal fellowship training was available. While these doctors were not formally trained in an integrative medicine fellowship program, many are highly skilled integrative medicine practitioners. It is important to take into account not only qualifications but also a practitioner's experience and your impressions before deciding to work with any healthcare provider. In summary, people interested in pursuing an integrative medicine approach to healthcare should choose a doctor who is knowledgeable and experienced in <u>both</u> conventional medicine and other healing disciplines.

Integrative Medicine and Chronic Hepatitis C

A typical visit to an integrative medicine doctor often begins much like a conventional medical visit. You will likely be questioned about your medical history, *symptoms*, and the specifics of your *hepatitis C* experience including recent laboratory studies (*genotype*, *viral load*, *liver enzymes*, etc.) and treatment to date.

An integrative medicine doctor is also likely to ask other questions about your life and experiences that may be <u>unlike</u> those you've been asked by other healthcare providers. The point of these questions is to help your doctor get to know you; who you are is more than the sum of your medical data and symptoms. Some topics often included in an integrative medicine interview include:

- your upbringing and parents
- the nature of your relationships (spouse, children, friends, etc.)
- aspects of your life that really matter to you
- sources of joy in your life
- stressors in your life and how you manage them
- your diet
- physical activities, exercise, and frequency
- the role of spirituality in your life
- what you do for relaxation

An integrative medicine practitioner uses the information you provide to help him or her tailor your treatments to suit your personal preferences, lifestyle, and personality. The information you provide can be particularly helpful in choosing mind/body interventions that are likely to be beneficial.

Following the initial interview, the review of your current symptoms and physical exam is generally much like a conventional medical visit. Practitioners skilled in traditional Chinese medicine may include a tongue and pulse examination, two diagnostic skills not used by conventional medical doctors. The doctor then reviews the information gathered during your visit along with your medical records (including *liver biopsy*, ultrasound, and laboratory results). After considering all of this information and discussing treatment options and goals with the client, a treatment plan is prepared.

Integrative medicine doctors may recommend many different healing techniques. The choice of recommendations varies with each patient. Taking into consideration a person's specific medical condition and goals, and a reasonable chance of success, an integrative medicine doctor may well recommend conventional interferon-based therapy. Both conventional and alternative techniques are often used to help decrease the occurrence and severity of side-effects for people on conventional therapy.

For a number of patients, *HCV viral clearance* may not be an immediate goal of integrative medicine therapy for *chronic hepatitis* C. Among these patients, the focus is typically on decreasing liver *inflammation* since it contributes to the *fibrosis* and scarring that can lead to *cirrhosis*. In addition, maintaining liver functions such as detoxification and making nutrients is a high priority. If a person's functional capabilities can be maintained and disease progression can be prevented or slowed with minimal side-effects, then the goals of integrative medical therapy for HCV have been accomplished.

Before exploring some of the healing techniques integrative medicine doctors commonly use in treating chronic hepatitis C, I want to address the topic of liver biopsies. In our practice, we often propose liver biopsies – but only if the results may influence future management. For example, if a patient is adamant about not using interferon-based therapy under any circumstances, a liver biopsy will not provide the patient with more management choices. However, for a patient who is considering conventional therapy, a liver biopsy provides very useful information that may well influence the timing and/or decision to treat. For a person who would like to delay treatment until such time as there is marked deterioration in liver status, a liver biopsy gives a baseline assessment of the current state of the liver and enables the treatment team to monitor for disease progression.

Postponing therapy is a personal choice. However, we try to make sure a patient has all of the facts needed to make an informed decision. Eligibility for future treatments is a factor in some patients' decision to postpone conventional treatment. Say a remarkable new therapy with great preliminary success in the laboratory is discovered tomorrow. The new treatment will most likely be available first to "treatment naïve" people in *clinical trials*. Someone who is treatment naïve has not received prior treatment for the condition being studied in a clinical trial. Allowing only people with no prior treatment into a trial eliminates the possibility that previous treatment effects will influence response to the new therapy. Thus, the first people who are most likely to receive new therapies are those with previously untreated hepatitis C. Typically, if a new therapy is successful in treatment naïve people, it will then be studied in people whose prior therapy failed. The timeframe between these two types of testing is variable. Thus, this issue may not be as clear-cut as it first appears.

Healing Techniques That May Be Used in an Integrative Medicine Treatment Plan for Hepatitis C

A wide range of healing techniques may be used by integrative medicine doctors for the management of chronic hepatitis C. The treatment plan is typically tailored to match a person's unique personality, needs, attributes, and goals. A few of the more common healing techniques used by integrative medicine for the management of HCV are briefly discussed in this section. Other chapters offer additional details about many of the topics mentioned here.

MIND/BODY MEDICINE
This broad area of healing takes advantage of the fact that the immune system is subject to controls both within our awareness (conscious) and outside our awareness (subconscious). A field of study called "psychoneuroimmunology" is devoted to discovering and understanding the complex interactions between the mind and the immune system.

Meditation, yoga, and numerous other mind/body systems have been found to influence immune function. I commonly recommend a formal meditation sitting practice for patients. I prefer a simple program such as the one established by Jon Kabat-Zinn at the University of Massachusetts. He calls his program, "Mindfulness-Based Stress Reduction." It is taught in classes throughout the United States, as well as in self-study books and tapes. Although the program is loosely based on Buddhist meditation techniques, it does not promote any particular religious denomination.

Clinical hypnosis is another mind/body technique that has been useful in people with hepatitis C. Hypnosis uses subconscious suggestions given during a trance state. A hypnotic trance is nothing more than a daydream state. There is no loss of control during the induction of a trance. A trance is simply a form of deep relaxation. A hypnosis session will leave you relaxed yet invigorated. You need not fear that you will quack like a duck or sing like Elvis. Clinical hypnosis is not a form of entertainment but a genuine healing technique. We recommend people work with a practitioner certified by the American Society for Clinical Hypnosis (www.asch.net).

TRADITIONAL CHINESE MEDICINE
Both traditional Chinese medicine and acupuncture are addressed in *Chapter 11, Chinese Medicine*, so I refer you to there for details about these forms of treatment.

In our clinic, the majority of people with chronic hepatitis C have normalized their liver enzymes and lowered their viral loads using these techniques. However, I need to add another fact to keep in mind. There is insufficient evidence to prove that lowering liver enzyme levels has any effect on liver inflammation or disease progression in people with chronic HCV infection. We have seen good outcomes in our clinic with Chinese medicine, but there have been no rigorously controlled studies to determine if there is a relationship between the normalization of laboratory values and the level of liver inflammation in chronic hepatitis C. One study supports the intuitive notion that maintaining normal liver enzyme levels is preferable to having markedly high levels. In a 12-month trial of people with viral hepatitis, a high dose of milk thistle (420 milligrams of silymarin) resulted in a reversal of liver cell damage as seen on liver biopsy. Participants also showed increased blood *proteins* and lowered liver enzyme levels. Common symptoms of hepatitis such as abdominal discomfort, decreased appetite, and *fatigue* also improved.[3]

NUTRITION

We give individualized nutritional advice to people with hepatitis C. However, some of the following generalities may be useful to you.

- We recommend a low-protein, low-fat diet with approximately 15% of the total daily calories coming from protein. By lowering the need to digest protein, the liver's workload is reduced. Similarly, we recommend avoiding extremely low *carbohydrate* diets such as the Atkins' diet, and concentrated protein and *amino acid* supplements.

- Increase your fiber intake. Fibers are great at binding toxins in the intestine and speeding their excretion from the body. This reduces the liver's workload by reducing the amount of detoxification needed. We also recommend that patients take a small amount of psyllium (for example, Citrucel®) daily.

- Increase your starch, fruit, and vegetable intake to about eight servings daily. If possible, eat organic products to decrease your exposure to *hormones* and potentially toxic chemicals. Washing all fruits and vegetables before eating (even organic produce) also helps decrease your exposure to chemicals.

- Eliminate saturated fats as much as possible. Cutting down on meat, and palm and coconut oils will help accomplish this. Margarine and most vegetable oils contain large amounts of polyunsaturated fats that should also be limited.

- Increase your intake of omega-3 essential fatty acids. These fatty acids have been found to help decrease inflammation. In some studies, they also showed anti-cancer properties. It is important that you limit your intake of certain fish that may be "naturally" contaminated with heavy metals, such as tuna, shark, swordfish, king mackerel and bluefish. More information may be found on the web at www.edf.org/page.cfm?tagID=1521.

- Limit your *iron* intake, including in multivitamins. Iron can accumulate in liver cells and tax the liver. Further, elevated iron levels have been associated with increased severity of viral hepatitis infections.[4]

HERBS & NUTRITIONAL SUPPLEMENTS

Certain herbs and plant (botanical) preparations have a long history of use in liver diseases. An excellent discussion of medicinal herbs can be found in *Chapter 14, Naturopathic Medicine*. Three botanicals we use frequently in our practice are presented in this section.

MILK THISTLE (SILYBUM MARIANUM)

Milk thistle contains silymarin, a mixture of natural chemicals (flavonoids) that help protect the liver by reducing inflammation. Silymarin also promotes regeneration of liver cells and helps them become more efficient at detoxifying the blood. Conventional medicine uses silymarin to treat Amanita phalloides (death cap mushroom) poisoning because of its liver-protective effects. It is thought to act by inhibiting the uptake of amatoxin by liver cells and interfering with the delivery of the toxin from the intestine to the liver.[5] Milk thistle also has potent *antioxidant* activity.

Nonetheless, evidence regarding the possible therapeutic effects of milk thistle remains lacking. A review of all the published literature on this topic in 2007, the authors concluded that there is no evidence that milk thistle is harmful, but there is also not conclusive evidence that it is beneficial.[7] The authors also noted that high quality scientific studies were few and encouraged further research into this topic. See *Chapters 14 and 16* for additional information about antioxidants and their role in the liver.

SCHIZANDRA (SCHIZANDRA CHINENSIS)

The dried berries of the schizandra plant contain substances called "lignins" that help prevent liver damage from hepatitis. Schizandra has been shown to normalize liver enzyme levels and increase the liver's ability to detoxify the blood. It also contains an anti-inflammatory substance (gomisin A) that seems to act specifically on the liver. Schizandra is a nontoxic plant and is very safe. It is backed by over 1,000 years of use in China. However, schizandra may affect the circulating levels of some drugs that are processed by the liver.

OLIVE LEAF EXTRACT

Olive leaf extract is a nontoxic herb that may lower the HCV viral load. The active component is thought to be a substance called oleuropein. Most commercial preparations are standardized to contain specific amounts oleuropein.

OTHER INTERVENTIONS THAT MAY BE USED TO MANAGE CHRONIC HEPATITIS C

GREEN TEA

Several clinical studies support the use of green tea for the treatment of hepatitis. In a study of 124 patients with viral hepatitis, 3 grams of catechins (the active component of green tea) daily significantly lowered alanine aminotransferase (*ALT*), *aspartate aminotransferase (AST)*, and *bilirubin* compared to an inactive substance (*placebo*).[6] Patients with hepatitis C had the best response.

AVOIDANCE OF LIVER TOXINS

We advise patients to avoid any medications or herbal supplements that are processed by the liver. For example, we recommend avoiding Tylenol® (*acetaminophen*) and Advil® (*ibuprofen*). In addition, we encourage all patients with hepatitis C to eliminate all alcohol consumption.

IMMUNIZATIONS

We immunize our hepatitis C patients against *hepatitis A* and *hepatitis B*. These vaccines protect against the potentially serious complications that can arise from infection with two or more hepatitis viruses.

Summary

Integrative medicine is a relatively new approach to healthcare that incorporates the best of both conventional medicine and CAM. Broad ranges of healing techniques are used by integrative medicine practitioners to treat chronic hepatitis C. Treatment plans are tailored to meet the unique needs, goals, attributes, and personality of the individual. People interested in an integrative medicine approach to managing chronic hepatitis C should seek well-trained, qualified practitioners who are willing to work with you and your *gastroenterologist* or *hepatologist*.

References

1. Ader R, Cohen N. Behaviorally conditioned immunosuppression. *Psychosom Med.* 1975;37:333-40.
2. Smyth JM, Stone AA, Hurewitz A, Kaell A. Effects of writing about stressful experiences on symptom reduction in patients with asthma or rheumatoid arthritis: a randomized trial. *JAMA.* 1999;281(14):1304-9.
3. Berenguer J, Carrasco D. Double-blind trial of silymarin vs. placebo in the treatment of chronic hepatitis. *Munch Med Wochenschr.*

1977;119:240-60.
4. Cotler SJ, Emond MJ, Gretch DR, et al. Relation between iron concentration and hepatitis C virus RNA level in liver tissue. *J Clin Gastroenterol.* 1999;29:322-6.
5. Floersheim GL. Treatment of human amatoxin mushroom poisoning: myths and advances in therapy. *Med Toxicol.* 1987;2:1-9.
6. Rambaldi A, Jacobs BP, Gluud C. Milk thistle for alcoholic and/or hepatitis B or C virus liver diseases. *Cochrane Database Syst Rev.* 2007;(4):CD003620.
7. Piazza M, Guadagnino V, Piciotto G, et al. Effect of (+)-cyanidanol-3 in acute HAV, HBV, and non-A non-B viral hepatitis. *Hepatology.*1983;3:45-9.

Other References

Maizes V, Caspi O. The principles and challenges of integrative medicine: more than a combination of traditional and alternative therapies. *West J Med.* 1999;171:148-9.

Maizes V, Koffler K, Fleishman S. Revisiting the health history: an integrative approach. *Advances.* 2002;18(2):31-4.

Ayurvedic Medicine

Shri K. Mishra, MD, MS, Bharathi Ravi, BAMS and Sivaramaprasad Vinjamury, MD

Introduction

Ayurveda is a natural system of medicine that has been practiced in India for more than 5,000 years. It was developed by seers (rishis) through centuries of observation, experimentation, discussion, and *meditation*. The origins of Ayurvedic medicine are recorded in the Atharva Veda, one of the four Vedic scriptures.[1] For several thousand years, Ayurvedic teachings were passed down orally from teacher to student. The first summary of these teachings was put into writing around 1500 B.C. The main sources of knowledge are the three Vedic classics Charaka Samhita, Susruta Samhita, and Ashtanga Hridaya.[2]

Ayurveda is a Sanskrit word made up of two components, ayush meaning life, and veda meaning knowledge or science. Hence, Ayurveda is the "science of life." The teachings of this ancient system of medicine are written in Sanskrit, the ancient language of India and Hinduism. It is based on Indian (Vedic) philosophy. Ayurveda was the first holistic system of diagnosis and treatment integrating nutrition, hygiene, rejuvenation, and herbal medicine. Ayurvedic medicine considers the human body to be in balance with nature. The body is believed to be a dynamic and resilient system that can cope with all stresses from its environment while maintaining the ability to heal itself.[3, 4]

The main objectives of Ayurveda are:

- to maintain and promote health by preventing physical, mental, and spiritual ailments
- to *cure* disease through natural medicine, diet, and a regulated lifestyle

Ayurveda tries to help us live a long and healthy life, achieve our fullest potential, and express our true inner nature on a daily basis.[4] The Ayurvedic classic Charaka Samhita defines Ayurveda as, "the knowledge that indicates the appropriate and inappropriate, happy or sorrowful conditions of living, what is auspicious or inauspicious for longevity, as well as the measure of life itself."[5]

Basic Concepts of Ayurveda

It will be helpful to understand a few important concepts and some Ayurvedic terminology before deciding whether you want to include Ayurveda in your *hepatitis C* treatment plan. The next few pages provide a brief overview of Ayurvedic concepts on which the diagnosis and treatment of all ailments are based.

Pancha-Maha-Bhoota Theory

According to Ayurvedic philosophy, the entire cosmos is made up of the energies of five elements: earth, water, fire, air, and ether (space). Even the human body and herbs are made up of these elements. Collectively, these elements are called pancha-maha-bhootas or material particles. The material particles and the anti-material particles (the spirit) form the cognitive aspect of a living being.

The predominance of a particular element(s) determines the characteristics of a thing, whether it is an animal, a person, or an herb. The medicinal properties of a drug or an herb are determined by the characteristics it exhibits. Similarly, depending upon the relative amounts of the elements, each of us exhibits a unique set of physical and mental characteristics. A disease state changes these characteristics. This change is the basis for the diagnosis and treatment of disease. In prescribing a remedy, the doctor chooses a treatment with the opposite characteristics of the disease to counteract the *symptoms*.

Tri-Dosha Theory

According to Ayurvedic theory, there are three humors in the body called doshas. These determine the constitution of a person and also the life processes of growth and decay. The doshas are genetically determined. The three doshas are vata, pitta, and kapha. Each dosha is made up of the five fundamental elements. Each dosha is responsible for several body functions. When the doshas are healthy and balanced, this is the state of good health. Imbalances cause disease. Ayurveda recognizes that different foods, tastes, colors, and sounds affect the doshas in different ways. For example, very hot and pungent spices aggravate pitta. Cold, light foods such as salads calm it down. This ability to affect the doshas is the underlying basis for Ayurvedic practices and therapies.

VATA

Vata is composed of space and air. It is the subtle energy associated with all voluntary and involuntary movement in the human body. It governs breathing, blinking, muscle and tissue movement, and the heartbeat. It is also responsible for all urges. Creativity, flexibility, and the ability to initiate things are seen when vata is in balance. Indecision, restlessness, anxiety, and fear occur when vata is out of balance. Vata is the motivating force behind the other two humors. In modern medicine, the *physiological* role of vata is in the central and peripheral nervous systems.[6-8] Vata has a tendency to expand indefinitely and to disturb the nervous activity or the vital forces in the body.

PITTA

Pitta is composed of fire and water. It is responsible for all digestive and metabolic activities. It governs body temperature, complexion, visual perception, hunger, and thirst. In a balanced state, pitta promotes intelligence, understanding, and courage. Out of balance, pitta produces insomnia, burning sensations, *inflammation*, infection, anger, and hatred. Pitta is the humor involved in liver disorders.[6-8] Pitta has a tendency to become more liquid and to weaken the digestive and biochemical processes in the body.

KAPHA

Kapha is composed of water and earth. It provides the strength and stability for holding body tissues together. Kapha is the watery aspect of the body. It provides lubricants at the various points of friction in the body. In balance, kapha is responsible for wisdom, patience, and memory. Out of balance, kapha causes looseness of the limbs, *lethargy*, greed, and generalized sluggishness or *hypoactivity*. This dosha maintains body resistance to disease.[6-8] Kapha has a tendency to thicken and obstruct the passages of the body and damage the process of lubrication.

Sapta-Dhatu Theory

Ayurvedic theory states the human body is composed of seven tissues called dhatus.

- plasma and *interstitial* fluids (rasa)
- blood (rakta)
- muscle (mamsa)
- fat or adipose tissue (medas)
- bone (asthi)
- bone marrow (majja)
- reproductive tissue (sukra)

Kapha is specifically responsible for plasma, muscle, fat, marrow, and semen. Pitta creates blood. Vata creates bone. Diseases of the humors are usually reflected in the tissues they govern. When out of balance, the humors can enter any tissue and cause disease.[6-8]

MALAS
The quantities and qualities of the three excreta from the body, sweat (sweda), feces (mala), and urine (mutra), and other body waste products play an important role in the diagnosis and treatment of disease. The Sanskrit word for these waste products is malas.[6-8]

TRIPOD
Tripod includes the doshas, dhatus, and malas. They maintain health when they are in equilibrium and produce disease when they are not.

SROTAS
The human body has numerous channels to allow the flow of energy, nutrients, and waste products. These channels are called srotas. Some of the srotas such as the alimentary canal (the digestive channel that runs from the mouth to the anus) are very large. Some are small such as arteries and veins. Others are very minute such as the capillaries, nerve terminals, and the lymphatics. Some srotas carry nutritional materials to the tissues of the body. Other srotas carry waste materials out of the body. The three doshas are present in every part of the body and move through every srota. Blockage or improper flow within the srotas produces ailments. The physical channels are similar to the different systems of western medicine such as the digestive, respiratory, and *cardiovascular* systems. Diseases are classified according to the systems they involve.[9]

AGNI AND AAMA
Poor functioning of the digestive system leads to many diseases. The digestive fire or agni controls the activities of digestion. According to Ayurveda, digestion is the cornerstone of good health. Good digestion nourishes the body. Eating the correct foods makes a big difference in your well-being. Agni helps the body produce secretions and generates the metabolic processes necessary to create energy, and maintain and repair the body.[10] Agni is also part of the *immune system* since its heat destroys harmful organisms and toxins. There are 13 agnis. The activity of agni varies throughout the day. A natural ebb and flow of your digestive fire is necessary for good digestion and immune function, and resistance to disease.[11]

The opposite of this process is aama. Aama is defined as imperfectly metabolized food or drugs. In other words, an aama is a toxin that needs to be eliminated from the body. Aama is usually generated in the body because of weak digestive fire or jatharagni.[12] It is also believed that aama is produced by out of balance doshas. Aama is mixed up with the tissues and causes disease by clogging the channels. Out of balance pitta, dosha, and poor agni play important roles in the symptoms of liver disorders.

OJAS
Ojas is the essential energy of the immune system. It is a unique concept of Ayurveda that embodies a subtle essence of all the tissues in the body. In other words, ojas is the glue that cements the body, mind, and spirit together, integrating them into a functioning individual. Proper agni is required for proper production of ojas. Ojas decreases with age. Low ojas levels cause chronic degenerative and immunological diseases.[13] In western medicine, ojas would be similar to *immunoglobulins* and other *immunomodulators* like *cytokines*. Abnormalities of ojas lead to decreased *immunity*, making a person more vulnerable to infections including hepatitis.

PRAKRUTI AND GUNAS
The proportion of the humors varies from person to person. One humor is usually predominant and leaves its mark on a person's appearance and disposition. Based on the predominant humor, every person is born with a unique mind-body constitution called prakruti. Gunas denote a person's mental make up and are of three types: satva (perfect), rajas (semi-balanced), and tamas (unbalanced). A person's prakruti is determined at the time of conception. Every person has specific physical, mental, and emotional characteristics. These characteristics are called a person's constitution. Prakruti must be considered in determining natural healing approaches and recommendations for daily living.[14]

Ayurvedic Definition of Health

Ayurveda defines health as, "the equilibrium of the three biological humors (doshas), the seven body tissues (dhatus), proper digestion, and a state of pleasure or happiness of the soul, senses, and the mind."[15] This definition dates back to 1500 B.C. and is described in Sushruta Samhita, the surgical compendium of Ayurveda.

A balance among the three doshas is necessary for health. Together, the three doshas govern all metabolic activities. When their actions in our mind-body constitution are balanced, we experience psychological and physical wellness. When they go slightly out of balance, we may feel uneasy. When they are more obviously unbalanced, symptoms of sickness can be observed and experienced.[16, 17]

Pathogenesis of Disease

Ayurveda asserts that each person is unique, made up of specific characteristics that are his or her own. This means that in order to protect or preserve your health, you need to follow a diet and lifestyle that create balance with your constitution or internal environment. Such a lifestyle keeps the humors at normal levels.

Aggravating factors such as diet, climate, seasons, emotions, and lifestyle can make the humors go out of balance. Imbalance weakens the digestive fire and increases the production of toxins. The toxins along with the out of balance humor(s) block the channels and disrupt the energy and nutrition flow to that particular tissue. The result is that the tissue involved in the process becomes diseased.[17] This happens in six *stages*: accumulation, aggravation, overflow, relocation, manifestation, and diversification.[18]

Classification of Diseases

Various diseases are produced by imbalances of specific humors in specific tissues. Diseases are classified as vata, pitta, or kapha disorders, and combinations of these three. Based on the predominant humor, 80 vata, 40 pitta, and 20 kapha disorders have been identified. There is further classification of the disorders based on the physiological systems or srotas involved. Most diseases of the organ systems are further sub-classified and are named after the predominant humor, tissue, or organ involved in the disease process.[19]

Diagnosis of Disease

Diagnosis in Ayurveda is done in eight parts. Disease is diagnosed by taking a detailed history of the causative factors, *prodromal symptoms*, *cardinal signs* and symptoms, and the aggravating and relieving factors.[20] The affected humor and tissue are identified for treatment.

Various methods are used to help acquire information during an assessment. These methods are very similar to other medical disciplines and include questioning, observation, *palpation*, direct perception, and *inference*. Techniques such as taking the pulse, observing the tongue and eyes, noting physical symptoms, and examinations of urine and stool are employed during an assessment.[21] The pulse is one of the important tools in diagnosing the constitution of an individual and the humors involved in a disease. In some cases, the pulse can identify the stage of the disease. Pulse diagnosis gets more accurate as the Ayurvedic practitioner gains experience.[22]

Prognosis of Diseases

Ayurveda is not a *cure* for all ailments and all stages of disease. Diseases are classified based on their *prognosis*.

- Easily curable: recent onset, one humor involved
  - example - digestive disorders
- Difficult to cure: chronic, one or two humors involved
  - example - most skin disorders

- Chronic with maintenance therapy: two or more humors involved, or chronic and metabolic diseases
    - examples - diabetes and hepatitis C
- Incurable: all three humors involved with associated complications
    - example - cancer
- Terminally ill: the chance of continued life is very bleak

If the first two stages of a disease are not treated properly, they can progress to become a chronic disease with maintenance therapy or could end up as incurable.[23]

Principles of Ayurvedic Treatment
The first goal of Ayurveda is health promotion and disease prevention. The second goal is to treat physical, mental, and spiritual illness. Ayurveda teaches that separating mind and spirit from the body creates physical imbalance, the first step in the disease process. It naturally follows that reintegration of mind, spirit, and body is the first step toward healing.

The goal of treatment for any disease is to restore the balance of the humors to reestablish a person's original constitution. This is achieved by adjusting the factors responsible for causing disease. A combination of herbs, bodywork, and lifestyle changes are suggested for the treatment of a disease or ailment. Dietary advice is also an important component of Ayurvedic treatment. The practitioner will suggest a specific diet that helps eliminate or slow the progression of disease.

Finally, yoga and meditation are advised because they are integral to Ayurvedic treatment. Treatment recommendations are based on a person's constitution, current health imbalances, and the time of year.[15, 24]

The humors are balanced and toxins are eliminated from the body through cleansing therapies known as panchakarma. Panchakarma is another hallmark of Ayurvedic treatment. Panchakarma is comprised of five parts: emesis, purgation, cleansing enemas, retention enemas, and cleansing nasal medication.[2]

After panchakarma, rasayana (rejuvenation therapy) is recommended. This helps enhance immune function and also helps the person have a longer, healthier life.

Ayurvedic Medicine and Hepatitis C

The liver is called yakrit in Ayurveda. Pitta is the predominant humor of the liver. Most liver disorders are aggravated conditions of pitta. Excessive *bile* production or a blockage in the flow of bile usually indicates high pitta, which in turn affects the agni or *enzyme* activities responsible for absorption, digestion, and *metabolism*.

Diet and lifestyle activities that aggravate pitta include:
- alcohol abuse
- red meat
- spicy, oily, heavy foods
- lack of sleep
- too much direct exposure to the sun
- smoking

Aggravation of the pitta causes such liver diseases as *fatty liver*, *cirrhosis*, and hepatitis. All types of viral hepatitis are of relatively recent discovery, so there is obviously no mention of them in the classic Ayurvedic texts. Nevertheless, one can find similar symptoms described under kaamala.[26, 27]

Ayurveda describes two basic types of kaamala (hepatitis or *jaundice*).

- Shakhasrita is caused by the minimal aggravation of pitta and kapha, and is easily curable.
- Kumbha kaamala results from very high pitta and is difficult to cure. It can become incurable if not attended to immediately.

Panaki and haleemaka are two other types of hepatitis or jaundice that are explained in Ayurvedic texts. Panaki is late stage kaamala. Haleemaka is an advanced stage of *anemia* that occurs when both the vata and pitta are out of balance.[26]

Pathogenesis

Excessive intake of alcohol, and hot, spicy, sour, or contaminated food or water aggravate pitta. When pitta is out of balance, the liver causes disease in the blood, muscle tissue, and biliary system. This manifests as kaamala or jaundice. It is believed that an anemic and/or immunocompromised person is more prone to this ailment.

Symptoms of kaamala include:

- loss of appetite and taste
- generalized weakness
- yellowish discoloration of the eyes, nails, oral cavity, and urine
- vague body pains
- burning sensation
- weakness in all sensory organs

In extreme cases, *emaciation* (extreme thinness) is also seen. All these symptoms signify the involvement of the immune system in infectious hepatitis. Ayurveda teaches that hepatitis involves the *gastrointestinal* system, cardiovascular system, musculoskeletal system, and the skin.[26-28]

Symptoms such as generalized *edema* (shotha), excessive thirst (atitrishna), bloody stools (krishna varna mala mutra), vomiting blood (rakta yukta chardi), red eyes (rakta netra), dizziness (bhrama), drowsiness (tandra), total loss of appetite (teevra agni mandya), and *hepatic* coma (nashta sanjna) indicate that the liver disease is at an incurable stage, and the patient is believed to be terminally ill.[29]

Diagnosis of Liver Disorders and Hepatitis C

A diagnosis of liver disease is suggested by signs and symptoms such as loss of appetite, *fatigue*, jaundice, occasional vomiting, and mild fever. The determination of the type of liver disease is made according to the severity of the symptoms. The magnitude of pitta aggravation is diagnosed through pulse reading, observing the eyes and tongue, and palpating the abdomen. Important parts of the examination include assessments of the person's constitution, physical strength, and mental state. Other information is also gathered such as a person's lifestyle and whether he or she lives or has lived on the coast, far inland, or in the mountains.[29, 30]

Treatment of Liver Disorders and Hepatitis C

Ayurveda promotes a specific treatment for every ailment. The objective of any treatments is to return balance to the affected dosha. Reestablishing a person's constitution is always an important component of therapy. The method used to achieve constitutional balance could be elimination, palliation, or both.

The treatment of liver disorders usually involves a combination of herbs, body work, dietary advice, lifestyle changes, yoga, and meditation. It is important to follow a specific diet and curtail excessive activities. Depending on the person's physical state, treatment begins with a mild laxative, which is either limited to the start of treatment or taken daily. If the person is unable to tolerate the laxative, it is stopped and treatment proceeds to the next step.

After cleansing, oral medications are given two or three times daily. These medications can be herbal concoctions, powders, pills, fermented syrups, and/or herbs processed in clarified butter (ghee). The dosage, form, and combination of medications are selected depending upon the patient's constitution, stage of disease, and physical condition. Only an experienced Ayurvedic healthcare provider can make appropriate medication recommendations. Though special emphasis is placed on agni in all instances, it is given more importance when treating liver disorders.[26-28, 31]

Medicinal plants (botanicals) have been used for the management of liver diseases by Ayurvedic and other traditional healers for thousands of years. Numerous plants and herbal formulations containing several botanicals are reported to have liver protective (*hepatoprotective*) properties. Nearly 150 chemicals from 101 different plants have been claimed to have liver protecting activity.[23] Most studies on hepatoprotective plants are carried out using chemically induced liver damage in rodents. Several plants have been reported as hepatoprotective in animals by investigators from India during the last decade.[23]

For descriptions of the herbs used to treat liver disorders in Ayurvedic medicine, see *Appendix II, Ayurvedic Medicine*. The appendix also contains sample panchakarma and rasayana *protocols* for patients with liver disease. However, recall that Ayurvedic therapy is individualized according to each person's unique characteristics. If you are interested in pursuing Ayurvedic therapy for hepatitis C, you are urged to consult a qualified Ayurvedic practitioner.

Ayurvedic Dietary Guidelines for Liver Disorders

Pitta is the primary humor involved in liver disorders. It influences digestion, metabolism, and biological transformations in the body. Therefore, it is important to follow a diet and lifestyle that reestablishes the balance of pitta.

In general, Ayurvedic medicine promotes a vegetarian diet for liver disorders. Bitter, sweet, and astringent tastes are favored. It is recommended that you consume starchy foods such as vegetables, grains, and beans. Salads are also good.

Excesses of salty, sour, and/or spicy food items are harmful. Avoid processed and fast foods as they tend to have excessive salt and sour tastes. You are urged to reduce your consumption of oil, butter, and fats. Avoid doughnuts, fried foods, pickles, yogurt, sour cream, cheese, egg yolks, coffee, alcohol, and fermented foods. Try to avoid vinegar in salad dressings by using lemon juice. A detailed list of recommended food items for people with liver disorders is given in Table 1.

Table 1. Ayurvedic Dietary Recommendations by Food Group

Food Group	Favor	Reduce or Avoid
Vegetables - sweet and bitter vegetables	asparagus, broccoli, Brussels sprouts, cabbage, cauliflower, celery, cucumbers, green beans, green sweet peppers, leafy green vegetables, whole mung beans	beets, carrots, eggplant, garlic, hot peppers, mushrooms, okra, onions, radishes, parsley, peas, potatoes, sprouts, squash, spinach, sweet potatoes, tomatoes, tofu, zucchini, other soy products
Fruits - all fruits should be sweet and ripe	apples, avocados, cherries, coconut, figs, dark grapes, mangoes, melons, oranges, pears, pineapples, plums, prunes, raisins	apricots, bananas, berries, sour cherries, cranberries, grapefruit, papayas, peaches, persimmons, green grapes*, oranges*, pineapples*, plums* *unless they are sweet and ripe
Grains	barley, oats, wheat, white rice (preferably basmati rice)	brown rice, corn, millet, rye
Dairy	butter, buttermilk, egg whites, ice cream, milk	cheese, egg yolks, sour cream, yogurt

HERBS AND SPICES

Spices should generally be avoided as they aggravate pitta. In small amounts, cardamom, cilantro (green coriander), coriander seed, dill, fennel, mint, saffron, and turmeric are good for protecting the digestive fire and helping remove blockages.[28]

Lifestyle, Yoga, and Meditation

Your lifestyle is as important as your diet in preserving health. Our changing lifestyles have been a major cause of many ailments. If you have a liver disorder, you should avoid sleeping in the afternoon, exposure to hot sun, exertion, anxiety, alcohol abuse, smoking, eating at irregular intervals and times, and staying up late at night.

YOGA

The literal translation for yoga is "union." Yoga is an excellent way to take care of both your body and your mind. Yoga helps improve your energy level and immune function, calms mood swings, and helps alleviate the "brain fog" that some *HCV*-infected people experience.

A yoga posture or asana is a dynamic position in which the person is perfectly poised between activity and inactivity. A corresponding mental balance exists between movement and stillness. In yoga, each posture reflects a mental attitude. Yoga strengthens the elimination system and helps detoxify the body. A few stimulating postures help disperse stagnation and congestion, and get energy flowing again to strengthen the digestive system and liver function.[32]

Vajraasana, shalabhasana, halasana, padahastasana, savasana, abdomen lift, and stomach lift are some of the yoga postures that are very helpful in liver disorders.[32] Yoga postures cause a squeezing action on a specific organ or gland resulting in the stimulation of that body part. Slow, deep breathing during yoga practice increases the oxygen and prana (life force) supply to the target organ or gland. Focusing attention on the target organ or gland brings the mind into play and greatly increases the circulation and prana supply to the organ or gland.

It is best to practice yoga in the early morning or early evening. However, yoga can be practiced at any time. You should not eat right before practicing yoga. However, it is a good idea to eat something about thirty minutes after finishing your yoga session. Wait at least one hour after getting out of bed before doing yoga because you will be too stiff. Avoid taking a hot shower or bath immediately after yoga because it draws blood away from the internal organs and glands. A shower that is just warm will not counteract the benefits of yoga. It is important to drink plenty of water after yoga practice. The water will help flush the toxins released by the body during yoga.

Yoga is advised only for individuals who can withstand mild exercise and whose liver function is not compromised. If you are interested in adding yoga to your hepatitis C treatment *protocol*, you should first talk it over with your primary care practitioner to be certain it is safe for you. If your healthcare provider gives permission to proceed, we urge you to look for a well-trained, experienced yoga instructor. Be sure to tell your instructor that you have hepatitis C, and let him or her know if you have any other medical conditions. *Appendix II, Ayurvedic Medicine* has descriptions of some yoga postures that are frequently recommended for people with liver disorders. This is provided for your information only. We strongly recommend you do not begin yoga practice unless you have discussed it first with your primary care provider.

Pranayama is a systematic breathing exercise that helps increase blood supply and oxygen to the affected part of liver and helps liver regeneration.[32] There is no restriction for this exercise unless you are very weak and/or suffer from fluctuations in blood pressure. Pranayama provides relaxation and relieves anxiety. There are various methods for pranayama, which consists of inhalation, retention, and exhalation.

A simple method for performing pranayama is to close the right nostril using the right thumb and close the left nostril using the right little and ring finger. Breathe in through the left nostril while closing the right nostril. Hold the breath as long as you can tolerate. Exhale through the right nostril thus completing one cycle. Next, breathe in through the right nostril and breathe out through the left nostril. Repeat this process ten to twelve times.

MEDITATION
Meditation is an important part of yogic practice. It has various stages. The first stage is dharana, meaning concentration. It is accomplished by sitting in a quiet place, closing your eyes, and chanting mantras. Focus your mind on an inner object, look at the tip of your nose, or focus on a picture of your choice. Continue this process until you are able to focus your mind. You try to concentrate by bringing your mind to the desired object.

The second stage of meditation is dhyana, which means contemplation. During this stage, you attempt to advance to a deeper stage of meditation. In this stage, you increase your concentration for a long period through practice.
The third stage of meditation is only for very advanced practitioners. It is known as samadhi. This form of meditation has the ability to control vital functions such as the heartbeat, breathing, etc. This is beyond the scope of the majority of yogic practitioners.

BENEFITS OF YOGA AND MEDITATION
Yoga and meditation are used in Ayurveda to promote health and well-being. Research suggests yoga practice may decrease symptoms such as anxiety, *depression*, and pain. Yoga and meditation have been reported to increase physical endurance, fitness, mental well-being, and quality of life.

Yoga and meditation may help people with hepatitis C overcome physical stress and fatigue. They may also help ease anxieties and tensions during treatment.

Research Data on the Efficacy of Herbs Used in the Ayurvedic Treatment of Liver Disorders and Hepatitis C

Despite tremendous advances in allopathic medicine, there are no effective hepatoprotective medicines. Plant-derived drugs (botanicals) play a vital role in the management of liver diseases in several non-western medical disciplines including Ayurveda, traditional Chinese medicine, and naturopathy. Numerous plants and polyherbal formulations claim to have hepatoprotective activities.[23]

The hepatoprotective effects of individual herbs or herb combinations are tested using experimental animals. The animals are given chemicals known to be toxic to the liver along with the substance being tested. Animals given substances that are hepatoprotective show less liver injury than animals given the toxic chemicals alone. However, if a substance is not hepatoprotective, the level of injury is the same regardless of the addition of the test substance.[20, 22, 27] In most studies of polyherbal formulas, marginal to moderate levels of hepatoprotective effects were observed.

The *antiviral* activities of only a few traditional botanicals have been tested in experimental animals. This is primarily because animal models for hepatitis C have only recently been developed.

ANDROGRAPHIC PANICULATA (KALAMEGH)

A. paniculata belongs to the plant family Acanthaceae and is also known as chirayata. Preparations containing Andrographic paniculata only and formulas containing this plant product have been described as being potent hepatoprotectants.[24]

Administration of *A. paniculata* has been shown to protect the activity of several important enzymes in the liver (superoxide dismutase, catalase, *glutathione* peroxidase, and glutathione reductase). It has also been shown to protect liver glutathione. (See *Chapter 14, Naturopathic Medicine* for information about the role of glutathione in the liver.) These findings support the *antioxidant* and *hepatoprotective* effects of *A. paniculata*.[25]

CURCUMA LONGA (HARIDRA)[4]

C. longa is commonly known as turmeric. It has a long tradition of use in both Chinese and Ayurvedic medicine. The anti-inflammatory and hepatoprotective characteristics of turmeric and its constituents have been widely researched.[33-36]

Reasons for Using Ayurvedic Medicine and Who May Benefit

Ayurvedic medicine emphasizes disease prevention and health promotion. Periodic cleansing of the system, and a review of lifestyle practices and diet are the most important parts of treatment.

Ayurvedic treatments support liver function and have some antiviral properties. The use of antiviral, time-tested hepatoprotective herbs and cleansing provide additional benefit to a person with hepatitis C.

Newly diagnosed patients with normal liver function and only moderately elevated *liver enzymes* may derive great benefit from Ayurvedic treatment. Non-alcoholics and those in younger age groups who are otherwise healthy respond well to the Ayurvedic approach. Because the mind and body are interconnected, people with a positive attitude toward Ayurveda benefit more from this approach than those who are skeptical.

Anecdotal Story of Treatment Success with Ayurvedic Medicine

A 54-year-old male presented to our clinic for evaluation. He was an alcoholic and a diabetic on oral diabetes medicine. He was diagnosed with hepatitis C in July 1999. He was being evaluated for painful swelling in the abdomen, legs, and feet. On physical exam, an inflamed left lobe of the liver was felt which was associated with mild tenderness. *Ultrasound* revealed a moderately enlarged liver. Laboratory tests showed a moderate increase in liver enzymes, but were otherwise normal. *Liver biopsy* showed *grade* II inflammation and stage II *fibrosis*. The man was treated with interferon plus *ribavirin* for more than two months, but he did not respond to treatment. Liver enzyme levels did not drop significantly and other liver blood tests were unchanged.

In our clinic, the patient's hepatitis C infection and associated changes in liver biochemistry were treated as an excess of pitta humor. However, because this patient had edema and abdominal discomfort, the involvement of kapha humor was also considered. After analyzing the man's physical constitution, it was decided that he was a vata prakruti person.

The following treatment plan was designed in three stages for five, one, and 45 days, respectively. The selection of herbs for this patient was based on the assessment of his unique condition.

- Elimination of toxins with panchakola choornam in a powder formula

- Elimination of aggravated pitta through purgation, after preparation of the patient with avipatti choornam in a powder formula. This was repeated every two weeks as long as the patient could tolerate it.

- Rejuvenation of the liver with herbs and diet with Piper longum in a powder formula, and in a graded dose called vardhamana pippali rasayana.

A fat-free diet with softly cooked old rice, porridge, non-citrus fruits, sugar cane juice, boiled vegetables, lentils, and freshly made buttermilk was advised for the patient. The patient was also advised to avoid non-vegetarian foods including fish, eggs, and ice cream. The patient was told to avoid cold drinks and sleeping for long periods of time during the day to prevent aggravating the humors.

At the end of 56 days, the patient experienced reduced symptoms. His abdomen became soft and non-tender. Ultrasound revealed the liver was of normal size. His alkaline phosphatase (a liver enzyme), which had been high, returned to normal. The patient was advised to continue the rejuvenating herbs. His *viral load* could not be measured because of financial constraints.

Reasons for Not Using Ayurvedic Medicine

People with *acute hepatitis* C or *chronic hepatitis* C with multiple complications and a severely cirrhotic liver may not benefit from Ayurvedic medicine. Those who cannot tolerate bitter medicines and/or who have reservations about Ayurvedic medicine are also unlikely to benefit. *Ascites* (an accumulation of fluid in the abdomen) is an incurable condition according to Ayurveda. People presenting with ascites cannot be helped by Ayurvedic medicine, nor can those who are highly debilitated.

Anecdotal Story of Treatment Failure with Ayurvedic Medicine

A 70-year-old male came to our clinic with mild jaundice, elevated liver enzymes, ascites, loss of appetite, *shortness of breath*, and fatigue. He had been diagnosed with HCV five years earlier when he developed jaundice after a blood transfusion during abdominal surgery. His liver blood tests were consistently abnormal. *Serum bilirubin* remained between 1.5-3.5mg/dL (a significant elevation above normal). He had no major symptoms and was able to carry out his normal activities. He had been treated with rest and polyunsaturated fatty acids for the first two years of his illness, perhaps due to lack of awareness of other treatments. Later, his viral load was tested and he was put on interferon plus ribavirin. He completed his drug therapy but did not improve. A year later, he developed ascites. This is when he approached an Ayurvedic doctor for help.

Given this man's presenting symptoms, particularly his ascites, the Ayurvedic treatment options were limited. Detoxification and cleansing procedures, which are mandatory in Ayurveda, could not be used in this patient because of his poor health and nutrition. A symptomatic treatment was planned and he was put on concoctions of liver protecting herbs such as Tinospora cordifolia, Picorrizha curroa, Vitis vinifera, and Piper nigrum, and others. Mild laxatives such as avipatti choornam were given in small doses, and a pitta-pacifying diet and lifestyle were recommended. Initially, his appetite improved and his serum bilirubin returned to normal. His other liver blood tests remained abnormal. His *shortness of breath* came down from class three to class one.

His abdomen became soft and he was able to pass normal stools. Ultrasound showed cirrhosis and ascitic fluid in abdomen. Viral load testing was not repeated, as the patient could not afford it.

Though the patient is continuing treatment after more than six months, there has been no significant improvement in his liver health. This is not unexpected because of this patient's cirrhosis and ascites. According to Ayurveda, the onset of ascites indicates a poor *prognosis*. Age, time, and complications could also have worked against this patient.

Future Research Possibilities: Prevention and Treatment

Chronic hepatitis C presents in a number of different ways. The liver damage is due to both the direct effect of the virus and the inflammatory changes created by activation of the immune system. The effectiveness and potential liver toxicity of botanicals (herbs and other plant-derived supplements) used to treat chronic hepatitis have not been adequately studied. Research needs to continue on a large scale. Multi-center trials are needed to determine the role of botanicals in the prevention and treatment of hepatitis. We also need studies to determine the best dosage forms for botanicals. Finally, research is needed on the use of the total plant, rather than just what is believed to be the active ingredient(s).[37] Double-blind, randomized, controlled studies, the gold standard of *clinical* research, should be the ultimate goal of all future research.

Summary

Hepatitis C poses unique challenges for both patients and healthcare providers. Ayurveda, the holistic Indian system of medicine, provides a ray of hope. It emphasizes prevention of disease and promotion of health. There is a great deal of historical information about the drugs and plants used in Ayurveda. We have descriptions of how these treatments work to improve the health of people with liver disorders. Ayurvedic texts describe how treatments protect and detoxify the liver. To validate this traditional knowledge, Ayurveda is undergoing scientific inquiry to establish its efficacy in the treatment of liver disorders.

References

1. Chatterjee P. *Physiology of Gastrointestinal Tract: Human Physiology, Part I*. Calcutta, India: Popular Publishers; 1997.
2. Seef LB. The A, B, C, D, E's of viral hepatitis. Annual Postgraduate Gastroenterology Course, Section 2A: Liver. College of Gastroenterology 64th Annual Scientific Meeting. Phoenix, Arizona. 1999.
3. Thomas DL, Astemborski J, Rai RM, et al. The natural history of hepatitis C virus infection: host, viral, and environmental factors. *JAMA*. 2000;284:450-456.
4. Patrick, L. Hepatitis C: Epidemiology and review of complementary alternative medicine treatment. *Altern Med Rev*. 1999;4(4):220-238.
5. National Institutes of Health Consensus Development Conference Panel Statement: management of hepatitis C. *Hepatology*. 1997;26(3 Suppl 1):2-10S.
6. Laksmipathi A. History of Ayurveda. *Ayurvedic Encyclopaedia*, Vol 1, 16th Edition. Vavilla Ramaswamy Sastrulu and Sons. Madras, India. 1965.
7. Laksmipathi A. Treatises of Ayurveda. Ayurvedic Encyclopaedia, Vol 1. Vavilla Ramaswamy Sastrulu and Sons. Madras, India. 1965.
8. Sharma PV (Ed.). Charaka Samhita: Sutrasthanam, 23rd Edition. Chaukambha Orientalia. Varanasi, India. 1981. Chapter 30, stanza 23.
9. Sharma PV (Ed.). Charaka Samhita: Sutrasthanam, 23rd Edition. Chaukambha Orientalia. Varanasi, India. 1981. Chapter 30, stanzas 26, 47.
10. Sharma PV (Ed.). Charaka Samhita: Sutrasthanam, 23rd Edition. Chaukambha Orientalia. Varanasi, India. 1981. Chapter 30, stanza 41.
11. Varier, PS. Principles of Ayurveda, Chikitsa Samgraham. Arya Vaidya Sala, Kottakkal, India. 1989.
12. Sharma PV (Ed.). Charaka Samhita: Sutrasthanam, 23rd Edition. Chaukambha Orientalia. Varanasi, India. 1981. Chapter 12.
13. Vagbhata, D. Ashtanga Hridayam. Chaukambha Orientalia. Varanasi, India. 1980.
14. Vagbhata, D. Ashtanga Hridayam. Chaukambha Orientalia. Varanasi, India. 1980. Stanza 1-8.
15. Sharma PV (Ed.). Charaka Samhita: Sutrasthanam, 23rd Edition. Chaukambha Orientalia. Varanasi, India. 1981. Chapter 20, stanzas 11-13.
16. Sharma PV (Ed.). Charaka Samhita: Vimanasthanam. Chaukambha Orientalia. Varanasi, India. 1981. Chapter 5.
17. Susruta Samhita: Sutrasthanam. Motilal Banarasidas Publishers. New Delhi, India. 1983. Chapter 21, stanza 9.
18. Sharma PV (Ed.). Charaka Samhita: Vimanasthanam. Chaukambha Orientalia. Varanasi, India. 1981. Chapter 5, stanzas 6-10.
19. Vagbhata, D. Ashtanga Hridayam. Chaukambha Orientalia. Varanasi, India. 1980. Chapter 13, stanza 25.
20. Sharma PV (Ed.). Charaka Samhita: Sutrasthanam, 23rd Edition. Chaukambha Orientalia. Varanasi, India. 1981. Chapter 30, stanzas 6-11.

21.   Sharma PV (Ed.). Charaka Samhita: Vimanasthanam. Chaukambha Orientalia. Varanasi, India. 1981. Chapter 8, stanzas 112 -115.
22.   Susruta Samhita: Sutrasthanam. Motilal Banarasidas Publishers. New Delhi, India. 1983.
23.   Susruta Samhita: Sutrasthanam. Motilal Banarasidas Publishers. New Delhi, India. 1983. Chapter 24, stanza 10.
24.   Susruta Samhita: Sutrasthanam. Motilal Banarasidas Publishers. New Delhi, India. 1983. Chapter 21.
25.   Sharma PV (Ed.). Charaka Samhita: Sutrasthanam, 23rd Edition. Chaukambha Orientalia. Varanasi, India. 1981. Chapter 20.
26.   Sharma PV (Ed.). Charaka Samhita: Nidanasthanam. Chaukambha Orientalia. Varanasi, India. 1981. Chapter 1, stanzas 6-11.
27.   Yogaratnakara: Vol ume I, Pradhamakanda. Chaukambha Prakashan. Varanasi, India. 1989. Verse 35.
28.   Sarangadhara Samhita.. Chaukambha Orientalia. Varanasi, India. 1987. Chapter 1, verses 1-3
29.   Susruta Samhita: Sutrasthanam. Motilal Banarasidas Publishers. New Delhi, India. 1983.
30.   Sharma PV (Ed.). Charaka Samhita: Vimanasthanam. Chaukambha Orientalia. Varanasi, India. 1981. Chapter 7, stanzas 33, 43.
31.   Vagbhata, D. Ashtanga Hridayam. Chaukambha Orientalia. Varanasi, India. 1980. Chapter 13.
32.   Sharma PV (Ed.). Charaka Samhita: Sutrasthanam, 23rd Edition. Chaukambha Orientalia. Varanasi, India. 1981. Chapter 2.
33.   Deshpande UR, Joseph LJ, Samuel AM. Hepatobiliary clearance of labeled mebrofenin in normal and D-galactosamine HCl-induced hepatitis rats and the protective effect of turmeric extract. Indian J Physiol Pharmacol. 2003;47(3):332-6.
34.   Thapliyal R, Naresh KN, Rao KV, Maru GB. Inhibition of nitrosodiethylamine-induced hepatocarcinogenesis by dietary turmeric in rats. Toxicol Lett. 2003;139(1):45-54.
35.   Song EK, Cho H, Kim JS, et al. Diarylheptanoids with free radical scavenging and hepatoprotective activity in vitro from Curcuma longa. Planta Med. 2001;67(9):876-7.
36.   Anon. Curcuma longa (turmeric). Monograph. Altern Med Rev. 2001;6 Suppl:S62-6.
37.   Mishra,Shri K. Recent advances in liver diseases in Ayurvedic medicine in complementary and alternative medicine in chronic liver disease. National Institutes of Health Conference on Complementary and Alternative Medicine in Chronic Liver Diseases. Bethesda, Maryland. 1999;p.67. Chatterjee P. Physiology of Gastrointestinal Tract: Human Physiology, Part I. Popular Publishers. Calcutta, India. 1997.

CHINESE MEDICINE

Misha Cohen, OM, LAc

TRADITIONAL CHINESE MEDICINE AND HEPATITIS C

Introduction

Many people with the *hepatitis C virus (HCV)* turn to traditional Chinese medicine (TCM) for treatment. In the western world, TCM is often considered "alternative" medicine; however, in mainland China, Taiwan and other areas with Chinese origin, TCM is widely considered an integral part of the healthcare system and is often used as a primary form of medicine.

The term "TCM" is often used specifically within the field of modern Chinese medicine to refer to the standardized set of theories and practices in an organized system of training and education that was developed in the People's Republic of China after the Chinese revolution in 1949. This term, TCM, is distinguished from the broader related traditional theories and practices preserved by Chinese people around the world. In this section, we will use the term TCM to refer to all the related practices of Asian-based medicines that have found their origin in China. Traditional Chinese medicine is the longest continually used and developed organized medical system in the world today.

TCM has a long history in the treatment of *chronic hepatitis. Hepatitis B* and C infections are prevalent throughout China, and the Chinese medical system has been dedicated to solving these problems for many years. The Chinese are working to eliminate sources of hepatitis and to develop treatments for chronic viral hepatitis using both TCM and western medicine.

At the International Symposium on Viral Hepatitis and AIDS held in Beijing, China in April 1991, more than 100 papers on viral hepatitis were presented. Several of these papers documented the positive results of studies involving Chinese herbal medicines. Studies on the use of herbal *antivirals*, and blood cooling and circulating herbs for liver damage repair were presented. These studies corroborated hundreds of years of treatment experience with Chinese herbs for the *symptoms* of hepatitis.[1-3] A 1995 literature review revealed there are at least 55 herbal formulas used to treat hepatitis.[4] Some recent herbal studies from China and Australia showed positive results in chronic hepatitis C using herbal formulas similar to those widely used in the United States.[5-7]

In the United States, TCM is a popular *complementary and alternative medicine (CAM)* therapy among people with chronic liver diseases. TCM uses nutrition, acupuncture, heat therapies (such as *moxibustion*), exercise, massage, *meditation*, and herbal medicine to treat people infected with HCV. *Protocols* have been developed that have successfully helped people infected with *HIV* and HCV decrease symptoms, normalize or lower *liver enzymes*, and slow the progression of liver disease. A 1995 pilot study conducted among people coinfected with HIV and viral hepatitis (B or C) at San Francisco ís Quan Yin Healing Arts Center indicated acupuncture alone might have an effect in lowering and/or normalizing liver enzymes.[8]

Chinese Medicine Philosophy

The primary goals of TCM are to create wholeness and harmony within a person thereby allowing the mind, body, and spirit to self-heal. Chinese philosophy states there are two opposing principles of life, yin and yang. Imbalances between yin and yang within a person can manifest as illness because the body is considered a microcosm of the world.

TCM defines the *physiological* components of illness using the concepts of *qi* (vital energy), *xue* (blood), *jin-ye* (body fluids), *jing* (essence), *shen* (spirit), and organ systems. Organ systems are domains within the body that govern particular body tissues, emotional states, and activities. TCM theory states the key to health is the internal ability of the body to remain strong. According to this theory, people are born with a certain amount of original qi (pronounced "chee"). The qi is easily depleted as the body uses energy and is not replaced.

It is difficult to increase the original qi. A person must work hard during life just to retain it. Exercise such as *tai chi* and *qi gong*, healthy eating, and good sleep habits are highly recommended for maintaining the original qi. If a person consistently lacks sleep, does not have a healthy diet, abuses drugs or *alcohol*, and/or has excessive or unsafe sex, he or she becomes qi deficient. When weakened and qi deficient, a person is more susceptible to infection by harmful external elements.[9]

Traditional Chinese Medicine and Hepatitis

According to TCM literature, people in China have experienced various *syndromes* associated with viral hepatitis for over 2000 years. This is because TCM diagnoses are based on *symptoms*, not on detection of *antibodies* to a specific virus. TCM treatments for these syndromes have been used over the past millennia and are generally considered safe and effective for all patients. Further, TCM recognizes that each person has a unique constitution and pattern of disease that exists in conjunction with the age-old syndromes. TCM contends that the best form of treatment is to modify, alter, or supplement base therapies to create an individualized treatment that meets each patient's unique characteristics and needs.

Chinese medical theory states that viral hepatitis is not a singular disease, but includes a combination of *stages* and syndromes. The diagnosis and staging of HCV are accomplished using tongue diagnosis, pulse diagnosis, and questioning to determine if the patient's initial western diagnosis is consistent with TCM theory.

According to TCM, the organ systems primarily disturbed in hepatitis are the liver and spleen. These disturbed organ systems affect digestion and energy. According to TCM, acute viral hepatitis is generally associated with excess damp heat or damp cold conditions. While a few people acutely infected with HCV may have symptoms, they are rare. The TCM stage at which one is diagnosed with hepatitis C is usually either the chronic stage of qi stagnation or the stage of qi and yin deficiency. Advanced chronic disease includes development of the patterns of xue stagnation and xue deficiency. All HCV infection is associated with *toxic* heat or the *li qi* or *yi qi* (the pestilence/epidemic factor).[10]

Traditional Chinese Medicine Therapy For HCV

In western medicine, extremely harmful external elements include severe bacterial or viral infections such as HCV and HIV. However, those terms are not used in TCM. Instead, traditional Chinese medicine, "... recognizes the existence of Pestilences called *li qi* or *yi qi*. These are diseases that are not caused by the climatic factors of Heat, Cold, Wind, Dampness, or Summer Heat dryness, but by external infectious agents... that are severely toxic because they strike directly at the interior of the body.î In the case of HCV, the particular pestilence is identified as toxic heat. Toxic heat is considered by TCM to be both an epidemic factor (something that is seen in a number of patients) and its own individual, treatable syndrome.[10]

The various modalities of TCM therapy include diet, massage, heat therapies, exercise, meditation, and acupuncture. Heat therapies include the use of moxibustion. Moxibustion is the burning of the herb mugwort over certain areas of the body to stimulate or warm these areas. Exercise therapy ranges from martial arts to more subtle forms of movement such as tai chi and qi gong.

Acupuncture is perhaps the most well known form of TCM in the United States. It is the art of inserting fine, sterile, metal filiform needles into acupuncture points on the body in order to control the flow of energy (qi). Acupuncture therapy can include electrostimulation and/or hand stimulation. This form of therapy is most appreciated for its ability to relieve pain. However, acupuncture is also able to help change body energy patterns, which promotes the body's ability to heal itself of disease syndromes and symptoms.

In these treatments, TCM often does not distinguish energetic effects from *physiologic* effects. The different modalities of TCM have different aims. Some focus on balancing the body's energy, while others focus on building the physical body and adding substances to both balance and change the body materially. For example, the Enhance® herbal preparation used in HCV, as well as HIV, contains herbs to tonify the spleen qi and build xue. Qi tonification increases the amount of energy available for certain bodily function. Qi tonic herbs often have the specific effect of increasing digestion and food absorption. This increases the quality of the blood (xue).

Acupuncture is associated with balancing the body's energy levels, while herbal substances are more like drugs or foods in that they have specific physical effects. Breathing exercises are known to strengthen qi. One meaning of the Chinese word qi is air. By learning how to breathe correctly, more oxygen is made available to enter the bloodstream. Specific Chinese traditional therapies are discussed below.

Chinese Herbal Medicine for HCV

TCM herbal treatment for HCV depends on the stage of the disease and the syndromes involved. In my clinic and in the Chinese herbal formulas I have designed for use in hepatitis C, we use a combination of western research into the cause of hepatitis and its manifestations in conjunction with TCM traditional knowledge of combining individual herb into herbal formulas. We choose herbs for the formulas that have specific western effects for herbal formula development as well as the traditional usage of herbs used for centuries for the patterns associated with hepatitis. The modern Chinese herb formulas we end up with are formulas designed with the traditional complex organization specific to Chinese traditional herbal medicine in conjunction with modern herbal *pharmacology*. This creates balance and harmony within the formulas as dictated by traditional principles yet is guided by contemporary herb principles.

In the last several decades, Chinese medicine has developed two herbal medicine modern principles, Fu Zheng and Jiedu/Qu Xie. Originally developed for use in cancer in the 1970's, they are now used in treating chronic viral infections and other infectious disease.[11] Fu Zheng uses treatments to support the body's natural disease-fighting systems (that is, the *immune system*). Jiedu/Qu Xie, focuses on eliminating External Pernicious Influences (outside *pathogens*). In western terms, Fu Zheng and Jiedu/Qu Xie can be called immune-regulating and anti-*toxin* therapies. As the body becomes stronger, the disease itself can be controlled and the body can return to balance.[9]

Herbal medications in conjunction with rest and dietary recommendations can treat the symptoms of *acute hepatitis* fairly rapidly. Chronic hepatitis C is more difficult to treat. Research and experience both from China and from TCM clinics in the United States suggest that a one-year course of TCM therapy is the minimum needed to alter the progression of hepatitis C.

In our clinics, TCM therapy for chronic hepatitis C usually includes combinations of herbal preparations, which are often specifically designed for the disturbed organ system patterns. For example, the combination of Enhance® and Clear Heat® herbal formulas were developed for the treatment of HIV and other chronic viral disease using the concepts of Fu Zheng and Jiedu/Qu Xie. These formulas were tested in an herbal study at San Francisco General Hospital.[12] Hepatoplex One®, Hepatoplex Two®, and other herbal formulas have been designed specifically for the treatment of chronic hepatitis and related problems.

A few Chinese medicine practitioners in the U.S. have developed specific treatments for HCV and HIV infections based on these principles. Two such practitioners are Dr. Subhuti Dharmananda of Portland, Oregon and Dr. Qing-Cai Zhang of New York, New York (See *Chapter 11. 2, Modern Chinese Medicine* for additional information on Dr. Zhangís protocol.) My own experience treating people with HIV and HCV led me to develop the following herbal formulas. The formulas shown in Table 1 can be recommended and prescribed by licensed TCM practitioners and qualified herbalists. Special additional training in these herbal formulas and certification in HCV is given to licensed practitioners through the Quan Yin Healing Arts Centerís Hepatitis C Professional Training Program along with the Misha Ruth Cohen Education Foundation.

Table 1. Examples of Chinese Herbal Formulas Used for HCV at Chicken Soup Chinese Medicine and Quan Yin Healing Arts Center, San Francisco, California

Indication	Herbal Formulas
Acute hepatitis C	Coptis Purge Fire® Clear Heat® Hepatoplex One® Ecliptex® Long Dan Xie Gan Tang
Chronic hepatitis C	Hepatoplex One® Hepatoplex Two® Ecliptex®
Immune disorders	Cordyseng® Cordyceps PS® Enhance® Tremella American Ginseng®
Toxic heat related to chronic viral inflammation	Clear Heat®
Digestive problems	Curing Pills Quiet Digestion®
Gallstones or gall bladder Inflammation	GB6®
Liver inflammation and chronic hepatitis	Milk Thistle 80® / Silymarin (Karuna)
Qi Stagnation with Xue deficiency	Women's Balance®
Other	Milk Thistle 80® / Silymarin (Karuna)

Hepatoplex One® is used for acute and chronic hepatitis symptoms. It may be used when liver enzymes are elevated. It can be used with Clear Heat® to increase the Clear Heat® toxin-cleaning effect. It is designed to regulate qi, vitalize xue, clear heat, and clean toxin.

While there are herbs to help protect the digestion in Hepatoplex One®, this formula is usually used in conjunction with formulas that protect the spleen and stomach, as there are a number of herbs that are cooling or cold and vitalize xue. For example, to increase the effects of tonifying qi and yin, this formula can be taken with Cordyseng® or Cordyceps PS®. If there is spleen dampness and deficiency with loose stools, add Shen Ling®. If there is liver invading spleen, a common scenario in chronic hepatitis patients, you may add Shu Gan®.

To protect the yin in liver disease and specifically in chronic hepatitis, you may use Ecliptex®. For *immunodeficiency* disorders, you may add Enhance® or Tremella American Ginseng®. For xue stagnation including liver *fibrosis, cirrhosis,* and decreased blood circulation, add Hepatoplex Two®.

For xue deficiency and xue stagnation, or to protect the bone marrow during *interferon* plus *ribavirin* treatment, *chemotherapy*, or radiation, add Marrow Plus®. This formula is used for pre-treatment and during interferon/ribavirin therapy.

Hepatoplex Two® is designed to vitalize xue. When used in chronic hepatitis, it should be used in conjunction with other herbal formulas. Its special uses are for liver fibrosis and cirrhosis, and to decrease the size of an enlarged liver. It may also have an effect on splenomegaly (an enlarged spleen). As Hepatoplex Two® is a formula designed to vitalize xue, it should increase circulation of the blood and improve microcirculation in the capillaries.

Cordyseng® and Cordyceps PS® is used as an adjunct to other herbal formulas to increase the function of qi tonification and increase energy. The formula tonifies both yin and yang. It primarily strengthens the spleen, stomach, kidney, and lung, and helps digestion. It is especially good for the chronic fatigue found in chronic hepatitis.

Case Study Examples

A person presents with chronic hepatitis C with stage III fibrosis and grade II *inflammation*. He is preparing to go on interferon treatment in three months. The patient is fatigued. The tongue and pulse configuration match the Chinese diagnoses of toxic heat, damp heat qi and xue stagnation, and possible qi and xue deficiency. The recommended herbal protocol for this patient could be:

- Cordyseng® or Cordyceps PS®
- Marrow Plus®
- Hepatoplex One® and/or Hepatoplex Two®

A person presents with hepatitis C with stage 0 fibrosis and grade I inflammation. She has a very high *viral load*. The patient generally feels well. She has been advised to wait to try interferon therapy. The tongue and pulse configuration match the Chinese diagnoses of toxic heat, and qi stagnation. The recommended herbal protocol for this patient could be:

- Hepatoplex One®
- Clear Heat®

A person presents with hepatitis C with stage one fibrosis and grade two inflammation. The patient has lots of gas and digestive problems and fatigue is worse after loose stools. The tongue and pulse configuration match the Chinese diagnoses of toxic heat, spleen deficiency with dampness and qi stagnation. The recommended herbal protocol for this patient could be:

- Hepatoplex One®
- Shen Ling®

Acupuncture Therapies for HCV

TCM uses acupuncture extensively in the treatment of chronic hepatitis. Though some of the herbal theories already discussed may apply to acupuncture, the primary goal of acupuncture treatment is to readjust the body's qi in order to enable the body to heal itself. Therefore, acupuncture treatment can be used to treat both specific symptoms and a general epidemic pattern.

After a TCM diagnosis is given for a patient infected with HCV, an acupuncture treatment plan is developed by considering the epidemic nature of the disease, the individual's complaints, and any underlying constitutional TCM patterns of illness. On a symptomatic level, acupuncture treatments for HCV infection address digestive functions, appetite, energy level, stress, anxiety, *depression*, pain, and skin complications. Acupuncture has also been used to lower elevated liver enzymes as part of a chronic hepatitis protocol using special acupuncture points.[8] Acupuncture can play a role in relieving side effects during interferon-based therapy.[13]

Moxibustion

An important part of TCM treatment in HCV is the use of moxibustion. Moxibustion is the burning of the herb mugwort (called moxa in Chinese) over certain points or areas of the body that correspond to acupuncture points. Moxa is rolled into a cigar-like stick or used loose over protected skin to create warmth and tonification. In Chinese studies, moxa has been shown to increase digestive function, *white blood cell* and *platelet* counts, and may have an effect on the transformation of *T cells* (one type of immune cell). Moxibustion is often used for pain syndromes and areas that appear or feel cold on the body. It is often prescribed for home use in treating both HIV and HCV infections.

Qi Gong for HCV

Qi gong meditation and exercise is a common practice in China. It is growing in popularity in the United States among people who have HCV, HIV and other life-threatening illnesses such as cancer. Many studies show the positive effects of qi gong on immune function.[14-16] Many locations around the United States offer medical qi gong classes specifically designed for people infected with HCV and/or HIV.

Dietary Therapy for HCV

A healthy diet is considered a key part of maintaining qi and harmony in the body. Most TCM practitioners recommend that people generally eat a cooked, warm diet in order to strengthen the spleen and stomach. Other recommendations are based on the specific organ pattern diagnosis. For example, those suffering from chronic diarrhea may be advised to eat white rice (not brown) or barley daily, especially in the form of an easy-to-make rice porridge called congee or jook.[17] A low *glycemic index* diet is also advised to control *insulin* resistance.[18]

Congee Recipes

Congee — or hot rice cereal — is often used in Chinese medicine for its curative powers and is often used by people during or after a long illness in which one is weak and may have difficulty eating. You can concoct many varieties using foods and herbs. Your Chinese medicine practitioner can prescribe those that are particularly suited for your constitution.

Basic Congee

Cook one cup of rice in seven to nine cups of filtered water for six to eight hours (with insulin resistance you may use whole barley as a substitute).

> **Variations**
> Add 1/4 cup of the following ingredients for every 1 to 1 1/2 cups of congee.
>
> > **Mung bean** - Mung bean congee cools fevers.
> >
> > **Aduki Bean** - Aduki bean congee removes dampness, helps ease swelling and edema, and aids in treatment of bladder-kidney problems.
> >
> > **Carrot** - Carrot congee eases indigestion.

Combining Eastern and Western Therapies

If you decide to use a combination of eastern and western therapies, you must discuss <u>all</u> of your treatment approaches with both your eastern and western practitioners. The use of some herbal therapies in conjunction with interferon-based therapy may be inappropriate.

In my experience, Chinese medicine can be highly effective for the management of side effects from medicines used in therapy. In my clinic, and through practitioners trained in the Hepatitis C Professional Training Program, we offer a special Optimum Interferon Protocol[10, 13] that can be used to prepare for and be used during interferon/ribavirin therapy.

Some people with HCV rely on both western and eastern diagnosis, are followed by their *hepatologist* for years, yet have only used Chinese medicine and other CAM therapies to manage their liver health as well as overall wellness.

Protecting your liver is key no matter what therapies you choose.

- Always tell <u>all</u> of your healthcare providers about each and every medication, herb, supplement, or other medicinal you are taking or using. This will ensure the safety of your overall health care plan, and will help you gain the greatest benefit from all of your treatment modalities

- Avoid anything that is toxic to the liver. A list of herbs and drugs that have known liver toxicity can be found in *Appendix IV*.

Summary

Many people with HCV are using TCM as either complementary or alternative treatment. TCM uses a number of therapies including acupuncture, moxibustion, Chinese herbs, qi gong, and dietary therapy. While these therapies have not undergone major *clinical trials* in the west, many of them have been used for centuries in China for hepatitis and other conditions. The results of modern Chinese research on herbs and other modalities are used in the development of current Chinese medicine treatments for HCV.

For recommended reading on traditional Chinese medicine, please see the *Resource Directory*.

References

1. Wang C, He J, Zhu C. Research of repair of liver pathologic damage in 63 cases of hepatitis with severe cholestatis by blood-cooling and circulation-invigorating Chinese herbs. International Symposium on Viral Hepatitis and AIDS. Beijing China. Abstract, p 5. 1991.
2. Chen Z, et al. Clinical analysis of chronic hepatitis B treated with TCM compositions Fugan No. 33 by two lots. International Symposium on Viral Hepatitis and AIDS. Beijing, China. Abstract, p 2. 1991.
3. Zhao R, Shen H. Antifibrogenesis with traditional Chinese herbs. International Symposium on Viral Hepatitis and AIDS. Beijing China. Abstract, p 20. 1991.
4. Ergil K. Fifth Symposium of the Society for Acupuncture Research Conference. Herbal safety and research panel. Society for Acupuncture Research Conference. Palo Alto, California.1998.
5. Batey RG, Benssoussen A, Yang Yifan, Hossain MA, Bollipo S. Chinese herbal medicine lowers ALT in hepatitis C. A randomized placebo controlled trial report. Cathay Herbal Laboratories. Sydney Australia. 1998. Available at: http://www.cathayherbal.com Accessed August 20, 2008
6. Li H, et al. Qingtui fang applied in treating 128 cases of chronic hepatitis C. *Chinese Journal of Integrated Traditional and Western Medicine for Liver Diseases.* 1994;4(2):40. [Note: This journal is not included in the National Library of Medicine's PubMed database.]
7. Wu C, et al. Thirty-three patients with hepatitis C treated by TCM syndrome differentiation. *Chinese Journal of Integrated Traditional and Western Medicine for Liver Diseases.* 1994;4(I):44-45. [Note: This journal is not included in the National Library of Medicine's PubMed database.]
8. Cohen M, Wilson CJ, Surasky, A. Acupuncture Treatment In HIV+ People With HCV/HBV Co-Infection And Elevated Transaminases, Abstract Book # 60211. XIIth International Conference on AIDS, Geneva Switzerland, 1998.
9. Cohen M. *The HIV Wellness Sourcebook: An East West Guide To Living Well with HIV/AIDS.* New York: Henry Holt; 1998
10. Cohen M. Doner K. *The Hepatitis C Help Book: A Groundbreaking Treatment Program Combining Western and Eastern Medicine for Maximum Wellness and Healing, Revised Edition.* New York: St. Martin's Griffin; 2007.
11. Mingji P. *Cancer Treatment with Fu Zheng Pei Ben Principle.* Fujian: Fujian Science and Technology Publishing House; 1992
12. Burack JH, Cohen MR, Hahn JA, Abrams DI. Pilot Randomized Controlled Trial of Chinese Herbal Treatment for HIV-Associated Symptoms. *Journal of Acquired Immune Deficiency Syndromes & Human Retrovirology.* 12(4):386-393, August 1, 1996.
13. Cohen MR. Optimum Interferon Protocol. Available at: http://www.docmisha.com/applying/hepatitis_help/06download.html#interferon.

CHINESE MEDICINE

Qing Cai Zhang, MD (China), LAc

SECTION

2

MODERN CHINESE MEDICINE THERAPEUTICS FOR HEPATITIS C

Introduction

One-third of the world's viral hepatitis carriers reside in China: over 150 million viral hepatitis patients. More than 30 million people in China are infected with the *hepatitis C* virus (*HCV*).[1] Thus, doctors in China have a great deal of experience treating hepatitis with Chinese medicine.

For the most part, China is still a developing country. Expensive drugs such as *interferon* and *ribavirin* are not readily available, nor are they affordable. In addition, the success rate of these drugs is not satisfactory and the side effects can be severe. This has prompted most Chinese hepatitis C patients to use traditional Chinese medicine (TCM), or integrated Chinese and western medicine known as modern Chinese medicine (MCM).

TCM serves more than one billion people in China and Southeast Asia. There are more than one million TCM practitioners in China alone. Five years ago, the Chinese government conducted a national survey on Chinese medicinal substances and found that 11,146 species of plants, 1,581 species of animals, and 80 minerals have been used as TCM remedies.[2] One-fourth of the world's population uses TCM, the second largest medical system in the world today. In Japan, there are more than 200,000 healthcare providers prescribing Chinese herbal medicines for their patients. TCM is used to treat almost every disease identified by western medicine. TCM is used in Europe, Canada, and the United States, especially in the western, eastern, and northern parts of the U.S.

As discussed in *Chapter 11.1, Traditional Chinese Medicine and Hepatitis C*, TCM is a very old and established healing system based on the restoration of the body's harmony and balance. TCM focuses on maintaining health rather than managing disease. TCM is an empirical medicine, which was mainly developed through *clinical* observation.

During the past five decades, there has been a new development in TCM. Practitioners have begun integrating TCM and western medicine. This combination of TCM and western medicine has created a new version of integrated medicine, modern Chinese medicine. The marriage of TCM and western medicine has brought great benefits to patients. Since the late 1950's, a modernization movement brought TCM into every medical school in China. TCM is taught along with western medicine. The majority of Chinese healthcare providers include both TCM and western medicine in their practices. For most clinical conditions, these two medical approaches are used together and the results are usually better than when either approach was used alone.[3] As part of this movement, many western healthcare providers have devoted large amounts of time and energy to the scientific study of TCM.

This section discusses the general principles of MCM treatments for hepatitis C, and also uses the *protocols* developed in Zhang's Clinic in New York City as an example of modern Chinese medicine. It is important to note that, because of differences in education and training, every qualified practitioner develops his/her own way of practicing MCM. This is only one example of how MCM can be applied to the treatment of people with *chronic hepatitis* C. Anyone considering MCM should compare different practitioners' approaches and make an educated decision about whom they should see for treatment.

Modern Chinese Medical Therapeutics for Liver Diseases

Modern Chinese Medical Therapeutics for Liver Diseases (MCMTLD) is a new branch of Chinese medicine developed from *integrative medicine* studies on liver diseases. It is the application of Chinese medicine to treat liver diseases such as viral hepatitis, nonalcoholic *steatohepatitis* (*NASH*), *jaundice*, *cirrhosis*, and *hepatocellular carcinoma* as defined by western medicine.

After a half century of practice and data accumulation, MCMTLD has succeeded in improving the clinical outcomes of liver diseases, especially in viral hepatitis C and B. Many effective herbal treatment protocols for liver diseases have been developed and put into practice. MCMTLD is the main *modality* for treating viral hepatitis in China today.[4]

In dealing with *chronic hepatitis* C, MCM uses western medical knowledge of how the disease originated, how the disease causes harm, and how to diagnose and monitor the disease. This knowledge is combined with TCM diagnostic tools and Zheng *symptom* pattern differentiation to individualize each patient's health status diagnosis and treatments accordingly. In MCM, herb use is based on both TCM principles and plant *pharmacology*. We now know the active ingredients of the herbs and their actions in the body. We have learned more about possible *toxicities* and side effects, proper doses, and treatment courses.

The main MCM treatments for hepatitis C are focused in two areas: controlling liver *inflammation* and *antifibrosis*.[5] The pathology of hepatitis C is similar to that of chronic *hepatitis B*, so many MCM treatment methods are the outgrowth of previously developed hepatitis B protocols.

Chinese medicine's approach to chronic viral infections is called fu zheng qu xie. The translation of this phrase is, "dispelling evil (the virus) by supporting righteous qi (normal function of the body)." The *immune system* is a major part of the righteous qi (pronounced chee). Therefore, supporting the immune system is an important part of Chinese medical treatment for hepatitis C. There are many Chinese therapies to help regulate and support the immune system.

Chinese medicine asserts that the body itself is the major healing force. Medications and procedures can help the body heal, but they cannot replace the healing function of the body. In treating chronic hepatitis C, Chinese medicine focuses on normalizing liver functions and restoring overall health to strengthen the body's immune functions. As the body becomes stronger, the disease itself can be controlled and the body can return to balance.

During the course of chronic *HCV* infection, many pathological changes occur in the body. Some of these changes are inadequate immune reactions, liver inflammation, *fibrosis*, and *portal hypertension*. All of these changes have significant effects on disease *prognosis*. Therefore, MCM treatment is a multiple target regulatory strategy that attempts to cover the full spectrum of the *pathogenesis*.

Multiple Target Strategy: Eight Goals of MCM Treatment for Hepatitis C

1. Reduce HCV *viral load* and/or suppress viral *replication*
2. Heal liver inflammation and restore liver function to halt disease progression (anti-inflammation)
3. Regulate immune functions
4. Improve *microcirculation* (blood flow to organs and tissues) and lower portal vein hypertension
5. Promote liver cell regeneration to restore liver structure
6. Suppress *fibroblastic* activity to reduce scarring (antifibrosis)
7. Facilitating *bile* flow to release bile retention
8. Treat hepatitis C peripheral symptoms and complications to improve overall health

---

MCM Antiviral Treatments

Since hepatitis C is an infectious disease, the eradication of the virus is an important goal of treatment. MCM herbal remedies do not eliminate the hepatitis C virus. If the patient is seeking total eradication of HCV, then *interferon- based therapy* is advised. MCM can be a complementary treatment to mitigate HCV symptoms. It is also used to alleviate the side effects of *interferon-based treatment*.

A healthier body is better able to control the virus and prevent it from causing further harm. Suppressing HCV is achieved by strengthening the immune system and using *antiviral* herbal remedies. Herbal treatments may be able to reduce HCV viral load, but cannot eliminate the virus. These include oleuopain (the purified extracts of the olive leaf) and glycyrrhizin (the active ingredient of Glycyrrhiza uralensis Fisch).

Glycyrrhizin has been found to have anti-*HBV*, anti-*HIV*, and anti-VSV (vesiculovirus) effects in the laboratory.[6-8] In our clinic, we use Olivessence Capsule® and Glycyrrhizin Capsule® for antiviral treatment of HCV.

MCM Anti-Inflammation Treatment

Liver inflammation causes fibrosis, which may lead to *cirrhosis*. In order to stop the progression of fibrosis, liver inflammation must be controlled. MCM has developed many herbal remedies for controlling liver inflammation, such as schizandrin B and C (active ingredients of Schizandrae Fructus), glycyrrhizin, oleanolic acid (active ingredient of Ligustrum lucidum Ait), silymarin (active ingredient of Silybum marianum), oxymatrine (active ingredient of Sophorae Subprostratae Radix), and Sedin (active ingredient of Sedi sarmentosi herba). These herbal substances can lower alanine aminotransferase (*ALT*) and *aspartate aminotransferase* (*AST*) levels, protect the liver cell membrane, and reduce inflammatory cell infiltration and liver cell *necrosis*.

The active ingredients of schizandra and schisandrin B and C have been tested in *clinical trials* in China. Studies involving 4,558 patients showed schisandrin B and C reduced and/or normalized ALT levels in 75% of the cases within 2 to 3 months. Of 153 patients treated with oleanolic acid, 110 (70%) experienced normalization of their ALT within 50 days.[9] The therapeutic effects of oleanolic acid was also studied in a multicenter clinical trial and found to have an efficacy rate of 69.8%.[10] Glycyrrhizin has been used to treat chronic viral hepatitis in China and Japan. Studies have shown that it was effective in normalizing ALT in 64% of patients in Japan, and 84.5% of patients in China.[11] The phytopharmacology and clinical studies of these herbal active ingredients were done on animal models, in liver cell cultures, and in multi-center clinical trials of patients.[12]

ALT is an important marker of liver inflammation and liver cell necrosis. After treatment, if three consecutive ALT tests (done 2 to 3 months apart) are normal, liver inflammation is considered as being well controlled. In a clinical observation done in our office in 2000, we found that 77% of our patients had their ALT level normalized and 93% improved their ALT level with our anti-inflammatory treatment.[13]

The liver is a complex organ and has hundreds of functions. Aside from laboratory markers that only test about a dozen parameters, the patient's general feeling of well-being and overall health status carries significant value in evaluating the results of liver inflammation control and liver function restoration. Patient reports of reduced *fatigue*, decreased liver area discomfort, improved appetite and digestion, improved bowel movements, fading of liver palm and spider moles, normalization of urine and stool color, and the *clearance* of jaundice are considered in MCM as indicators of controlled liver inflammation and liver function restoration.

MCM Antifibrosis Treatments

Fibrosis is the process that results in the majority of the liver damage in chronic hepatitis C. Serious complications of liver diseases are due to extensive fibrosis. Therefore, antifibrosis treatment has been an important focus of research on treatment for chronic liver disease. If fibrosis can be arrested or reversed, the prognosis for those with chronic hepatitis C can be greatly improved. MCM treatment goals to improve *microcirculation*, lower portal vein hypertension, promote liver cell regeneration to restore the liver structure, and suppress fibrosis are discussed in this section.

Liver fibrosis is the net result of the imbalance between synthesis and degradation of the *extracellular* matrix (ECM). Fibrosis progresses when ECM synthesis is active and its rate of decomposition is decreased.

Fibrosis can be halted or reversed if its driver, liver inflammation, is controlled. Chinese studies have found that with antifibrosis herbal treatment, it is possible to enhance the activity of collagenase. Collagenase is an *enzyme* that breaks down *collagen*, a component of scar tissue. Enhanced collagenase activity promotes the breakdown of ECM and may arrest fibrosis progression.

For many years, MCM antifibrosis studies have shown that fibrosis is reversible.[14, 15] In China, antifibrosis with Chinese medicine is an intensive field of research in the treatment of chronic viral hepatitis. From 1998 to 2001, more than 2,000 articles on liver fibrosis have been published in China and over half of these articles discuss antifibrosis treatments. In our clinic, of the seven patients that underwent before and after herbal treatment biopsies six found their fibrosis *stage* decreased.

Antifibrosis Treatments Based on TCM Theories

In China, most antifibrosis studies have been based on chronic hepatitis B or schistosomiasis (a parasitic worm infection). In TCM literature, fibrosis is discussed under the topics of Yu Xue (blood stasis) and Zheng Jia (abdominal masses), which are the main *pathogeneses* of liver fibrosis according to TCM theories. Typically, patients have the following symptoms and *signs*: liver palms (redness of the palms of the hands), spider moles, cold hands and feet, purplish tongue, dark lips, a dark ring around each eye, and/or an enlarged liver and spleen.[16]

The main treatment principle underlying antifibrosis treatments is based on Huo Xue Hua Yu (promoting blood circulation by removing blood stasis) and Ruan Jian San Jie (softening and resolving hard masses). The interpretation of the treatment principle is to remove hard masses by promoting the blood circulation. Promoting circulation involves:

- improving the liquidity of the blood

- reducing blood viscosity

- suppressing the clustering of *red blood cells* and *platelets*

- promoting the work of *white blood cells* in removing circulatory immune complexes

- promote microcirculation to increase blood delivery to the tissues

TCM herbal formulas used to treat liver fibrosis were evaluated from TCM treatments for other fibrotic diseases. The traditional formulas used for this therapy are:

- Xue Fu Zhu Yu Tang (*Decoction* for Removing Blood Stasis in the Chest)[17]

- Ge Xie Zhu Yu Tang (Decoction for Removing Blood Stasis Below the Diaphragm)[18]

- Shao Fu Zhu Yu Tang (Decoction for Removing Blood Stasis in the Lower Abdomen)[19]

In our clinic's protocols, we use Circulation P Capsule® as one of the major antifibrosis remedies. Circulation P Capsule® is a modification of above mentioned traditional formulas Xue Fu Zhu Yu Tang and Ge Xie Zhu Yu Tang. Chinese studies have found that after taking Xue Fu Zhu Yu Tang formula for three months, the levels of fibrosis markers (such as hyaluronic acid, laminin, collagen IV, and precollagen type III) are significantly reduced.[20] Our Circulation P Capsule® formula is composed of a combination of the two formulas mentioned above with the addition of more potent active ingredients, such as notoginsenoside, chuanxingzine, tanshinone, and ferulic acid. Circulation P Capsule® is the main formula we use for antifibrosis treatment by the "blood activating and stasis expelling" mechanism.

MCM Theories of Antifibrosis Treatments

The studies on MCM antifibrosis treatments were focused on suppressing the activities of *hepatic stellate cells* (HSC) and *cytokines*, reducing the synthesis of ECM, and restoring the equilibrium of the production and degradation of ECM.[21] Because fibrosis is complex process, antifibrosis therapy is a multipronged treatment.

PREVENT LIVER CELL INJURY, ANTI-OXIDATION, AND CONTROL INFLAMMATION

Liver cell injury sets off the liver fibrosis process. Treating the primary liver disease, such as chronic hepatitis C, to reduce the inflammation, eliminate *free radicals*, and prevent liver cell damage is the most important antifibrosis therapy.[22]

SUPPRESS HEPATIC STELLATE CELL ACTIVITY

Liver stellate cells are key players in fibrosis. Suppressing HSC activity and promoting its destruction is an important antifibrosis treatment. Studies using liver biopsies have shown herbal antifibrosis treatment can reduce the number and activity level of hepatic stellate cells.[23]

SUPPRESS THE SYNTHESIS AND SECRETION OF EXTRACELLULAR MATRIX

Serum markers such as hyaluronic acid, laminin, collagen IV, and pre-collagen III are frequently used as fibrosis markers as they are all components of the extracellular matrix (the "glue" between cells). Ginkgolides has the effects of inhibiting cytokines that promote collagen deposition in the ECM.[24] Salviolic acid B has shown suppressive effects on the secretion of TGF-β1 (which promotes ECM activity) by HSC, and also inhibits collagen synthesis in HSC.[25] Antifibrosis formula 861 has been shown to reduce the levels of total collagen and type I, III, and V collagen.[26]

PROMOTE THE DECOMPOSITION OF ECM

Fibroblastic (fiber making) and *fibrocatalytic* (fiber degrading) activities exist side by side. In the early stages of fibrosis, the levels of catalytic enzymes called matrix metalloproteinases (MMP) also increase. However, this increase is not enough to completely contain increased fibroblastic activities. In the late stage of liver disease, MMP activities decrease and results in significant decline of fiber catalytic activities. This in turn, causes the net increase of the ECM.

Chinese herbal treatments, such as formula 861, can increase MMP *gene* expression and activities, which strengthens the catalytic activities of collagen to reduce the ECM.[26] Herbal active ingredients ginkgolides, glycyrrhizin, cordyceps, extracts of Persicae Semen, and oxymatrine all promote the decomposition of ECM.[27]

PREVENT LIVER SINUSOID CAPILLARIZATION

The deposit of collagen IV and laminin triggers liver sinusoid capillarization. This is a very important *pathological* change during liver fibrosis and hinders the exchange of chemical substances between liver cells and the blood circulation. It also increases resistance to blood flow through the liver causing portal hypertension. Oxymatrine and Cordyceps sinensis may reverse the capillarization process and improve material exchange between liver cells and the blood circulation.[28]

Antifibrosis Herbs and Their Active Ingredients

Based on clinical and experimental research in China, the following herbs have been found to have antifibrosis effects [29]:

Cordyceps sinensis	*Bos Taurus demesticus*
Glycyrrhiza uralensis Fisch	*Gleditsia sinensis*
Salviae Miltiorrhziae Radix	*Stephania tetrandra*
Cnidii Rhizom	*Curcuma longa*
Sophorae Subprostratae Radix	*Notoginseng Sanchis Radix*
Rhei Rhizoma	*Angelicae Radix*
Persicae Semen	*Astragali Radix*

For detailed information on the action of these herbs, see *Appendix III*.

Antifibrosis Herbal Formulas

In recent years, there has been much progress in the field of antifibrosis treatment using herbal formulas.[30] Formulas can organize and combine the pharmacological actions of single herbs to address multiple targets and different areas of the fibrosis pathway. When designing formulas, anti-inflammatory and antifibrosis compounds are used as the main ingredients, while other herbs that are immune supportive, tonifying, and invigorating are used to enhance the formula's overall therapeutic effect.

Examples of these formulas include:

Xue Fu Zhu Yu Tang	*Fu Zheng Hua Yu Fang*
Ge Xie Zhu Yu Tang	*Bu Yang Huan Wu Tang*
Herbal Formula 861®	

Treating Hepatitis C-Related Complications and Symptoms to Improve Quality of Life

Control Bile Retention and Jaundice

Chronic viral hepatitis patients often exhibit thickened bile that may become blocked by inflamed liver tissue. This can cause jaundice, gall bladder inflammation, and gallstones. Bile retention can also injure the liver and further promote fibrosis. This leads to a rise in *liver enzymes* and *bilirubin* level in the blood. Therefore, improving bile secretion is an important treatment goal in hepatitis. The following formulas can be used to release blocked bile and clear jaundice:

> Gall No. 1 Capsule®
>
> Capillaris Combination (*Yin Chen Hao Tang*)

They can also be used to treat gallbladder inflammation and to eliminate small gallstones.[31]

Lower Portal Vein Pressure

Portal hypertension is the main cause of many complications in advanced chronic liver disease. Portland hypertension is usually present in people with cirrhosis and can lead to *ascites* (accumulation of fluid in the abdomen), *edema* (accumulation of fluid in the feet and lower legs), spleen enlargement, and *varices* (abnormal expansion of veins). Thus, reducing portal pressure is important for patients with advanced liver disease. To lower *portal vein* pressure, we use Red Peony Capsule®, which can lower pressure in the portal vein, spleen, mesenteric, and esophagus veins. This formula also has antifibrosis effects.

Improve Fatigue

The liver is the major powerhouse of the body. When liver function deteriorates, the patient often experiences fatigue. The improvement of fatigue symptoms relies mainly on the improvement of liver function. If fatigue is the major problem, it can be treated with the Cordyceps Capsule®. This formula can improve energy level and has antifibrosis effects.

Insomnia

Sleep disorders are a common complaint among hepatitis C patients. Prescription sleep medications can be addictive and cause side effects such as morning drowsiness. In addition, prescription medications may also be toxic to the liver. The herbal formula, HerbSom Capsule® addresses this problem without harmful effects on the liver and is not addictive.

Control Autoimmune Reactions Such as Joint Pain, Skin Rashes, Vasculitis, Psoriasis, and Sjögren Syndrome

Patients with hepatitis C often exhibit *autoimmune* symptoms and syndromes. Our treatment strategy is to regulate the body's autoimmune response. In our clinic, we use the AI #3 Capsule® and Circulation P Capsule®.

Stabilize Blood Sugar

One of the liver's functions is assisting in *blood sugar* regulation. The amount of sugar in the blood increases after eating. Excess sugar is turned into *glycogen* and is stored in the liver. When blood sugar drops, glycogen in the liver is broken down into *glucose* and is released into the blood. This process is sometimes disrupted in chronic hepatitis C patients, causing blood sugar abnormalities. We use the BM (Bitter Melon) Capsule® formula to treat HCV-related blood sugar abnormalities.

Prevent External Infections

During the course of chronic hepatitis C, patients may become ill with other infectious diseases such as colds, sinusitis, and bronchitis. Antimicrobial herbs can be used to fight external infections. The most important herbal remedy we use for infections is the Allicin formula®. The Coptis Capsule® may also be used to fight infections.

Control Fluid Retention: Ascites and Edema

Ascites (fluid accumulation in the abdomen) and edema (fluid accumulation in the feet and legs) can occur with cirrhosis and *liver failure*. We use Red Peony Capsule® to lower portal pressure and Cordyceps to raise the albumin level. At the same time, an herbal formula such as R-788 Capsule® can be used to expel excess water from the body.

Control Bleeding

Cirrhotic patients may be at risk for *bleeding varices*. Bloody vomiting and/or passing of black, tar-like stools may accompany the bleeding. Bleeding from varices is a medical emergency. If this happens, the patient should go the emergency room immediately. Bleeding from the gums or nose are more common and less serious forms of bleeding that occur in cirrhotic patients. The classic herbal formula Yunan Bai Yao Capsule is used to treat less serious types of bleeding.

Control Gastrointestinal Irritation and Diarrhea

Diarrhea is a common complaint of people with chronic hepatitis C. Diarrhea often improves as liver function improves. If diarrhea lasts and becomes severe, the following formula can be used: Ginseng and Atractylodes Formula.

Control Nausea And Vomiting

Nausea is more common than vomiting in people with chronic hepatitis C. It can occur when bile secretion is blocked. If these complaints become persistent, the following formula can be used: Pinellia and Hoelen Combination.

MCM Treatment of Postviral Hepatitis Syndrome

After successful clearance of HCV, some people may still experience lingering symptoms. This is called post viral hepatitis syndrome (PVHS), a concept recently coined by viral hepatitis medical researchers in China. PVHS is a clinical condition in which the patient complains discomfort in the liver area, nausea, vomiting, stomach distension, indigestion, fatigue, mental fog, and joint pains. These symptoms may persist for a few months to a few years.

From the western medical standpoint, if the virus has been eradicated, the patient is considered *cured*. However, according to the Chinese medical definition of cure, if the patient has not returned to a healthy state, he or she is not considered fully cured. In PVHS, despite abnormal symptoms, the virological, biochemical, and *histological* examination are normal. Thus, there is no diagnosis or treatment in conventional medicine.

In our clinic, we have seen a few dozen patients who were sustained virological responders to interferon-based therapy, but still exhibited liver disease symptoms. This is usually caused by the accumulation of liver and other systemic damage over the years of infection.

One study observed 36 cases of PVHS (22 males, 14 females). The symptom patterns were recorded among the patients were:

100% (36/36) liver area discomfort
61% (22/36) joint pain
47% (17/36) fatigue
36% (13/36) nausea
31% (11/36) stomach broadness
6% (2/36) vomiting

These patients were examined thoroughly with biochemical, histological, immunological, and virological tests and the findings were all negative. However, the symptoms persisted and hospitalization was required for several patients with severe symptoms.[32]

The exact cause of PVHS is not clear. Chronic viral hepatitis patients often exhibit *immune globulin* disorders (such as the presence of rehumatoid factor, *ANA*, and *cryoglobulins*), which can cause symptoms outside the liver. The pathology of PVHS may also be related to circulating immune complex (CIC) deposits in tissues. The CIC deposits can cause inflammatory reactions and is known to be responsible for causing rehumatoid arthritis-like symptoms. Another possible cause of PVHS is that the functions of the liver have not been completely restored after previous viral infection. These conditions demonstrate that chronic viral hepatitis is not just a standalone viral infection, it is a systemic disease. Thus, a comprehensive treatment strategy is required to cover multiple areas of the pathology.

Herbal formulas such as Minor Bupleurum Combination (Xiao Chai Hu Tang), Bupleurum and Rehmannia Combination (Chai Hu Qing Gan Tang), Siler and Platycodon Formula (Fang Feng Tong Sheng San), Tang-kuei and Bupleurum Formula (Xiao Yao San) and Bupleurum and Evodia Combination (Shu Gan Tang) can be used for PVHS. Some single herbs and their active ingredients can also be used, such as glycyrrhizin, ligustrin, schisandrin, and silymarin to restore liver functions. AI #3 Capsule® can be used to reduce the globulin production, and Circulation P Capsule® can be used to promote the removal of CIC deposits.

We use the following herbal formulas to treat PVHS patterns: Hepa F. #2 Capsule®, Glycyrrhizin Capsule®, Ligustrin Capsule®, Circulation P Capsule®, AI #3 Capsule® and Cordyceps Capsule®. The treatment should last at least a few months until all symptoms have resolved. In addition to herbal treatment, psychological counseling, a balanced diet, and proper physical exercises are also important to promote recovery from PVHS.

Intended Endpoints of MCM Treatment: "Cure" With MCM

Chinese medicine defines cure as the body's return to balance and normal functioning. According to Chinese medicine, the ultimate goal of healthcare is to restore a person's health, body functions, and a normal life expectancy.

The goals of MCM treatment for hepatitis C are to arrest and reverse the impact of HCV infection. In turn, quality of life improves and there is a reasonable expectation for a normal life span. Long-term and ongoing treatment may be required but as the patient is able to live a normal quality of life and prolong life expectancy, they have sufficient time to wait for more effective and safer treatments in the future.

The Advantages and Shortcomings of MCM Treatments for Hepatitis C.[33]

The Advantages of Using MCM to Treat Hepatitis C:

- MCM is an individualized treatment system based on patient's health status and disease status. It is a holistic and multilevel treatment strategy.

- It can improve and release the subjective symptoms and objective physical signs and improve the patient's life quality.

- It can control liver inflammation, improve liver functions, and release jaundice. These effects can be tested and measured by laboratory examinations.

- It can improve immune function and the overall health of the patient.

- It has virtually no side effects and is easily accepted by patients.

The Shortcomings of MCM Treatment for Hepatitis C

- As of now, MCM cannot eradicate HCV. Therefore, it is not a curative treatment.

- In clinical outcomes, assessment of efficacy mainly relies on biochemical tests. Major clinical events such as cirrhosis and the development of *liver cancer* as prognostic markers were not frequently used as assessment tools.

- Due to financial limitations, most MCM clinical trials are not strictly controlled and do not adhere to the standards of conventional western clinical trials. MCM relies primarily on clinical observation and the experience of the practitioner.

Reasons for Using MCM Therapies and Who May Benefit

Chinese herbal treatments for HCV have many positive features.

- effective

- time-honored

- easy to take

- affordable (15-20 times less expensive than western medication)

- virtually nontoxic

- largely side effect free

- work life-long

However, MCM remedies do not eradicate HCV. It provides an alternative solution for people who are unwilling or unable to use conventional medicine. For these people, TCM or MCM may be a viable alternative. "In the US, it is likely that more patients with hepatitis C use nonprescription agents of unproven effectiveness than interferon-based therapy."[34]

For the approximately 50% of people who do not respond to conventional treatment, MCM can be used to help improve liver function, slow down the development of fibrosis, and improve overall quality of life. MCM used together with western treatments usually yields better results than either one used alone. Ideally, these two systems can be used together to complement each other. Patients on interferon-based therapy may wish to use MCM herbal treatments to mitigate treatment side effects.

Reasons for Not Using MCM

Common reasons given for not using TCM or MCM include:

- It is not intended to eradicate HCV, so it is not a "cure." The concept of "cure" in TCM and MCM is different than it is in western medicine.

- TCM and MCM herbal remedies are unproven. They have not gone through rigorous scientific testing. Most TCM and MCM remedies are customized to meet the specific needs of the client, taking into account other conditions and limitations. It is very difficult to conduct clinical trials with herbal remedies because TCM and MCM do not subscribe to the "one size fits all" approach of western medicine. In many cases, this means clinical trials would be invalid because they would be comparing "apples to oranges."

  The National Center for *Complementary and Alternative Medicine* (NCCAM) Internet page "Hepatitis C: Treatment Alternatives" labeled TCM and MCM as having "no research to a limited amount of research." Because most of the published research on TCM and MCM is in Chinese, this issue is further complicated.

- The FDA does not regulate herbal products, so using herbs can be dangerous. You may not get what you are supposed to get.

  This can be true, especially if the herbalist is not well versed in the plant pharmacology and toxicity data. Because of this potential danger, it is important to verify the credentials of any herbalist you decide to consult.

  The Internet site at www.consumerlab.com is a privately owned, and monitors the quality of *nutritional supplements* and herbs. You may find this site useful. If you choose to take herbal products, it is very important to confirm the quality of the herbs or products.

- Herbal medicines are not stable with respect to their active essence because species, collecting seasons, and production sites vary.

  The method of preparation (drying, steaming, and decocting) can dilute the active essence of an herb. It is also argued that herbal medicines are inconvenient to prepare for ingestion. Finally, herbal medicines can be perceived to be bitter and unpleasant to ingest.

  These drawbacks can be alleviated through scientific preparation procedures to achieve a consistent amount of active ingredients. In addition, herbal extracts can be concentrated so that the daily dosage is small and requires no special preparation. Since capsule, tablet, and granular forms of herbal preparations are placed on the tongue and swallowed with a large glass of water, poor taste need not be a deterrent.

- The numbers of different chemicals in herbs make it hard to control their interactions with conventional drugs.

**If you are taking any herbal products, you need to tell your western doctor.
He or she will be able to advise you about any possible interactions.
Your herbalist can also advise you about this.**

Anecdotal Stories of Treatment Success With MCM

An *anecdotal* story is one that is not based on a controlled, clinical trial, but on an individual's personal experience. Whether or not the results of anecdotal stories have value is up to you.

On the next page are two stories of success and two stories of failure based on cases from my clinic in New York City. Patient names have been changed.

Joseph V.

Joseph V. is a New Jersey firefighter. He was diagnosed with hepatitis C in 1996. When he saw me in 1997, he was on disability and his ALT was quite high (above 300). He felt tired and could not work. Two months after herbal treatment, his liver enzyme levels normalized, and he went back to active duty as a firefighter.

His western healthcare provider convinced him to try interferon, and he did not want to lose the chance to try this FDA-approved therapy. He stopped taking herbs and went on interferon for eight months. During this time, he went back on disability and felt very sick. When the treatment was finished, his ALT went up to 380. At that point, his western doctor suggested the combination of interferon and ribavirin. He refused. He came back to me for treatment and resumed herbal therapy. Within two months, his *liver function tests* normalized. He has since returned to active duty as a firefighter and has married. He told me the herbal treatment helped him to put his life together and gain the confidence to build a family.

Lorraine D.

Lorraine D., 41, works for a large pharmaceutical company that produces interferon. She was diagnosed with hepatitis C in 1997. She might have contracted the virus seven years earlier. In March 1998, she stopped a seven-month course of interferon treatment. At that time, her liver function tests were normal. However, the side effects of interferon forced her to discontinue treatment. Her platelet count dropped to a dangerously low level. She often had bruises on her skin. She was diagnosed with idiopathic thrombocytopenia *purpura* (ITP), an autoimmune disease. She was put on steroids to treat the ITP. Her *thyroid gland* was also not functioning well. She was given synthetic thyroid *hormone* to correct her thyroid function. The steroids helped her platelet count increase in two months, but they triggered a *relapse* of liver inflammation. She came to see me in May 1998 after this relapse. Her ALT and AST were both abnormal. Her viral load was at 27 million, much higher than before interferon treatment. Lorraine was very tired and had pain in her liver area and joints, dark urine, and occasional diarrhea with pale stool. Her skin and *conjunctiva* (the skin around the inside of the eyes) were yellowish. In addition, she had a *pituitary tumor* as an underlying condition, which made her situation quite complicated. Her western healthcare provider recommended interferon and ribavirin, but she refused.

I first focused on her liver inflammation. Her ITP and thyroid gland abnormality showed that her liver inflammation had autoimmune involvement. I emphasized anti-autoimmune therapy. She began taking Hepa Formula No. 2®, Glycyrrhizin Capsule®, Ligustrin Capsule®, AI Capsule No. 3®, Circulation Tablet No. 1®, and Formula R6379® (for *hypothyroidism*). One month later, her blood tests showed that all liver enzyme levels had normalized. Her platelet count increased and her thyroid tests normalized. She was ecstatic because the treatment had normalized her ITP and rid her of hypothyroidism and liver inflammation in only one month. Her liver enzyme levels have been normal since that time, except once in reaction to a drug treatment for edema in her ankles. She is now on a maintenance protocol. All of her symptoms are gone.

More than 3,000 patients at Zhang's Clinic in New York City have used the protocols described. I n January 2000, we had test results on file for over 400 patients. A scientific analysis was conducted by reviewing the medical records of 75 patients for whom both pre- and post-treatment ALT levels were available. ALT was used to determine whether the protocols were effective. The average before treatment ALT level was 128 (±114), and the average after-treatment ALT level was 47(±42). Of these 75 patients, 77% experienced normalization of their ALT, and 93% experienced ALT improvement. All patients reported improvement in their symptoms. Four patients had *liver biopsy* results available before and after herbal treatment. Three of the four patients experienced regression of liver fibrosis from stage III to stage I after herbal treatment.

Anecdotal Stories of Treatment Failure With MCM

About 10% of the patients using Chinese medicine protocols do not get favorable results.

Doug F.

Doug F., 50, visited my office in August 1999. He was first diagnosed with non-A, non-B hepatitis (hepatitis C) in 1977 after a blood transfusion. He was a heavy drinker from age 17 to 29. His liver enzymes were very high (ALT 426, AST 155). His viral load was 48,000. He had *genotype* 1a HCV. He occasionally felt fatigued, his urine was golden yellow, and he sometimes had diarrhea. After approximately one month on the herbal treatments Hepa F. #2®, Ligustrin®, Glycyrrhizin, AI #3®, and Circulation #1®, his ALT and AST decreased, but his viral load went up to 200,000. He was very happy with these results. Approximately one month later, his ALT and AST levels went back up. Although his ALT level went back down approximately one month later, his AST continued to rise. He was very depressed and felt more fatigued. From then on, the results on his liver enzyme tests were continuously worse. In January 2000, he had a liver biopsy and found that his inflammation *grade* was II and the fibrosis stage was II. His ALT and AST continued to be markedly elevated, and his viral load was greater than one million. I tried using second-line herbal remedies and switched the Hepa F. #2® to Hepa F. #1a®. In March 2000, his ALT and AST dropped, but he lost confidence in herbal treatment and went on western therapy.

Bruce D.

Bruce D., 61, was diagnosed with hepatitis C in 1984 as non-A, non-B hepatitis. He might have become infected in 1975. His HCV genotype was 1b. Before he started an herbal protocol in December 1998, his baseline liver function tests were ALT 389, AST 192, and viral load 2.6 million. His liver biopsy showed stage II-III fibrosis with marked active ongoing inflammation (grade III). His blood clotting studies were slightly abnormal. He had been an alcohol drinker, but stopped drinking four years earlier. Clinically, he had a gassy stomach, loose stools, and slightly yellowish skin, but no other obvious symptoms.

He started a first-line protocol of Hepa F. #2 Capsule®, Ligustrin Capsule®, Glycyrrhizin Capsule®, AI#3 Capsule®, and Circulation #1 Capsule®. In the first year (1999), his ALT levels improved. Once in July 1999, when his ALT went up to 276, I added a new herb, Paniculate Tablet, which brought the ALT back down. His viral load was sometimes very high. In 2000, his ALT shot up again. Beginning in March 2000, I switched him to a second-line protocol, which included using Hepa F. #1a® to replace Hepa F. #2®. This change did not generate any significant positive effect.

Summary

TCM and MCM have been used for thousands of years by millions of people to promote health and provide therapy when health is impaired. Chinese medicine doctors are treating one third of world's viral hepatitis patients and they have great deal of experiences and skill in treating viral hepatitis.

TCM and MCM provide an effective and well-documented treatment methodology for patients with hepatitis C, which is a multilevel, regulatory treatment. The main goal of treatment is to control liver inflammation and halt or reverse the progression of fibrosis.

Each practitioner of TCM or MCM uses his or her own herbal formulations and methods to treat hepatitis C based on his or her training background. If you are currently seeing a TCM practitioner or are considering TCM or MCM as a treatment option, be sure to check your practitioner's training and qualifications. The Resource Directory at the back of this book provides information on locating a TCM practitioner.

Regardless of what options you decide to pursue in the treatment of your hepatitis C, be sure to inform all of those in whom you entrust your healthcare of all the approaches you are using.

References

1. Peng WW, et al. *The Studies of Viral Hepatitis*. Guangzhou, China: Guong Dong Science and Technology Press; 1999.
2. Chen KJ. Some thoughts on Advancement of Chinese Medicine. *Chinese J of Integrated Traditional and Western Medicine*. 2000;20(4):294.
3. Ji ZP, Review and prospect of integration of traditional Chinese and western medicine in past 30 years. *Chin J Integr Me*. 1988;8:88-89.
4. Jian J. Some Thoughts on traditional Chinese medical Hepatology. *Chinese J of Integrated Traditional and Western Medicine on Liver Diseases*. 2005;15(2):65.
5. Wang CB. Integrated TCM-WM research of viral hepatitis. *Chin J Integr Med*. 1988 8(2):152-156.
6. Su XS et al. Clinical observation and laboratory studies on glycyrrhizin treatment for acute and chronic viral hepatitis. *TCM Journal*. 1982; 11:33-36.
7. Li TM, et al. The antiviral effects of extracts of licorice roots. *TCM Herbology*. 1994;25(12):655-658.
8. Nakashima H, et al. A new anti-HIV substance glycyrrhizin sulfate. *Jpn J Cancer Res*. 1987;78(8):767-771.
9. Jie YB. *Pharmaceutical Action and Application of Available Composition of Chinese Materia Medica*. Harbin, China: Helongjian Science and Technology Press, 1992.
10. Oleanolic acid study Group. *Pharmaceutical Bulletin*. 1980;(12):46.
11. Wang JT, et al. A Review on Treating Hepatitis B with Chinese Medicinal Herbs. *Chinese J. of Infectious Diseases*. 1991;9(4):208.
12. Zhang Z et al. Anti-HBV Effects of 60 Chinese Medicinal Herbs. *Academic J of Beijing Medical University*. 1988;20(3):211.
13. Zhang QC. The efficacy of Zheng's Chinese herbal protocol in treating hepatitis C patients – A retrospective analysis of its clinical practice. In: *Healing Hepatitis C with Modern Chinese Medicine*. New York, NY. Sino Med Research Institute, 2000, New York
14. Wang BH. *The Progression of Hepatology*. Shanghai Science and Technology Press; 1991.
15. Wang BH, The reversibility of liver fibrosis and cirrhosis. *CJITWM on Liver Diseases*. 2000;10(supplement):2.
16. Tang ZM, et al. Expounding on the relationship between liver-blood-stasis and hepatic fibrosis. *Chin J Basic Med TCM*. 1996;2(3):14-17.
17. Song JW, et al. Effects of different component in decoction Xue Fu Zhu Yu decoction on anti-hepatofibrosis. *CJITWM on liver diseases*. 1995;5(2):23-25.
18. Zhang JY, et al. Ge Xie Zhu Yu Tang's effects on the expression of rat TMP-1/2. *J of TCM Information*. 2004;21(3):66-68.
19. Zheng ML, et al. The basic study and clinical research on hepatic fibrosis. People's Health Press; 1996.
20. Chinese Society of Integration of Chinese and Western Medicine ed. *Studies of Blood Stasis and Blood Circulation Promoting and Stasis Expelling*. Beijing: Xuewan Press; 1990.
21. Gao CF, et al. Hepatic stellate cells and the liver fibrosis. *Clinical J of the Liver and Gallbladder Disease*. 1994;10(3):125.
22. Paradis V, et al. In situ detection of lipid peroxidation byproducts in chronic liver diseases. *Hepatology*. 1997;26(1):135-142.
23. Yu H. et al., Herbal Compound 861 on apoptosis of hepatic stellate cells. *CJITWM on Liver Disease*. 2000;10 (6):32-33.
24. He Ming, et al. Clinical study on treatment of pulmonary interstitial fibrosis with Ginkgo Extract. *CJITWM*. 2005;25(3):222-224.
25. Hu YY, et al. Effects of salvianolic acid A on collagen type I and its gene expression of experimental rats with hepatic fibrosis. *Chin J Tradit Med Sci & Technol*. 1999;6(4):235-236.
26. Jia JD et al. TCM therapy for hepatic fibrosis. *Chin J Hepatol*. 2001;9(4):120-121.
27. Wang Li, et al. The extracts of gingko's effects on the MMP-2 of experimental liver fibrosis. *Medical J of Snan Dong*. 2004;44(1):27-29.
28. Lu LG, et al. Oxymatrine's effects on the expression of type I, III, IV collagen in carbon tetrachloride induced rat liver fibrosis. *World J of Chinese on Digestion*. 2003;11(10):1488-1491.
29. Chen Y, et al. The progress of the studies on the mechanisms of antifibrosis Chinese materia medica in recent three years. *CJITWM on Liver Diseases*. 2005;15(4):249-252.
30. Chen J, et al. Recent progress on the studies of anti-liver fibrosis herbal formulas. *CJITWM on Liver Diseases*. 2004;14(4):252-254.
31. Fu JY. *Chinese Medical J*. 1956;42(10):930.
32. Li WW, et al. Report on 36 post-hepatitis syndrome. *Chin J Integra Tradi & Western Med on Liver Diseases*. 2004;14(1):15.
33. Huang YZ. The advantages and shortcomings of MCM treatments for hepatitis C. *CJITWM on Liver Diseases*. 2005;15(2):120-121.
34. Schiff ER, et al. *Schiff's Diseases of the Liver, Eighth Edition*. 1999.

Homeopathic Medicine

Sylvia Flesner, ND

Introduction

Homeopathy is a *nontoxic* form of medicine that was developed approximately 200 years ago by Dr. Samuel Hahnemann. The word homeopathy is derived from two words: *homoios* meaning similars and *pathos* meaning suffering. Homeopathy is a form of medicine that uses highly diluted *pathogens* or other potentially toxic substances as remedies. These remedies provoke healing responses in a person's *immune system*, or provoke other body responses to treat the root causes of illnesses.

The theory behind homeopathy is based on the law of similars. "Like *cures* like." In the 1700's, Peruvian bark (also known as chincona or china) was used to treat malaria. The healing power of Peruvian bark was thought to be due to its bitter taste. Dr. Hahnemann disagreed with this conclusion and experimented on himself. He ingested the bark to evaluate its effects. Eventually, he developed fevers and chills, *symptoms* typical of malaria. Dr. Hahnemann theorized that because the bark produced symptoms similar to malaria, taking a small amount of the bark would stimulate the body to heal itself of malaria.

The law of similars dates back to the time of Hippocrates, but it also has present-day applications. For example, many *vaccines* involve giving a small dose of the *microorganism* that causes a specific disease. This stimulates an immune response against that microorganism thereby protecting the person from the disease.

The theoretical basis of the homeopathic approach is as follows. Symptoms of a disease that result when large doses of a homeopathic drug are given to healthy subjects under controlled conditions (called "provings") will be eliminated when the homeopathic drug is given in extremely small doses to someone who actually has the disease.

Practitioners of homeopathy come from a variety of healthcare disciplines, as well as the lay public. Naturopaths, chiropractors, psychologists, nurses, and even some western doctors practice homeopathy. A homeopath can also be a layperson that has knowledge of homeopathy. Currently, there are no certification or licensure requirements to practice homeopathy. However, because homeopathic remedies are safe and nontoxic when used appropriately, there is virtually no danger in using them.

Principles of Homeopathy

Homeopathy requires that drugs be tested, or proved, in healthy subjects. Proving is necessary because the homeopathic drug can only express itself in its pure form in a healthy person that is unaffected by interactions with a disease process. The quest for knowledge about homeopathic drugs through provings on healthy subjects has yielded a fascinating body of literature. This is particularly true in Europe where homeopathy is a more common form of therapy than in the United States.

One double-blind study that evaluated the effect of a homeopathic remedy on people with the flu found almost twice as many flu sufferers recovered within 48 hours after receiving the homeopathic remedy compared to patients who received *placebos* (inactive pills).[1] In another study, hay fever sufferers experienced six times as much symptom relief after taking a homeopathic remedy compared to those who took placebos.[2] An evaluation of 89 *clinical trials* of homeopathic remedies was recently conducted by seven health professionals in the United States and Germany.[3] They found homeopathic medicines were more than twice as effective as placebos in the evaluated trials.

Symptoms as the Basis for Homeopathic Treatment

One of the biggest differences between the homeopathic medicine and western medicine is in the emphasis on making a diagnosis.

Western medicine groups patients according to the diagnosis they share. Patients who have the same diagnosis generally receive the same or similar treatments, even if there are striking differences in their symptoms. One of the major goals of western treatment is to suppress symptoms. This has resulted in a large market for products that reduce pain, fever, and other common symptoms.

Homeopathic treatment is determined by looking at the whole patient as a unique individual rather than categorizing his or her illness based on symptoms that are similar to those of other patients. According to homeopathic thought, the body's symptoms of illness are an expression of the body trying to heal itself and should not be suppressed. This individual expression of symptoms is of utmost importance in determining homeopathic prescriptions, since the remedy must perfectly match the symptoms. It is like finding the correct key for a specific lock. Homeopathic treatment can begin based on symptoms alone even if an underlying diagnosis has not been made.

For record-keeping purposes and/or to make it easier to discuss a person's ailment, homeopathic practitioners might say that a person is suffering from a certain kind of flu or ulcerative disease. However, such names by themselves do not determine a patient's treatment.

Homeopathic remedies do not eliminate the cause of disease, nor do they cure disease. They do not provide immediate relief of symptoms. Rather, homeopathic remedies help establish balance in the body, and promote its ability to heal itself. In order to treat seriously ill people, the practitioner must effect a profound change at the deepest levels boosting the immune system. Homeopathy intervenes at the level of a person's reactive, self-curative powers, with or without the person's fully conscious cooperation. The goal is to bring about a change in the total functioning of the body. Although homeopathic treatment can be supplemented by other holistic therapies, practitioners believe such a change can be brought about by homeopathic treatment alone.

Homeopathy and Hepatitis C

Hepatitis C is a very serious disease. Everyone who has hepatitis C should be under the care of a western doctor (an MD or DO) on a regular basis. If you are experiencing any of the symptoms listed below, you should consult an MD or DO who can provide appropriate testing and treatment as these symptoms may indicate disease progression.

- extreme *fatigue*
- low-*grade* fever
- disinterest in food and queasiness
- heavy, painful, and/or tender liver
- very light-colored stools and very dark-colored urine

Homeopathic Treatments for Symptoms of Liver Disease

Some homeopathic medicines require a prescription while others can be purchased over-the-counter. While homeopathy is ideal for self-treatment of conditions that are generally self-limited such as colds, influenza, and headaches, the treatment of *chronic hepatitis* C is best accomplished by a trained professional.

Aconite is sometimes used to treat the high fever, restlessness, and fearful anguish that can occur in the earliest *stage* of acute liver disease. Belladonna, chelidonium, lycopodium, mercurius, nux vomica, and the herb china may be used to treat shooting pain in the region of the liver.

The herb *china* is also useful for treating symptoms such as sensitivity to pressure in the liver, the tendency to become chilled, and sensitivity to open air. It is also used to treat feelings of heaviness or fullness in the stomach and abdomen, especially after eating.

I use an immune stimulator in my practice to help patients handle viral infections such as hepatitis C more effectively. The stimulator is a combination remedy that includes *Triffolium pratense, Echinacea purpurea, Asclepias tuberosa, Ferrum Iodatum, Vaccinum, Euphrasia off., Thuja occidentalis, Camphora, Calcarea arsenica, Ichthyolum, Vaccinotoxinum, Morbillinum, Variolinum, Influenzinum, Vincetoxicum, Coxsackievirus, Encephalitis, Calmette-Guerin, Cytomegalovirus, Viscum mali (Iscador®)*, and isotonic plasma.

Ensuring the Safety of Homeopathic Remedies

According to federal law, homeopathic remedies are considered drugs. To be considered an official homeopathic medicine, a product must meet the guidelines described in the *Compliance Policy Guide* (CPG) developed by the American Homeopathic Pharmacists Association and the Food and Drug Administration (FDA). A remedy must have known homeopathic provings and/or known effects that mimic the symptoms, *syndromes*, or conditions for which it is given. It must also meet the manufacturing specifications established by the Homœopathic Pharmacopœia of the United States (HPUS). HPUS is the official compendium of homeopathic medicines recognized by the FDA. The HPUS contains all of the official manufacturing procedures for homeopathic medicines. This includes procedures for dosing, labeling, and administration information for users. Currently, there are over 1,300 official HPUS substances. The HPUS initials on a product label identifies it as a homeopathic medicine, and insures that the legal standards for strength, quality, purity, and packaging have been met for that product.

The standards applied to products seeking HPUS approval are established by the Homœopathic Pharmacœpœia Convention of the United States (HPCUS). HPCUS is a nongovernmental, nonprofit, scientific organization. HPCUS members are experts in the fields of medicine, art, biology, chemistry, and *pharmacology* who have appropriate training and demonstrated knowledge, and an interest in homeopathy.

The Role of Diet in Homeopathic Medicine

A good diet that stimulates your immune system is an important companion to homeopathic remedies. Good nutrition can help you obtain and maintain good health. It can also help improve the health of your liver.

The following yeast-free diet was designed to help clean your system, reduce stress on your liver, and maintain good health.

Recommended Foods and Liquids	
Fish, Lamb, Wild Game	preferably organic, not smoked, and without the skin
Poultry	chicken and turkey – preferably organic, not smoked, and without the skin eggs
Dairy Products	butter - preferably brands that are *pesticide*- and *hormone*-free such as Horizon® sheep and goat milk, yogurts, and cheeses
Fresh Vegetables	preferably organic, wash thoroughly

Starchy Vegetables	potatoes
	sweet potatoes
	yams
	pumpkin
	acorn and butternut squash
Fresh Fruits	citrus fruits
	kiwi
	melons
	apples
	pears
	peaches
Beverages	unsweetened juices
	filtered water (not distilled water)
	soy drinks such as Eden Soy Original®
	herbal teas such as Take-a-Break®
	Pero Coffee® is a good, *caffeine*-free substitute for coffee
	It is *very* important to drink at least 8 glasses of water daily.
Foods To Be Eaten in Moderation	
Legumes	pumpkin seeds
Grains Limit white flour and wheat products.	air-popped popcorn
	muffins
	biscuits
	cornbread
	pancakes (made with soymilk or water and honey)
	pastas
	potatoes
	rice and rice cakes
	grains (such as couscous, quinoa, millet)
	grits
	yeast-free breads made with baking powder and limited white flour
	tortillas and tortilla chips (not fried)

Condiments	homemade mayonnaise - made without vinegar or sugar
	guacamole - made without mayonnaise or vinegar; instead of vinegar, use lemon
	honey, maple syrup, apple butter - all in moderation and in very small quantities
	nuts and nut butters such as peanut butter and almond butter

Some suggested food substitutes include:

- Crispini® crackers for crackers made with yeast
- Eden Soy Original® for animal milk
- Bragg's Liquid Amino® for soy and teriyaki sauces
- Rice Dream® for ice cream
- Jeannie Macaroons® for cookies

After 21 days on the yeast-free diet, the following foods CAN BE ADDED	
Fresh Fruits	strawberries – in moderation
Legumes	lentils
	lima beans
	pinto beans
	split peas
	black eyed peas
Rice and grains Limit white flour and wheat products.	sourdough rye Essene bread
Condiments	carob
Foods and Liquids To Avoid on This Diet	
Red Meats	beef
	veal
	pork

After 21 days on the yeast-free diet, the following foods CAN BE ADDED	
Fruit	grapes raisins bananas plums all dried fruits glazed with sugar
Vegetables	mushrooms
Cow Dairy Products	milk milk products: cheese, margarine, yogurt, cottage cheese, ice cream, etc.; butter is acceptable if it is pesticide- and hormone-free
Grains	breads made with yeast
Beverages	*alcohol* - including all beer, wine, hard liquor, or anything fermented caffeinated or decaffeinated coffee tea soft drinks
Specific Condiments	ketchup mustard mayonnaise (unless homemade) vinegar (except apple cider vinegar) yeast pickles olives soy, teriyaki, barbecue sauce, and hot sauces such as picante and Tabasco® margarine
Sweeteners	sugar artificial sweeteners such as Sweet-n-Low® and NutraSweet®
Other Food Rules	no fried foods no chocolate no canned fruits or vegetables no chemicals or preservatives, including MSG

Read all food labels. Many products contain yeast, sugar, vinegar, and/or preservatives that you should eliminate from your diet.

All artificial sweeteners, such as NutraSweet® and Sweet-n-Low® should be permanently eliminated from your diet. Margarine should also be permanently eliminated from your diet.

Antibiotics, birth control pills, prescription drugs, steroids, and *hormones* should be avoided unless you and your doctor believe they are necessary.

Your Environment

Your environment is important to your health. I recommend keeping a clean house to minimize exposure to dust, mites, fungi, and molds. Two molds are particularly dangerous to your health, Aspergillus penicillium and Stachybotrys chartarum. These molds can deplete the immune system, and attack the liver and lungs. In extreme cases, exposure to these molds can be life-threatening.

Reasons for Using Homeopathic Medicines and Who Might Benefit

Homeopathic medicine can be very effective for treating some of the symptoms of hepatitis C. It can also be effective for some of the side effects from western drug-based treatments. Homeopathic remedies are safe when taken as directed because they are virtually nontoxic. However, hepatitis C is a very serious disease. Homeopathic remedies are best provided under the direction of a trained *complementary and alternative medicine* (*CAM*) practitioner.

Anecdotal Story of Success Using Homeopathic Medicine

David J. is a 36-year-old husband and father of two. He was overweight and a heavy drinker when he came to me for care of hepatitis C. I started him on the yeast-free diet, liver detoxification, and homeopathic remedies. I advised him to eliminate the use of *alcohol*. He followed all of my instructions. One month after his initial visit, his ALT and AST levels were almost normal. One year later, he experienced a *relapse* when his *liver enzymes* became elevated again. A *liver biopsy* was done and showed normal liver tissue. We decided he needed to resume the yeast-free diet. He also began taking a different group of homeopathic drugs. His liver enzymes returned to and remain at normal levels.

Reasons for Not Using Homeopathic Medicines

Homeopathy does not claim to be able to eliminate the hepatitis C virus (*HCV*). If your primary treatment goal is to eliminate HCV, homeopathic remedies are probably not the right choice for you. Unless they are also MDs or DOs, homeopathic practitioners cannot conduct certain tests such as liver biopsies that are needed to monitor HCV disease progression. Only MDs or DOs can order these tests.

Homeopathic medicine requires a significant commitment from the patient to make necessary lifestyle changes. Many people find they cannot make the commitment and/or required changes if they are drastically different from their current lifestyle.

Anecdotal Story of Failure Using Homeopathic Medicine

Joe S. is a 42-year-old Vietnam veteran. He is married with children and has a stressful job. When he came to see me, he smoked cigarettes, drank moderate amounts of alcohol, and large quantities of coffee daily. Having been recently diagnosed with hepatitis C, he consulted me to see how I could help him. He had elevated liver enzymes, moderate *viral load*, and some *fibrosis* on liver biopsy. I advised him to stop smoking cigarettes, and to give up alcohol and coffee. I prescribed a yeast-free diet to cleanse his liver. After completing the liver cleansing process, I planned to prescribe some homeopathic remedies to help improve the health of his liver. He was able to make most of the changes I recommended, but did not give up drinking coffee. Rather than put a greater effort into eliminating coffee from his diet, Joe chose to return to many of his previous behaviors. His liver health has not improved.

Summary

Homeopathy has the potential to alleviate the symptoms of hepatitis C and to help the body reestablish internal balance at the deepest levels. When cure is possible, homeopathy may help the body maintain a lasting cure.

If you have hepatitis C, get as much rest as you feel you need and eat a well-balanced, low-fat diet with moderate amounts of *protein*. Try to eat well even if you are not hungry. Avoid eating irritating spices, oily foods, and coffee. You should also avoid unnecessary drugs. You must abstain entirely from drinking alcohol.

Homeopathic medicines are inexpensive and often do not require a prescription. Over-the-counter homeopathic medicines are available in health food stores, pharmacies, grocery stores, and other outlets. Product labels that contain the HPUS initials mean that the products were manufactured according to the guidelines of the Homœopathic Pharmacopœia of the United States.

As with all forms of medicine, no one *modality* is right for everyone all the time. We need to continue to conduct research into the causes and cures of illness, and to use the least toxic and most effective systems of treatment.

References

1. Ferley JP, Zmirou D, D'Adhemar D, Balducci F. A controlled evaluation of a homoeopathic preparation in the treatment of influenza-like syndromes. *Br J Clin Pharmacol.* 1989;27(3):329-335.
2. Reilly DT, Taylor MA, McSharry C, Aitchison T. Is homoeopathy a placebo response? Controlled trial of homoeopathic potency, with pollen in hayfever as model. *Lancet.* 1986;2(8512):881-886.
3. Linde K, Clausius N, Ramirez, et al. Are the clinical effects of homeopathy placebo effects? A meta-analysis of placebo-controlled trials. *Lancet.* 1997;350(9081):834-843.

Other References

Wagner H, Wiesenauer M. *Phytotherapie and Pflazliche Homoopathika.* Jena, New York: Fischer-Verlag; 1995.
Boericke, W. *Homeopathic Materia Medica with Repertory, 9th Edition.* Philadelphia, Pennsylvania: Boericke and Runyon; 1927.
Clarke, JH. *The Prescriber.* Essex, United Kingdom: The CW Daniel Company; 1987.
Johnson, J. *Homeopathic Family Guide.* Philadelphia, Pennsylvania: Boericke & Hahnemann Publishing House; 1886.

Mind-Body and Spiritual Healing

Sharon D. Montes, MD

Introduction

For thousands of years, mind-body and spiritual practices have been an integral part of worldwide healing traditions. A European worldview described by Sir Isaac Newton and René Descartes led to a medical system that looked at the physical body independent of consciousness. Descartes' philosophy formed a belief that mental and physical health are separate domains, and the physical laws described by Newton still guide the teaching and practice of modern medicine.

Our modern medical system focuses on understanding the chemistry and physical components of the body. Modern medicine as taught and practiced in the United States frequently regards physical health as a combination of parts. If we know enough about the individual parts, we can "fix" the whole. We have one set of healthcare providers to care for the mind and another to care for the body. So fixed is this division in our medical system that insurance will not reimburse providers if they provide treatment for or use diagnostic codes from the other's domain.

As limitations of this way of engaging in caring for people have become more evident, many providers and consumers are advocating for a more holistic medical system that integrates treating disease and maximizing wellness. As the field of *integrative medicine* evolves, it is clearer that the goals of "fighting disease" and promoting a great quality of life, regardless of specific disease diagnosis, are not at odds. Proof of this evolving view of healthcare is in the creation of this book that you are now reading.

In my *clinical* experience, the areas of mind-body medicine and spiritual healing are among the most powerful practices in improving life quality in patients who are living with the diagnosis of *chronic hepatitis* C. Research confirms that adults in the United States also frequently choose to use these modalities. In 2002, prayer was used by more than 50% of the U.S. population, and relaxation techniques, imagery, *biofeedback* and hypnosis were used by more than 30% of the population.[1] In 1992, the National Institutes of Health created an Office of Alternative Medicine. In 1998, this office increased in size and became the National Center for *Complementary and Alternative Medicine* (NCCAM). NCCAM organizes the study of integrative medicine into five fields as shown in Figure 1.

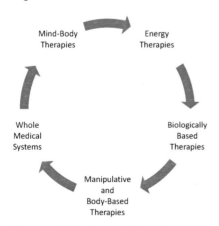

Figure 1. Major Types of Complementary and Alternative Medicine

Mind-Body Therapies

Energy Therapies

Whole Medical Systems

Biologically Based Therapies

Manipulative and Body-Based Therapies

This chapter will discuss some of the NCCAM descriptions of mind-body practices and then focus on some of the mind-body practices that I have found useful in my clinical practice. There will then be a discussion of NCCAM descriptions of energy therapies and conclude with some specific practices that I have found most useful in working with people who have chronic hepatitis C.

Mind-Body Fields of Practice

Mind-body practices can be an integral part of a treatment plan for any medical diagnosis. While the use of a mind-body practice may not make a medical condition disappear, it frequently improves the quality and/or quantity of life. As part of an effort to understand and research how altering mental health can affect physical health, NCCAM defines mind-body medicine to include the following practices.

Relaxation Techniques

The goal of relaxation techniques is to guide the body towards a state of balanced nervous system activity. This area includes a wide variety of techniques and is divided into deep and brief methods. Deep methods include *meditation*, progressive muscle relaxation, and autogenic training. There are many forms of meditation and this practice is discussed in much greater detail later in this chapter. Progressive muscle relaxation focuses on relaxing muscles from head to toe. Muscles are tensed and then relaxed in a sequence either from head to toe or from toe to head. Autogenic training helps a person produce comforting body sensations such as, warmth and consistently visualizing a peaceful environment. Brief methods are usually abbreviated forms derived from deep methods.

Hypnosis and Imagery

Hypnotic techniques promote a state of relaxation to achieve a desired clinical outcome. The hypnotic state may be self-induced or induced by another. Hypnosis practices include three phases: presuggestion to promote relaxation, suggestion to promote desired therapeutic goal, and postsuggestion to integrate the suggestion. The presuggestion component may include imagery, progressive muscle relaxation, or any other technique to promote muscle relaxation. During the hypnotic phase, a suggestion is offered such as decreased craving for nicotine or experience less pain postoperatively. The postsuggestion phase involves incorporating the suggestion into one's life.

Imagery is frequently thought of as closing one's eyes and seeing a desired image. Effective imagery actually uses a combination of senses. The image is more powerful and easy to create, if it is moving and involves other senses (e.g., the smell of pine trees, the feel of warm sun and a cool breeze on the skin, or the sound of a bubbling brook). Preferred imagery is a personal choice. Once while performing a small office procedure, I encouraged the patient to take a mini vacation in her mind and offered her the possibility of a trip to the ocean. Her response was, "I have left the state once in my life. That was enough. I prefer to stay home." Her preferred relaxation image was to be at home sewing while sitting on her living room sofa. One study showed the effects that hypnosis and imagery can have positive effects on immune function. Twenty-one patients who suffered from recurrent infection with genital herpes were taught self-hypnosis combined with imagery. After 6 weeks of using these practices, disease recurrence was reduced by almost 50%.[2]

Meditation

Meditation has three basic forms. One form is to focus the mind. The object of focus can be your breath, a candle flame, a word or a sound. The second type of meditative practice is to widen the view to observe the activity of the mind. Termed "mindfulness," the object of this practice is to observe as the mind leaps from past to future, stirring emotions as it travels back and forth. The third type of meditative practice is done to cultivate within oneself a desired quality. The quality can be compassion, harmlessness, or the ability to express unconditional love. This type of meditation may be used within religious tradition and beings who express this quality may be called upon for assistance (e.g. Quan Yin, Jesus or Krishna).

Biofeedback

This practice uses machines or other devices to provide audible, visual, or tactile information about body processes that frequently are under subconscious influence. This feedback can be as simple as holding a piece of tape that changes color when someone successfully practices a relaxation technique and warms their hands. In contrast, some very sophisticated computer programs allow a person to proceed in a computer game when their brain waves shift in a certain manner. Somewhere between these levels of technology are machines that provide light or sound feedback when a person successfully relaxes a muscle, lowers blood pressure, or lessens nervous system stress measured through changes in electrical conductance of the skin.

Yoga, Tai Chi, and Qi Gong

These forms of movement therapy are integral parts of the Ayruvedic (medicine from India) and Oriental medical systems. They involve slow movement combined with deep slow breathing. This combination of slow movement and breathing have been used for thousands of years to both prevent and treat disease. A recent article in Orthopedic Nursing compares it to western exercise programs and encourages nurses to promote its use.[3] A systematic review looking at several studies showed *tai chi* to promote both physical and *psychosocial* benefits. Physical benefits include improved balance, flexibility, and *cardiovascular* fitness.[4]

Although much of the research of tai chi focuses on its health benefits for elders, there is also evidence to support its use in improving immune function. Studies looking at changes in immune function related to fighting viral infections may be more pertinent to people with *HCV*. Two studies have measured changes in blood cells associated with improved *immune system* health. One study looked at 21 practitioners of tai chi. Before and after class, participant stress was assessed and their blood was drawn. After class, a significant number of students showed increased number and activity of *natural killer cells* as well as a significant decrease in stress.[5]

Another study showed evidence of immune changes that would keep elders from developing a late complication of chicken pox known as shingles. Usually the chicken pox virus (acquired during childhood) remains dormant in the body because our immune system keeps it from replicating. With age or certain medications, a portion of our immune system becomes weak and the virus may begin to replicate. Growing in the nerves, frequently along the rib cage, the virus leads to pain and sores causing a condition called shingles. A group of elders was instructed to practice tai chi. Blood samples were drawn that showed that they had a significant improvement in the type of immune response that keeps the chicken pox virus from replicating and later causing shingles.[6]

Cognitive-Behavioral Therapies and Group Support

Once considered "alternative," these methods are now part of mainstream medical treatments. In 1996, the National Institutes of Health organized a panel to examine the integration of behavioral and relaxation approaches into the treatment of chronic pain and insomnia. Cognitive-behavioral techniques we found to be moderately effective for relieving chronic pain.[7]

Art, Music, and Dance Therapy

In many traditional societies, art, music, and dance are integrated into everyday life. In this culture, many people only participate in these activities when they interact with children. Creative activities provide an outlet for expression of subconscious beliefs or feelings. Once these beliefs are mobilized or brought to a conscious level, they can be modified or used to promote a healing response. Art, music, and dance are considered essential activities for all humans by some cultures, regardless of medical condition. These therapies can be done individually or in group settings.

Spirituality

Spirituality is defined by NCCAM as a mind-body practice; this area has been granted significantly more attention by NCCAM within the last few years. The winter 2005 issue of the newsletter "CAM at the NIH" focused on prayer and spirituality in health. In response to criticism that it is inappropriate for NIH to fund studies of religion, the research focus is shifting from prayer and spirituality to positive meaning and personal growth. NCCAM's Deputy Director and Director of the Division of Extramural Research and Training, Margaret A. Chesney, PhD stated in the newsletter, "The advantage of focusing our research on positive psychological states, such as positive meaning, is that people can be trained to increase these states, and the subsequent effects on well-being and health can be directly measured. By advancing the focus of research from prayer and spirituality to positive meaning and personal growth, NCCAM will be in a far better position to apply scientific rigor to this domain and to make discoveries that will be applicable to the widest range of people."

Most NIH-funded research focuses on influencing the mind to improve physical health, decrease *symptoms*, or promote a sense of well-being. A more recent research development is to look at how practices focused on the physical body affect mental and emotional health. In one study, a group of nurses was offered a 15-minute massage weekly for five weeks. The self-reported stress levels showed a more significant decrease than the physical measure correlated with stress, urinary cortisol, and blood pressure.[8]

As the western mind better understands the nature of mind-body integration, more research will focus on how affecting the physical body – through a variety of practices that include massage, the Alexander technique, chiropractic, and others – leads to mental and emotional changes as well.

Specific Mind-Body Practices I Have Found Especially Useful In My Clinical Practice

Meditation

While many different meditative practices are used, three specific practices have been significantly researched in the United States. These practices include: transcendental meditation (TM), the relaxation response, and mindfulness-based stress reduction (MBSR). TM and the relaxation response are examples of focused meditation.

TM was introduced in the United States in the 1970s. Derived from the Ayruvedic medical tradition, people are given a one-syllable sound, based on their year of birth. This sound, repeated silently, is particularly matched to the constitution of the practitioner. More information about this type of meditation is available from www.tm.org.

The relaxation response was popularized and researched by physician Herbert Benson. Contrasting health benefits he found in regular meditators with the adverse health effects described by Hans Selye's "stress response," Dr. Benson used the term relaxation response to emphasize that we have choices in how we respond to external stressors. In a practice similar to TM, people are encouraged to sit quietly each day and focus their thoughts on a word. For this form of meditation people are encouraged to chose a word that has particular meaning for them (for example, love, peace, joy, soft belly). More information about this form of meditation is available from www.mbmi.org.

MBSR is a form of mediation that combines components from different meditative traditions and relaxation techniques. Established by Jon Kabat-Zinn at the University of Massachusetts, the Center for Mindfulness Internet site provides a wealth of information about courses and research (see www.usmassmed.edu/cfm). Emphasizing a focus on the breath, MBSR also includes a tolerant observation that the mind has a tendency to "chatter" and jump from past to future. Emotions are frequently attached to thoughts. Thinking about the future may trigger feelings of anxiety or desire, while thinking about the past may trigger feelings of guilt or anger. MBSR practice emphasizes gentle acceptance of that experience and return to focus on the breath. In addition, MBSR emphasizes bringing this state of mindfulness into one's everyday affairs. A review of 20 studies of MBSR showed that it successfully improved physical and emotional well-being in people with a variety of clinical conditions.[9]

Energy Psychology or Emotional Body Clearing

Over the last 15 to 20 years, a field of mind-body medicine has emerged that emphasizes nonverbal ways of releasing toxic emotions or beliefs from the body. Developed by psychologist Francine Shapiro, one of the best researched of these practices is eye movement desensitization and reprocessing (EMDR). Dr. Shapiro observed that moving her eyes from side to side could decrease the anxiety associated with stress-filled memories. She observed similar results in working with her patients. EMDR has gained international recognition as an effective technique to assist people suffering from posttraumatic stress disorder. Further information about research and application of this practice can be found at www.emdr.com.

The American Psychiatric Association has recognized EMDR as effective as cognitive behavioral therapy for decreasing symptoms of acute and chronic post-traumatic stress disorder. An analysis comparing EMDR with other therapies for the treatment of post-traumatic stress disorder found that EMDR was more efficacious than medication and required a lesser number of treatments than cognitive-behavior therapy.[9, 10]

Another practice to assist in removal of negative emotions is the emotional freedom technique (EFT). EFT combines asking people to be aware of a belief and feeling, express unconditional positive regard for themselves (regardless of the negativity of the feeling), and tap on specific acupuncture points. Many energy psychology practices use acupuncture *meridians* or points. It is believed that these locations allow access to the emotional body and facilitate emotional healing.

An integration of the EMDR and EFT techniques is found in another practice known as the WHEE technique (Whole Health, Easily and Effectively) developed by psychiatrist Dr. Daniel Benor. The WHEE technique combines the rapid stimulation physical stimulation of both sides of the body of EMDR along with the EFT practices of quantifying distress and accepting self despite negative beliefs, and if necessary, using meridian points to facilitate release of negative emotions or beliefs. The advantage of the WHEE technique is that as the emotions are released, there is less anxiety than with EMDR and the practice takes less time to learn and do than EFT. How to practice the WHEE technique is discussed later in this chapter.

Acupuncture

In 1997, a National Institutes of Health consensus panel agreed that there is good research evidence to support the use of acupuncture for treatment of nausea and tooth pain.[7] Most of the published research done in the western world focuses on the use of acupuncture for pain relief. Research also shows acupuncture to be particularly effective in relieving back and arthritis pain. Looking at acupuncture as practiced within the context of Oriental medicine, it also has applications for preventing disease and assisting with mental or emotional pain. Acupuncture relieves physical pain by changing the chemistry and electrical patterns in the nervous, hormonal, and immune system. It also affects emotional and mental health.

Very small needles, placed mostly in locations below knees and elbows, cause the deep part of the brain to produce chemicals that travel to the rest of the body. Some of these chemicals, known as *endorphins*, promote a deep sense of well-being. Other chemicals encourage the ad*renal* glands to release less stress *hormones*. Many people seek acupuncture care regularly as a preventive medicine practice during change of seasons or as a "tune-up." A recent review article on acupuncture supports this use of acupuncture. Acupuncture "will not change the amount of stressors a person is subject to but will change the *physiological* response to them. When the nervous system is in homeostatic balance, individuals will report enhanced feelings of well-being, be more effective in coping with their conditions of living, and therefore, be less susceptible to illness."[11]

Spirituality as a Mind-Body Practice

When discussing spirituality, frequently the concepts of religion and prayer come to mind. For the purposes of this chapter, spirituality is defined as the unique connection between an individual and what they define as the source of healing.

Religion includes activities that people engage in as a group. Those activities may be organized to promote spiritual or social goals. The two most commonly described prayer forms include petitionary (to ask for oneself) and intercessory (to ask something for others). Many other types of prayer, such as confession or expressions of gratitude, exist and this complicates the process of studying the effects of prayer. In a large survey of U.S. adults that asked about their use of different complementary or alternative medicine practices (CAM), only petitionary or intercessory forms of prayer were asked about. Prayer was the most common practice used of all the CAM techniques that were asked about. Forty-three percent of the people interviewed had prayed for their own health, almost 25 % had asked others to pray for them, and nearly 10% had participated in a prayer group.[12]

In my job as a physician, I am careful to respect each person's connection with the source of healing and work to honor their vocabulary and concept of what that is. In this country, there is sometimes a danger of equating mental/emotional or spiritual health with a disease-free physical body. There may be an unstated judgment, by self or others, that if people would just fix something within themselves their disease would go away. My clinical observation does not support this belief. Many people of great mental, emotional, and spiritual health suffer from chronic disease or experience traumatic accidents. Also, I have known a fair share of people who abuse the body through consumption of nicotine, excess food or alcohol, and who live to be healthy elders.

After spending thousands of hours studying different medical systems in attempt to gain a complete understanding of all the factors that can lead to disease and can be mobilized to promote health, I have learned to be at peace with the unknown. (This isn't to say that my busy, inquisitive mind stops searching for answers and solutions. Now, a wiser voice allows me to be at peace, knowing that my knowing will always be incomplete.) With everyone, there is some mystery as to exactly why they have a combination of symptoms and what path will best lead to the removal of obstacles to best allow an individual's healing to occur.

It is through a regular spiritual practice that many people may return to a state of unknowing or connection with something grander than themselves. In finding or returning to that state, important healing perspectives are gained. A spiritual practice can be spending time in nature, being of service to others, reading poetry or inspirational literature, communing with ancestors, meditating, choosing to practice harmlessness. One purpose for engaging in a practice is to gain a different perspective about everyday life activities. In one study, 40 people diagnosed with HCV were asked to complete questionnaires that assessed their spirituality and personal experience in dealing with the infection. The respondents who were described as being spiritually oriented defined treatment success as having the "ability to manage HCV symptoms, the medical system, and the HCV-imposed life limitations and to approach life with an accepting, positive attitude."[13]

Energy Medicine

Also known as vibrational medicine, energy medicine can be described as either veritable or putative.

Veritable energy medicine can be measured and includes vibrations such as sound and electromagnetic waves such as light, magnetism, laser beams, and other frequencies from the electromagnetic spectrum. Frequently this type of energy medicine involves the use of specific, measurable wavelengths and frequencies in providing care.

Putative energy fields or biofields are not yet consistently measurable. These practices are based on a belief that there is a bioenergetic field of energy that animates the biochemical and biomechanical parts of our being. Imbalance in this bioenergetic field can be corrected through the use of intercessory prayer, homeopathy, or passing healing energy through the body of one human to another without providers necessarily touching the person receiving the healing. Examples of this type of energy medicine practice include Reiki, therapeutic touch, healing touch, and polarity therapy.

Light and Sound Therapy

One well-researched use of light therapy is exposing people who become lethargic or depressed in the fall and winter months to high-intensity light. This form of light therapy has been shown to balance serotonin levels. Other forms of light therapy, lacking strong scientific proof, include using low-level light on acupuncture points, wounds, or painful areas.

Sound therapy includes more than listening to or creating music. It may involve the use of drums, tuning forks, metal or crystal bowls, or the human voice to create sounds that set up healing, harmonic resonances in the body. Author Ted Gioia describes the area of sound healing as consisting of two extremes. The shamanic provider of healing sounds (with generations of tribal history contributing to the power of the healing sound) is contrasted with the music therapist (who gains their credentials through earning a degree and a requisite certification). Ted Gioia proposes that it is in our role as creators, not consumers, of sound therapy that we have become unbalanced. "Our instinctive need to move in rhythm, to dance, to drum, to sing: these find almost no outlet in modern society."[14] Whether created by voice (our own or others), instruments, drums, bowls, or tuning forks, sound waves promote healing by creating order in their surrounding environment. In the late 18th century Ernst Chaldni created complex beautiful figures in sand by exposing the grains to violin music. This work was further developed by family physician Hans Jenny who published two volumes describing the effects of vibration on different materials. His photographs demonstrate the effects of sound on liquid, quartz, glycerin and various powders.[14] This work may help explain the current popularity of "singing bowls." Originally brought to the United States by Tibetan monks, metallic bowls that are an amalgam of several metals create complex resonant sounds. The last decade has seen the creation of crystal bowls pitched to create specific notes that are purported to heal specific physical or emotional disharmonies.

Electromagnetic Pulse and Low-Voltage/Power Generators

A standard use for pulsating electromagnetic therapy has been to promote healing of nonunion fractures. This therapy has also been used to treat multiple sclerosis, osteoarthritis, migraine headaches, and sleep disorders. Although the mechanism of low power, millimeter wave therapy is not completely understood, this practice is commonly integrated in patient care in Eastern Europe and Russia. This type of therapy is used for a variety of diseases. Clinical conditions said to respond to this therapy include cancers, cardiac disease and skin diseases.

One proposed mechanism of action is that by offering the physical body the specific electromagnetic frequencies associated with healthy tissue, the body uses the information as a stimulus to heal. The idea is that everything in the universe has a unique resonance. From water molecules to bacteria to liver tissue, if offered the correct electromagnetic frequency, the cells can remember their "health" program.

Homeopathy

As described in *Chapter 12, Homeopathic Medicine*, homeopathy was established in the early 1800s by German physician Dr. Samuel Hahnemann. Homeopathy lost its place within western medicine when it came to the preparation of the remedies. To create each medicine, Dr. Hahnemann took a remedy, shook it up, diluted it again, and shook it up again. This process is repeated many times so that by the time a "high" potency remedy is created, it lacks any physical molecules of the original remedy.

To look at a mechanism of action we have to look to energy medicine. Maybe one day our physicist colleagues, with their ability to measure more precisely than most current biological/lab measures, will show us that each remedy has a different energetic signature.

Local and Distant Healing

The theory with these methods of healing is that humans, as bioenergetic beings, can create energy fields that heal others. This healing can happen while people are in the same place or across great distance. Therapeutic touch, healing touch and Reiki are examples of local energy healing. Frequently working in an area 2 to 12 inches away from the body, practitioners of these therapies will use their hands to scan the client's energy field for areas of imbalance. Using intention to restore balance to a person's bioenergetic field, a practitioner may continue to treat with hands off or they may gently touch the client. Therapeutic touch is frequently taught and researched within the nursing community. It has been used in treating anxiety, migraine headaches, osteoarthritis pain, and to promote wound healing. One study reviewed 11 therapeutic touch studies and found seven of the studies showed that patients receiving the therapeutic touch treatments responded more favorably than patients not receiving the treatments.[19]

Forms of therapy that are purported to promote healing across distance include qi gong and prayer. *Qi gong* is a form of movement therapy done to cultivate increased vitality within one's body. In the Chinese literature there are several reports of qi gong masters using this energy to promote health in the body of someone located a long distance from the practitioner.

While the scientific data about the efficacy of intercessory prayer is mixed, it is still recommended by many healthcare providers as a practice for family of hospitalized patients, if such a recommendation is consistent with their belief system. A report that reviewed 23 studies of "distant healing," which included therapeutic touch because it does not involve physically touching the patient found 13 of the studies showed significant positive treatment effects. Nine studies showed no effect over control interventions, and one study showed a negative effect from treatment.[20]

Specific Practices to Improve Your Mind-Body Health

Change the inner dialogue about what your diagnosis means. Many people with the diagnosis of hepatitis C live long, productive lives. Infection does <u>not</u> equal disease. As the stress created by the diagnosis that you have hepatitis C fades, it becomes easier to gain perspective.

> Your essential self is not the infection you have, it is not hepatitis C disease, but is rather something much more powerful that is able to choose a life-affirming response.

I have seen many people confronted with a diagnosis of hepatitis C who, after the emotional dust settles, use that diagnosis as an opportunity for personal growth and transformation.

Practice forgiveness each day.

Cited to be a significant force in promoting well-being, the practice of forgiving self and others has special importance to anyone diagnosed with actual or potential liver disease. Within the wisdom of the Oriental medical system, it is believed that anger is particularly harmful to the liver and that liver disease predisposes towards imbalance in the expression of anger. This imbalance can be either expressing too much anger or denying and suppressing all anger. To practice forgiveness is frequently very difficult, because it seems an irrational act. Of course, there is a reason to be angry. Deciding to release the reason and <u>choose</u> to forgive requires effort. Many people draw upon their religious faith to make this effort less of a struggle. Sometimes it is only after repeatedly practicing forgiveness that people are truly able to appreciate that forgiving really does improve the quality of their own life. Forgiveness of self and others is recommended as a daily practice to help keep the liver healthy.

Be clear about what you desire from your support team.

Many healthcare providers are trained to ask "What is wrong with you?" This question and focus creates a very different response than "What do you want?" Sometimes achieving clarity to that question takes time and the answer changes with time. Many years ago, I created a complex chart to guide patients in their choice of healthcare providers. With questions for patients to ask potential healthcare providers, the chart included characteristics such as whether a provider was directive or collaborative in style, regularly practiced self-care such as exercise or healthy nutrition, and whether the provider believed in something greater than information or technical skill to be as important to the healing process. As I became older, the chart became simplified to one question:"Do you leave the visit feeling good about yourself and the treatment plan?"

> As you think about your healthcare, it is helpful to ask yourself "What do I want?" Having clarity about this central question will help you greatly in actually achieving your health-related goals – whatever they may be.

Sometimes it takes training to be clear about knowing what you want from your support team. This may be especially true for women who are sometimes more adept at being clearer about others' feelings than their own. The body gives very clear messages. Once someone has mastered listening to the body's language of "yes" and "no," life becomes simpler. Yes, this feels good, this is an opening in life, this path is one of alignment. No, this feels tight or tense, less joyful, less light. I am going to choose the <u>yes</u> option.

Also, in relations from family and friends, have you clearly identified your needs and negotiated a way to have them met in a way that works for all? This sounds simple but can be complex. However, it is worth the effort for your health and well-being, and that of those around you.

Belly Breathing

Frequently taught as part of yoga practice, belly breathing changes the tone of the nervous system allowing someone to respond to stress in a more balanced way. While an infant naturally breaths this way, many adults have forgotten how. To remember you can practice the following:

- Start by thinking of the trunk of your body as a bottle, filling with your favorite drink – grape juice, sparkling mineral water, chocolate milk. (Calories are nonexistent in this image.) You fill the bottle from the bottom up and empty from the top down. Attach the same enthusiasm for filling your body with air as you would for drinking your favorite beverage if you were very thirsty. Many people's bodies are starved for adequate oxygen. Know that each breath of light filled air is sustaining and improving your health. By increasing the amount of air in the lungs through deep belly breathing, you are better nourishing each of body cell with oxygen.

- Lie face up in bed.

- Place your hands or a small bag of rice on your belly.

- Inhale through your nose and push your belly out, away from your back.

- Exhale through your mouth, pulling belly towards back.

After you have mastered belly out with inhale and belly in with exhale (possibly overcoming years of encouragement to "suck in the gut"), you are ready to proceed to the next phase.

- Move one hand off the belly to the middle of your chest.

- Imagine that as the belly moves out, it is making room for the lungs to hold more life-sustaining air. You start filling the body with air from the belly up. First belly, then the middle of the chest, then the top of chest.

- As you exhale, empty your body of air in the reverse fashion. Air out from top, then the middle of chest, followed by the belly coming in to the back.

Once you have mastered belly breathing lying down, you can try it standing and sitting. While belly breathing is great to do early in the morning before arising and late at night before bed, it becomes even more effective in promoting well-being when practiced throughout the day. Link doing a belly breath with something you do at least 20 times throughout your waking hours – walk through a door, look at a watch, hit CTRL-ALT-DEL on the computer, answer the phone. Those of us reading this chapter are all breathing on a regular basis. The goal is to maximize the quality of the breathing we do.

WHEE Technique
WHOLISTIC HYBRID OF EYE MOVEMENT DESENSITIZATION AND REPROCESSING (EMDR) AND EMOTIONAL FREEDOM TECHNIQUE (EFT)

This is a practice that combines the emotional body healing practices of EMDR and EFT, allowing efficient release of feelings without having to relive the trauma of whatever originally created the feelings. One of the advantages of this specific practice is that it can be learned quickly and practiced almost anywhere by adults and children.

Following are instructions for how to practice the WHEE technique as presented by the developer of this method, Dr. Daniel J. Benor, in 2005.

- Describe how strong the negative feeling is that you want to address. Rate your feelings about something, someone, some event on a scale from 0 (not bothering you at all) to 10 (the worst it could possibly feel).

- Create an affirmation to transform the feeling. One generic affirmation adapted from the Emotional Freedom Technique is as follows:

   "Even though I have this [name the feeling - anger, anxiety, panic, fear] when I think about [name something, someone, some event] I completely and totally love and accept myself and know that God loves and accepts me unconditionally."

   This is just an example. Use whatever strong positive statement suits you best at the time you need it.

- Tap alternately on right and left sides of your body. For example, your pat right then left thigh, back and forth. Alternate touching teeth on right and left with your tongue. Tap your right and left eyebrows with a finger.

- EMDR suggests the use of a "butterfly hug" as one of its self-treatment interventions, particularly for children. Cross your arms and rest your hands on your biceps muscles. Alternately tap each bicep with each hand. Many find this self-hug comforting, as well as highly effective when combined with the affirmation.

- Holding one hand over the heart/chest center while the other hand does the alternate side tapping can enhance the effects. A deep breath following the affirmation facilitates releases.

- After tapping for a few minutes, re-rate the feeling again. The rating usually decreases. Repeat the assessing and tapping until the rating of the negative feeling is zero. Then you can build up a positive affirmation to replace the negative, simply stating the positive as you tap, followed by the strong positive statement.

- If the numbers do not shift after you have tapped, you can give yourself a gentle massage on the releasing spot located just below the outside portion of the collar bone (the lung 2 acupressure point). No affirmation is needed here. Then return to tapping.

For more information about Dr. Daniel J. Benor and the WHEE technique, go to www.WholisticHealingResearch.com.

Castor Oil Packs

Originally described and prescribed by healer Edgar Cayce, castor oil packs have been used for a variety of medical and pain conditions for at least 60 years.[21] A castor oil pack uses a cloth soaked in castor oil which is placed on the skin. It is used to enhance circulation and promote healing of the tissues and organs underneath the skin. It is also used to improve liver function, relieve pain, reduce *inflammation*, and improve digestion.

There are two proposed mechanisms of action. One is that the castor oil contains a variety of anti-inflammatory compounds that are absorbed by the skin. The immune cells in the skin then use these anti-inflammatory compounds to promote the health of the body. Another proposal is that the combination of white (which contains all colors) flannel cloth combined with the healing properties of castor oil offer the body different frequencies of energy from which it is able to select what it needs to promote healing. Regardless of mechanism of action this is a practice I have found useful for a variety of conditions.

How to Make a Castor Oil Pack

Materials Needed: castor oil
3 layers of un-dyed cotton flannel large enough to cover
         the affected area
soaking container
plastic wrap
hot water bottle (optional)

Instructions

1. Place the flannel in the container and soak it in warm castor oil. You want the fabric to be saturated, but not dripping.
2. Place the pack over the area to be treated.
3. Cover the oil-soaked area with plastic wrap.
4. Place hot water bottle over the pack. (This is optional.)
5. Leave the pack in place for 30 minutes to 2 hours. Rest comfortably.

Oil that may get on clothing or bed linens can be cleaned by washing with baking soda. The pack can be stored in a covered container in the refrigerator and can be reused up to 30 times.

Summary

Mind-body practices are an integral part of regaining and maintaining health. The nervous system is woven throughout the body, and the human body is a greater creation than the sum of its individual physical systems.

Modern medicine is integrating new and traditional ways to look at health. Many of the world's traditional medical systems never lost the perspective that mind and body are one – different forms of energy. An exciting vision of 21st century medicine is to combine the technology and science of this culture with the wisdom of medical traditions that have thousands of years of experience in promoting health at all levels of being.

Modern physics has changed its Newtonian worldview with the incorporation of Einstein's theory of relativity and the demonstration that energy and matter are different forms of the same stuff. Although slower in adapting to this new view of the universe, modern medical science is also changing.

In the 1990's, Dr. Larry Dossey described three different eras in medicine. Era I medicine, most influential from the mid 1800's to the mid 1900's, was described as being the era of extremely materialistic medicine. Because the body is perceived as being an organized like a machine, effective therapies are based on this materialistic worldview. Many of the diagnostic practices and therapies that dominate modern medicine are based on this assumption (for example, drugs, surgery, and radiation). Era II medicine began in the 1950's with the initial studies and practices showing that emotions, beliefs, and thoughts can significantly affect physical health. The majority of this chapter has focused on looking at these practices. Over the last 20 years many of these practices that once were considered "alternative" have been incorporated into mainstream medicine.

Era I and era II medicine are frequently complementary in that they both emphasize the individual mind operating in an individual body. In this way, they are consistent with a Newtonian organizational view of universal order. In contrast, era III medicine takes into account the organizational view proposed by modern physics. "Mind" is viewed not just as residing within the bones of the skull, but is a consciousness that transcends time and space. Physicists know that just by turning their attention to studying a phenomenon, they have changed that phenomenon. With their greater comfort with uncertainty, physicists make great collaborators in the investigation of this frontier of modern medicine.[22]

As we move forward in our search for understanding, and as you move forward in your journey with hepatitis C, we all seek the same thing: healing that leaves us with a sense of well-being regardless of circumstance.

References

1. Wolsko P. M., Eisenberg D.M., Davis R.B., et al. Use of mind-body medical therapies. *J Gen Intern Med.* 2004;19:43-50.
2. Ursano R. J., C. Bell, S. Eth, et al. Practice guideline for the treatment of patients with acute stress disorder and posttraumatic stress disorder. *Am J Psychiatry.* 2004;161:3-31.
   Notes: CORPORATE NAME: Work Group on ASD and PTSD
3. Adler, P. A., Roberts B.L. The use of Tai Chi to improve health in older adults. *Orthop Nurs.* 2006;25:122-6.
4. Wang C., Collet J.P., Lau J. The effect of Tai Chi on health outcomes in patients with chronic conditions: a systematic review. *Arch Intern Med.* 2004;164:493-501.
5. Kimura H., Nagao F., Tanaka Y., et al. Beneficial effects of the Nishino breathing method on immune activity and stress level. *J Altern Complement Med.* 2005;11:285-91.
6. Irwin M. R., Pike J.L. , Cole J.C., et al. Effects of a behavioral intervention, Tai Chi, on varicella-zoster virus specific immunity and health functioning in older adults. *Psychosom Med.* 2003;65:824-30.
7. Integration of behavioral and relaxation approaches into the treatment of chronic pain and insomnia. NIH Technology Assessment Panel on Integration of Behavioral and Relaxation Approaches into the Treatment of Chronic Pain and Insomnia. *JAMA.* 1996;276:313-8.
8. Bost N., Wallis M.. The effectiveness of a 15 minute weekly massage in reducing physical and psychological stress in nurses. *Aust J Adv Nurs.* 2006;23:28-33.
9. Grossman P., Niemann L., Schmidt S. et al. Mindfulness-based stress reduction and health benefits: A meta-analysis. *J Psychosom Res.* 2004;57:35-43.
10. Irwin, M. R., Pike J.L., Cole J.C. et al. Effects of a behavioral intervention, Tai Chi, on varicella-zoster virus specific immunity and health functioning in older adults. *Psychosom Med.* 2003;65:824-30.
11. Walling, A. Therapeutic modulation of the psychoneuroimmune system by medical acupuncture creates enhanced feelings of well-being. *J Am Acad Nurse Pract.* 2006;18:135-43.
12. Barnes, P. M., Powell-Griner E., McFann K. et al. *Complementary and alternative medicine use among adults: United States, 2002.* Adv Data. 2004;1-19.

13. Humphrey, SSITPU. *Body/mind/spirit integration and healing hepatitis c: Is spiritual integration a factor in treatment choice and efficacy?* Dissertation Abstracts International: Section B: The Sciences and Engineering; 2004.

14. Gioia, T. *Healing Songs*. Durham, NC: Duke University Press; 2006.

15. Jonas, W. B., Kaptchuk T.J., and Linde K. A critical overview of homeopathy. *Ann Intern Med*. 2003;138:393-9.

16. Linde, K., Hondras M., Vickers A., et al. Systematic reviews of complementary therapies - an annotated bibliography. Part 3: homeopathy. *BMC Complement Altern Med*. 2001;1:4.

17. Cucherat, M., Haugh M.C., Gooch M. et al. Evidence of clinical efficacy of homeopathy. A meta-analysis of clinical trials. *HMRAG* Homeopathic Medicines Research Advisory Group. *Eur J Clin Pharmacol*. 2000;56:27-33.

18. Linde, K., Clausius N., Ramirez G. et al. Are the clinical effects of homeopathy placebo effects? A meta-analysis of placebo-controlled trials. *Lancet*. 1997;350:834-43.

19. Winstead-Fry, P., Kijek J. An integrative review and meta-analysis of therapeutic touch research. *Altern Ther Health Med*. 1999;5:58-67.

20. Astin, J. A., Harkness E., Ernst E.. The efficacy of "distant healing": a systematic review of randomized trials. *Ann Intern Med*. 2000;132: 903-10.

21. McGarey, WA. *The Oil That Heals: A Physician's Successes With Castor Oil Treatments*. Virginia Beach, Virginia: A.R.E. Press; 1996.

22. Dossey, L. *Healing Words: The Power of Prayer and the Practice of Medicine*. New York, NY: Harper-Collins; 1997.

Naturopathic Medicine

J. Lyn Patrick, ND

Introduction

The philosophy of naturopathic medicine can best be described as the utilization of the healing power of nature. Several basic thoughts are at the core of this philosophy. Naturopathic healthcare providers approach health with prevention and education foremost in their minds. If disease enters the picture, the approach is to treat the whole person so that the natural healing powers of the body are able to resolve the root cause of the illness.

There are four accredited naturopathic medical colleges in the United States. If you choose to include naturopathic medicine in your *hepatitis C* treatment plan, it is important that you see a licensed naturopathic doctor. Naturopathic medicine is currently licensed in 14 states. Licensed or licensable naturopaths also practice in states where they may not hold licenses. The American Association of Naturopathic Physicians provides information on well-trained, naturopathic doctors in the United States (see the *Resource Directory*).

The Principles of Naturopathic Treatment for Hepatitis C

Naturopathic healthcare providers use many different tools in the care and treatment of patients. These include botanical medicines (herbs), acupuncture, *nutritional supplements*, traditional Chinese medicine, homeopathic remedies, nutrition counseling and diet therapy, massage and/or spinal *manipulation*, exercise, and other forms of therapy.

The section discusses the naturopathic approach to hepatitis C management and the options a naturopathic provider might consider for someone with hepatitis C.

The Liver as an Organ of Detoxification

The liver is a large organ. It weighs about 3½ pounds and filters almost two quarts of blood every minute. Filtering the blood is essential to survival because the liver receives blood directly from the intestines. The liver filters *proteins* and other nutrients and chemicals from the food we eat. The liver regulates blood sugar levels, stores fat-soluble *vitamins*, activates and breaks down *hormones* and drugs, and aids in the elimination of pollutants and *toxins*. The liver also manufactures nutrients, *enzymes*, and *hormones*.

For the liver to function well, it needs certain nutrients for the detoxification and *immune systems*. The liver requires B vitamins (B_2, B_3, B_6, B_{12}, and folic acid), magnesium, zinc, copper, choline, betaine, and the *amino acids* methionine, taurine, and cysteine to break down medications, pollutants, and chemicals found in air, water, and food.[1]

GLUTATHIONE
Glutathione is one of the most important chemicals needed for liver health. The body cannot function without glutathione. Loss of glutathione can cause kidney and *liver failure*. Low glutathione levels can be found in people with cataracts, *HIV* infection, *chronic hepatitis* C, and *cirrhosis*.[2] People with cirrhosis of the liver may have difficulty making glutathione. This may explain why glutathione levels 30% below normal have been found among people with cirrhosis of the liver.[3]

Glutathione is an *antioxidant*, a chemical that protects the liver from damage by other chemicals called *free radicals* and oxidants. Glutathione is produced in the liver and elsewhere in the body from some of the nutrients listed above. Glutathione is a sulfur-based substance that helps eliminate free radicals and *metabolize* (break down) medications and chemicals.

Glutathione is used by many types of cells as the main defense against *oxidative stress* (an overabundance of free radicals). *Iron* can cause oxidative stress, and damage from liver iron can be a contributing factor in the process of fibrosis. Because glutathione protects against damage from oxidants such as iron, it may slow the *fibrosis* process.

Glutathione is also a crucial activator of certain immune system cells called *cytotoxic T-cells*. Cytotoxic T-cells kill viruses and cancer cells.[4] Glutathione has been shown to have direct *antiviral* effects. Levels of reduced glutathione (the most important form of glutathione) can be significantly below normal in people who have alcoholic hepatitis or hepatitis C.[5, 6]

Studies have shown that people with hepatitis C who had the lowest glutathione levels also had the highest *viral loads* and more evidence of liver damage.[6] Although no research has been done with the hepatitis C virus (*HCV*), glutathione has been shown to inhibit HIV in the test tube.[7] While this research does not prove that raising glutathione levels leads to lower viral loads, it does indicate that optimal levels of glutathione may be an important factor in controlling HCV infection.

Limiting Exposure to Liver-Damaging Substances and Situations

People with HCV should avoid exposure to anything that may cause damage to the liver. Following are examples of substances that may place stress upon and possibly damage the liver.

ALCOHOL

Alcohol consumption is a significant risk factor for liver cirrhosis. Chronic alcohol drinkers who do not have HCV are actually at a <u>higher</u> risk of developing cirrhosis than those who <u>do</u> have hepatitis C but do not drink.[8] Among people with HCV, the risk of developing cirrhosis is about 16 times higher in drinkers than in those who do not drink alcohol. It is important to remember that one study has shown, low levels of drinking (less than six ounces per week) are related to higher HCV viral loads and increased liver fibrosis.[9] National consensus conferences of doctors and scientists in France and the United States have recommended that people with hepatitis C refrain from drinking <u>any</u> alcohol.[10]

> **Alcohol consumption is a significant risk factor for liver cirrhosis.**

The breakdown products of alcohol have direct *toxic* effects on liver cells and cause *inflammation*, which can also damage the liver. In addition, alcohol damages the liver by depleting it of glutathione. Even people who have HCV without *symptoms* and only mild elevations in *liver enzymes* can have liver damage that may be worsened by loss of glutathione from alcohol use. For more information on this topic see *Chapter 2, Alcohol and Hepatitis C*.

ACETAMINOPHEN

The over-the-counter medicine *acetaminophen* (APAP, Tylenol®) can deplete the liver of glutathione.[11] Because glutathione levels may already be low in people with HCV, risking even lower levels with long-term acetaminophen use may be unwise. Use of acetaminophen for a headache every now and then will <u>not</u> affect liver glutathione levels. But frequent or daily use of this medicine may deplete glutathione stores.

Acetaminophen is the active ingredient in many over-the-counter pain relievers. It is also found in many cold remedies and prescription pain medications. If you need a pain reliever, ask your healthcare provider about alternatives to acetaminophen that provide similar pain relief. Naturopathic doctors prescribe botanical medicines for pain relief such as food extracts and herbs. Examples include Bromelain (an enzyme extracted from pineapples), *Picrorhiza kurroa* extract, *Boswellia serrata* extract, *Curcuma longa* (a turmeric root extract), and *Salix alba* (white willow bark).

TOBACCO AND RECREATIONAL DRUGS

The liver breaks down all the toxic and *carcinogenic* compounds found in tobacco, marijuana, and other recreational drugs. Tobacco smoke contains more than 4,000 different chemicals, and marijuana contains many of the same carcinogenic compounds.

Research data clearly show that daily marijuana smoking significantly increases the risk of hepatitis C disease progression.[12-14] A recent study found that daily marijuana use was associated with a significantly higher rate of fat in the liver (*steatosis*),[15] which has been linked to more rapid disease progression in chronic hepatitis C. Similarly, higher levels of liver damage have been reported in association with cigarette smoking.[16, 17] Both tobacco and marijuana use increase the risk of *liver cancer* for people infected with HCV.[14, 18-20]

Daily marijuana use is strongly associated with moderate to severe fibrosis.

In general, recreational drugs and tobacco products should be avoided as they may damage your overall health and your liver health. If you are having difficulty with pain or loss of appetite, talk with your healthcare provider about alternatives to marijuana use to control these symptoms.

OCCUPATIONAL EXPOSURES

Exposure to *pesticides*, *herbicides*, and other chemicals can cause liver damage and elevation of liver enzymes.[21-23] If your job exposes you to chemicals, solvents, fumes, pesticides, or herbicides, it is very important that you use *OSHA*-approved protective gear to prevent breathing the fumes or having physical contact with these chemicals. This includes exposure to paint and lacquer, solvents such as dry cleaning fluid, glues and epoxy, fabric coatings, and many others. If you have a history of chemical exposure and are concerned about the effects on your liver, there are proven ways to reduce the burden of these toxic compounds on your body. Elimination of these toxic compounds requires the supervision of a trained doctor. Naturopathic doctors and medical doctors trained in environmental medicine can supervise programs designed to eliminate these substances from the body. The Encyclopedia of Natural Medicine was written by licensed naturopathic doctors and is a good resource for information about naturopathic support for detoxification.[24]

Diet and Hepatitis C

SUGAR

One of the basic concepts of a naturopathic diet is the inclusion of only minimal amounts of processed foods and simple sugars (sucrose, glucose, corn syrup, etc.). This recommendation is based on research that examined the effect of large amounts of simple sugars on the immune system. In the study, eating 2.5 to 3.5 ounces of white sugar, honey, or fruit juice appeared to reduce the ability of specific *white blood cells* to attack foreign viruses and bacteria.[26] This immune suppressing effect started 30 minutes after eating and lasted for five hours afterward. Since the average American consumes over six ounces of sugar daily, the potential effect on the immune system is considerable.

The immune system is an important factor in hepatitis C. We know that those who clear HCV appear to have *lymphocytes* (white blood cells) that are better able to kill the virus than those who become chronically infected.[27]

DIETARY FAT

A study that examined how dietary fat, *carbohydrate*, and protein levels affect liver disease progression found that a high fat diet coupled with low protein and carbohydrate intake increased the risk of progression to cirrhosis.[28] People who are overweight or obese tend to have more fat in their diet, which may lead to steatosis (fat in the liver cells). Steatosis can accelerate the progression of liver disease in people with chronic hepatitis C.[29] For more information on steatosis see *Chapter 4.1, Understanding Hepatitis C Disease – Liver Disease Progression*.

As explained in *Chapter 15, Nutrition and Hepatitis C*, not all fats are bad. Some types of fat actually appear to be beneficial for people with hepatitis C.

- Omega-3 fatty acids actually have helpful immune regulating effects and should always be included in a nutritional plan for optimizing the immune system.

- Studies of *phosphatidylcholine*, a type of fat found in fish and soybeans, showed it has a beneficial effect in reducing liver enzymes and increasing the response rate to *interferon*.[30] People who were given polyunsaturated phosphatidylcholine (1.8 grams/day) during treatment with interferon and for six months following treatment had significantly fewer *relapses* than those who did not take the fat supplement. Forty-one percent of the patients in the phosphatidylcholine group had a *sustained response* compared to 15% who received only interferon. Different forms of phosphatidylcholine have been used in hepatitis resulting from alcoholism, and have been effective in decreasing fibrosis.[31]

For a thorough discussion of the fundamentals of a naturopathic approach to eating a healthy diet, see *Chapter 15, Nutrition and Hepatitis C*.

COFFEE

Studies on the consumption of coffee and its effects on liver disease have arrived at mixed conclusions over the years. However, recent studies have reported beneficial effects of filtered coffee on abnormal liver biochemistry, cirrhosis, and *hepatocellular carcinoma*.[32-35] The reason for this effect remains unclear, as does the amount of coffee consumed daily to achieve these benefits.

Research indicates that the effects of unfiltered coffee may be different from filtered coffee.[32] This difference may be due to the fact that there are other substances in unfiltered coffee that have been shown to increase liver enzyme levels in healthy people. Research has been conducted on two compounds found in coffee beans: cafestol and kahweol (called diterpenes). One study found these compounds increased ALT levels by 80% in 46 healthy subjects who were drinking 5 to 6 cups of strong, French press (unfiltered) coffee daily.[36] ALT levels dropped to 45% above normal 24 weeks after the study participants stopped drinking unfiltered coffee. Other studies have shown that cafestol and kahweol raise blood *cholesterol*, *triglyceride*, and low-density *lipoprotein* (a harmful fat) levels, and increase other risk factors for heart disease.[37] However, separate laboratory research indicates these same two compounds (cafestol and kahweol) may have protective effects with regard to the development of liver cancer.[38, 39]

In summary, the effects of coffee and its many components on the human body remain the focus of much clinical and laboratory research. The fact that coffee contains many different chemicals and that what may be present changes depending on how the coffee is prepared surely complicates this research. In addition, health considerations must always take into account the effects on all the body's organ systems, not just a single effect on a single organ system. Overall, people living with hepatitis C are best advised to err on the side of caution. So with respect to coffee, especially because the sum total of its effects remain unclear at this time, it may be safest to avoid coffee if possible. If you are a coffee drinker, filtered coffee is a better option than unfiltered. Filtering coffee eliminates both cafestol and kahweol. Water-processed, decaffeinated, filtered coffee decreases the potentially harmful effects coffee may have.[40]

Nutritional Supplementation

A nutritious diet, nutritional supplementation, and botanical medicines are the foundations of the naturopathic approach to managing chronic hepatitis C. The nutritional supplements listed in *Chapter 16, Nutritional Supplementation* are mostly antioxidants. They work to decrease liver inflammation and raise glutathione levels. Glutathione is an important antioxidant and immune system regulator. The supplements listed in *Chapter 16, Nutritional Supplementation* are meant to be taken together as a total *protocol*, not as substitutes for each other or as choices that can be taken individually. As stated in *Chapter 15, Nutrition and Hepatitis C*, neither diet alone nor supplements alone are enough to help the body effectively manage chronic hepatitis C.

Drug-Herb Interactions

Most active substances in medicines and botanicals are processed (metabolized) by either the liver or the kidneys. It is important to realize that whenever you are taking more than one medication or botanical, there is a potential for interaction between the active ingredients. The potential for interactions applies to <u>all</u> medications (prescription drugs and over-the-counter formulations) and <u>all</u> botanicals (supplied by a healthcare practitioner or purchased over-the-counter).

For the purposes of this discussion, all prescription medications, over-the-counter remedies, individual herbs, and botanical preparations are considered and will be referred to as "drugs."

Drug-herb interactions fall into four categories:

- **altered absorption**
  Drugs taken by mouth must be absorbed into the blood through the stomach and intestines. Two or more substances taken together can affect absorption in several different ways. Drugs taken together may bind to one another and decrease the overall absorption of both substances. Substances that affect the acidity in the stomach can also alter the absorption of other drugs. Any drug that has a laxative effect may decrease the absorption of other drugs taken by mouth. The important concept to understand is that two or more substances taken together may alter the amounts of active ingredients absorbed by the body.

- **altered renal (kidney) elimination**
  Some drugs are eliminated from the body primarily by the kidneys. They are excreted in the urine. When two or more medicinal substances that are eliminated by the kidneys are taken at the same time, the kidneys may be overwhelmed. Toxic amounts of one or more substances may build up in the bloodstream, especially if there is underlying kidney damage or if one of the drugs decreases normal kidney function.

- **additive effects or toxicities**
  Medicinal substances often have similar effects on the body. Some of these effects are beneficial, but others are toxic. Two medicinal substances that interact with one another in a similar way are said to have pharmacodynamic interactions. These interactions can be additive or neutralizing (see Figure 1). For example, *ribavirin* and certain anti-HIV medicines can cause *anemia*. When ribavirin is given along with one of these anti-HIV medications, anemia is more likely to occur than when either drug is given alone. Herbs and drugs can also have pharmcodynamic interactions. Even when two medicinal substances have the same beneficial action individually, combining the two may be detrimental. For example, a mild laxative may be helpful if you are having trouble moving your bowels. But combining a mild laxative with an herb that also has a laxative effect may cause diarrhea. Two medicinal substances with opposite actions may cancel out the effectiveness of one another. Many drug-herb interactions fall in this category.

Figure 1. Pharmacodynamic Interactions

anti-viral ✚ anti-viral ➡ Improved Anti-Viral Activity				Additive Effects
laxative ✚ laxative ➡ Diarrhea				
lower BP ✚ increase BP ➡ Unchanged Blood Pressure				Neutralizing Effect

- **altered hepatic (liver) metabolism**
  Some of the most complicated drug interactions and potentially serious drug-herb interactions for people with chronic hepatitis C are those involving altered liver metabolism. Much of the processing of medicinal substances in the liver is done by a group of enzymes called the cytochrome P-450 system. The activity of these liver enzymes that break down medicinal ingredients can be increased or decreased by drugs and herbs. When the activity of cytochrome P-450 enzymes is increased, drugs are broken down more quickly than expected. Circulating blood levels may be too low to bring about the desired effects. Conversely, when cytochrome P-450 activity is decreased, drugs may not be eliminated from the body as quickly as expected. Toxic levels of drugs may build up.

The effects of medicinal substances on liver metabolism are further complicated by the fact that a substance may increase the activity of some P-450 enzymes while decreasing the activity of others. The reactions of people with underlying liver disease such as chronic hepatitis C to substances metabolized by the liver are also somewhat unpredictable. A drug that is well tolerated by one person may cause serious problems in another person despite the fact that they appear to have similar *stages* of disease.

In summary, the potential for drug-herb interactions in people with liver disease is complex and often unpredictable. Substances with very different uses may well be processed by the same liver enzymes and interact in potentially serious, undesired ways. For example, you may not think there is any potential for interaction between an herb used to improve mood and a blood thinner since they have such different actions in the body. However, substances with these actions have been known to interact and cause very serious problems. (See the section on St. John's wort later in this chapter for additional information).

> **Keep all of your healthcare providers informed about all medicines, herbs, and supplements you are taking!**

The potential for undesired and serious interactions is the reason you <u>must</u> keep all of your healthcare providers informed about all medicines, botanicals, and supplements you are taking. People with chronic hepatitis C should always be cautious about taking any medicinal substances. Always check with a healthcare provider before taking anything new. Also keep in mind that many over-the-counter formulas marketed to people with hepatitis C contain several different herbs. Keeping your providers informed about all of the prescription and over-the-counter substances you are taking is one of the most important responsibilities you have in your healthcare.

> **Never take any medicinal product if you are uncertain about what it contains.**

Now that you have been cautioned about taking and combining medicinal substances (including herbs), we can discuss some of the potential benefits of botanicals for people with chronic hepatitis C.

Botanicals Used to Treat Hepatitis C Liver Problems

SILYBUM MARIANUM (MILK THISTLE)

Silybum marianum (milk thistle) has been used medicinally in Europe since the 13th century to treat liver-related diseases. It is available in Germany in both injectable and oral forms.[41]

Milk thistle is commonly used by people with liver disease. A 1999 survey evaluating the use of *complementary and alternative medicine* (CAM) among hepatitis C patients in liver clinics found that 42-73% of all patients who used other alternative therapies were also taking milk thistle. All participants who used only herbs to treat their liver disease (63%) identified milk thistle as one of the herbs taken.[42]

The active ingredients in milk thistle are contained in the extract silymarin. Silymarin is a mixture of active plant materials that includes silybinin, a plant compound known as a *flavinoid*. Although silybinin has not been shown to have any antiviral activity against HCV, some flavinoids do have antiviral properties.

Silymarin has specific effects on liver cells that have been seen in laboratory animal studies. Silymarin appears to stabilize or strengthen liver cells' ability to withstand the effects of substances that are toxic to the liver including recreational drugs, some medications, poisonous mushrooms, and chemicals. It prevents the damage that occurs when free radicals attack the fatty layer of liver cell membranes.[43] Silymarin also appears to inhibit the process of inflammation of liver cells that eventually leads to cirrhosis.[44] Silymarin increases glutathione levels in the liver. Some studies of hepatitis C patients have found abnormally low levels of glutathione.[45, 46]

A 2005 review of the published research on the effects of milk thistle for alcoholic and/or *hepatitis B* or C liver diseases concluded that:

> Milk thistle does not seem to significantly influence the course of patients with alcoholic and/or hepatitis B or C liver diseases. Milk thistle could potentially affect liver injury. Adequately conducted randomized clinical trials on milk thistle versus *placebo* may be needed.[47]

While there are no published studies on the effects of silymarin among large populations of hepatitis C patients, there have been several studies on the effects of silymarin among people with liver disease. In people with *acute hepatitis* (both A and B), silymarin was found to decrease the number of complications, speed recovery time, and improve *liver function test* scores.[48] In chronic liver disease (both alcoholic and chronic hepatitis), silymarin has been shown to decrease symptoms of *fatigue* and abdominal pain, and to significantly decrease liver enzyme levels.[49] Silymarin has also been shown to improve the survival rates of people with cirrhosis. Those with histories of alcohol-related liver damage fared better than those who had cirrhosis from drug use.[50] These studies were done prior to widespread testing for hepatitis C, so it is not known how many of the people in these studies were actually infected with HCV.

Not all studies with silymarin have shown a clear benefit in liver disease. A study of 125 patients with alcoholic cirrhosis who took 450 mg of silymarin per day for two years did not find any improvement associated with silymarin use.[51] Whether these results were influenced by the effects of alcohol abuse is not known.

A study on the effects of silymarin and liver damage in baboons found silymarin was effective in preventing fibrosis in alcohol-related liver damage.[52] The animals were given both alcohol and silymarin along with a nutritionally adequate diet for 3 years. The average dose of silymarin given to the baboons was the equivalent of 2,800 mg per day for a 150-pound person. This is significantly higher than the doses of silymarin used in previous human studies. The study found silymarin prevented fat accumulation in the liver and significantly decreased free-radical related damage to the liver, both of which can occur in people with chronic hepatitis C. This study does not mean taking silymarin will protect you from the damaging effects of alcohol. Only 2 of the 6 baboons getting alcohol and silymarin escaped liver damage. The point of this study is that the positive effects from silymarin were achieved at a dosage much higher than what has been used in human studies with silymarin to date. This dosage level does not appear to be harmful in animals or humans, although, diarrhea may result from increased bile secretion.

Researchers have also looked at using silymarin instead of standard treatment with interferon/ribavirin in hepatitis C. At doses of 420 to 1,260 mg per day, those on silymarin had no improvements in their liver enzymes or viral load.[53] Although higher doses of silymarin were used (1,260 mg) in seven patients, it is not clear how long each patient was actually taking the silymarin; the total time patients were on any dose of silymarin was somewhere between 7 to 29 weeks. Whether this is enough time for an effect to be seen is not clear.

Silymarin therapy has also been compared to a combination of ribavirin and two other drugs: ursodeoxycholic acid and amantidine, in order to see which therapy would be more effective in normalizing liver enzymes.[54] The group that received the drugs had a much higher chance of normalizing their liver enzymes: 58% of them had normal liver enzymes by the end of 24 weeks while only 15% those in the silymarin group had normal liver enzymes.

Another form of silymarin called silipide or silybin-phosphatidylcholine has also been studied. This form is more easily absorbed than other forms of silymarin. In a small study with eight patients (five had hepatitis C), liver function tests and markers that reflect cell damage in the liver were significantly improved in patients who had been taking the equivalent of 120 mg of silybin twice daily between meals for two months.[55]

Milk thistle is available over-the-counter in standardized extracts that contain 70% silymarin. The active ingredients of milk thistle are not water-soluble. Therefore, a tea made from milk thistle seeds is not useful. If the label for milk thistle does not list the silymarin content, there is no guarantee there is any silymarin in it. Standard dosages used in studies range from 400-1,140 mg per day of the standardized extract. The common dosage for active liver disease is 200 mg of standardized extract (containing 70% silymarin) taken three times daily. Silipide (the phosphatidylcholine form) is commonly dosed at 100 mg taken three times daily.

Silymarin is safe and has no known *toxicity*, though doses over 1,500 mg per day may cause diarrhea because of increased *bile* secretion. Silymarin is safe to use in pregnancy and while breast feeding.[56] Silymarin has been shown to alter the activity of some P-450 enzymes. Although there have been no studies to determine if taking silymarin along with ribavirin and interferon alters the levels of these drugs in the body, that possibility does exist.

GLYCYRRHIZA GLABRA (LICORICE ROOT)

Glycyrrhiza glabra (licorice root) preparations have been used for over 20 years in Japan to treat both hepatitis B and C.[57] Glycyrrhizin, an extract made from the Glycyrrhiza glabra plant, is used as an intravenous injection on a daily basis for eight weeks. The preparation can be given at that frequency or reduced to several times a week, and can be continued for as long as 16 years.

A study of 193 hepatitis C patients being treated with intravenous glycyrrhizin for 2 to16 years showed decreased risk of developing cirrhosis. Those on treatment were about half as likely to develop cirrhosis (21% compared with 37%).[57] The rate of liver cancer was also less than half in those who were treated compared to those who were untreated. Twelve percent of the treated patients and 25% of the untreated patients developed liver cancer. German studies with intravenous glycyrrhizin showed that, when given daily, glycyrrhizin was as effective an antiviral agent as interferon alone without ribavirin.[58]

The intravenous form of glycyrrhizin is not readily available in the United States, but the oral form is easily available over-the-counter. The effectiveness of the oral formulation of glycyrrhizin against hepatitis B was studied in China. Significant numbers of patients who had taken 7.5 grams of licorice root (concentrated to 750 mg licorice root extract) twice daily for 30 days experienced a normalization of liver enzyme levels. Twenty-five percent of the patients fully recovered from hepatitis B, while no one in the control group recovered.[59] Again, it is important to remember that hepatitis B and hepatitis C are caused by two different classes of viruses, so it is difficult to say whether licorice root has any effect on the hepatitis C virus.

Licorice root does have a potentially problematic side effect. A breakdown product of glycyrrizin alters the production of the hormone aldosterone. This can cause increased blood pressure, water retention, and a reduction in blood *potassium*. The injectable form of glycyrrhizin has two amino acids (glycine and cysteine) added to prevent this side effect, but pure licorice root does not. If you are taking doses higher than 400 mg of glycyrrhizin daily, have your blood pressure monitored regularly. If you have a history of high blood pressure and/or have kidney failure, you should avoid taking licorice root.

OTHER BOTANICAL MEDICINES

Catechin is an extract of the Unicaria (cat's claw) plant that has been researched extensively in England for its ability to improve liver function in people with hepatitis B.[60] Although study results were positive, the research on catechin was discontinued in the late 1980's because the use of the synthetic form of catechin resulted in a serious form of anemia in six patients.[61]

Recently, research in Africa has identified similar plant compounds in the Garcinia species that have antiviral activity and are used by native people to treat hepatitis.[62] The active compound is a flavinoid (a vitamin-like compound in many plants, fruits, and vegetables) and will continue to be the subject of research in treating both hepatitis B and C.[63] Other plant medicines used by native people in areas where hepatitis is common, such as those from the Phyllanthus amarus plant, have been shown to have direct antiviral effects on the hepatitis B virus.[64] Picrorhiza kurroa also has activity against hepatitis B, though neither of these plants have been tested specifically with hepatitis C.[65].

Botanicals Used to Treat Extrahepatic Hepatitis C Problems

The serious effects of HCV on the liver are well known. HCV also has serious effects on other parts of the body. The fatigue, *depression*, and lack of energy reported by hepatitis C patients may be related to an effect of HCV on the central nervous system.[66] In one study, researchers found problems with memory and concentration were not necessarily due to a history of intravenous drug use, depression, or fatigue, but were more closely related to HCV infection and some changes in brain function that were measured by a brain scan. A recent study found similar problems with higher brain function in 32 people with chronic hepatitis C.[67] These studies bring to light a possible cause of what hepatitis C patients have long described as "brain fog." The changes seen in the brain scans were similar to changes seen in the brains of people with HIV infection. Although the way that HIV can damage the brain is still being studied, one of the mechanisms seems to involve the immune system found in the brain. When immune cells in the brain are stimulated by HIV infection, they produce free radicals that damage brain cells.[68] Treating the HIV-infected brain cells with *vitamin E* stopped damage and death in the affected brain cells.

Symptoms of forgetfulness and brain fog are common complaints of people with hepatitis C. Research data showing that changes can be seen in the brain tissue of people with hepatitis C is evidence that HCV infection has an effect on brain tissue. Although we do not know if these changes occur in the same way as HIV-induced brain cell damage, we do know that free radical damage is a factor in many brain diseases such as Parkinson's disease,[69] Alzheimer's dementia,[70] and many others. While it is reasonable for a person with HCV to take antioxidants for liver health, there are antioxidants that have been tested specifically for treating damage to brain cells and the symptoms of memory loss and lack of attention that result.

GINGKO BILOBA

Gingko biloba extract has been shown to protect brain cells from damage due to aging and oxidative stress. Over 250 research studies have been published on gingko and brain function. *Ginkgo biloba* extract has been shown to be effective at improving blood supply to the brain. It also has a beneficial effect on attention span and brain function in elderly patients, resulting in significant improvements in memory, alertness, and mood.[71] Studies in those with Alzheimer's dementia have shown beneficial effects on alertness, concentration, and memory.[72] When Gingko biloba extract was compared to four medications called cholinesterase-inhibitors that are used to treat mild to moderate dementia from Alzheimer's disease, gingko was as effective as all four drugs with very few side effects.[73]

Depression is another common symptom of hepatitis C, even among people who are not being treated with western drug therapy (see *Chapter 5, Signs and Symptoms That May be Associated with Hepatitis C*). In one study, 28% of people being seen in a clinic for hepatitis C were diagnosed with depression.[74] *Gingko biloba* has been studied by one research group among older adults who had not responded to standard antidepressants.[75] The group that stayed on antidepressant medication without gingko experienced little improvement in their depression. However the group that took antidepressant medication plus gingko experienced significant improvement.

Gingko is an approved prescription drug in Europe, and has been proven safe and *nontoxic.*[76] All the published studies with gingko used an extract that contains 24% gingko heterosides. The extract was given in doses of 40-80 mg three times daily. A few case reports have been published in the medical literature of people who were diagnosed with bleeding in the brain who were also using high amounts (up to 1,200 mg per day) of gingko. It is not clear if the gingko was related to the bleeding. There are no *contraindications* (situations in which it should not be used) to ginko use stated by the German Commission E (a group that studies the uses and safety of herbs and nutritional supplements) if it is taken in prescribed doses of 120-240 mg per day.

HYPERICUM PERFOATUM (ST. JOHN'S WORT)

St. John's wort (*Hypericum perfoatum*) is a plant product that has been studied for its antidepressant action. A 2007 review published research studies on the use of herbal medicines to treat psychiatric disorders concluded that there is high-quality data to support the use of St. John's wort for depression.[77] An earlier review of 27 human studies also indicated St. John's wort is effective for mild to moderate depression. The St. John's wort in these studies was given as a 0.2% hypericin-based preparation (one of the active ingredients).[78] The studies examined St. John's wort alone and in comparison to the popular antidepressants fluoxetine (Prozac®) and imipramine (Tofranil®). The authors concluded that the studies clearly demonstrated St. John's wort was equally effective with significantly fewer side effects than the standard antidepressants. However, it was also clear that St. John's wort is not effective for severe depression. Prescription drugs work better for severe depression.

Harmful side effects have been reported from use of St. John's wort, although they appear to be uncommon. Over eight million people were given prescriptions for St. John's wort in Germany from 1990 to 2000. In this time period, 70 people complained of negative side effects including allergic reactions, stomach complaints, rashes after sunlight exposure, breakthrough bleeding on birth control pills, prolonged *prothrombin* (clotting) *time*, and interactions with the drug cyclosporin (given to organ transplant recipients).[79]

St. John's wort has been shown to affect the speed at which the liver breaks down certain drugs. This may lower levels of certain drugs in the bloodstream. Following is a list of drugs that are known to interact with St. John's wort. If you are taking any of these drugs, it is very important to talk with your healthcare provider before taking St. John's wort.

Drugs That Interact with St. John's wort
prescription antidepressants
oral contraceptives
anticoagulants (Coumadin)
theophylline
indinavir
digoxin
cyclosporin

Reasons for Using Naturopathic Medicine and Who May Benefit

Naturopathic treatment options may benefit those who are motivated to adopt the following healthy lifestyle practices including:

- a nutritious diet low in sugar, red meat, and processed foods

- avoidance of smoking, alcohol, and recreational drugs

- regular exercise

- stress management

While these practices are helpful with any therapeutic approach, they are vital to the success of naturopathic treatment. If you choose a naturopathic approach, you need to be willing to take nutritional supplements and botanicals such as those mentioned in this chapter and in the chapter on nutritional supplementation (*Chapter 16, Nutritional Supplementation*), or those prescribed by your naturopathic doctor. You must also be willing to eat a healthy diet (see *Chapter 15, Nutrition and Hepatitis C*).

If cost is a concern, you need to be aware that most health insurance policies do not cover nutritional supplements and botanicals.

Helen: A Person for Whom the Naturopathic Approach was Appropriate

Helen had been diagnosed with hepatitis C six years prior to coming to our office. She had no idea how she had been infected, and had not experienced any symptoms that she knew were related to hepatitis C. Although her viral load was low and her *liver biopsy* showed only mild inflammation, her gastroenterologist encouraged her to start *interferon-based treatment*.

Helen was resistant to interferon-based treatment because she was a single mother of three children, had a demanding job, and was supporting an ailing mother. She was afraid the potential side effects of treatment could make it hard for her to keep up with her responsibilities. She worried about being able to care for her children and provide financial support for her mother. Helen did not have a strong support system of friends and family who could step in and take care of her children if treatment made her tired or depressed.

Helen was willing to change her diet and she had given up alcohol when she was first diagnosed. She was also willing to find time to exercise with her children. She committed to taking the antioxidant protocol and botanicals. Her gastroenterologist agreed to follow her liver enzymes and repeat the liver biopsy to see if any improvement had occurred. Helen was relieved that she could do something other than watch and wait, and that the treatment approach she was taking fit into her belief system.

Her liver enzymes normalized and Helen had a repeat liver biopsy three years later. The biopsy showed that the level of inflammation had normalized to that of someone without hepatitis. Her *hepatologist* agreed that standard interferon-based treatment was not necessary for Helen as long as her laboratory tests remained normal and she continued to get liver biopsies every five years.

Reasons For Not Using Naturopathic Medicine

The appropriate treatment for people with end-stage liver failure is western medical care including possible liver transplantation. Alternative medicine, including naturopathic medicine, cannot effectively treat end-stage liver failure. Without a firm commitment to the necessary lifestyle changes, you probably will not benefit from a naturopathic approach. From the naturopathic perspective, it is difficult for the liver to heal when it is under siege from tobacco smoke, alcohol, recreational drugs, and/or the chemicals found in processed foods. For naturopathic treatment to work, you need to be willing to "clear the way" before you can expect any changes from of a naturopathic treatment protocol.

Robert: A Person for Whom the Naturopathic Approach Alone Was Not Appropriate

Robert is a 43-year-old lawyer who contracted hepatitis C during a brief period of intravenous drug use when he was in his twenties. He was diagnosed when a yearly physical showed his liver enzymes were elevated 10-15 times above the normal level. His viral load was high and his liver biopsy revealed cirrhosis.

Robert had not experienced symptoms other than some intestinal bloating and a little fatigue after work. He blamed these symptoms on his heavy work schedule, eating on the run, and the stress of his demanding job. Robert was interested in treating his hepatitis C, but wanted to use an alternative approach. He wanted to take an herbal pill that would "get rid of the virus once and for all without the side effects that the drugs have." He wanted to continue working full time. He also drank alcohol often and smoked a pack of cigarettes per day.

Robert was quite willing to take supplements and antioxidants, but when it came to lifestyle changes, he was not so sure. He did not want to make any drastic changes, though he was willing to cut down on his alcohol and nicotine use and "maybe start eating a little better." However, he was not willing to give up anything altogether. He was aware that he was not dealing with stress very well. He had high blood pressure and daily tension headaches. He did not have time to exercise or do anything that would take him away from his work. Robert was also seeing a gastroenterologist who had warned him that his condition was serious and he needed treatment, but Robert wanted an "easier" route to recovery.

It was suggested to Robert that he pursue western antiviral therapy in addition to a naturopathic approach for several reasons. It was crucial that Robert quit drinking and his naturopathic doctor knew that. She also knew that Robert would not be able to get western treatment if he continued to drink. She hoped that with the support of Robert's gastroenterologist, they could convince Robert to stop using alcohol and begin treatment.

Robert's situation was dangerous. He had significantly elevated liver enzymes and cirrhosis. He was at risk for advanced hepatitis C including the possibilities of liver transplant and/or liver cancer. Robert did not have a lot of time to waste, so a combined approach was probably the best approach for him. This would have allowed him to use supplements and some botanicals to help his liver while undergoing western treatment for the hepatitis C. With a combined treatment approach, he could have a positive response to treatment.

After a serious talk with his gastroenterologist and his naturopathic provider, who both urged him to consider interferon-based treatment to stop the progression of his cirrhosis and possibly save his life, Robert agreed that he needed to do something more serious than take a botanical. He started going to AA meetings with a friend who had stopped drinking and was able to stay sober for 6 months. Robert then started interferon and ribavirin along with antioxidants and botanical medicines that would not interfere with the effects of interferon. He was also able to quit smoking with the aid of an acupuncturist and changed his diet, cutting out red meat and fast food.

Robert continued to receive acupuncture for the duration of his treatment. He was encouraged when his doctor told him his viral load was undetectable just 12 weeks after starting treatment. Although Robert was not able to work full-time during treatment, he was able to work part-time for the duration of treatment.

Six months after treatment was completed, Robert was still virus negative and decided that his 60-hour work schedule was a thing of the past, and that he would continue to stay sober one day at a time.

Summary

Naturopathic medicine offers people with HCV another tool in their efforts to manage their disease. Many people infected with HCV who include naturopathic medicine in their treatment protocol use it primarily as a way to enhance the body's ability to heal itself. Many feel that by doing this, they can keep the virus under control until more is known about it and better treatment options are available. Other people infected with HCV use naturopathic medicine as their primary care option. If and how naturopathic care fits into your treatment protocol is up to you

If naturopathic care is something you are interested in, it is important that you find out as much as you can about it. Many books and Internet sites are available that can help you better understand what naturopathic medicine has to offer. Some of these are listed in the *Resource Directory*.

References

1. Pizzorno J. *Total Wellness*. Rocklin, California: Prima Communications; 1996.
2. Droge W, Pottmeyer-Gerber C, et al. Glutathione augments the activation of cytotoxic T lymphocytes *in vivo*. *Immunobiology*. 1986;172(2):151-156.
3. White AC, et al. Glutathione deficiency in human disease. *J Nutr Biochem*. 1994;5:218-226.
4. Burgunder JM, Lauterburg BH. Decreased production of glutathione in patients with cirrhosis. *Eur J Clin Invest*. 1987;17:408-414.
5. Loguercio C, Blanco FD, De Girolamo V. Ethanol consumption, amino acid and glutathione blood levels in patients with and without chronic liver disease. *Alcohol Clin Exp Res*. 1999;23(11):1780-1784.
6. Barbaro G, Di Lorenzo G, Soldini M. Hepatic glutathione deficiency in chronic hepatitis C: quantitative evaluation in patients who are HIV positive and HIV negative and correlations with plasmatic and lymphocytic concentrations and with the activity of the liver disease. *Am J Gastroenterol*. 1996;91(12):2569-2573.
7. Staal FJ, Roederer M, Anderson MT, et al. Glutathione deficiency and human immunodeficiency virus infection. *Lancet*. 1992;339:909-912.
8. Alter H, Seef L. Recovery, persistence and sequelae in hepatitis C infection: a perspective on long-term outcome. *Sem Liver Disease*. 2000;20(1):17-35.
9. Pessione F, Degos F, Marcellin P. Effect of alcohol consumption on serum hepatitis C virus RNA and histological lesions in chronic hepatitis C. *Hepatology*. 1998;27(6):1717-1722.
10. Dienstag JL. Management of hepatitis C: a consensus. *Gastroenterology*. 1997;113(2):375.
11. McClain CJ, Price S, et al. Acetaminophen hepatotoxicity: an update. *Curr Gastroenterol Rep*. 1999;1(1):42-49.
12. Hézode C, Roudot-Thoraval F, Nguyen S, et al. Daily cannabis smoking as a risk factor for progression of fibrosis in chronic hepatitis. *Hepatology*. 2005;42(4):975-976.
13. Ishida JH, Peters MG, Jin C, Louie K, Tan V, Bacchetti P, Terrault NA. Influence of cannabis use on severity of hepatitis C disease. *Clin Gastroenterol Hepatol*. 2008;6(1):69-75.
14. Mallat A, Hezode C, Lotersztajn S. Environmental factors as disease accelerators during chronic hepatitis C. *J Hepatol*. 2008;48(4):657-665.
15. Hézode C, Zafrani ES, Roudot-Thoraval F, et al. Daily cannabis use: a novel risk factor of steatosis severity in patients with chronic hepatitis C. *Gastroenterology*. 2008;134(2):432-439.
16. Pessione F, Ramond MJ, Njapoum C, et al. Cigarette smoking and hepatic lesions in patients with chronic hepatitis C. *Hepatology*. 2001;34(1):121-125.
17. Hézode C, Lonjon I, Roudot-Thoraval F, et al. Impact of smoking on histological liver lesions in chronic hepatitis C. *Gut*. 2003;52(1):126-129.
18. Mori M, Hara M, Wada I. Prospective study of hepatitis B and C viral infections, cigarette smoking, alcohol consumption, and other factors

associated with hepatocellular carcinoma risk in Japan. *Am J Epidemiol.* 2000;151(2):131-139.

19. Hara M, Tanaka K, Sakamoto T, et al. Case-control study on cigarette smoking and the risk of hepatocellular carcinoma among Japanese. *Cancer Sci.* 2008;99(1):93-97.

20. Zhu K, Moriarty C, Caplan LS, Levine RS. Cigarette smoking and primary liver cancer: a population-based case-control study in US men. *Cancer Causes Control.* 2007;18(3):315-321.

21. Michalek JE, Ketchum NS, Alchtar FZ. Postservice mortality of US Air Force veterans occupationally exposed to herbicides in Vietnam: 15-year follow-up. *Am J Epidemiol.* 1998;148(8):786-792.

22. Longnecker MP, Rogan WJ, Lucier G. The human health effect of DDT and PCBs and an overview of organochlorines in public health. *Annu Rev Public Health.* 1997;18:211-244.

23. Redlich CA, Beckett WS, Sparer J, et al. Liver disease associated with occupational exposure to the solvent dimethylformamide. *Ann Int Med.* 1988;108(5):680-686.

24. Pizzorno J, Murray M. *Encyclopedia of Natural Medicine.* Rocklin, California: Prima Communications; 1998.

25. Sanchez A, Reeser J, Lau HS, et al. Role of sugars in human neutrophilic phagocytosis. *Am J Clin Nutr.* 1973;26(11):1180-1184.

26. Ringsdorf W, Cheraskin E, et al. Sucrose, neutrophil phagocytosis and resistance to disease. *Dent Surv.* 1976;52(12):46-48.

27. Lirussi F, Sanchez B, et al. Natural killer cells in patients with chronic hepatitis C (CHC). *Gut.* 1998;42 (Supp 1):A32.

28. Corrao G, Ferrari PA, Galatola G. Exploring the role of diet in modifying the effect of known disease determinants: application to risk factors of liver cirrhosis. *Am J Epidemiol.* 1995;142(11):1136-1146.

29. Hu KQ, Kyulo NL, Esrailian E, et al. Overweight and obesity, hepatic steatosis, and progression of chronic hepatitis C: a retrospective study on a large cohort of patients in the United States. *J. Hepat.* 2004 Jan;40(1):147-54.

30. Niederau C, Strohmeyer G, Heintges T, et al. Polyunsaturated phosphatidylcholine and interferon alfa for treatment of chronic hepatitis B and C: a multi-center, randomized, double-blind, placebo-controlled trial. Leich Study Group. *Hepatogastroenterology.* 1998;45(21):797-804.

31. Lieber CS. Alcoholic liver disease: new insights in pathogenesis lead to new treatments. *J Heptatol.* 2000;32(1 Suppl):113-128.

32. Cadden IS, Partovi N, Yoshida EM. Review article: possible beneficial effects of coffee on liver disease and function. *Aliment Pharmacol Ther.* 2007;26(1):1-8.

33. Larsson SC, Wolk A. Coffee consumption and risk of liver cancer: a meta-analysis. *Gastroenterology.* 2007;132(5):1740-1745.

34. Bravi F, Bosetti C, Tavani A, et al. Coffee drinking and hepatocellular carcinoma risk: a meta-analysis. *Hepatology.* 2007;46(2):430-435.

35. Klatsky AL, Morton C, Udaltsova N, Friedman GD. Coffee, cirrhosis, and transaminase enzymes. *J Hepatol.* 2007;46(5):980-982.

36. Urgert R, Meyboom S, Kuilman M, et al. Comparison of the effect of cafetiere and flitered coffee on serum concentrations of liver aminotransferases and lipids: six-month randomized controlled trial. *BMJ.* 1996;313(7069):1362-1366.

37. Urgert R, Schultz AGM, Katan et al. Effects of cafestol and kahweol from coffee grounds on serum lipids and serum liver enzymes in humans. *Am J Clin Nutr.* 1995;61(1):149-154.

38. Huber WW, Teitel CH, Coles BF, et al. Potential chemoprotective effects of the coffee components kahweol and cafestol palmitates via modification of hepatic N-acetyltransferase and glutathione S-transferase activities. *Environ Mol Mutagen.* 2004;44(4):265-276.

39. Higgins LG, Cavin C, Itoh K, Yamamoto M, Hayes JD. Induction of cancer chemopreventive enzymes by coffee is mediated by transcription factor Nrf2. Evidence that the coffee-specific diterpenes cafestol and kahweol confer protection against acrolein. *Toxicol Appl Pharmacol.* 2008;226(3):328-337.

40. Etherton GM, Kochar MS. Coffee. Facts and Controversies. *Arch Fam Med.* 1993;2(3):317-322.

41. Flora K, Hahn M, Rosen H, et al. Milk thistle (Silybum marianum) for the therapy of liver disease. *Am J Gastroenter.* 1998;93(2):139-143.

42. Strader D, Bacon B, Hoofnagle J, et al. Use of CAM by patients in liver disease clinics. NIH Conference on Complementary and Alternative Medicine in Chronic Liver Disease. Bethesda, Maryland. 1999.

43. Bosisio E, Benelli C, Pirola O. Effect of the flavanolignans of Silybum marianum L. on lipid peroxidation in rat liver microsomes and freshly isolated hepatocytes. *Pharmacol Res.* 1992;25:147-154.

44. Boigk G, Stroeder L, Herbst H, et al. Silymarin retards collagen accumulation in early and advanced biliary fibrosis secondary to complete bile duct obliteration in rats. *Hepatology.* 1997;26:643-649.

45. Campos R, Garrido A, Guerra A, et al. Silybin dihemisuccinate protects against glutathione depletion and lipid peroxidation induced by acetaminophen on rat liver. *Planta Med.* 1989;55:417-419.

46. Bernhard MC, Junker E, Hettinger A, et al. Time course of total cysteine, glutathione, and homocysteine in plasma of patients with chronic hepatitis C treated with interferon-alfa with and without supplementation with N-acetylcysteine. *J Hepatol.* 1998;28(5):751-755.

47. Rambaldi A, Jacobs BP, Iaquinto G, Gluud C. Milk thistle for alcoholic and/or hepatitis B or C liver diseases--a systematic cochrane hepato-biliary group review with meta-analyses of randomized clinical trials. *Am J Gastroenterol.* 2005 Nov;100(11):2583-91.

48. Magliulo E, Gagliardi B, Fiori GP. Results of a double blind study on the effect of silymarin in the treatment of acute viral hepatitis, carried out at two medical centres. *Med Klin.* 1978;73(28-29):1060-1065.

49. Feher J, Deak G, Muzes G, et al. Hepatoprotective activity of silymarin (Legalon) therapy in patients with chronic liver disease. *Orv Hetil.* 1989;130(51):2723-2727.

50. Ferenci P, Dragosics B, Dittrich H, et al. Randomized controlled trial of silymarin treatment in patients with cirrhosis of the liver. *J Hepatol* (Netherlands). 1989;9(1):105-113.

51. Pares A, Planas R, Torres M, et al. Effects of silymarin in alcoholic patients with cirrhosis of the liver: results of a controlled, double-blinded, randomized and multi-center trial. *J Hepatol.* 1998;28:615-621.

52. Lieber CS, Leo MA, Qi C, et al. Silymarin retards the progression of alcohol-induced hepatic fibrosis in baboons. *J Clin Gastroenterol.* 2003;37:336-339.

53. Huber R, Futter I, Ludtke R. Oral silymarin for chronic hepatitis C- a retrospective analysis comparing three dose regimens. *Eur J Med Res.* 2005;10:68-70.

54. El-Zayadi AR, et al. Non-interferon-based therapy: am option for amelioration of necro-inflammation in hepatitis C patients who cannot afford interferon therapy. *Liver Int.* 2005;25:746-751.

55. Moscarella S, Giusti A, Marra F. Therapeutic and antilipoperoxidant effects of silybin-phosphatidylcholine complex in chronic liver disease: preliminary results. *Curr Ther Res*. 1993;53:98-102.

56. Alschuler L. Milk thistle: goals and objectives. *Int J Integrative Med*. 1999;1:29-34.

57. Arase Y, Ikeda K, Murashima N, et al. The long-term efficacy of glycyrrhizin in chronic hepatitis C patients. *Cancer*. 1997;79(8):1494-1500.

58. Wildhirt E. Experience in Germany with glycyrrhizinic acid for the treatment of chronic viral hepatitis. In: Nishioka K, Suzuki H, Mishiro S. (Eds.). *Viral Hepatitis and Liver Disease*. Springer-Verlag. Tokyo, Japan. 1994:658-661.

59. Xianshi S, Huiming C, et al. Clinical and laboratory observation on the effect of glycyrrhiza in acute and chronic viral hepatitis. *J Tradit Chin Med*. 1984;4:127-132.

60. Susuki H, Yamamato S, Hirayama C. Cianidanol therapy for HBe-antigen-positive chronic hepatitis :a multicentre, double-blind study. *Liver*. 1986(1);6:35-44.

61. Salama A, Mueller-Eckhardt C. Cianidanol and its metabolites bind tightly to red cells and are responsible for the production of auto- and / or drug-dependant antibodies against these cells. *Br J Haematol*. 1987;66(2):263-266.

62. Iwu M. Dietary botanical supplements with antiviral and anti-inflammatory properties used in the treatment of liver disorders in traditional African medicine. Complementary and Alternative Medicine in Chronic Liver Disease Conference. National Institutes of Health. Bethesda, Maryland. 1999.

63. Ferrea G. In vitro activity of a combretum micranthim extract against herpes simplex virus types 1 and 2. *Antiviral Res*. 1993;21:317-25.

64. Ott M, Thygarajan SP, Gupta S. Phyllanthus amarus suppresses hepatitis B virus by interrupting interactions between HBV enhancer I and cellular transcription factors. *Eur J Clin Invest*. 1997;27(11):908-915.

65. Mehrotra R, Rawat S, Kulshreshta DK, et al. In vitro studies on the effect of certain natural products against heptitis B virus. *Indian J Med Res*. 1990;92:133-138.

66. Forton, DM, Thomas HC, Murphy CA, Allsop, et al. Hepatitis C and cognitive impairment in a cohort of patients with mild liver disease. *Hepatology*. 2002;35:433-439.

67. [Neuropsychological function in Greek patients with chronic hepatitis C. Karaivazoglou K, Assimakopoulos K, Thomopoulos K, Theocharis G, et al. *Liver Int*. 2007 Aug;27(6):798-805.]

68. Viviani B, Corsini E, Binaglia M, et al. Reactive oxygen species generated by glia are responsible for neuron death induced by human immunodeficiency virus-glycoprotein 120 in vitro. *Neuroscience*. 2001;107(1):51-58.

69. Fahn S. The endogenous toxin theory of the etiology of Parkinson's disease and a pilot trial of high-dose antioxidants in an attempt to slow the progression of illness. *Ann NY Acad Sci*. 1989;570:186-196.

70. Floyd RA, et al. Neuroinflammatory diseases: an hypothesis to explain the increased formation of reactive oxygen and nitrogen species as major factors involved in neurodegenrative disease development. *Free Rad Biol Med*. 1999;26(9/10):1346-1355.

71. Curtis-Prior P, Vere D, Fray P. Therapeutic value of *Ginkgo biloba* in reducing symptoms of decline in mental function. *J Pharm Pharmacol*. 1999; 51(5):535-41.

72. Ramassamy C, Clostre F, Christen Y, Costentin J. In vivo Gingko biloba extract (EGb 761) protects against neurotoxic effects induced by MPTP: investigations into its mechanisms of action. In: Christen Y, Costentin J, Lacour M (Eds.). Effects of Gingko biloba extract (EGb 761) on the central nervous system. *Elsevier*. Paris, France. 1992:27-36.

73. Wettstein A. Cholinesterase inhibitors and gingko extracts: are they comparable in the treatment of dementia? Comparison of published placebo-controlled efficacy studies of at least six months duration. *Phytomedicine*. 2000;6(6):393-401.

74. Dwight MM, Kowdley KV, Russo JE, et al. Depression, fatigue, and functional disability in patients with chronic hepatitis C. *J Psychosom Res*. 2000;49(5):311-317.

75. Schubert H, Halama P. Depressive episode primarily unresponsive to therapy in elderly patients: efficacy of Gingko biliba extract (EGB 761) in combination with antidepressants. *Geriatr Forsch*. 1993;3:45-53.

76. Gaby A. Gingko biloba extract: a review. *Altern Med Rev*. 1996;1(4):236-242.

77. Linde K, Ramirez G, Mulrow C, et al. St. John's wort for depression. An overview and meta-analysis of randomized clinical trials. *BMJ*. 1996; 313(7052):253-258.

78. Sarris J. Herbal medicines in the treatment of psychiatric disorders: a systematic review. *Phytother Res*. 2007 Aug;21(8):703-16.

79. Schulz V, Hansel R, Tyler VE. *Rational Phytotherapy: A Physician's Guide to Herbal Medicine*. 4th Ed. New York, NY: Springer; 2000.

Nutrition and Hepatitis C

Lark Lands, PhD

Introduction

Good nutrition is very important for anyone living with *hepatitis C*. Nutrients provide the building blocks for the body's physical structure—its cells, tissues, and organs. This includes that all-important organ, the liver. Wide varieties of nutrients are also needed to support the body's immune response to infection. While both of these roles are important for anyone, they are particularly crucial for someone living with hepatitis C.

The ongoing presence of the hepatitis C virus (*HCV*) means the *immune system* is always responding to it. Since an active immune system requires energy, there must be a steady intake of nutrients to provide that energy. In addition, the immune system must be able to create a constant flow of immune cells and chemicals to fight the virus. Those cells and chemicals, fundamental components of the body's immune response to HCV, are created from nutrients. This means that a steady supply of nutrients is absolutely necessary for viral control.Any damage done to the body by HCV must be repaired. This also requires a constant intake of the nutrient building blocks needed to make new cells. Finally, having proper amounts of nutrients may actually help prevent liver damage. There is also evidence that certain nutrients may help prevent *liver cancer*, a major risk for those living with *chronic hepatitis C*.[1]

There are two sources for the nutrients that meet all these needs: the foods we eat and drink, and micronutrient supplements including *vitamins,* minerals, amino acids, and fatty acids. It is important to know that supplements cannot substitute for a healthy diet. Gulping down handfuls of pills will not make up for eating a bad diet. On the other hand, even the best diet may not provide the amount of certain nutrients needed to protect and repair the liver in someone living with hepatitis C.

Only a steady intake of nutritious foods can provide the body with the nutrients it needs. Research continues to show us that newly discovered nutrients play critical roles in the body's immune function and in maintaining overall health. It is safe to say there are probably many nutrients yet to be discovered. You cannot depend on supplements to provide your basic nutrition needs because manufacturers cannot put into a tablet or capsule ingredients that have not yet been discovered. To ensure good health, it is critical to take in all the nutrients Mother Nature designed, not just the ones we have studied. In addition, whole foods contain countless components that help nutrients work better in the body.

Many studies have shown that certain vitamins, minerals, amino acids, and fatty acids may help improve the health of people living with hepatitis C. Although supplements can help provide higher than normal levels of certain nutrients that may be needed for liver protection and repair, only a healthy diet can provide the nutrient base that is absolutely necessary for good health. See *Chapter 14, Naturopathic Medicine* and *Chapter 16, Nutritional Supplementation* for more information on supplements.

Healthy Food for a Healthy Body

The first step toward ensuring you are getting all the nutrients you need is to make the most of what you eat. This means eating a wide variety of whole foods every day, along with plenty of the water and other healthy liquids your body needs to function at its best. The most nutritious food is usually that which is closest to its natural state. Too much processing, refining, and overcooking can chip away at any food's nutrients. Eating the following types of nutritious food every day will help build good health into every cell of your body.

Table 1. Nutritious foods for good healh

fresh or lightly cooked vegetables and fruits
raw or lightly toasted nuts and seeds
whole grains such as brown rice and barley
whole wheat breads, pastas, cereals, and crackers
mixed grain/nut/seed/bean combinations, eggs, poultry, fish, lean meat, and dairy products for good quality protein

Instead of struggling to follow complex dietary rules, it is easier for most people to just look at the overall picture and try to always choose healthy foods, while avoiding those that adversely affect health. Here are some simple guidelines to help you accomplish that.

Carbohydrates

When you're choosing foods that are high in carbohydrates for your meal—breads, cereals, rice, pastas, and so on—choose mostly complex carbohydrates that have been refined as little as possible. These are the good kinds of carbohydrates that, along with the carbohydrates you get from fruits and vegetables, can provide a substantial portion of the energy you need every day.

Fruits and Vegetables: Add a wide variety of the vegetables and fruits to your meals that will help you get all the nutrients and fiber needed for healthy body function—including immune function. Try to eat at least 3 to 5 servings of vegetables and 2 to 4 servings of fruit each day.

- One serving of vegetables is approximately one cup of raw vegetables or one-half cup of cooked vegetables.

- One serving of fruit is approximately one-half cup of fresh, chopped, or canned fruit.

Protein

Make sure you get plenty of the *protein* you need for a healthy body and a competent immune response. You can choose from a wide variety of foods that will contribute to your *total protein* intake, including lean meat, poultry, fish, beans, eggs, nuts, seeds, milk, yogurt, and cheese.

Good Fats

Try to make sure that you get a moderate amount of only good fats every day, but keep the overall fat content of the diet relatively low. Researchers have shown that high fat intake is tied to an increased risk of progression to *cirrhosis* in those with chronic hepatitis C.[2]

Sweets and Snacks

Last but not least, although an occasional sweet treat or snack food can be fun, most sweets and other "junk" foods contain few nutrients and often substitute for more healthy foods you might otherwise be eating. Limiting your intake of sweets and white-flour snack foods is a good way to improve your chances for a total daily intake of nutrients that is supportive of your good health.

An important and easy way to increase your daily nutrient intake is to go for variety and color. Each food is rich in certain nutrients, but not in others. Choosing a wide variety of foods will help ensure intake of all the nutrients nature can provide. You run the risk of limiting your nutrient intake if you tend to eat the same foods over and over.

Emphasizing color when you select a wide variety of foods is additional nutritional insurance. Think of it as "the rainbow theory of shopping." When you are in the bread, pasta, cereals, and cracker aisles, choose brown, whole grain varieties instead of white. White varieties contain processed grains, and processing removes most of the important nutrients found in the whole grain. When you are in the produce section, pick up a variety of colors: red, purple, green, orange, yellow, blue, etc. Any time you see natural color, you are seeing nutrients. The more your shopping basket looks like a rainbow of color, the better your diet will be.

Adjusting Your Diet to Meet Individual Needs

Any dietary recommendations may need to be modified based on your individual needs and your current physical condition.

Total Calorie Needs

Both your *metabolism* (the rate at which your body uses energy) and your lifestyle can significantly affect your calorie requirements. These individual characteristics make it difficult to come up with generic recommendations on how many calories someone needs each day. You may have a high rate of metabolism and an energy-demanding job such as construction work or an intensive daily exercise schedule, all of which increase your calorie needs. On the other hand, you may have been born with a very low rate of metabolism and have a sedentary desk job or a lifestyle that does not include much exercise, all of which lessen your calorie needs. Regardless of these individual variables, the total intake of food that you need daily is somewhat increased by chronic hepatitis C. Your immune system has an ongoing response to the virus and this response is constantly burning up calories.

Protein Intake Adjustment

Since adequate protein is generally so important, it is easy to jump to the conclusion that more is better. However, in the presence of serious liver disease, too much protein can actually be dangerous. A damaged liver cannot process protein as well as a healthy liver. Too much protein can result in protein overload that may lead to *encephalopathy*, a brain condition that causes mental confusion and, in advanced *stages*, coma. If you have significant liver damage, it is very important for you to discuss your dietary needs with your healthcare provider to ensure that your nutritional needs are met without placing undue stress on your liver.

Salt Intake Reduction

Another dietary change that may be very important for some people is salt reduction. *Ascites* is a complication of cirrhosis in which fluid accumulates in the abdomen. Too much salt in the diet can significantly worsen ascites.

Adjustments for Those with HCV/HIV Coinfection

People coinfected with HCV and *human immunodeficiency virus* (*HIV*), may require additional dietary adjustments. For example, many people living with HIV have lactose intolerance, an inability to properly digest the milk sugar lactose. This results in gas and/or diarrhea when dairy products are eaten. People with lactose intolerance often need to reduce or eliminate milk and milk products (cheese, yogurt, ice cream, etc.) from their diet.

A reduced ability to digest and absorb fats is also common in HIV disease. This can be another cause of gas and/or diarrhea. Therefore, people living with both viruses may need to keep the fat content of their diets even lower than those who have HCV alone.

Finally, some of the drug regimens taken by many coinfected people require additional dietary adjustments.

For all these reasons, it is very important to discuss the details of your personal situation with your healthcare provider, and ask for advice about dietary adjustments that may be needed. You and your healthcare provider will need to consider your health history, laboratory results, the state of your liver, and any other conditions such as diabetes or heart disease that may require dietary adjustments. For those who are coinfected, you will also want to discuss all aspects of your HIV disease. Your healthcare provider may want you to make an appointment with a nutritionist or dietitian who specializes in hepatitis C. A qualified nutrition counselor can help you create an individualized dietary program. Just make sure your counselor is truly knowledgeable about the nutritional needs of people living with HCV.

All that can be offered to you in this book is a generalized look at what we know about nutrition for those living with hepatitis C. Consider the information presented here to be a base of knowledge that must be modified by your healthcare provider based on all aspects of your current health status. A diet that has been adjusted to precisely meet your current health status and individual needs is ideal.

Making the Best Choices in Each Food Category

With this in mind, we will now provide some specific suggestions on healthy choices for each of the important food categories.

Carbohydrates

Carbohydrates are the main source of your body's energy so making good choices of *carbohydrate*-rich foods is very important. Carbohydrates are classified according to their structure as either simple or complex. Simple carbohydrates are found in sweet foods and sweeteners such as fruit, fruit juice, sugar, and honey. Complex carbohydrates are found in root vegetables such as carrots, beans, peas, winter squashes, and grains such as wheat, rice, corn, and oats. Most of the carbohydrates you eat should be the complex variety, along with a reasonable amount of simple carbohydrates, mostly from fiber-rich fruit.

Whole grains (those that are largely unrefined) provide vitamins, trace minerals, and fiber, all of which are important to the immune system and your overall health. One of the best ways to improve your nutrient intake is to substitute whole grains for the "white" foods that are common in our society. Although both are in the category of complex carbohydrates, the heavily refined white foods provide little nutrition.

Good complex carbohydrate choices are important to get the most from the foods you eat. For example, use brown rice instead of white. Eat whole grain bread instead of white bread. Be sure to read the label and make sure your bread is all or mostly whole grain, such as whole wheat or whole rye. If the label says, "enriched flour," "white flour," or "wheat flour," be aware that this really means nutrient-poor white flour. Use whole-grain pasta instead of spaghetti, macaroni, or noodles made from white flour. Eat whole grain rye, wheat, or rice crackers instead of white flour saltines. Again, do not be tricked by the name on the box; read the label carefully. Whole grain flaked cereals and whole grain hot cereals such as oatmeal have far more nutrients than the usual cold breakfast cereals.

Beans of all varieties are also excellent sources of complex carbohydrates and low-fat protein. Do not think of beans as a boring side dish. Make up a spicy bean dip, add them to a pasta dish, or sprinkle a tasty variety on your salad. And do not forget about corn and winter squashes. They are loaded with nutrients and can be a tasty source of complex carbohydrates from breakfast (whole corn grits) to dinner (baked spaghetti squash used in place of pasta in your favorite Italian dish).

Don't be confused by the recent controversy about carbohydrates created by the widespread promotion of high-protein, low-carbohydrate diets. Many people have been confused and developed the mistaken belief that carbohydrates, in general, are a problem. That is simply not true. Carbohydrates provide a large part of the fuel that powers your physical activity and keeps your organs functioning properly. Carbohydrates will always be an important part of the human diet. What is true is that all carbs are not created equal. The key for health is to choose carbohydrates wisely from the whole grains, fruits, and vegetables that truly support health rather than from the highly processed foods loaded with white flour and white sugar that provide little nutritional value.

By choosing the "good" carbohydratess, you will not only increase your intake of nutrients and fiber, but also generally be focused on foods with a moderate to low. The glycemic load is a measure that looks at the amount of carbohydrates in a particular food, combined with how rapidly those carbohydrates are broken down and, thus, the ultimate effect that they have on your *blood sugar*. When carbohydrates are broken down, they will all have some effect on your blood sugar. Foods that are broken down the most rapidly raise your blood sugar the highest and are the ones of most concern. Diets with large amounts of such "high glycemic" foods have been tied to an increased risk for diabetes and heart disease. The "*glycemic load*" classifies foods according to their effect on blood sugar, and there are online lists available that show the specific *glycemic index* for many foods (www.glycemicindex.com). However, the end effect on your blood sugar will be a result of not only a food's glycemic index but also the total amount of carbohydrate in an average serving, and this is reflected in the glycemic load.

By choosing foods with medium or low glycemic loads, you can improve your chances for keeping your blood sugar at healthy levels. The Harvard School of Public Health provides a list of foods and their glycemic load at www.hsph.harvard.edu/nutritionsource/carbohydrates.html#glycemicload. However, if you simply focus your food choices on whole foods while avoiding the highly processed foods made from mostly white flour and white sugar, you will end up with a diet where most of the foods have moderate effects on blood sugar.

Other than potatoes (which have a high glycemic load), most fruits and vegetables are low glycemic load foods. Most whole grains (including whole-grain breads and pastas, oatmeal, and brown rice) are medium glycemic load foods. And unsurprisingly, most highly processed foods (candy, sugar-loaded drinks, and white-flour breads, cereals, and pastas) are high glycemic load foods. By avoiding the high-glycemic, nutrient-poor foods, those who are already living with chronic liver disease can significantly reduce the risk that they might also have to deal with other serious diseases such as heart disease and diabetes.

Fruits and Vegetables

Fruits and vegetables are nature's most abundant source of most vitamins and minerals, including the *antioxidant* nutrients that are particularly important for protecting the liver. In addition, they provide a great deal of the fiber that is important for your health. Including a variety of vegetables and fruits in your diet every day is one of the most important things you can do for good health.

Most experts recommend eating 5 to 9 servings of fruits and vegetables every day, with the high end of that considered optimal. Many people do not even come close to that amount. That makes fruits and vegetables an important area to emphasize for improving nutrient intake.

Fresh fruits and vegetables, lightly steamed or sautéed vegetables, and fresh-squeezed fruit and vegetable juices (preferably made with a juicer that retains the nutrient-loaded pulp) are the most nutrient-rich choices in this group because there has been little or no processing to degrade the nutrients. These fruit and vegetable options contain all of the vitamins and minerals nature intended. Cooking at high temperatures destroys *enzymes* and some nutrients. Therefore, including fresh or lightly cooked fruits and vegetables in your daily diet can be a particularly potent source of nutrients.

Whether raw, steamed, sautéed, or cooked into soups or sauces, the greater the variety of vegetables you eat, the better your chances of getting all the important nutrients you need. Avoid eating the same vegetables day after day. Choose from the entire produce section and include several helpings each day. Your choices are many! If you cook vegetables with onions, garlic, ginger, peppers, and/or tomatoes, you will add the healing nutrients of these ingredients to your body's health store, too.

Several helpings of fruit each day are also important for your diet. Take advantage of the wide variety of fruits available in modern supermarkets. It is important to eat fresh fruit rather than just drinking fruit juice since juice often does not contain the fiber and pulp that provide many of the fruit's most important nutrients. Do not forget that fruit is the best and most healthy dessert you can eat. Fruit is also a far healthier snack food than the common sugar and salt-loaded varieties.

> **Increasing your fruit and vegetable intake to optimal levels can seem impossible to some people, but it may not be as difficult as you think.**
>> **One serving of fruit equals ½ cup of fresh chopped fruit.**
>>> To reach the recommended 2 to 4 servings of fruit, just think in terms of trying to eat 1 to 2 cups of fruit each day.
>> **One serving of vegetables equals 1 cup of raw vegetables or ½ cup of cooked vegetables.**
>>> To get your 3 to 5 servings of vegetables, think in terms of a mixture of raw and cooked vegetables that equals about 1 quart per day.

Eating the recommended amount of fruits and vegetables is not very difficult if you concentrate your food choices appropriately. Have a piece of fresh or stewed fruit as a dessert and for some of your between-meal snacks. Eat a couple of servings of vegetables with your main meal of the day, and include at least one or two other vegetable servings at another meal or as a snack. In the morning, sauté a mixture of vegetables such as onions, spinach, mushrooms, tomatoes, and potatoes and stir them into an omelet for a nutrient-loaded breakfast. Add a variety of vegetables to rice, barley, couscous or any other grains you are cooking. Bake some carrots or winter squash along with the chicken you're cooking for dinner.

Vegetables cooked into soup count as a serving or two, depending on how many vegetables you put into the soup and how much of it you eat. Making up a big pot of hearty vegetable soup can help provide vegetables for a number of meals. You can eat the soup over several days or freeze individual portions to use when other vegetable preparation feels too difficult. If you add beans, chicken, or fish to your soup, you will also be getting lots of protein. For days when eating seems like a difficult chore, getting good nutrition can be made easier by pureeing or blending soup in a blender or food processor so that it becomes an easily drinkable, liquid meal.

Protein
Your body cannot survive without adequate protein. You need protein to:

- build and maintain cells
- keep muscles and organs healthy
- produce enzymes and *hormones*
- make the *hemoglobin* that carries oxygen to your cells
- maintain your immune system

When your protein intake is too low to maintain your protein stores, the immune system cannot function normally. A loss of immune function created by protein deficiency can cause a lowered resistance to infections, improper wound healing, and a lessened ability to control viruses including HCV. Too little protein can also result in weight loss, *fatigue*, and a decreased ability to respond to drug therapy.

The risk of getting too little protein in North America is quite low. Researchers from the Harvard School of Public Health note that almost any reasonable diet will provide the daily protein requirement. If you want to get technical, the average adult needs about nine grams of protein for every twenty pounds of body weight. For the average adult, that's about 70 grams of protein daily. You can look up the protein content of various foods. Many lists are available online including a very extensive list available for browsing or download from the USDA at www.nal.usda.gov/fnic/foodcomp/Data/SR20/ nutrlist/sr20a203.pdf. But again, it's highly likely that with adequate intake of food, you will get the level of protein you need for health.

In fact, in an era where high-protein diets have been heavily promoted, the greater risk may be getting too much protein. As already discussed, this is a case where more is not necessarily better, especially for those with advanced liver disease for whom processing too much protein may be harmful. The same is true for those with impaired kidney function. If you have any of these concerns, it is best for a healthcare provider who knows the details of your health status to prescribe the exact amount of protein you need each day.

In general, the best recommendation is to eat moderate amounts of protein from a wide variety of foods each day. Proteins are made of building blocks called amino acids. When making protein choices, it is important to remember that we require all of the amino acids necessary for the body to build the proteins it needs. The eight so-called essential amino acids are those the body cannot make on its own. They must be obtained from your diet. The so-called non-essential amino acids are those your body can manufacture for itself, provided it has the necessary materials. To manufacture non-essential amino acids, the body uses other amino acids, vitamins, minerals, and enzymes. If any of these are in short supply, even the non-essential amino acids may become deficient.

Complete proteins contain all of the essential amino acids. Complete proteins are found in animal foods such as eggs, dairy products, meats, fish, and poultry. Essential amino acids can also be obtained through complementary proteins created by combining grains, nuts, seeds, and legumes such as beans, peas, and nuts. However, building tissue from complementary proteins requires more energy than building it from complete proteins. Therefore, if you have already experienced muscle loss and/or your appetite is low, it may be better for you to concentrate on eating animal foods that contain complete proteins.

On the other hand, plant foods are generally less expensive than animal foods. If cost is a concern, remember that including some combination of beans, peanut butter, peas, rice, corn, nuts, seeds, and other grains in your daily diet will give your body the protein it needs. Small amounts of animal proteins added to a mostly plant-based diet can ensure that such combinations work without increasing the cost too much. Always remember that eggs top the list for high quality, inexpensive protein.

Some good, concentrated sources of protein are:

- eggs
- poultry - skinless to lower the fat content
- fish - preferably deep-water, cold-ocean varieties since these are less likely to contain the liver-stressing toxins that fish from polluted waters may have
- complementary proteins found in mixed grain/nut/seed/bean combinations
- lean meat

Unless lactose intolerance is a problem, cheese and other dairy products can add to your protein intake. But remember that many such foods are high in fat. Adding things such as alfalfa sprouts, chickpeas or other beans, or sesame seeds to your salad or having beans as part of your meal can increase your protein intake substantially. Snacking on sunflower seeds will do the same. Just be careful not to overdo on seeds or nuts since they also contain substantial amounts of fat. With a reasonable combination of such protein foods in your three daily meals and occasional snacks, you should easily be able to eat the amount of protein you need.

Fat

A moderate intake of good fats is necessary for your health. But fat intake should be limited in people living with hepatitis C. Fats should come from healthy sources, which means focusing on natural fats. The best fat choice is monounsaturated fat such as that found in extra-virgin, cold-processed olive oil (which is probably the best overall choice), as well as in canola oil, avocadoes, peanuts, cashews, almonds, and most other nuts;. Cold water fish (such as wild salmon and sardines) contain the heart-healthy omega-3 fatty acids that are another good kind of fat. Eating modest amounts of fish can provide the natural anti-inflammatory effects of fish oil, although it's important to avoid fish that may be high in mercury (swordfish, tilefish, shark, and king mackerel). It's best to limit saturated fats by choosing lean cuts of meat or low-fat dairy products.

Perhaps most important of all is to avoid the bad fats that are common in the North American diet. In particular, it is very important to eliminate partially hydrogenated fats from your diet. Hydrogenation is a process that uses heat and chemicals to change the structure of fatty acids in vegetable oils so that the oils are solid at room temperature. For example, hydrogenation is how liquid corn oil is converted into solid margarine. You will see partially hydrogenated fats referred to as trans fats. Trans fatty acids may contribute to blocking some of the body's normal chemical processes, including those related to fat metabolism. Trans fats have many negative health effects. In 1994, a group of Harvard researchers stated, "Federal regulations should require manufacturers to include trans fatty acid content in food labels and should aim to greatly reduce or eliminate the use of partially hydrogenated vegetable fats."[3] The U.S Food and Drug Administration recently acknowledged the importance of this issue. All foods are now required to have the trans fat content listed on the nutrition label.

Partially hydrogenated fats are found in countless foods. These include margarine, shortening, most standard breads, crackers, cookies and other baked goods, many condiments such as mayonnaise, most commercial salad dressings, and some processed meats and snack foods such as potato chips, corn chips, ice cream, and French fries. It is crucial to read labels carefully in order to eliminate these unhealthy fats from your diet. If the words "partially hydrogenated" appear anywhere on the label, do not eat that food. Seek out brands of foods that have eliminated these bad fats in favor of healthy, natural ones. When eating out, be aware that many fast-food establishments use partially hydrogenated oils in their cooking processes. If you just have to have a burger and fries, you are better off making them at home from healthy ingredients. Even in better restaurants, it is a good idea to ask what kinds of fats they use in cooking and what is in the bread they put in front of you.

In general, try to make sure that you are consuming fats that nature made. Green, cold-processed olive oil not only makes great salad dressing, it is also a wonderful spread on bread. You can even use it for sautéing garlic, onions, or vegetables, as long as you keep the temperature fairly low since it has a low smoke point. Nut and seed butters are another source of healthy and tasty fat, whether they are spread on bread or used in salad dressing. If you want a more traditional fat for cooking or spreading on your toast, plain old-fashioned sweet cream butter is definitely preferable to a partially hydrogenated margarine. Just be careful not to eat too much of any of these foods since your overall fat level needs to be moderately low to help reduce your chance of disease progression to cirrhosis.

When looking at possible ways to reduce fat, remember that much of it is hidden. Most meats (other than very lean varieties) and dairy products (other than those made from skim milk) are loaded with fat. Bacon, sausage, hot dogs, luncheon meats, and other similar products are very high in fat content. Almost all snack foods are also loaded with fat. This includes most chips, peanuts, nuts, many types of crackers, cookies, granola bars, candy bars, and many others. The fats found in salad dressings, peanut butter or other nut butters, and many sauces can add huge amounts of fat calories to your diet. Fried foods of all kinds (such as hamburgers, French fries, fried chicken, fried fish, fried or deep-fried vegetables) are often incredibly high in fat. Finally, the addition of fatty products such as butter, vegetable oils, mayonnaise, whipping cream, and sour cream can dramatically increase the fat content of any dish.

Relatively simple dietary and food preparation changes can significantly reduce the fat content of your diet. Some useful tips are noted in the following list. Any one of these can go a long way in increasing both the appetite-stimulating smell and flavor of foods while at the same time reducing the fat in your diet.

- Bake, broil, or grill your meats, poultry, and fish instead of frying.

- Use skim milk and skim milk cheeses and yogurt instead of whole milk and whole milk products.

- Avoid high-fat bread products such as croissants, doughnuts, muffins, and most cornbread. Use whole-wheat pita bread or low-fat whole grain breads instead. If you are making your own baked goods or sauces, use unsweetened condensed skim milk in place of cream.

- Avoid high fat sauces, gravies, and butter. Substitute herbs and other seasonings to improve the flavor of foods.

- Unfortunately, removing the fat from dishes often seems to remove a lot of the flavor to which we are accustomed. Try using salsas, roasted garlic or shallots, flavored vinegars, chicken broth, and various hot sauces to spice up low fat dishes.

- Thicken sauces or soups with pureed white beans, instant mashed potatoes, or cornstarch and skim milk instead of heavy cream.

- Make mashed potatoes using fat-free chicken broth instead of butter and milk.

- Avoid fried potatoes or other vegetables, substituting steamed or baked versions.

- Sauté foods like onions, garlic, mushrooms and so on using water or poultry broth instead of butter or oil. Alternatively, just "sweat" such foods by placing the chopped onions or garlic in a frying pan. Use moderate heat just until they begin to brown around the edges, and then pour in stock or vinegar to deglaze the pan.

- Prepare your own popcorn using grated skim-milk cheese and various seasonings instead of butter as the topping.

- Use toasted sesame oil or other strongly flavored oils when you want a little fat for flavor.

One caution in this discussion of fat is that you should not carry fat avoidance to an extreme. You want a whole foods diet that includes moderate amounts of good fats. You do not want a diet with no fat at all. In our concern to educate people about the need to lower dietary fat content, it is sometimes forgotten that fat is necessary at appropriate levels and in appropriate forms. Essential fatty acids are just that, essential. Both the omega-3 and omega-6 fatty acids are very important for human health.

When fat intake drops so low that the levels of essential fatty acids in the body are compromised, many negative health consequences can result. These consequences include skin problems, *neurological* problems, energy problems, and suppressed *immunity*. Fat provides the body's storehouse of energy. Fat in the diet is required for the absorption of the fat-soluble *vitamins A, D, E,* and *K*. In your attempt to decrease your intake of unhealthy fats, be sure you do not eliminate the good ones in the process. Moderate amounts of healthy fats are essential for a nutritious diet. Both too much and too little fat are unhealthy.

Sweets and Treats

A healthy diet involves limiting the amount of concentrated sweets, white-flour products, and high-fat nutrient-poor fast foods and snack foods in your diet. Many people consume too many junk foods and desserts that are often loaded with excessive sugar and fat. Then they are not hungry for all the nutrient-rich foods that they really need for health. The end result is a diet loaded with empty calories that does not promote good health. Try to make both sweets and fatty junk foods occasional treats instead of a major part of your diet.

Healthy Liquids

Drinking plenty of healthy liquids is just as important as eating nutritious foods. Water is a dietary essential. Your diet must include plenty of water. The old adage about drinking eight large glasses of water per day (approximately two quarts) is actually a good beginning. However, because your size affects how much water you need, a better and simpler rule is to divide your body weight in pounds in half, and then drink at least that number of ounces of water every day. For example, if you weigh 140 pounds, divide that in half and drink at least 70 ounces of water (almost nine cups) each day. Many people drink far too little water thinking that they can substitute other water-based beverages like soft drinks and coffee. However, these drinks are not a substitute for pure water.

You need to drink plenty of fresh, pure water every day because without sufficient water, the body simply cannot function properly. Anytime you are running a fever, have diarrhea, are suffering from nausea and vomiting, or have daytime or nighttime sweats, you run the risk of *dehydration*. Dehydration describes the state your body is in when it does not have enough water. Under these circumstances, you should put drinking plenty of fluids at the top of your list of priorities.

It is especially important for those who are coinfected with HIV to remember that the water you drink must be free of all disease-causing organisms. It is crucial for those with seriously compromised immunity (CD4 cells below 100) to ensure the safety of water by boiling it or using a water purifier that is designed to kill or filter out bacteria, protozoa, and other disease-causing organisms. The risk of water-borne infections is too high to ignore this.

Many people find herbal teas to be an enjoyable addition to their list of healthy liquids. Make sure you consult with your pharmacist or healthcare provider to make sure the herbs you are drinking have no potential for liver toxicity and will not interact with any of your medications. Fresh fruit and vegetable juices are also healthy liquids. However, remember that many of the nutrients in vegetables and fruits are in the pulp. If you are preparing fresh juice, it is best to use a juicer that retains the pulp so that you get the most nutrient value from your juice.

Bottled fruit juices are another source of good liquids and are widely available. Be sure to pick the varieties with no added sugar. There are also canned or bottled juice spritzers that are sweet, cold, and carbonated. They have no added sugar and none of the chemicals that most sodas contain, but taste great and are just as fizzy as carbonated soft drinks. These spritzers do contain simple fruit sugars so they shouldn't be consumed in excess, but they are definitely preferable to standard soft drinks or so-called sports drinks.

Soups can also contribute to your fluid intake. Warm liquids such as soups, herbal teas, and roasted-grain coffee substitutes are not only nutritious, but are also less demanding on the body than icy cold drinks. Anything that is drunk icy cold requires some of your body's energy to warm it up. Drinking large quantities of very cold beverages can actually drain away calories your body needs.

Diet Dangers

There can be hidden dangers lurking in certain foods and liquids. Both alcohol and salt (especially if ingested in excess) are bad for people with hepatitis C. The facts are simple.

Alcohol is highly *toxic* to the liver and can cause serious disease and/or death, even in those with no active viral infection. In people with HCV, alcohol intake has been linked to increased risk of cirrhosis, a more advanced degree of liver *fibrosis*, and a higher death rate. If you are considering *interferon-based therapy*, you should know that alcohol consumption has been associated with a decreased response to treatment.[4, 5]

Another hidden dietary danger is the large amount of salt (*sodium*) contained in the typical American diet. High salt intake is not healthy for anyone, but for those with cirrhosis, it can be particularly dangerous since it can lead to or worsen ascites. Anyone with ascites must be on a salt-restricted diet. It is estimated that every 1,000 mg of sodium consumed can result in the accumulation of approximately 1 cup (200 mL) of ascitic fluid. The more the salt content of the diet can be reduced, the better the chances of avoiding this excessive fluid accumulation. For people with advanced disease, liver experts recommend limiting sodium intake to no more than 500 mg to 1,000 mg daily.[6] This level of salt restriction requires careful shopping and scrupulous attention to food labels. Most fast foods and snack foods (especially chips, pretzels, and crackers) are dangerously loaded with sodium and must be avoided if you are on a salt-restricted diet. Even foods that might otherwise be considered healthy can be dangerously loaded with salt. For example, one cup of chicken noodle soup may contain an amazing 1,108 mg of sodium.

The only way to cut salt intake is to look at the sodium content of all the foods you are eating. Use food labels on prepared foods and a chart that shows sodium levels for other food ingredients to determine your total daily intake of sodium. One easy way to cut sodium intake is to avoid prepared foods. Since many people with high blood pressure are placed on low sodium diets, there are many cookbooks and dietary plans available to help you avoid salt. People with hepatitis C who have not developed ascites usually do not need severe sodium cutbacks, but moderating your salt intake is likely to be beneficial.

Another possible dietary danger is eating too many *iron*-containing foods. This is a particular concern for those who have had a *liver biopsy* showing an abnormal accumulation of iron. Iron is stored in the liver and is used by the body for many different processes such as producing *red blood cells*. Iron is also a very important component of the enzymes involved in energy production and the manufacture of *DNA*, the building block of life. Therefore, the human body requires some amount of iron. However, because of its ability to act as a source of substances called *free radicals*, iron can cause liver damage in people with hepatitis C. This damage can lead to *inflammation* and scarring. See *Chapter 14, Naturopathic Medicine* and *Chapter 16, Nutritional Supplementation* for discussions of free radical damage.

Studies have shown that excessive iron may contribute to liver damage in people who have hepatitis C. A study in India with *hepatitis B* and C patients showed that a low-iron diet significantly lowered blood iron and *ALT* (a *liver enzyme*), especially in those who started with high iron levels.[7] Many iron-rich foods are also high in protein. Although it is not a good idea to sacrifice protein for the sake of a low-iron diet, it is fairly simple to avoid foods that contain very high amounts of iron or are fortified with iron while still getting enough protein.

In general, dietary iron is poorly absorbed. The iron from meats is better absorbed (10% to 20%) than the iron from plants (2% to 5%). If you already have a high iron level in your liver, it may be advisable to decrease your animal protein intake as a way to lower your intake of iron. You can substitute plant proteins for the animal proteins. Be aware that many processed foods are fortified with iron and can significantly increase your iron intake. Unless your physician has recommended iron supplements, it is best to avoid iron supplements.

As a final cautionary note, people with hepatitis C should avoid raw fish and shellfish. These foods can be contaminated with the *hepatitis A* virus. The chance of contracting hepatitis A from raw fish or shellfish is not worth the risk for people already infected with HCV, as the complications can be severe.

Summary

A summary of dietary guidelines for people living with hepatitis C is rather simple. Try to avoid junk food and fast food. Avoid other nutrient-poor foods that are made with white flour or white sugar, deep-fried in chemically altered oils, overcooked, or loaded with chemicals.

Create your meals from whole foods using a wide variety of properly prepared fruits and vegetables, whole grains, and high quality protein. Include plenty of healthy liquids.

Put care and thought into what you put into your body so that every mouthful adds nutrients and increases your capacity to heal. If you have created each cell in your body from healthy foods and liquids, then there is no question that you will have dramatically increased your body's ability to resist the assault of any disease, including hepatitis C.

References

1. Yu MW, Horng IS, Hsu KH, et al. Plasma selenium levels and risk of hepatocellular carcinoma among men with chronic hepatitis virus infection. *Am J Epidemiol*. 1999;150(4):367-374.
2. Corraro G, Ferrari PA, Galatola G. Exploring the role of diet in modifying the effect of known disease determinants: application to risk factors of liver cirrhosis. *Am J Epidemiol*. 1995;142(11):1136-1146.
3. Willett WC, Ascherio A. Trans fatty acids: are the effects only marginal? *Am J Public Health*. 1994;84(5):722-724.
4. Alter H, Seef L. Recovery, persistence and sequelae in hepatitis C infection: a perspective on long-term outcome. *Sem Liver Disease*. 2000;20(1):17-35.
5. Pessione F, Degos F, Marcellin P. Effect of alcohol consumption and serum hepatitis C virus RNA and histological lesions in chronic hepatitis C. *Hepatology*. 1998;27(6):1717-1722.
6. Palmer BF. Pathogenesis of ascites and renal salt retention in cirrhosis. *J Investig Med*. 1999;47(5):183-202.
7. Tandon N, Thakur V, Guptan RK, Sarin SK. Beneficial influence of an indigenous low-iron diet on serum indicators of iron status in patients with chronic liver disease. *Br J Nutr*. 2000;83(3):235-239.

Nutritional Supplementation

Lark Lands, PhD and J. Lyn Patrick, ND

Introduction

There are two sources of liver damage with *chronic hepatitis* C. One is from the infection itself. The other is from the *immune system*'s attempt to fight the virus. Even if you eat a healthy, balanced diet that provides a broad spectrum of nutrients, there is may still be an important role for *nutritional supplements*. *Antioxidants*, *amino acids*, and fatty acids may help moderate liver damage in people living with *hepatitis C* .

A process called *oxidative stress* plays a role in the progression of chronic hepatitis C. Oxidative stress occurs when *free radicals* (unstable electrons and oxygen molecules) move through the liver causing *inflammation* and scarring. Free radicals form naturally in the body, especially when the immune system attacks an invader. The process is accelerated in chronic viral infections. The amount of damage caused by oxidative stress is linked to both the *grade* of liver *fibrosis* and the overall level of liver damage.[1, 2]

The level of *glutathione* (an antioxidant) can be significantly depressed in many people with hepatitis C.[1] Insufficient amounts of glutathione can reduce the liver's ability to break down drugs, chemicals, and other *toxins*. This can result in liver damage.

Antioxidant Supplements

A study of people chronically infected with the *hepatitis C virus* (*HCV*) found their blood levels of the antioxidants glutathione, *vitamin A*, *vitamin C*, *vitamin E*, and selenium were much lower than those of people the same age and sex who did not have HCV.[3] Low levels of antioxidants were accompanied by high levels of blood markers that indicate oxidative stress (damage from free radicals). The levels of these markers were closely correlated to the amount of liver fibrosis. The higher the level of oxidative stress, the more advanced the fibrosis. Fibrosis was also related to low blood levels of the same antioxidants.

These findings applied not only to people with significant fibrosis and *cirrhosis* on *liver biopsy*, but also to those with minimal fibrosis and no cirrhosis (Ishak scores of 0-2, please see *Chapter 4.1, Liver Disease Progression*). Higher levels of oxidative stress were associated with lower levels of antioxidants and more severe liver damage. The most important information this research reveals is that even in the beginning *stages* of hepatitis C, antioxidants are important. Although this information does not prove antioxidants prevent liver damage, the authors of this research suggested that antioxidants might play an important role in slowing the progression of HCV and delaying the onset of cirrhosis.

Nutritional antioxidants can counteract the damage caused by oxidative stress and low glutathione levels. Many different antioxidants work in many different ways in the body. These include vitamins A, E, and C, the family of carotenoids (including beta-carotene), the minerals zinc and selenium, alfa-lipoic acid, N-acetyl cysteine, and SAMe.

The antioxidants vitamin E, N-acetyl cysteine, SAMe, and selenium have been studied in people with hepatitis C to determine their effect on liver inflammation. The process of inflammation involves the accumulation of fat in the liver. Fatty cells are susceptible to damage, which can cause fibrosis and, ultimately, cirrhosis.[4, 5]

Vitamin E, selenium, zinc, and N-acetyl cysteine (NAC) have also been studied for their potential to inhibit fibrosis in chronic hepatitis. Of particular importance are the antioxidants and nutrients that work together to increase glutathione. The use of supplements to normalize glutathione levels may be very important for preventing liver damage. The nutrients that contribute to glutathione production are alfa-lipoic acid, vitamin C, vitamin E, NAC, and glutamine. The *B vitamins* and the mineral selenium also contribute to the antioxidant defense system.

Following are descriptions of several nutritional supplements, their effects in the body, and their roles in maintaining or improving liver health.

Alfa-Lipoic Acid

Alfa-lipoic acid (ALA) is a fatty acid and an antioxidant. It is very important in liver cell *metabolism*. ALA is rapidly depleted when the liver is under stress. ALA has a long history of use in Europe where it is used to treat liver disorders because of its apparent ability to help the liver repair itself.[6] ALA's effectiveness in raising cellular glutathione levels is thought to be very important for liver repair with diseases like hepatitis C and *HIV* since both can cause glutathione deficiency.

Unlike most other antioxidant nutrients that work in either the fatty parts of the body (including the outer layers of cells) or the watery parts (including the blood), ALA works in both. This allows ALA to provide protection to cells throughout the body. ALA also helps recycle and regenerate other antioxidants including vitamins E and C. This helps maintain optimal levels of these nutrients in the body. ALA has been given in doses up to 1,200 mg intravenously without *toxicity*. The only side effect reported was nausea and vomiting, and this was reported infrequently. No side effects have been reported with oral doses up to 1,000 mg daily.[7, 8] Oral ALA doses of 500 mg to 1,000 mg have been well tolerated in *placebo*-controlled studies.[9]

Glutamine

Glutamine is an amino acid normally found in greater abundance in the body than any other free amino acid. It is crucial to many body functions including maintenance of optimal antioxidant status, intestinal health, and immune function. Glutamine powers immune cells and is therefore in high demand in the bodies of people living with chronic viral infections.

Some researchers believe that among people with chronic hepatitis C, the body's demand for glutamine can exceed the amount that can be supplied in the diet.[10] Lack of glutamine can result in inadequate production of glutathione, which is needed to counteract the oxidative stress of chronic hepatitis C. The reason is somewhat complex, but simply stated, glutamine is the factor that determines how much glutathione the body can produce if a sufficient amount of cysteine is available (see the discussion of NAC and cysteine production for additional information). If glutamine stores are depleted by ongoing immune system demands, glutathione production will be inadequate. This situation is particularly important for people coinfected with HCV and HIV because their immune systems are fighting two chronic infections instead of one.

Glutamine is an important nutritional supplement. It is given to support the liver and its glutathione production. Research suggests doses of at least 10 grams of powdered glutamine daily for people coinfected with HCV and HIV (J. Shabert, personal communication).

N-Acetyl Cysteine

N-acetyl cysteine (NAC) is a form of the amino acid cysteine found in plants and animals. Like all amino acids, cysteine is a building block of proteins. NAC has been used to treat lung diseases and *acetaminophen* poisoning. It is used in acetaminophen poisoning to increase glutathione in the liver. NAC has been shown to increase blood glutathione in HIV-infected patients.[11] One study of 24 hepatitis C patients who had low glutathione showed that 600 mg of NAC taken three times daily along with *interferon* led to a normalization of *ALT* in 41% of patients.[12] The *viral loads* of patients who were on NAC were significantly lowered. NAC appeared to have the important effect of bringing glutathione levels back to normal inside *white blood cells* after six months of the combined therapy. NAC alone had no effect.

However, the results of studies using NAC in hepatitis C are conflicting. A study of NAC (1,200 mg daily) along with 600 IU per day of vitamin E and interferon found no effect on *liver enzymes*.[13] Similar studies using 1,800 mg daily doses of NAC and interferon also found no effect on liver enzymes. Researchers found no changes in glutathione levels in the blood or white blood cells.[14] A separate study that included NAC at 1,800 mg per day had no effect when it was given along with selenium and interferon.[15]

It is unclear whether NAC has no influence on the effectiveness of interferon or if larger doses are needed to have an effect. In one study, the doses necessary to raise glutathione levels in HIV-infected people appeared to be 3,200 mg to 8,000 mg daily.[11] Unfortunately, doses that high often cause nausea. The authors of this research have speculated that doses of approximately 2,000 mg may be capable of achieving the same effect. However, the dose of 1,800 mg used in some studies with hepatitis C patients was very close to that amount and still had no effect.

Studies of HIV-infected people who improved on a combined antioxidant *protocol* of NAC, glutamine, vitamin C, vitamin E, selenium, and beta-carotene indicate that antioxidants may need to be given together to have an effect.[10] Antioxidants work in different ways in different places in the body, and interact with each other in many positive ways. It is not surprising that better results are seen in people given a broad spectrum of antioxidant nutrients rather than one alone. In the case of NAC, people with hepatitis C may be deficient in glutamine. Those who are coinfected with HIV have an even higher risk of glutamine deficiency. Although the cysteine in NAC is initially the limiting factor in how much glutathione can be produced, when enough cysteine is present, glutamine becomes the limiting factor. Thus, if people are deficient in glutamine, all the NAC in the world will not raise glutathione levels and, therefore, will not provide liver protection.

Another important factor that can influence the results of NAC supplementation is its form. To maintain its antioxidant capacity, NAC must be manufactured with care and packaged in a way that prevents oxidation. Products that are not manufactured and packaged carefully can oxidize over time, losing their antioxidant capacity. It is best to choose products made from pharmaceutical grade NAC and packaged in vacuum-sealed containers known as blister packs, which protect against oxidation. NAC should always be taken with meals. It should be avoided if you have active stomach ulcers.

Selenium

Selenium is a mineral that has been investigated for its potential to improve immune function and decrease cancer risk. Selenium provides powerful antioxidant protection to the body via the selenium-containing *enzyme* glutathione peroxidase. This enzyme helps the body maintain sufficient levels of glutathione in the liver and all other glutathione-containing cells of the body. Selenium is one of the most crucial of all nutrients for maintaining effective immune responses. Many cancer researchers believe it is one of the most important nutrients in preventing cancer.[16]

Selenium is one of the antioxidant nutrients that can be significantly reduced among people with HCV.[3] One study found people with hepatitis C who did not have cirrhosis had selenium levels 20% below normal, and those with cirrhosis had levels 40% below normal.

Selenium is very important both as an antioxidant and as a cancer prevention agent. Therefore, low selenium levels in people with hepatitis C could contribute to progressive liver damage and the development of *liver cancer*. One study looked at selenium levels in 7,342 men with chronic *hepatitis B* and C and their risk of developing liver cancer (*hepatocellular carcinoma*).[17] For analysis, the participants were divided into four groups based on their selenium levels. The study found selenium levels were lowest in the men with chronic hepatitis C. Participants in the group with the highest selenium levels were 38% less likely to get liver cancer than those in the group with the lowest selenium levels. This decreased risk of liver cancer was greatest in the men with chronic hepatitis C who smoked and had low levels of vitamin A or carotenoids. Carotenoids are vitamin A-like compounds including beta-carotene. Although this study does not prove that selenium is the reason people developed less liver cancer, other studies have shown that selenium does play a protective role against liver cancer in people with chronic hepatitis.

Another selenium study conducted in China, an area with high rates of chronic hepatitis B and liver cancer, involved 130,471 people. Participants were given table salt that had been supplemented with selenium and were followed for eight years.[18] The rate of liver cancer in people taking supplemental selenium was found to be one third lower than the usual liver cancer rate observed in that area. The same study included 226 people with chronic hepatitis B. Participants were given either 200 mcg of selenium daily or a placebo (an inactive substance), and were followed for four years. No one in the group that took selenium (113 people) developed liver cancer. Of the 113 who took placebo, seven developed liver cancer. The selenium was then taken away, and both groups were followed for another four years. The incidence of liver cancer in people no longer taking selenium rose to a rate similar to those who never took selenium. This indicates the supplemental selenium may have had a preventive effect on the development of liver cancer in this group of chronic hepatitis B patients.

A study that examined selenium levels in HIV-positive people showed people coinfected with HCV and HIV had lower levels of selenium than those who had only HIV.[19] HIV infection is more likely to be fatal in a person who is selenium deficient.[20] Clearly, having HCV, HIV, and low selenium is not a good combination.

Studies on selenium supplementation have used 50 mcg to 400 mcg (micrograms) daily of different forms of selenium. Selenomethionine appears to be one of the safest and most absorbable forms of selenium. Other forms of selenium can be *toxic* at high doses.[1]

Selenium provides general antioxidant protection and immune defense. Selenium in doses of 200 mcg to 400 mcg daily may also provide protection against the development of potentially life-threatening liver cancer.

S-Adenosyl-L-Methionine

S-adenosyl-L-methionine (SAMe) is another compound that aids glutathione production in the liver. SAMe is an amino acid that can be made in the liver. It helps cell membranes (the outside layer of a cell) function normally. It also assists in detoxifying drugs and other compounds the liver processes.[21]

SAMe is used as a medication to treat liver disease in Europe. SAMe is usually called AdoMet in Europe. It has been shown to delay the need for liver transplantation in people with alcoholic cirrhosis.[22] Recent research revealed that SAMe has the ability to protect normal liver cells while causing liver cancer cells to die.[23] Although this research does not mean that SAMe alone can prevent or treat liver cancer, it does suggest that SAMe may provide some protection against developing liver cancer.

Other research involving liver disease and SAMe centers around its ability to normalize *bile* secretion by the liver, a process commonly affected by chronic liver diseases. SAMe has been used in multiple studies to treat the chronic skin irritation and resulting itching (*pruritus*) that is a common *symptom* of hepatitis C and many other chronic liver diseases. Studies in hepatitis B and C, and other chronic liver conditions found that SAMe helps reduce the symptoms of itching, *jaundice*, and *fatigue*, and lowers liver enzymes and *bilirubin* levels in as little as 16 days.[24, 25] Doses of SAMe in these studies were either 800 mg intravenously, or 800 mg to 1,600 mg by mouth. No side effects were reported in any of the studies with SAMe in chronic liver disease. More studies with SAMe are needed in the United States since all of the current studies were done in Europe or Russia.

SAMe is sold without a prescription. It is usually packaged in bottles or vacuum-sealed containers known as blister packs because it oxidizes (loses its potency) easily. SAMe is expensive, so some people take a combination of the amino acid methionine, tri-methyl glycine (betaine), vitamin B12, and folic acid to help the body make its own SAMe. The dosages for this combination are 500 mg methionine, 500 mg betaine, 800 mcg folic acid, and 500 mcg to 3,000 mcg of vitamin B_{12} daily. Whether this combination results in the same effect as taking supplemental SAMe is unknown. However, betaine, folic acid, and vitamin B_{12} are nontoxic and do not have any harmful side effects at these doses.

Vitamin C

Vitamin C (ascorbic acid) is a powerful antioxidant and natural anti-inflammatory agent. Both characteristics are crucial for people with hepatitis C since much of the damage caused by HCV comes from a combination of oxidative stress and inflammation in the liver. One recent study examined the relationship of blood levels of vitamin C to ALT levels in people living with hepatitis C . The researchers found that higher ALT levels were associated with lower levels of circulating vitamin C . They concluded this relationship may indicate greater consumption of vitamin C with increasingly severe oxidative stress in the liver.[26]

Vitamin C is also very important for immune function. The white blood cells that perform many of your immune functions are dependent on vitamin C. Therefore, vitamin C is a crucial nutrient for control of any viral infection. Individual needs for vitamin C vary. For this reason, recommended dosages can range from 1,000 mg to 6,000 mg or more per day. Amounts in excess of individual tolerance of vitamin C can result in gas and/or diarrhea.

Vitamin E

Vitamin E is an antioxidant that works in the fatty parts of the body, including the outer layers of cells called cell membranes. Vitamin E is important for the protection of liver cell membranes.

In one study, 24 people with hepatitis C undergoing *interferon-based therapy* were divided into three treatment groups. Group 1 took interferon alone. Group 2 took interferon plus 1,800 mg of NAC and 400 mcg of selenium per day. Group 3 took 544 IU of vitamin E per day in addition to interferon, NAC, and selenium.[15] Liver enzyme levels, HCV viral load, and response to interferon were similar in the first two groups. Those who received the complete combination that included vitamin E had a significantly greater response to treatment and achieved significantly greater drops in viral load. Although the study was small and the *relapse* rate was equal in all groups, the effect of the combination that included vitamin E was significant. It is unclear whether the vitamin E alone should be credited with the improved results or, perhaps more likely, the improvement was the result of using an effective combination of nutrients. It is always important to remember that nutrients interact in many ways and places in the body. Thus, combinations often work better than an individual nutrient.

Another study of 23 hepatitis C patients on 800 IU of vitamin E found almost half the participants experienced improvement of liver enzyme levels.[27] Liver enzymes went back up almost immediately after stopping the vitamin E. This suggests that vitamin E was neither combating the viral infection nor permanently stopping the process of inflammation in the liver, but was directly affecting inflammation in the liver while it was being taken. In other words, vitamin E only works while you take it. Other studies looking at the use of vitamin E and other antioxidants along with interferon have found similar results. It appears that vitamin E taken with interferon does not reduce viral levels long term and therefore does not make interferon more effective.[13] However, it may slow the process of fibrosis.[1]

Vitamin E appears to work by interrupting the biochemical pathway that leads to fibrosis in the liver. Fibrosis can lead to cirrhosis. A study of six patients on 1,200 IU of d-alfa tocopherol (a form of vitamin E) per day for eight weeks resulted in a complete interruption of this pathway, but had no effect on viral loads.[28] Animal studies have shown d-alfa tocopherol inhibits the genetic mechanisms that lead to cirrhosis.[29]

Vitamin E and vitamin C supplementation was recently examined in a study of people with *NASH* but without HCV. NASH stands for non-alcoholic *steatohepatitis*. NASH is a disease in which increased liver fat can lead to fibrosis and cirrhosis. It occurs in people with and without HCV who do not drink large amounts of alcohol. The study participants took 1,000 IU of vitamin E and 1,000 mg of vitamin C daily along with a low-fat diet and weight loss plan. After six months, participants' liver biopsy results improved significantly.[30] It is unclear whether the same results would occur in someone with NASH <u>and</u> chronic hepatitis C. But these vitamin dosages are safe, and we know vitamin E has a measurable effect in chronic hepatitis C. Therefore, it seems reasonable that this combination may be helpful in someone with both conditions. However, a larger *clinical trial* is needed to determine this with certainty.

A dose of 800 IU to 1,200 IU of vitamin E daily is safe, unless you are on a blood-thinning drug such as coumadin or suffer from a *vitamin K* deficiency.[31] Talk with your doctor to be sure the dose you are taking is safe in combination with your other medications.

Zinc

Patients with chronic liver disease can have low levels of several minerals including zinc.[32] Zinc deficiency is known to suppress the immune system. A small study of 40 people undergoing interferon plus *ribavirin* therapy for HCV found zinc levels among those with hepatitis C were significantly lower in those with HCV compared to healthy control subjects.[33] These levels were further depressed during interferon-based therapy, but were restored to normal by supplemental zinc. No difference in viral response to the interferon-based therapy was found between those receiving zinc supplementation and those who did not receive supplemental zinc.

Researchers have begun to examine whether supplemental zinc may enhance response to interferon-based therapy for HCV . One small study (34 patients) conducted in 2000 looked at the effect of zinc supplementation in people with HCV *genotype* 1b undergoing standard interferon *monotherapy*.[34] Participants were given interferon alone (10 patients), interferon plus daily doses of zinc sulfate (9 patients), or interferon plus a zinc-containing product called polaprezinc (15 patients) . Sustained viral response was significantly higher in those receiving interferon + polaprezinc compared to those receiving interferon + zinc sulfate or interferon alone. However, the implications of this study remain unclear. Another small study (75 patients) of polaprezinc added to standard interferon monotherapy among patients with genotype 1b found no advantage in viral response with polaprezinc supplementation among those with high pretreatment viral loads, but improved response rates in those with "moderate" pretreatment viral loads.[35]

Polaprezinc does not seem to have the same advantage when added to *combination therapy* (interferon plus ribavirin). A study published in 2006 also conducted among patients with HCV genotype 1b (102 participants) found no enhancement in viral response with the addition of polaprezinc to interferon plus ribavirin therapy.[36] In another small study (23 participants), the addition of zinc to *pegylated interferon* plus ribavirin treatment was found to provide no advantage in terms of viral response.[37]

Polaprezinc is an approved drug in Japan, but is not available in the United States. However, both zinc and carnosine are available as supplements. It is not known whether taking zinc and carnosine as separate supplements has the same effects as polaprezinc itself.

Nutritional Supplement Combinations

Antioxidants and other nutrients interact with each other in positive ways. Therefore, it comes as no surprise that positive results occur in trials in which people are given a combination of nutrients rather than any single nutrient.

A combined antioxidant approach has been used in research conducted at the Integrative Medical Center of New Mexico in Las Cruces, New Mexico.[38] Three patients with progressive hepatitis C and moderate to severe cirrhosis were treated with a combination of 600 mg of lipoic acid daily, 400 mcg of selenium daily, 900 mg of silymarin daily, 100 mg of vitamin B complex twice per day, 400-800 IU of vitamin E daily, 1,000-6,000 mg of vitamin C daily, 300 mg of coenzyme Q-10 daily, and one multiple vitamin and mineral supplement daily. In addition to the supplements, participants were advised to eliminate *alcohol*, sugar, and caffeine, to decrease their meat intake to a few times weekly, to increase intake of purified water to eight glasses daily, and to begin a modest exercise program. The nutrients in this protocol were chosen because of their ability to protect the liver from free radical damage, to increase the levels of other important antioxidants, and to interfere with the progress of HCV infection. There were reductions in ALT of at least 60% in all three patients, and reported improvements in overall health and well-being.

A *phase I clinical trial* of 47 patients with chronic hepatitis C looked at changes in liver enzymes, viral load, and liver biopsy results while on a protocol of antioxidants . Oral daily doses of glycyrrhizin, schisandra, silymarin, ascorbic acid, lipoic acid, L-glutathione, and alfa-tocopherol were given for 20 weeks along with intravenous preparations of glycyrrhizin, ascorbic acid, L-glutathione, and B-complex given twice weekly for the first 10 weeks.[39] The antioxidants used in the study included oral daily doses of glycyrrhizin, schisandra, silymarin, ascorbic acid, lipoic acid, L-glutathione, and alfa-tocopherol, and twice weekly intravenous preparations of glycyrrhizin, ascorbic acid, L-glutathione, and B-complex. At the end of 20 weeks, 44% of the patients (15 out of 34) who started the study with elevated ALT levels had reductions to normal levels. Thirty-six percent of those in the study had an overall improvement in their liver biopsy results. Interestingly, those patients in the study who had not responded to previous trials with interferon/ribavirin did not show any improvement in liver biopsy results. While there is some indication that antioxidants may slow the progression of liver disease in hepatitis C, this specific antioxidant therapy cannot replace standard treatment as a means of eliminating the hepatitis C virus. However, the researchers suggest that the combination of antioxidants with *antiviral* therapy might improve the overall response rate.

Nutritional Supplements for Patients With Cirrhosis

In chronic hepatitis C infection that has progressed to cirrhosis, one of the concerns is an increased risk for liver cancer. The chances of developing liver cancer are estimated to be about 2% to 7% over the first 20 years of infection.[40] There are no drugs that specifically prevent liver cancer . However, sustained *viral clearance* as a result of interferon-based therapy has been shown to reduce the risk of future development of liver cancer.[41-44] Nonetheless, there are still many people who remain chronically infected with HCV with long-term risks for cirrhosis and liver cancer .

Retinol (a form of vitamin A) and vitamin K2 may have a role in reducing the risk for development of liver cancer among those with cirrhosis. A small study of 40 women with viral hepatitis cirrhosis evaluated the long-term risk of developing liver cancer between those taking 45 mg of vitamin K2 daily compared to those not taking supplemental vitamin K. The researchers found those taking vitamin K2 were significantly less likely to develop liver cancer compared to those who did not take supplemental vitamin K2.[45] The authors concluded, "There is a possible role for vitamin K2 in the prevention of hepatocellular carcinoma in women with viral cirrhosis." NOTE: If you are taking coumadin or are on any kind of anticoagulant therapy, you should not take vitamin K in any form.

A large study of men (213 patients and 1,087 controls) examining the level of circulating retinol with the risk of developing liver cancer found that higher levels of retinol (a specific form of vitamin A) were associated with reduced risk for liver cancer. This effect was most pronounced in men who also had hepatitis B.[46] Although the men in this study were more likely to develop liver cancer as a result of their hepatitis B than are people with hepatitis C, the way that vitamin A prevents liver cancer is the same in both forms of viral hepatitis. Interestingly, serum levels of alfa-carotene, beta-carotene, beta-cryptoxanthin, lutein, lycopene, zeaxanthin, alfa-, gamma-, and delta-tocopherols, and selenium were not found to independently affect the risk of liver cancer in this study.

Hepatic *encephalopathy* (see *Chapter 5*) can occur along with liver failure. When the liver is no longer able to break down *ammonia* or efficiently filter toxins from the intestinal tract, toxins build up that affect brain function. Symptoms of hepatic encephalopathy include sleep problems, confusion, depression, and disorientation. A study of 100 patients with hepatic encephalopathy found that treatment with the amino acid L-carnitine (2 grams twice daily) resulted in decreased levels of circulating ammonia and improved brain function.[47]

Summary

There is strong evidence that nutritional supplements such as antioxidants can play an important role in limiting the chronic inflammatory effects of HCV in the liver. Antioxidant supplements may counteract the damage caused by increased free radical activity in the body.

Other nutrients such as glutamine are important in the production of glutathione, an antioxidant used by the liver to break down toxins, drugs, and chemicals.

Adding appropriate nutritional supplements may have a positive effect on the health of your liver and on slowing the progression of hepatitis C.

References

1. Badamaev V, Majeed M, Passwater R. Selenium: a quest for better understanding. *Altern Ther Health Med*. 1996;2(4):59-67.
2. Bernhard MC, Junker E, Hettinger A, et al. Time course of total cysteine, glutathione, and homocysteine in plasma of patients with chronic hepatitis C treated with interferon-alfa with and without supplementation with N-acetylcysteine. *J Hepatol*. 1998;28(5):751-755.
3. Jain SK, Pemberton PW, Smith A, et al. Oxidative stress in chronic hepatitis C: not just a feature of late stage disease. *J Hepatol*. 2002;36(6):805-811.
4. Reeves HL, Burt AD, Wood S, Day CP. Hepatic stellate cell activation occurs in the absence of hepatitis in alcoholic liver disease and correlates with the severity of steatosis. *J Hepatol*. 1996;25(5):677-683.
5. Day CP, James OF. Hepatic steatosis: innocent bystander or guilty party? *Hepatology*. 1998;27(6):1463-6.
6. Bustamante J, Lodge JK, Marcocci L, et al. Alfa-lipoic acid in liver metabolism and disease. *Free Rad Biol Med*. 1998;24(6):1023-1039.
7. Biewenga GP, Haenen GR, Bast A. The pharmacology of the antioxidant lipoic acid. *Gen Pharmacol*. 1997;29(3):315-331.
8. Zeigler D, Hanefeld M, Ruhnau KJ, et al. Treatment of symptomatic diabetic peripheral neuropathy with the anti-oxidant α-lipoic acid. A 3-week multicentre randomized controlled trial (ALADIN Study). *Diabetologia*. 1995;38(12):1425-1433.
9. Bustamante J, Lodge JK, Marcocci L, et al. Alfa-lipoic acid in liver metabolism and disease. *Free Rad Biol Med*. 1998;24(6):1023-1039.
10. Shabert J, Winslow C, Lacey JM, Wilmore DW. Glutamine-antioxidant supplementation increases body cell mass in AIDS patients with weight loss: a randomized, double-blind controlled trial. *Nutrition*. 1999;15(11-12):860-864.
11. Herzenberg L, DeRosa SC, Dubs JG, et al. Glutathione deficiency is associated with impaired survival in HIV disease. *Proc Nat Acad Sci USA*. 1997;94(5):1967-1972.
12. Beloqui O, Prieto J, Suarez M, et al. N-acetyl cysteine enhances the response to interferon-alfa in chronic hepatitis C: a pilot study. *J Interferon Res*. 1993;13(4):279-82.
13. Ideo G, Bellobuono A, Tempini S, et al. Antioxidant drugs combined with alfa-interferon in chronic hepatitis C not responsive to alfa-interferon alone: a randomized, multicentre study. *Eur J Gastroenterol Hepatol*. 1999;11(11);1203-1207.
14. Bernhard MC, Junker E, Hettinger A, et al. Time course of total cysteine, glutathione, and homocysteine in plasma of patients with chronic hepatitis C treated with interferon-alfa with and without supplementation with N-acetylcysteine. *J Hepatol*. 1998;28(5):751-755.
15. Look MP, Gerard A, Rao GS, et al. Interferon/antioxidant combination therapy for chronic hepatitis C-a controlled pilot trial. *Antiviral Res*. 1999;43(2):113-122.
16. Garland M, Stamper MJ, Willett WC, Hunter DJ. The epidemiology of selenium and human cancer. In: Balz Grei, Balz Frei (Eds.). Natural Antioxidants in Human Health and Disease. San Diego, California: Academic Press; 1994.
17. Yu MW, Horng IS, Hsu KH, et al. Plasma selenium levels and risk of hepatocellular carcinoma among men with chronic hepatitis virus infection. *Am J Epidemiol*. 1999;150(4):367-374.
18. Yu SY, Zhu YJ, Li WG. Protective role of selenium against hepatitis B virus and primary liver cancer in Qidong. *Biol Trace Elem Res*. 1997;56(1):117-124.
19. Look MP, Rockstroh JK, Rao GS, et al. Serum selenium, plasma glutathione (GSH), and erythrocyte glutathione peroxidase (GSH-Px) levels in asymptomatic versus symptomatic human immunodeficiency virus-1 (HIV-1) infection. *Eur J Clin Nutr*. 1997;51(4):266-272.
20. Baum MK, Shor-Posner G, Lai S, et al. High risk of HIV-related mortality is associated with selenium deficiency. *J Acquir Immune Defic Syndr Hum Retrovirol*. 1997;15(5):370-374.
21. Osman E, Owen JS, Burroughs AK. Review article: S-adenosyl-L-methionine- a new therapeutic agent in liver disease? *Aliment Pharmacol Ther*. 1993;7:21-28.
22. Mato JM, Camara J, Fernandez de Paz J, et al. S-adenosylmethionine in alcoholic liver cirrhosis: a randomized, placebo-controlled, double-blind, multi-center clinical trial. *J Hepatol*. 1999;30(6):1081-1089.
23. Ansorena E, Garcia-Trevijano E, Martinez-Chantar M, et al. S-adenosylmethionine and methylthioadenosine are antiapoptotic in cultured rat hepatocytes but proapoptotic in human hepatoma cells. *Hepatology*. 2002;35(2):274-280.
24. Podymova SD, Nadinskaia MI. Clinical trial of heptral in patients with chronic diffuse liver disease with intrahepatic cholestasis syndrome. *Klin Med* (Mosk). 1998;76(10):45-48.
25. Gorbakov VV, Galik VP, Kirillov SM. Experience in heptral treatment of diffuse liver diseases. *Ter Arkh*. 1998;70(10):82-86.
26. Souza dos Santos RM, de Bern AF, Colpo E, et al. Plasmatic vitamin C in nontreated hepatitis C patients is negatively associated with aspartate aminotransferase. *Liver Int*. 2008;28(1):54-60.
27. von Herbay A, Stahl W, Niederau C, Sies H. Vitamin E improves the aminotransferase status of patients suffering from viral hepatitis C: a randomized , double-blind, placebo-controlled study. *Free Radic Res*. 1997;27(6):599-605.
28. Houglum K Venkataramani A, Lyche K, Chojkier M. A pilot study of the effects of d-alfa-tocopherol on hepatic stellate cell activation in chronic hepatitis C. *Gastroenterology*. 1977;113(4):1069-1073.
29. Chojkier M, Houglum K, Lee KS, Buck M. Long- and short-term D-α-tocopherol supplementation inhibits liver collagen α1(I) gene expression. *Am J Physiol*. 1998;275(6 Pt 1):G1480-1485.
30. Harrison SA, Torgerson S, Hayashi P, et al. Vitamin E and vitamin C treatment improves fibrosis in patients with nonalcoholic steatohepatitis. *Am J Gastroenterol*. 2003;98:2485-2490.
31. Kappus H, Diplock AT. Tolerance and safety of vitamin E: a toxicological position report. *Free Rad Biol Med*. 1992;13(1):55-74.
32. Takagi H, Nagamine T, Abe H, et al. Zinc supplementation enhances the response to interferon therapy in patients with chronic hepatitis C. *J Viral Hepatitis*. 2001;8(5):367-371.
33. Ko WS, Guo CH, Hsu GS, Chiou YL, Yeh MS, Yaun SR. The effect of zinc supplementation on the treatment of chronic hepatitis C patients with interferon and ribavirin. *Clin Biochem*. 2005;38(7):614-620.
34. Nagamine T, Takagi H, Takayama H, et al. Preliminary study of combination therapy with IFNα and zinc in chronic hepatitis C patients with genotype 1b. *Biol Trace Element Res*. 2000;75(1-3):53-63.
35. Takagi H, Nagamine T, Abe T, et al. Zinc supplementation enhances the response to interferon therapy in patients with chronic hepatitis C . *J Viral Hepat*. 2001;8(5):367-371.

36. Suzuki H, Takagi H, Sohara N, et al. Triple therapy of interferon and ribavirin and zinc supplementation for patients with chronic hepatitis C: a randomized, controlled trial. *World J Gastroenterol*. 2006;12(8):1265-1269.

37. Murakami Y, Koyabu T, Kawashima A, et al . Zinc supplementation prevents the increase of transaminase in chronic hepatitis C patients during combination therapy with pegylated interferon alfa-2b and ribavirin. *J Nutr Sci Vitaminol* (Tokyo). 2007;53(3):213-218.

38. Berkson B. A triple antioxidant approach to the treatment of hepatitis C using alfa-lipoic acid (thioctic acid), silymarin, selenium and other fundamental nutraceuticals. *Clin Prac Alt Med*. 2000;1(1):27-33.

39. Melhem A, Stern M, Shibolet O, et al. Treatment of chronic hepatitis C virus infection via antioxidants: results of a phase I clinical trial. *J Clin Gastroenterol*. 2005;39(8):737-742.

40. Di Bisceglie AM . Hepatitis C and hepatocellular carcinoma. *Hepatology*. 1997;26(3 Suppl 1):34S-38S.

41. Shiratori Y, Ito Y, Yokosuka O, et al . Antiviral therapy for cirrhotic hepatitis C: association with reduced hepatocellular carcinoma development and improved survival. *Ann Intern Med*. 2005;142(2):105-114.

42. Yoshida H, Shiratori Y, Moriyama M, et al . Interferon therapy reduces the risk for hepatocellular carcinoma: national surveillance program of cirrhotic and noncirrhotic patients with chronic hepatitis C in Japan. *Ann Intern Med*. 1999;131(3):174-181.

43. Pradat P, Tillmann HL, Sauleda S, et al. Long-term follow-up of the hepatitis C HENCORE cohort: response to therapy and occurrence of liver-related complications. *J Viral Hepat*. 2007;14(8):556-563.

44. Yu ML, Lin SM, Chuang WL, et al . A sustained virological response to interferon or interferon/ribavirin reduces hepatocellular carcinoma and improves survival in chronic hepatitis C: a nationwide, multicentre study in Taiwan. *Antivir Ther*. 2006;11(8):985-994.

45. Habu D, Shiomi S, Tamori A, et al . Role of vitamin K2 in the development of hepatocellular carcinoma in women with viral cirrhosis of the liver. *JAMA*. 2004;292(3):358-361.

46. Yuan JM, Gao YT, Ong CN, Ross RK, Yu MC . Prediagnostic level of serum retinol in relation to reduced risk of hepatocellular carcinoma. *J Natl Cancer Inst*. 2006;98(7):482-490.

47. Malaguarnera M, Pistone G, Elvira R, Leotta C, Scarpello L, Liborio R . Effects of L-carnitine in patients with hepatic encephalopathy. *World J Gastroenterol*. 2005;11(45):7197-7202.

Products Marketed to People with Hepatitis C

J. Lyn Patrick, ND

Introduction

Many over-the-counter products are marketed to people living with *hepatitis C*. A number of claims are made about these products. At times, it can be hard to determine what to believe. Your western doctor may not be able to provide you with guidance because he or she may not be familiar or experienced with these products. Making a decision about whether to use one or more of these products can be challenging. In addition, there is no way to be sure how any one person will react to a product.

One of the most common complaints from western doctors about alternative products is there are little or no data to support their claims of effectiveness. The data that do exist is often from studies that were poorly designed. Claims based on such studies are considered invalid by most western doctors. For the most part it is true that many alternative products have not been adequately studied, but this situation is beginning to change. Manufacturers of some alternative products realize that in order to gain credibility in the western medical community, they need valid evidence that their products are safe and useful.

Some of the most common products marketed to people with hepatitis C are reviewed in this section. Many more are available that do not appear here. The inclusion or exclusion of any product should not be considered to deny or affirm its existence or effectiveness. The products we have selected are those people with hepatitis C seem to be most aware of and therefore ask about most frequently.

Ultimately, it is up to you to do whatever research is necessary to make an informed decision about whether to try a given product. This is especially important in deciding whether to take a product that has little or no study data available. We have included references to *clinical trial* data where applicable. We independently researched each product discussed. We also contacted the manufacturers of the products discussed to request information directly from them. In some cases, we did not receive the information we requested. Therefore, this information may not be complete.

> **Be sure to tell each of your healthcare providers about all the products you are taking.**
> **This will help ensure coordinated and safe healthcare.**

Bee Propolis

Propolis is a sticky material produced by bees from plant parts. It is used as sealing material for the hive. Because it has significant antibacterial and antifungal activity, it has been used as a topical medicine for skin, ear, nose, and throat problems.[1] Propolis has *antiviral* activity, specifically to influenza and herpes viruses.[2] This antiviral activity is thought to be due to the *flavinoids* in propolis. These *vitamin*-like substances come from the plant materials picked up by the bees. Flavinoids also appear to be the active ingredients in the plant-based folk remedies used by traditional African medicine practitioners for the treatment of hepatitis.[3] No animal or human studies have been conducted on propolis as a treatment for hepatitis.

Colloidal Silver

Silver is a precious metal with many industrial uses. It has also been used medicinally for a variety of ailments for several centuries. Prior to the introduction of modern day antibiotics in the 20th century, silver-containing medicinals were used to treat a variety of infections. Some prescription silver products are still used to treat skin and eye ailments such as burns, warts, and eye infections. However, there are currently no prescription silver products that are meant to be taken internally (that is, ingested). Colloidal silver products consist of tiny bits of silver in a liquid base. Most colloidal silver products are intended to be taken by mouth, but some injection forms are available as well.

In 1999, the U.S. Food and Drug Administration (FDA) issued a ruling banning colloidal silver sellers from claiming any therapeutic value for the product. According to the U.S. National Center for *Complementary and Alternative Medicine*[4]: Colloidal silver products are not considered by the FDA to be safe or effective.

- Silver has no known function in the human body.

- The human body has no need for silver. Therefore, claims that people may have a "silver deficiency" condition are unfounded.

- There is no scientific evidence to support the many claims made about the effectiveness of colloidal silver for a variety of conditions.

Ingesting or injecting colloidal silver may cause serious side effects including seizures, kidney damage, stomach irritation, headaches, *fatigue*, and skin irritation. Equally important, colloidal silver may interfere with the body's absorption of certain medications including several antibiotics and thyroid *hormone* replacement medicine.

There is no evidence that colloidal silver has any benefits for people living with hepatitis C. But there is evidence that ingesting or injecting colloidal silver may cause physical harm.

Eurocel™

Eurocel™ is a proprietary herbal formula specifically marketed for the treatment of *chronic hepatitis* C by Allergy Research Group, a company that markets supplements to doctors and the public.

Eurocel™ contains the herbs Patrina villosa, Artemesia capillaris, and Schizandra fructus; the exact amounts of each ingredient are not disclosed. These common Chinese and Korean herbs have been used historically for the treatment of liver disease. The company cites unpublished data that the formula has been tested for toxicity in mice and found to be essentially nontoxic and non-mutagenic (it did not cause genetic changes in the animals tested).

The Allergy Research Group Internet site reports data from a small, unpublished pilot study involving ten people with hepatitis C. The participants were recruited from a clinic in South Korea. The patients were in different *stages* of the disease (between 3 and 20 years after diagnosis). All had elevated *ALT* levels and *HCV viral loads*. Participants were given two capsules (500 mg each) of Eurocel™ twice daily for a period of 6 to 24 months. Apparently, the herbal combination was stopped after HCV viral load dropped to 1,000 copies/mL in five patients who were followed with viral load testing for a period of six months. The follow-up data was not included in the report this author received.

No specific data was provided about ALT levels or other markers that were said to have improved. The report did not contain information about how many patients had low viral loads six months after stopping the herbal combination, or whether their ALT levels remained stable after stopping the product. If that data exist, it was not supplied by the company. However, they do state that the response to Eurocel™ is "an individual response."

This author was referred to a Korean physician, Dr. Ba, when Allergy Research Group was contacted. In speaking with Dr. Ba, he said he knew nothing about the study, nor that it was conducted in Korea. He did not have contact information for the healthcare providers who conducted the study.

Without the missing information, it is difficult to assess the effect of this herbal combination. Research data exists on the use of specific extracts of schizandra for hepatitis C (see *Chapter 11.2, Modern Chinese Medicine Therapeutics*) for Hepatitis C. However, there is no way of knowing whether Eurocel™ capsules contain significant quantities of schizandrin B and C since the ingredients are not listed by quantity. Eurocel™ is expensive ($149 for a 30-day supply as of April 2008). Incomplete information on ten patients is not enough to back the company's claim that, "Hepatitis C viral titers plummet with Eurocel™."

God's Remedy

God's Remedy is a group of products advertised for the treatment of hepatitis C. The products are alcohol-based liquid extracts of plants. The company Internet site describes a "two step system" with certain products for "first time users" and others for "continued use." Products in the group include Pure Herbal Remedy™, Milk Thistle™, Hepacure™, and Immune Booster™.

The Pure Herbal Remedy™ formula is advertised as an *antioxidant* supplement. It is said to contain 14 herbs including burdock root, nettle, red clover bloom, ginseng root, echinacea root, yellow dock root, dandelion root, blessed thistle, schizandra, astragalus root, olive leaf, plantain, Oregon grape, psyllium, and milk thistle. The advertising language explains the chemicals found in these plants are potent antioxidants and stimulate the human immune system. Although this statement is true in that plant chemicals called flavinoids are highly potent antioxidants, not all plants contain flavinoids. With the exception of schizandra, astragalus, and milk thistle, the plants contained in Pure Herbal Remedy™ are not known for their high flavinoid content. There are no published studies looking at the effects of these plant-derived flavinoids on chronic hepatitis C.

The God's Remedy milk thistle product is available as a liquid extract or in capsules. Information about the silymarin or silybin content is not provided, so it is difficult to know the potency of these products. Silymarin is the active ingredient in milk thistle, and all the clinical trials involving milk thistle specify of the dose of silymarin. See *Chapter 14, Naturopathic Medicine* for additional information on silymarin.

Hepacure™ is another product sold by this manufacturer. It is claimed to be an "extract version of Hepatico™." (See Hepatico™ listing in this chapter for information about this product.) The advertising text for Hepacure™ refers to clinical trials with Hepatico™ in the Republic of Georgia and Russia quoting, "complete healing and restoration of all organs and functions" in 91% of 300 test subjects. They site further states, "Recovery from *cirrhosis* took place over 1 to 7 months depending on the complexity and stage of the disease." The text goes on to say the product has been researched and is safe for treatment of acute and chronic forms of *hepatitis A*, B, and C, cirrhosis, and *liver cancer*. However, there is no reference to the source of this information. It is also unclear where this product was researched and how it was determined to be safe.

As mentioned in the section under Hepatico™, none of the references mentioned were published studies. The only published study we found was an animal study looking at the toxicity of the plants in Hepatico™. The ingredients listed for Hepacure™ are very different from the original Hepatico™ formula. Hepacure™ is said to contain nettle, plantain, horsetail, yarrow, golden rod, chamomile, feikhoa batsu, fern, ekala, pau d'arco, cleaver, and mayapple in a base of milk thistle, dandelion, and turmeric root.

The Immune Booster™ formula contains goldenseal root, red clover blooms, yellow dock root, burdock root, witch hazel bark, wild American ginseng root, Capsicum fruit, pau d'arco bark, spirulina, and Echinaccea augustifolia root in an alcohol base. The Immune Booster™ formula text states, "Numerous studies have shown that these remarkable natural substances stimulate our immune system's ability to recognize and surround foreign matter and eliminate it at a cellular level." The only actual published data looking at the immune stimulating effects of these plants have been with echinacea, berberine (the active ingredient in goldenseal), burdock root, and pau d'arco (Tecoma curialis). The relative amounts of each botanical in the formula are not given, so it is difficult determine the immune stimulating activity of the formula.

The Energy Formula™ is no longer advertised as part of the two-step God's Remedy hepatitis C system, but it is still available. The online text describing the product states, "It replenishes the nutrients which are drained from your body from hepatitis C and [a] weakened immune system." It is said to "diminish fatigue." The Energy Formula™ contains American, Korean, Siberian and Tienchi ginsengs, kola nut, damiana, and wild ginger root in an alcohol base. Kola nut contains *caffeine*. Various over-the-counter products that contain kola nut have been found to contain high amounts of caffeine. Because this is a liquid formula, the amount of caffeine in the product would be hard to regulate and difficult to label. If high amounts of caffeine are the ingredient producing the "needed boost throughout the day," green tea or another inexpensive source of caffeine may provide an economical alternative.

Hepatico™

The trademarked product Hepatico™ that had been marketed by Alta Natural Herbs & Supplements, Ltd. appears to be off the market at the time of this writing (Spring 2008). However, it may still be available through some Internet sites, so it is included here for your information.

Hepatico™ is a botanical compound producers claim has been used in Russia "for more than 150 years." It is a combination of three common plants (plantain, nettle, and immortelle) in a base of three other plants (turmeric, milk thistle, and dandelion root). Each capsule is said to contain 250 mg of a combination of the first three plants in 250 mg of a combination of the base herbs.

None of the three primary plants is commonly known to have any action on the liver or gall bladder. The base botanicals are known to have effects on the liver and *bile* ducts, but the doses in Hepatico™are low. The amount of Hepatico™ used in an unpublished study (discussed below) was one to two capsules three times daily. This means the amounts of the botanicals involved in the study were below the amounts commonly used in published research that has examined the individual action of turmeric, milk thistle, and dandelion root.

The information previously made available by the manufacturer includes a study done in Canada with 23 patients who had either *hepatitis B* or C, or both. The majority had chronic hepatitis C. Study participants were given one or two capsules of Hepatico™ three times daily (depending on the patient's weight) for a period of 20 to 40 days. At the end of the study period, four of 23 participants had normalization of their ALT levels, and three of 23 participants had normalization of their *AST* levels. Participants who experienced normalization of their *liver enzymes* had varying histories of hepatitis C infection from 2 to 24 years duration. There is no information about their individual disease progression. A second group of ten hepatitis C patients took Hepatico™ for the first month of a 7-month trial. Two had normalization of their blood ALT levels. The investigators reported the participants in this study had relief from digestive *symptom*s and insomnia, but they did not document when or for how long this occurred. The study gave incomplete information about the patients' medical conditions. The only other liver test conducted on participants was *GGT* levels, which did not change significantly during treatment. *Liver biopsy* results were not available.

It is unknown whether the claims for this product could be reproduced in clinical trials conducted in the United States. According to a study done in Canada (unpublished), improvement (normalization of ALT levels) occurred in only a small minority of patients.

Hepato-C™

Hepato-C™ is a botanical combination marketed by Pacific BioLogics. It contains 15 powdered herbs in capsule form. The manufacturer states, "Hepato-C™ is intended to be used to balance the total diet to help promote the strengthening of the liver." The manufacturer previously publicized a study of 11 hepatitis C patients on Hepato-C™ for nine months. Information on viral load levels and liver enzymes in these 11 people is inadequate to allow evaluation of the effects of the product. Follow-up viral loads were unavailable for seven of the 11 study participants. Ten people in the study were taking other substances (vitamins and other herbs) and receiving acupuncture treatments during the study. Liver enzyme levels were normal in five people at the end of the study period, but all of these people were taking other herbs and vitamins that were not specified. Three of these people had been on interferon or interferon plus *ribavirin* prior to taking Hepato-C™. According to product literature (May 2000), a few private practice and university-based healthcare providers have agreed to conduct clinical studies with this product. As of April 2008, no information is available on the Pacific BioLogics Internet site to indicate whether these studies were conducted.

IP-6

Myoinositol hexaphosphate is a B vitamin combined with phytic acid, a naturally occurring substance found in certain plant fibers (grains such as rice are particularly high in phytic acid). As a naturally occurring substance, IP-6 is present in a number of foods including beans, brown rice, corn meal, and wheat bran.

Abulkalam M. Shamsuddin MD, PhD holds the U.S. patent for supplemental IP-6 (inositol and myoinositol hexaphosphate). IP-6 is also known as phytic acid or phytate. Dr. Shamsuddin's research has demonstrated immune enhancing and anticancer actions of IP-6 in the laboratory. IP-6 is the subject of several published studies on cancer in animals and cultured cell lines, but this author found only one study on the use of IP-6 in liver disease.[5] A study in rats that included IP-6 in their diet appeared to prevent the accumulation of fat in the liver that would otherwise have occurred because of a high-sugar diet. Whether this finding has any relationship to viral hepatitis is questionable because different factors are responsible for liver damage in chronic hepatitis C.

Regarding safety, IP-6 has been shown to reduce the activity of *platelets* (circulating substances that help form plugs to stop bleeding). Therefore, people with low platelet counts, or who are taking aspirin or other blood thinning medications should avoid using IP-6. Supplemental forms of IP-6 may also bind with *calcium*, magnesium, copper, *iron* and zinc and should, therefore, not be taken with food.

There is no evidence to date that IP-6 has any direct effect on chronic viral hepatitis.

Liv.52™ and LiverCare™

Liv.52™ is an Ayurvedic formula of herbs first introduced in the 1950's. It is currently produced and marketed under several names including LiverCare™. Although the LiverCare™ manufacturer's Internet site states there are over 168 clinical papers published on the use of Liv.52™, only 50 clinical and experimental (animal) studies were found by this author in a search of the medical literature.

The main ingredients of Liv.52™ are capers (Capparis spinosa), wild chicory (Cichorium intybus), black nightshade (Solanum nigrum), arjuna (Terminalia arjuna), yarrow (Achillea millefolium), Negro coffee (Cassia occidentalis), and tamarish (Tamarix gallica). All of these plants are recognized in the writings of traditional Ayurvedic herbal medicine as treatments for liver problems. The combination of these medicinal plants has been widely used and researched in India for over 30 years.

The animal studies reviewed showed clear evidence that Liv.52™ has an antioxidant-like effect on the liver. It prevented damage from chemical toxins in animals, and from alcohol in both animals and humans. However, only three studies appeared to have been done in people with hepatitis, and none of these involved people with chronic hepatitis C.[6, 7]

One clinical study evaluated 24 people with chronic active hepatitis B who were taking Liv.52™.[8] A significant number of patients in this study had *jaundice*, *ascites*, and cirrhosis, all of which are *signs* of liver damage resulting from long-term infection. After treatment with Liv.52™, 58% of the study participants had significant decreases in their liver enzymes. The researchers considered this an improvement in symptoms. However, we cannot assume that Liv.52™ would have the same effect in people with chronic hepatitis C. First, HCV is a very different virus from the hepatitis B virus. Second, improved biopsy results need to be seen to prove improvement with chronic hepatitis C. Decreases in liver enzymes alone are not enough to prove efficacy. The authors cite an older published study that showed long-term improvement in people with chronic hepatitis who took Liv.52™ for nine months. However, this study was unavailable for review.

A separate study examined the effects of Liv.52™ on 188 patients with alcoholic cirrhosis. Study participants took Liv.52™ for two years. Among patients with the worst cirrhosis, those taking Liv.52™ had a higher death rate than those not taking the supplement (23 deaths versus 11 deaths). It is unclear if Liv.52™ was related to this observed increase in death rate. An increased death rate was not seen in study participants with less severe cirrhosis.[9]

Because Liv.52™ has been extensively tested in animals and has been used clinically for many years, its lack of toxicity has been proven. There has been concern about the levels of the *toxic* metal lead found in certain Ayurvedic preparations. However, an independent laboratory analysis has shown that the level of lead in Liv.52™ is low, and the compound is generally considered safe.

Liv.52™ appears to be beneficial in treating liver disease and may play a role as an antioxidant herbal preparation in supporting the liver function of people with chronic hepatitis C. However, there is no clinical evidence (that is, no human studies have been done) that Liv.52™ has an antiviral effect on the hepatitis C virus (HCV), or that it can prevent or treat cirrhosis.

The standard dosage of Liv.52™ suggested by Ayurvedic practitioners is two tablets twice daily with meals. However, each individual's dosage should be adjusted by a qualified Ayurvedic practitioner.

Liverite™ Liver Aid

Liverite™ Liver Aid is a *nutritional supplement* containing vitamin B12, *phospholipids*, cysteine, and bovine liver hydrolysate (cow liver that has been broken down by enzymes). Many studies examining the effects of these preparations on liver cells have been published in the European and Japanese medical literature. However, human studies have failed to show any clear benefit in hepatitis.[10, 11]

Liverite™ Liver Aid contains an unlisted amount of *phosphatidylcholine*, a type of fat found naturally in food. Approximately 20 years of medical research exists on the effects of phosphatidylcholine on the liver. Phosphatidylcholine has been shown to have a protective effect on liver tissue in alcoholics and people who are exposed to toxins, large doses of liver-damaging pharmaceuticals, and viruses.[12] Most studies used a combination of intravenous preparations of phosphatidylcholine and oral doses of 450mg to 700 mg. Other studies used only oral doses of 1,350 mg to 2,350 mg per day for alcoholic liver damage or hepatitis. Studies of chronic hepatitis B patients taking phosphatidylcholine and steroid therapy showed improved liver biopsy results. *Acute hepatitis* B resolved more quickly in those taking 1,350 mg phosphatidylcholine daily compared to those not taking the supplement. Phosphatidylcholine has also been studied in people with severe liver disease. In these studies, phosphatidylcholine used both intravenously and orally produced a reversal of *fibrosis* or scarring of the liver and a return to normal *liver function tests*.[13] Whether Liverite™ Liver Aid is the best dose or source (practically or economically) of phosphatidylcholine is unclear.

Microhydrin™

Microhydrin™ is a liquid suspension of minerals (silica, *potassium* carbonate, and magnesium sulfate) and safflower oil in a base of purified water. The manufacturer claims this product lowers the surface tension and raises the pH of water (makes it more alkaline), and increases the absorption of nutrients from drinking water. The developer of Microhydrin™, Dr. Patrick Flanagan, claims its effect comes from the fact that the product carries extra hydrogen atoms and "acts as a powerful antioxidant." He has published studies with athletes showing the product has the effect of lowering lactic acid levels after heavy exercise. The manufacturer publicizes this product as part of a regimen to improve nutritional status and hepatitis C. Individuals with hepatitis C have given personal testimonials supporting this claim. At this time, there is no evidence from human, animal, or cell studies that indicates Microhydrin™ has any direct effects on hepatitis C.

Mannatech™

Mannatech™ is a proprietary (secret) formula discovered by Terry Pulse, MD and Reg McDaniel, MD while they were working with AIDS patients. Mannatech™ is distributed by a multilevel marketing firm. It is based on a group of complex sugars called acemannan derived from the aloe vera plant that are known to have immune stimulating and antiviral properties.[14, 15] The manufacturers also use a product called arabinogalactan, a type of fiber that has been demonstrated to have an immune stimulating effect in humans.[16]

In a study published in 2000 in the "Proceedings of the Fisher Institute for Medical Research" (an entity that sells informational papers about Mannatech™ products), a group of eight chronic hepatitis C patients received "glyconutritional powder and an antioxidant supplement."[17] The patients in the study had declined interferon therapy or had experienced interferon treatment failure before entering the study. Participants were given the "glyconutritional powder and an antioxidant supplement" twice a day for six months. After six months on this *protocol*, ALT levels normalized in three out of eight patients, and four reported improvements in energy level. Liver biopsy was done on all eight patients at the beginning of the study, but no information is given about follow-up biopsy results. Viral loads were not available.

Although this small pilot study is interesting because there is reason to think that the ingredients in this proprietary formula may be useful, a much larger and more detailed study would is needed to determine if these plant nutrients have any antiviral or immune stimulating effect in hepatitis C.

MGN-3™

MGN-3™ is a molecule called an arabinoxylane that is extracted from rice bran. It has been tested in cancer studies and in small trials. The studies showed MGN-3 has the ability to enhance the immune response of cancer patients and to decrease the side effects of *chemotherapy* in studies with rats.[18, 19] There is clear evidence from papers published by Mamdooh Ghoenum, PhD and others that this compound increases blood levels of *natural killer cells* (a special type of immune cell). It also increases levels of gamma-interferon and another substance called tumor necrosis factor. Although the boost in *immunity* may possibly be useful in cancer therapies, hepatitis C is a different condition. In chronic viral infection, the immune system already makes too much tumor necrosis factor, which may be a large part of the problem in hepatitis C. To date, any direct effects of MGN-3 on hepatitis C are unproven.

MTH-68/B Vaccine

The Newcastle disease virus is found in chickens. It can be up to 100% fatal in fowl, but has no effect on humans. Dr. Laszlo Csatary developed a *vaccine* made from this virus, MTH-68/H. The vaccine has been used to treat a specific type of human brain cancer called glioblastoma.[20]

Beginning in the mid to late 1990's, Dr. Csatary and his associates have been conducting studies with another virus vaccine in people with hepatitis B and C. The vaccine contains an attenuated (weakened) form of the bursal disease virus and is called MTH-68/B. A study published in 1998 on MTH-68/B involved two groups of acute hepatitis patients, 43 with hepatitis B and 41 with hepatitis C. Half were treated with conventional treatment. The other half were given injections of the vaccine. Of those HCV patients on conventional treatment, 26% went on to develop chronic active (symptomatic) hepatitis. Of those given the vaccine, only 9% went on to develop chronic active hepatitis C. Of those who recovered, 79% on conventional treatment *relapsed* while only 32% of those who received the vaccine relapsed.[21]

In another study published in 1999, MTH-68/B was given to three patients with end-stage hepatitis B and C. All three patients experienced significant improvement that could only be attributed to the vaccine.[22] A search of the published medical literature conducted in 2008 found no additional publications on MTH-68/B since 1999.

Given that the research with the live virus vaccine (MTH-68/H) in cancer patients has proven to be free of toxicity, the attenuated virus vaccine (MTH-68/B) used in hepatitis research is also likely to be free from side effects. The MTH-68/B vaccine is not approved for use in the U.S.

Phlogenzym™

Phlogenzym™ is an oral enzyme therapy manufactured in Germany by Mucos Pharma. It contains proteolytic (*protein digesting*) enzymes and a vitamin from the flavinoid family called rutosid. It is primarily promoted as an arthritis remedy, but has also been promoted to treat kidney stones and cancer.

A 1997 clinical trial with hepatitis C patients in Egypt compared Phlogenzym™ to alfa-interferon and ribavirin.[23] Patients in the study were divided into four groups: 20 took ribavirin, 20 took interferon, 20 took Phlogenzym™, and 20 took a liver support protocol that consisted of vitamins and antioxidants. After four months, the researchers compared the results of the four groups. Phlogenzyme™ was reported to be more effective than interferon or ribavirin at lowering liver enzymes (ALT, AST, and GGT). It was also reportedly associated with a 50% reduction in symptoms including appetite loss, weight loss, fever, itching, fatigue, jaundice, and spider nevi (small broken blood vessels in the skin). Tolerance of Phlogenzym™ was rated as "good" in 14 patients.

A subsequent 2005 look-back study conducted in Germany to examine the effects of on Phlogenzym™ on the liver enzymes of patients with chronic hepatitis C reported very different results. Twenty-two hepatitis C patients were included in the study. They were taking six tablets of Phlogenzym™ per day for an average of 77 days. The researchers found that AST, ALT, and GGT did not change significantly during treatment. They further reported that 5 out of the 22 patients had to stop treatment because of side effects.[24]

With these conflicting results, it is unclear what (if any) beneficial effects are associated with Phlogenzym™ for hepatitis C. With no information about viral loads, the antiviral activity of this product is also unknown.

Sho-Saiko-To (SST)

Sho-saiko-to (also known by the trade name Liver Campo or by the Chinese name xiao chai hu tang) is distributed in the United States primarily through Honso U.S.A, Inc. This over-the-counter product contains a multitude of ingredients including "bupleurum root, pinellia tuber, scutellaria root, ginseng, jujube, licorice root, ginger, baicalin, baicalein, glycyrrhizin, saikosaponins, ginsenosides, wogonin, and gingerols" (as listed on the Honso U.S.A. Internet site). The manufacturer states that this is a classic Chinese botanical formulation. It has been used extensively in Japan for a number of years.

The manufacturer's site lists a number of publications citing research conducted primarily in animal models. Several of these papers report *antifibrosis* activity in rodent liver models.[25-28] However, a search of the published medical literature conducted in April 2008 revealed no clinical studies (that is, conducted in humans) on the safety or efficacy of sho-saiko-to for chronic hepatitis C.

Importantly, there have been several case reports of serious side effects related to the ingestion of sho-saiko-to. The most common of these serious side effects is a condition called *interstitial* pneumonitis.[29, 30] This condition is an inflammatory condition of the lung that can be fatal.

> **Sho-saiko-to should never be taken while on *interferon-based therapy* because of the risk of interstitial pneumonitis, a potentially fatal condition.**

Also important for hepatitis C patients is a report of acute hepatitis (nonviral) caused by the ingestion of sho-saiko-to[31] and another report of a dramatic drop in platelet count (a condition known as thrombocytopenia *purpura*).[32] Sho-saiko-to is currently being studied in a phase II clinical trial in the U.S. to determine its safety and possible efficacy for patients with chronic hepatitis C.

Thymic Protein A

Thymic protein A was formulated by immunologist and research scientist Terry Beardsley, PhD. He currently holds the U.S. patent on this protein and is involved in research evaluating its use in immune disorders.

Thymic protein A is chemically identical to a protein produced by the human *thymus gland*. It was originally derived from the thymus tissue of calves, but is now produced with the technology of cell cloning (reproducing cells in the laboratory). It has been shown to be absorbed orally, a problem with other thymus proteins. It increase the body's production of CD4 cells (T-helper cells) and natural killer cells, the immune system's virus killing cells.[33]

One study evaluated the effect of thymic protein A on people with chronic fatigue syndrome (Epstein-Barr disease). Participants were treated with 12 mcg (micrograms) of thymic protein A daily for 60 days. Treatment resulted in significant Epstein-Barr viral load reductions of 50% or greater in 67% of patients.[34]

Thymic protein A has not been studied in hepatitis C. However, the use of another thymic protein, thymosin alfa-1, has been the subject of hepatitis C studies. In one study, people with HCV were treated with a combination of thymosin alfa-1 plus interferon or interferon alone for 26 weeks. A higher proportion of patients treated with the combined therapy cleared virus and had a normalization of ALT compared to patients treated with interferon alone.[35] Post-treatment liver biopsy results were better in the combined therapy group than in the interferon group. In the follow-up period, the biochemical response rate dropped to 14% and 8% in the combined therapy and interferon groups, respectively.

Thymosin alfa-1 is a 28 *amino acid* protein fragment and is much smaller than the 500 amino acid thymic protein A. Therefore, thymic protein A may work differently than the thymosin alfa-1. In general, a larger protein fragment (thymic protein A) would be expected to have a greater effect than a smaller protein fragment (thymosin alfa-1). Thymic protein A has been tested in mice, cats, and humans and has been found to enhance immune response to viral infections. To date, there are no published studies evaluating the effects of thymic protein A on hepatitis C infection. Thymic protein A is sold over-the-counter under the brand name of ProBoost™.

Ultraviolet Blood Irradiation

Ultraviolet blood irradiation (UBI) is not a product but rather a technique that was popular in the United States during the early 1930's as a treatment for poliovirus. UBI involves removing blood from the body and exposing it to ultraviolet light. After the discovery of the Salk vaccine for the prevention of polio and the advent of antibiotics in the 1950's, the use of UBI all but disappeared.

Recently, there has been a renewed interest in this technique. It has been now been reapproved by the Food and Drug Administration for the treatment of a specific type of cancer called cutaneous T-cell lymphoma.[36] This type of UBI is called photophoresis. It is currently being investigated in clinical trials for the treatment of *autoimmune* diseases such as arthritis. The UBI process is time-consuming (each treatment takes about five hours) and expensive. A 1959 published study described the use of this process to treat acute hepatitis A and B, but there have been no published studies on its use to treat hepatitis C.[37]

This process can destroy *white blood cells* if it is not done properly. Therefore, it should only be performed in a medical setting by a licensed doctor who specializes in this procedure. UBI is sometimes used outside of the United States for the treatment of chronic hepatitis.

Reasons for Using Over-The-Counter Products

People decide to pursue complementary and alternative medicine (*CAM*) treatments for a variety of reasons. You may have decided to decline western therapy at this time. On the other hand, you may have experienced a treatment failure. Or perhaps your doctor has advised you to follow a "watchful waiting" course (you are monitored for disease progression but are not being treated). The reason for your interest in CAM therapy is not nearly as important as making sure whatever you decide to do is safe. It is extremely important to seek safe, clinically tested CAM treatments.

As you look into your options, realize that any treatment should have proof that it is effective at improving liver function and/or quality of life in people with hepatitis C. A product that has not undergone safety studies in animals or humans may not be a wise choice. Many botanicals (both western and traditional Chinese) have been shown to be harmful to the liver. Your first concern should always be to do no additional harm to your liver.

If you are on treatment and are having side effects from your medications, there are ways to reduce these symptoms. A licensed CAM provider can help you use botanical medicines, acupuncture, and supplements that are specific for the side effects you are experiencing. Their guidance can also help insure that whatever CAM therapies you use do not interfere with your treatment's antiviral, and/or immune-enhancing activities. Unfortunately, none of the products mentioned in this chapter have been shown to reduce side effects from interferon-based therapy.

Reasons for Not Using Over-The-Counter Products

Essentially, it is not your personal situation but the product that is in question here. If the manufacturer or provider cannot provide a reference to a published study documenting a positive effect in hepatitis C, you are taking a chance that it may not be safe and/or may have no beneficial effects.

Before you take anything, we urge you to consider checking with a licensed CAM provider who treats people with chronic hepatitis C. Many botanicals (both western and traditional Chinese) have been shown to be harmful to the liver. It is best to have someone trained in complementary and alternative medicine oversee your alternative treatments. He or she can work with your primary care doctor or *gastroenterologist/hepatologist*. Check with the American Association of Naturopathic Physicians (AANP), the American College for Advancement in Medicine (ACAM), or the American Holistic Medical Association (AHMA) for help in finding a qualified CAM practitioner. (See the *Resource Directory* for contact information.)

Over-the-counter products marketed to people with hepatitis C can be very expensive, especially when taken for months or years. Very few (if any) of these products are covered by health insurance.

You also need to be aware that there are no regulations governing the manufacture of these products. Therefore, it is often difficult to know if you are actually getting what is listed on the product label. Further, there is no assurance that you will get the same product from one bottle to the next. It is sometimes challenging to find reputable distributors for these products.

Summary

Many over-the-counter products are marketed to people with hepatitis C. While some of these products may benefit the user, there are very few documented studies on the effectiveness of these products. It may be difficult to find reliable advice on which products are or are not appropriate for you. Many western healthcare professionals are unfamiliar with these products, and are generally skeptical about their possible benefits.

It is very important that you learn everything you can about over-the-counter products you are considering taking. Your first priority should be insuring that a product is safe and not harmful to the liver. If you are considering using one of these products, you may want to consult with a qualified CAM practitioner before you make a decision. Remember, it is very important to discuss your use of any of these products with all of your healthcare providers. This will help insure your safety and maximize the possibility of benefit from all your treatments.

References

1. Marcucci MC. Propolis: chemical composition, biological properties and therapeutic activity. *Apidologie*. 1995;26:83-99.
2. Amoros M, Lurton E, Boustie J, et al. Comparison of the anti-herpes simplex virus activities of propolis and 3-methylbut-2-enyl caffeate. *J Nat Prod*. 1994;57(5):644-647.
3. Iwu M, Duncan A, Okunji C. *Dietary botanical supplements with antiviral and anti-inflammatory properties used in the treatment of liver disorders in traditional African medicine*. Complementary and Alternative Medicine in Chronic Liver Disease Conference. National Institutes of Health. Bethesda, Maryland. 1999.
4. National Institutes of Health, National Center for Complementary and Alternative Medicine. Backgrounder: Colloidal Silver Products. Rockville, Maryland. Updated December 2006. Available at nccam.nih.gov/health/alerts/silver/index.htm. Accessed April 25, 2008.
5. Katamaya T. Hypolipemic action of phytic acid (IP6): prevention of fatty liver. *Anticancer Res*. 1999;19(5A):3695-3698.
6. Patney NL, Pachori S. A study of serum glycolytic enzymes and serum B hepatitis in relation to Liv.52 therapy. *Medicine and Surgery*. 1986(XXVI);4:9.
7. Chawhan, RN, Talib SH, Talib VH, et al. Viral hepatitis in children. *The Medicine and Surgery*. 1976; 3, 9. [Note: This information was provided by an herb manufacturer, but is not available through the National Library of Medicine's database PubMed.]
8. Mukerjee AB, Dasgupta M. Cirrhosis of liver. Results of treatment with an indigenous drug Liv.52. *J Ind Med Prof*. 1971; 12:7853.
9. Fleig WW, Morgan MY, Hölzer MA. The ayurvedic drug LIV.52 in patients with alcoholic cirrhosis. Results of a prospective, randomized, double-blind, placebo-controlled clinical trial [Abstract]. *J Hepatol*. 1997;26(Suppl 1):127.
10. Fujisawa K, Suzuki H, Yamamoto S, et al. Therapeutic effects of liver hydrolysate preparation on chronic hepatitis - A double blind, controlled study. *Asian Med J*. 1984;26:497-526.
11. Sanbe K, Murata T, Fujisawa K, et al. Treatment of liver disease - with particular reference to liver hydrolysates. *Jap J Clin Exp Med*. 1973;50:2665-76.
12. Kidd P. Phosphatidylcholine: a superior protectant against liver damage. *Altern Med Rev*. 1996;1(4):258-274.
13. Freidman LS, Martin P, Munoz SJ. Liver function tests and the objective evaluation of the patient with liver disease. In: Zakim D, Boyer TD, (Eds.). *Hepatology: A Textbook of Liver Disease*. WB Saunders. Philadelphia, Pennsylvania. 1996:791-833.
14. Kahlon JB, Kemp MC, Yawel N, et al. In vitro evaluation of the synergistic antiviral effects of acemannin in combination with azidothymidine and acyclovir. *Mol Biother*. 1991;3(4):214-23.
15. Womble E, et al. The impact of acemannan on the generation and function of cytotoxic T-lymphocytes. *Immunopharm*. 1992;14:3-67.
16. Kelly G. Larch arabinogalactan. Clinical relevance of a novel immune-enhancing polysaccharide. *Altern Med Rev*. 1999;4(2):96-103.
17. Sweeney BF, McDaniel CF. Glyconutritional and phytochemicals in eight HCV-positive patients. Proceedings of the Fisher Institute for Medical Research. 1999;1(3):6-7.
18. Ghoneum M, Jewett A. Production of tumor necrosis factor-alfa and interferon-gamma from human peripheral blood lymphocytes by MGN-3, a modified arabinoxylan from rice bran, and its synergy with interleukin-2. *Cancer Detect Prev*. 2000;24(4):314-324.
19. Jacoby HL, Wonorowski G, Sakata K, et al. The effect of MGN-3 on cisplatin and adriamycin induced toxicity in the rat. *Gastroenterology*. 2000;118(4):4962. [Note: This information is not available through the National Library of Medicine's database PubMed, but a synopsis of the article was available at the time of publication at: www.jafra.gr.jp/sis-e.html.]
20. Csatary LK, Moss RW, Beuth J, et al. Beneficial treatment of patients with advanced cancer using a Newcastle disease virus vaccine (MTH-68/H). *Anticancer Research*. 1999;19(1B):629-634.
21. Csatary LK, Telegdy L, Gergely P, Bodey B, Bakacs T. Preliminary report of a controlled trial of MTH-68/B virus vaccine treatment in acute B and C hepatitis: a phase II study. *Anticancer Res*. 1998;18(2B):1279-1282.
22. Csatary LK, Schnabel R, Bakacs, T. Successful treatment of decompensated chronic viral hepatitis by bursal disease virus vaccine. *Anticancer Res*. 1999;19(1B):629-633.
23. Stauder G, Kabil S. Oral enzyme therapy in hepatitis C patients. *Int J Immunother*. 1997; XIII (3/4):153-158. [Note: This information was provided by the product manufacturer, but is not available through the National Library of Medicine's database PubMed.]
24. Huber R, Futter I, Goedl R, Rostock M, Lüdtke R. [Oral enzyme therapy for chronic hepatitis C--a retrospective analysis. Article in German.] *Forsch Komplementarmed Klass Naturheilkd*. 2005;12(3):144-147.
25. Ono M, Miyamura M, Kyotani S, Saibara T, Ohnishi S, Nishioka Y. Effects of Sho-saiko-to extract on liver fibrosis in relation to the changes in hydroxyproline and retinoid levels of the liver in rats. *J Pharm Pharmacol*. 1999;51(9):1079-1084.
26. Egashira T, Takayama F, Yamanaka Y, Komatsu Y. Monitoring of radical scavenging activity of peroral administration of the Kampo medicine Sho-saiko-to in rats. *Jpn J Pharmacol*. 1999;80(4):379-382.
27. Inoue T, Jackson EK. Strong antiproliferative effects of baicalein in cultured rat hepatic stellate cells. *Eur J Pharmacol*. 1999;378(1):129-135.
28. Shimizu I, Ma YR, Mizobuchi Y, et al. Effects of Sho-saiko-to, a Japanese herbal medicine, on hepatic fibrosis in rats. *Hepatology*. 1999;29(1):149-160.
29. Tomioka H, Hashimoto K, Ohnishi H, et al. [An autopsy case of interstitial pneumonia probably induced by Sho-saiko-to. Article in Japanese] *Nihon Kokyuki Gakkai Zasshi*. 1999;37(12):1013-8.
30. Sato A, Toyoshima M, Kondo A, Ohta K, Sato H, Ohsumi A. [Pneumonitis induced by the herbal medicine Sho-saiko-to in Japan. Article in Japanese] *Nihon Kyobu Shikkan Gakkai Zasshi*. 1997;35(4):391-5.
31. Hsu LM, Huang YS, Tsay SH, Chang FY, Lee SD. Acute hepatitis induced by Chinese hepatoprotective herb, xiao-chai-hu-tang. *J Chinese Med Assoc*. 2006;69(2):86-88.
32. Kiguchi T, Kimura F, Niiya K, Katayama Y, Harada M. Acute thrombocytopenic purpura after ingestion of Sho-saiko-to for hepatitis. *Liver*. 2000 Dec;20(6):491.
33. Beardsley T, Hayes SM. Induction of T-cell maturation by a cloned line of thymic epithelium (TEPI). *Proc Nat Acad Sci USA*. 1983;80(19):6005-6009.

34. Riordan NH, Jackson JA, Riordan HD. A pilot study on the effects of thymus protein on elevated Epstein-Barr virus titers in human subjects. Project RECNAC Wichita State University. Townsend Letter for Doctors. 1998;175:78-89. [Note: This information was provided by the product manufacturer, but is not available through the National Library of Medicine's database PubMed.]

35. Sherman KE, Sjorem M, Creager RL, et al. Combination therapy with thymosin alpha1 and interferon for the treatment of chronic hepatitis C infection: a randomized, placebo-controlled double-blind trial. *Hepatology.* 1998;27(4):1128-1135.

36. Edelson R, Berger C, Gasparro F, et al. Treatment of cutaneous T-cell lymphoma by extracorporeal photochemotherapy. *N Eng J Med.* 1987;316(6):297-303.

37. Olney RC. Treatment of viral hepatitis with the Knott technique of blood irradiation. *Am J Surgery.* 1959;90:402-409.

WOMEN AND HEPATITIS C

Norah Terrault, MD and Jessica Irwin, PAC

Introduction

Approximately 1.3 million women in the United States are infected with the *hepatitis C virus* (*HCV*). Women differ from men in terms of their risk of *cirrhosis* and *liver cancer*, the effects of *alcohol* on HCV-related disease, and response to HCV treatment. There are also several life issues specific to women that are affected by HCV, such as pregnancy and menopause. This chapter addresses the differences in the HCV experience that specifically affect women.

Risk Factors for Acquiring HCV Infection

HCV is transmitted through blood or blood-contaminated objects. Among persons with chronic HCV infection in the United States, the two most frequent ways the virus is acquired is from use of contaminated needles or other drug paraphernalia, or from receiving a blood transfusion prior to 1992 (when screening of blood for HCV began). Other risk factors for HCV infection are listed in the Table 1.

Sex with a HCV infected person can be a means of acquiring infection, although the virus is not transmitted very efficiently by sex. Nonetheless, women are at risk of acquiring HCV through their sexual partners.

Studies have shown the following:

- An uninfected woman is more likely to getting HCV from an infected male than vice versa.[1]

- Women in sexual partnerships with injection drug users are at risk for acquiring HCV in the partnership by engaging in risky injection and sexual practices.[2]

- This increased risk of getting HCV is related to risky behaviors. Women in partnerships with injection drug users are more likely to:

  - Inject drugs with used syringes

  - Allow other persons to inject for them

  - Engage in sexual activities with partners who are injection drug users

- *HIV* infection increases the risk of acquiring HCV infection by sexual contact.

Table 1. Risk Factors for Hepatitis C
Blood transfusion before 1992
Injection drug use
Hemodialysis
Needle-stick injury
Hemophilia
Mother is HCV-infected
HIV infection
Solid organ transplants
Unprotected sex with multiple partners

What Is the Risk of a Woman Transmitting HCV by Sex?

For women infected with HCV and in *monogamous* relationships, the risk of transmitting the virus to an uninfected partner is less than 1%.[3] Because the risk is so low, it is not recommended that couples specifically change their sexual practices to include use of barrier methods. However, this decision will vary with each couple's comfort level with the predicted risk of transmitting HCV. Additional "common sense" recommendations (since HCV is transmitted in blood) are:

- If sexual activities cause trauma to the mucosa or skin (resulting in blood exposure), use barrier protection or abstain from sex.

- If having sex during menses, use barrier protection or abstain from sex.

- If one or more of the partners has herpes or other open or ulcerating lesions, use barrier protection or abstain from sex.

For women infected with HCV who are not in monogamous relationship, barrier methods should be used. This recommendation also applies to women without HCV to prevent acquisition of sexually-transmitted diseases.

HCV: Pregnancy and Child-Birth

Does Pregnancy Change the Course of HCV Disease in an Infected Woman?
Whether pregnancy itself has an adverse effect on HCV disease is controversial. Serum *aminotransferase* levels (*ALT*) tend to decrease in the first trimester through to the third trimesters and rebound after delivery.[4] These effects may be related to the immune-rebound seen after delivery in other diseases.

For women with more advanced liver disease (such as those with significant bridging *fibrosis* or cirrhosis), complications of liver *decompensation* may occur during pregnancy, especially if there is evidence of portal *hypertension* prior to pregnancy. Women with advanced stages of fibrosis should seek expert medical advice regarding the risks of pregnancy prior to conception. This recommendation is not unique to HCV-infected women but is applicable to all women with chronic liver disease and advanced fibrosis who wish to become pregnant.

Mother-Infant Transmission of HCV
The risk of transmission of HCV from mother to infant is approximately 5%.[4-8] The exact time of transmission is not known. There are no preventative therapies available to interrupt transmission between mother and infant. Mother-infant transmission of HCV is currently the most common mode of acquisition of HCV in children.

FACTORS ASSOCIATED WITH RISK OF HCV TRANSMISSION FROM MOTHER-TO-INFANT

- **Presence of HCV RNA in the mother's blood at the time of delivery.**[4, 7, 9]
  There is no risk of transmitting HCV infection if the mother is HCV RNA negative (even though *HCV antibody* is present). This provides the rationale for considering treatment of HCV infection in women who are considering future pregnancy.

- **HIV coinfection**
  The risk of transmission of HCV is two to seven times higher in infants born to HCV/HIV coinfected mothers compared to children born to mothers infected with HCV alone.[7-10] Receipt of HIV antiretroviral therapy during pregnancy may reduce the risk of HCV transmission in coinfected mothers.[10]

FACTORS THAT MAY BE LINKED WITH RISK OF HCV TRANSMISSION FROM MOTHER-TO-INFANT
More studies are needed to address this question, but what we know today is as follows:

- **Elevated serum aminotransferase levels in the mother**
  In some (but not all) studies, higher rates of mother-infant transmission are seen in women with higher ALT levels than in those with normal or mildly elevated ALT levels.[10,11]

- **HCV viral load in the mother**
  Some (but not all) studies show a relationship between high *viral load* and higher risk of transmission. However, a specific HCV viral load threshold for transmission has not been determined. Longer duration of membrane rupture[7, 8], invasive fetal monitoring[7], and volume of blood loss ≥500g during the delivery have been reported as possible factors contributing to mother-infant transmission.[11]

FACTORS <u>NOT</u> RELATED TO RISK OF TRANSMISSION FROM MOTHER TO INFANT

- **Mode of delivery**

  There is much debate about mode of delivery and risk of mother-infant transmission of HCV. The majority of studies report no difference in mother-infant transmission by route of delivery, including studies evaluating elective cesarean sections versus emergency cesareans and vaginal delivery.[7, 8, 10] Therefore, HCV-infected women should not undergo elective cesarean section due to their HCV status, but there may be benefit in minimizing invasive procedures and the duration of rupture of membranes.

- **Breastfeeding**

  Breastfeeding has not been found to be associated with transmission of HCV from mother to infant.[4, 7, 8]

Follow-Up of Infants Born to HCV-Infected Women

Most infants are HCV RNA negative at birth but become HCV RNA detectable by age 2 to 6 months if they have been infected.[7, 11] A proportion of infants who are initially HCV RNA positive will become HCV RNA negative with further follow-up. For this reason, it is recommended that testing of infants be delayed until age 12 to 18 months. Since HCV antibodies from the mother may remain detectable in the uninfected infant for more than 12 months, testing of infants for HCV antibody should not be performed until after age 18 months.[12]

Spontaneous clearance of HCV infection among infants infected at birth occurs in up to 20% within the first 3 years of life.[13] In the short term, these infants do not appear to have any serious complications of chronic infection but a subset of children may progress to cirrhosis over years.

Risk of Cirrhosis and Liver Cancer in Women with HCV

For the woman chronically infected with HCV, the serious risks of the disease are cirrhosis and liver cancer. These complications develop over several decades of infection and do not occur in all infected persons. Interestingly, most studies on the course of chronic HCV infection show a lower risk of cirrhosis liver cancer in women compared to men. Men have a two fold increased risk of their HCV infection progressing to cirrhosis than women.[14] Data suggest that the reason women are "protected" from these complications is related to estrogen's effect on liver diseases.[15] The "high states" of estrogen are associated with decreased risk of scarring in the liver (fibrosis). Higher estrogen states during a woman's life occur during pregnancy and with use of oral contraceptive or *hormone* replacement therapy.

Studies find that women that have had one or more pregnancies have less fibrosis in their liver than women who have never been pregnant.[15] Women on birth control for an average of 5 years were found to have a lower score of fibrosis in their livers compared to women who did not use birth control. This association was not as strong as that found with pregnancy, but still follows the same pattern that higher states of estrogen maintained during a lifetime are associated with less liver damage.[15]

The production of estrogen begins to decrease as women age and is at its lowest levels after menopause. The risk of progressive liver damage or fibrosis increases after women reach menopause. Replacement of estrogen through hormone replacement therapy in menopause has been associated with a decrease in the rate of progression and a lower risk of cirrhosis. Women that used hormone replacement therapy or estrogen therapy early in menopause were shown in studies to have a lower rate of fibrosis in their liver than women that did not participate in any hormone therapy.[15, 16]

HCV-infected individuals whose disease progresses to cirrhosis are at a higher risk for liver cancer or hepatocellular carcinoma.[17] Liver cancer is more common in men than in women. However, the difference in risk between men and women decreases once women reach menopause.[14] Menopause is associated with lower estrogen levels and the risk of liver cancer increases after a decline in estrogen occurs. This suggests that estrogen may be protective against the development of liver cancer.

There are several lines of evidence suggesting that estrogens may be important in reducing the risk of liver cancer in women with chronic HCV infection.

- As with the risk of cirrhosis, studies show that women with a higher lifetime of estrogen were at less risk of developing liver cancer.[18]

- Higher lifetime estrogen levels are associated with multiple pregnancies and natural menopause occurrence, in comparison to early menopause mostly occurring due to surgical removal of uterus and ovaries.[18]

- Hormone replacement therapy also decreased a women's risk of developing liver cancer.[18]

Is Hormone Replacement Therapy (HRT) Advised in Women with HCV?

Menopause in the United States occurs, on average, at age 50. However, the body starts decreasing its production of estrogen and progesterone several years before menses stop. As discussed above, there are studies that show hormone therapy replacement is associated with a decrease in the progression of fibrosis as well as the risk of liver cancer.[15,18] However, this does not mean that all women with chronic HCV infection should use hormone replacement therapy (HRT). The decision to use HRT requires a careful weighing of potential risks and benefits of estrogen use.

Women with HCV infection can safely take HRT if this is desired. Studies have found no worsening of liver function or evidence of liver toxicity in women on HRT.[19] Low doses combining estrogen and progesterone are safe to use.

Alcohol in Women with HCV

Alcohol can negatively affect the liver. Alcohol is processed by the liver and broken down into byproducts. These byproducts are toxic to the liver and accelerate liver damage. Regular alcohol usage can cause continuous damage to the liver, resulting in the development of progressive fibrosis and eventually cirrhosis. Drinking on average more than two alcohol beverages per day increases the risk of cirrhosis to a significant degree.[20, 21] Cirrhosis is approximately 20 times more likely to occur in individuals that drink greater than two drinks per day.[20]

Studies show that women are more susceptible than men are to liver damage from alcohol.[21-24] Women have a higher risk of developing alcohol-related liver damage and cirrhosis at any alcohol intake (see Figures 1 and 2).[21]

Figure 1. Relative risk estimated for the development of alcohol induced liver disease
based upon sex and consumption of alcoholic beverages per week.

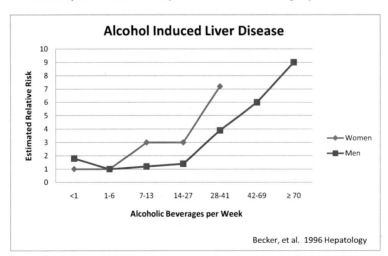

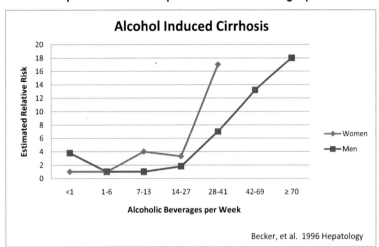

Figure 2. Relative risk estimated for the development of alcohol induced cirrhosis based upon sex and consumption of alcoholic beverages per week.

Excess alcohol consumption can worsen the course and outcomes of HCV infected individuals.[25] Data show that there is an increase in *inflammation* and fibrosis specifically in HCV-infected persons that consume more than 2 drinks per day.[26] When specifically addressing women's risk, data show that women drinking only one alcoholic beverage per day, still show an increase in inflammation and fibrosis.[26] The reason that women are at a higher risk of liver damage from drinking the same levels of alcohol as men is unknown. These are some of the possible factors.

FACTORS THAT MAY BE ASSOCIATED WITH INCREASED ALCOHOL DAMAGING EFFECT IN WOMEN

- Women have a lower body mass and fluid content, which corresponds to higher alcohol concentrations in their blood in comparison to men who have ingested the same amount of alcohol.[27, 28]

- Women have <u>decreased</u> *metabolism* of alcohol in the <u>stomach</u> and delayed gastric emptying, which increases the amount of alcohol that is absorbed into the blood.[24, 27]

- Women have <u>increased</u> metabolism of alcohol in the <u>liver</u>. This may increase the concentration of alcohol byproducts that can damage the liver.[24, 29]

- Estrogen, present in higher amounts in women, increases the presence of factors that cause injury and inflammation in the liver with alcohol byproducts present.[30]

Alcohol and hepatitis C are a dangerous combination, especially for women. Table 2 on the next page summarizes what is known about the effects of excess alcohol consumption on people living with HCV.

Table 2. Effects of Excess Alcohol Consumption in Persons Infected with HCV

HCV virus levels may increase by an average of 0.8 logs when consuming > 80g of alcohol a day.[31, 32]
There is significantly higher risk of progressing to cirrhosis in HCV patients who drink heavily when compared to those that do not drink.[21,33, 34]
Excess alcohol intake leads to a fatty liver and fat in the liver cells results in liver injury with inflammation and fibrosis.
Alcoholism increases the risk of liver cancer in HCV patients.[35, 36]
Alcohol use may reduce the effectiveness of HCV treatment.[32, 34, 37, 38] If the virus is cleared through treatment, alcohol usage may increases the risk of having a relapse or return of detectable virus after completing the treatment. [39]

THE TAKE-HOME MESSAGE:
Abstinence is the safest means of ensuring that alcohol does not contribute to the negative effects of HCV infection.
If alcohol is used, it is recommended that <u>no more</u> than 1 drink per day be consumed.
<u>12 oz of beer, 5oz of wine or 1oz of liquor = 14g of alcohol</u>

Fat in the Liver: Effect on HCV

There is an increasing rate of obesity in the United States. One way to evaluate obesity on a standard scale, is to identify a person's *body mass index* (BMI), which takes into account weight and height. The National Institutes of Health provides an online BMI calculator at www.nhlbisupport.com/bmi. Table 3 summarizes the interpretation of the BMI score.

Table 3. Interpretation of BMI

Under Weight	Healthy Weight	Overweight	Obese
BMI < 18.5	BMI is 18.6 – 24.9	BMI is 25 – 29.9	BMI > 30.0

Facts About Obesity and Women

- Women have a higher likelihood of developing obesity over their lifetime than men, even if their body weight was healthy during adolescence and young adulthood.

- Almost 63% of women in the United States are overweight and 33% are obese.[40, 41]

- Women have a 60% risk for obesity by age 35.[42] Obesity rates increase with age. Approximately 28% of adults aged 20 to 39 years were obese while 36.8% of adults aged 20 to 59 and 31% of those aged 60 years or older were obese.[41]

- As women age and progress through menopause their weight tends to increase, and there is high likelihood of being overweight or obese after menopause.[43, 44]

Being overweight or obese is associated with many health risks and diseases including liver disease. Excessive weight can cause a collection of fat to build up in the liver, a condition called *steatosis*. Steatosis can cause damage to the liver. Other conditions associated with the steatosis include type II diabetes, elevated levels of *triglycerides*, and certain medications.

Central or abdominal fat is associated with a higher rate of steatosis.[45] There are two ways fat is carried, either centrally (abdominally) or more evenly spread over the body. The body type that accumulates fat centrally has been described as "apple" shaped. The more generalized distribution is described as "pear" shaped. Figure 3 shows the differences between more central fat storage (apple shaped) and more generalize a spread over the body (pear shaped).

Figure 3. "Apple" and "pear" body types showing differences in excess fat storage

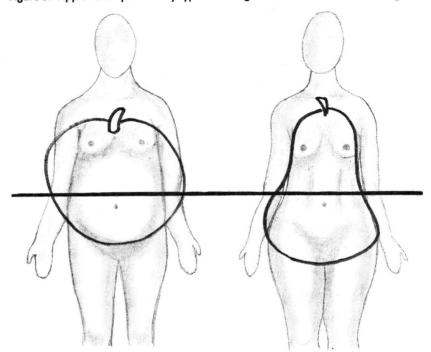

People with the "apple" body type (left) carry fat in the belly and upper body (in their middle). People with a "pear" body type (right) carry fat more below the waist in the hips, buttocks, and legs.

Several studies in HCV-infected persons have shown an association between the presence of steatosis and a higher degree of liver inflammation and fibrosis.[46, 47, 49, 50] It has been suggested that accumulated fat within a cell causes its early death, and is associated with increased inflammation and ultimately with increased damage to the liver and fibrosis.[51]

The cause of steatosis differs in individuals that are infected with different *genotypes* of HCV. There is a higher percentage of fat accumulation in the liver found with HCV genotype 3.[52] There has been an association with high virus levels in genotype 3, which indicates that the virus itself may be contributing to the fat collection.[49] In contrast, in individuals infected with HCV genotypes other than genotype 3, the fat in the liver is related to being overweight, having diabetes, or elevated triglycerides.

Obesity and steatosis in the liver can interfere with the effectiveness of hepatitis C treatment. With obesity, there is a greater body mass and this may reduce the amount of drug available in the body and impair the effectiveness of treatment.[52] There is a decreased rate of sustained virus clearance in individuals with excess fat in their liver (determined through *liver biopsies*) compared to those without excess liver fat.[47, 53, 54]

There is a higher risk for women to develop an unhealthy body weight with age, especially after menopause. Being overweight is a risk factor for worse disease outcome in HCV infection. Optimization of weight is an important issue for women infected with HCV. Data demonstrate that steatosis and inflammation in the liver can be reduced with even modest weight loss.[55] Individuals with a BMI greater than 30 are urged to actively participate in weight loss regimens or programs. Being at a healthy weight is important to prevent many diseases and to improve quality of life. However, it is crucial in an HCV-infected individual, since being at an unhealthy weight can worsen liver disease, increase the risk of complications, and affect treatment success.

HCV Treatment

The current standard treatment for *chronic hepatitis* C infection is a combination of *pegylated interferon* and *ribavirin*. Pegylated interferon is an injectable medication taken once a week. Ribavirin is an oral medication that is taken twice daily. These medications work by trying to stop the virus from entering into the liver cells and from making copies of themselves. The length of treatment depends on the HCV genotype. Studies have determined the appropriate length of treatment for different genotypes and the success rates of eliminating HCV.

The most important determinant of likelihood of success of treatment is HCV genotype. The most common genotypes in the United States are 1, 2 and 3. For genotype 1, 48 weeks of treatment is recommended. This provides a 40% to 50% chance of eliminating the virus. Genotype 2 and 3 HCV are more sensitive to current treatment and require a shorter duration of treatment, 24 weeks. The success rate of eliminating the virus is 70% to 80%. [56, 57]

Female sex has been associated with a higher likelihood of responding to HCV treatment in some but not all studies.[57-60] In those studies reporting a difference, women have a 10% to 20% higher likelihood of achieving viral clearance with pegylated interferon and ribavirin compared to men.[60]

There are several side effects associated with standard treatment and many patients report a temporary decline in their quality of life.[61] Once through treatment, individuals that have a *sustained viral response* report an improvement in their quality of life.[60, 62] The most common side effects of treatment include *fatigue*, muscle aches, joint aches, itchy rash, nausea, insomnia, and *depression*. The medication can also cause a decrease in blood cell counts, both *red blood cells* (*anemia*) and *white blood cells* (neutropenia). There are several ways to manage these side effects while on treatment.[64]

Certain side effects of the hepatitis C treatment affect women more frequently or severely than men.

- **Depression**
  Women are two times more likely to suffer from depression in the general population. HCV treatment is known to cause or worsen existing depression. It is more likely that women on treatment will have an issue with mood changes. Antidepressants are commonly used during HCV treatment to manage these symptoms.[63]

- **Sexual issues**
  Overall dryness is a common side effect of treatment - dry skin, dry eyes, dry mouth. Specifically for women, vaginal dryness can cause issues with sex. This can be managed with lubricating gels.[65]

- **Anemia**
  Women have a lower red blood cell count than men at the start of treatment and are therefore more likely to develop a decline in their blood counts that results in symptoms. Anemia can cause symptoms of fatigue, weakness, and *shortness of breath*. With the medication causing a decline in these counts, women can experience these symptoms earlier in treatment and more severely than men.

Special Considerations Related to Pregnancy and Treatment
HCV-infected women of childbearing age often seek guidance on the timing of *antiviral* therapy in the context of future pregnancy. The main reason for a woman to consider antiviral therapy prior to pregnancy is to eliminate the 5% risk of HCV transmission to the infant. However, antiviral therapy prior to pregnancy results in delays in the time to conception, and treatment is successful in at best a variable proportion of those treated. Most importantly, treatment cannot be taken during pregnancy or when breastfeeding.

Ribavirin is teratogenic (causes birth defects in the fetus) and its use in women and in their partners trying to conceive and in those pregnant is absolutely *contraindicated*. The effects of ribavirin are prolonged and it is necessary to wait six months after the last dose of ribavirin before trying to conceive.

Summary

Risk Factors for Acquiring HCV

- An uninfected woman is more likely to acquire HCV through sex from an infected man than vice versa.
- Women who are in sexual partnerships with injection drug users are at risk for acquiring HCV in the partnership by engaging in risky injection and sexual practices.
- There is a low risk of transmitting or becoming infected with HCV in monogamous partnerships.

Pregnancy

- There is a 5% chance that HCV can be passed from a HCV-infected mother to her child.
- There is no treatment to interrupt or prevent the transmission of HCV at the time of birth.
- Current HCV treatments <u>cannot</u> be taken while trying to conceive or during pregnancy as they are extremely harmful to the fetus.

Hormone Replacement Therapy

- Hormone replacement therapy can be taken by women with HCV.
- There are studies that suggest that estrogen use may be protective against developing cirrhosis and liver cancer.

Alcohol Usage

- Women are more susceptible to alcohol's effects on the liver and are at higher risk of developing cirrhosis than men drinking the same amounts of alcohol.
- It is recommended that women with HCV do not drink alcohol as it is not known if there is a safe level of alcohol intake. However, if a woman does drink, her intake should be a maximum of 1 drink per day.

Fatty Liver (Steatosis)

- Excess weight can lead to fat in the liver, which increases inflammation and liver damage. Fat in the liver is a risk factor for cirrhosis in HCV infected patients.
- Obesity and fat in the liver are associated with a decrease in the success rate of HCV treatment.

Hepatitis C Treatment

- Some studies suggest that women have a higher likelihood of achieving a sustained viral response to *interferon-based therapy*.
- Certain side effects of treatment (for example, depression and anemia) may occur more frequently or be more severe for women.

References

1. Thomas DL, Vlahov D, Solomon L, et al. Correlates of hepatitis C virus infections among injection drug users. *Medicine* (Baltimore). 1995;74(4):212-20.
2. Evans JL, Hahn JA, Page-Shafer K, et al. Gender differences in sexual and injection risk behavior among active young injection drug users in San Francisco (the UFO Study). *J Urban Health*. 2003;80(1):137-46.
3. Terrault NA. Sexual activity as a risk factor for hepatitis C. *Hepatology*. 2002;36(5 Suppl 1):S99-105.
4. Conte D, Fraquelli M, Prati D, et al. Prevalence and clinical course of chronic hepatitis C virus (HCV) infection and rate of HCV vertical transmission in a cohort of 15,250 pregnant women. *Hepatology*. 2000;31(3):751-5.
5. Dal Molin G, D'Agaro P, Ansaldi F, et al. Mother-to-infant transmission of hepatitis C virus: rate of infection and assessment of viral load and IgM anti-HCV as risk factors. *J Med Virol*. 2002;67(2):137-42.
6. Hillemanns P, Dannecker C, Kimmig R, et al. Obstetric risks and vertical transmission of hepatitis C virus infection in pregnancy. *Acta Obstet Gynecol Scand*. 2000;79(7):543-7.
7. Mast EE, Hwang LY, Seto DS, et al. Risk factors for perinatal transmission of hepatitis C virus (HCV) and the natural history of HCV infection acquired in infancy. *J Infect Dis*. 2005;192(11):1880-9.
8. European Pediatric Hepatitis C Network. A significant sex--but not elective cesarean section--effect on mother-to-child transmission of hepatitis C virus infection. *J Infect Dis*. 2005;192(11):1872-9.
9. Zanetti AR, Tanzi E, Romano L, et al. A prospective study on mother-to-infant transmission of hepatitis C virus. *Intervirology*. 1998;41(4-5):208-12.
10. Marine-Barjoan E, Berrebi A, Giordanengo V, et al. HCV/HIV co-infection, HCV viral load and mode of delivery: risk factors for mother-to-child transmission of hepatitis C virus? *AIDS*. 2007;21(13):1811-5.
11. Hayashida A, Inaba N, Oshima K, et al. Re-evaluation of the true rate of hepatitis C virus mother-to-child transmission and its novel risk factors based on our two prospective studies. *J Obstet Gynaecol Res*. 2007;33(4):417-22.
12. MMWR. Recommendations for prevention and control of hepatitis C virus (HCV) infection and HCV-related chronic disease. Centers for Disease Control and Prevention. *MMWR Recomm Rep*. 1998;47(RR-19):1-39.
13. Resti M, Jara P, Hierro L, et al. Clinical features and progression of perinatally acquired hepatitis C virus infection. *J Med Virol*. 2003;70(3):373-7.
14. Poynard T, Mathurin P, Lai CL, et al. A comparison of fibrosis progression in chronic liver diseases. *J Hepatol*. 2003;38(3):257-65.
15. Di Martino V, Lebray P, Myers RP, et al. Progression of liver fibrosis in women infected with hepatitis C: long-term benefit of estrogen exposure. *Hepatology*. 2004;40(6):1426-33.
16. Codes L, Asselah T, Cazals-Hatem D, et al. Liver fibrosis in women with chronic hepatitis C: evidence for the negative role of the menopause and steatosis and the potential benefit of hormone replacement therapy. *Gut*. 2007;56(3):390-5.
17. Kumar A, Sharma KA, Gupta RK, et al. Prevalence & risk factors for hepatitis C virus among pregnant women. *Indian J Med Res* 2007;126:211-5.
18. Yu MW, Chang HC, Chang SC, et al. Role of reproductive factors in hepatocellular carcinoma: Impact on hepatitis B- and C-related risk. *Hepatology*. 2003;38(6):1393-400.
19. Gitlin N, Korner P, Yang HM. Liver function in postmenopausal women on estrogen-androgen hormone replacement therapy: a meta-analysis of eight clinical trials. *Menopause*. 1999;6(3):216-24.
20. Bellentani S, Saccoccio G, Costa G, et al. Drinking habits as cofactors of risk for alcohol induced liver damage. The Dionysos Study Group. *Gut*. 1997;41(6):845-50.
21. Becker U, Deis A, Sorensen TI, et al. Prediction of risk of liver disease by alcohol intake, sex, and age: a prospective population study. *Hepatology*. 1996;23(5):1025-9.
22. Muller C. Liver, alcohol and gender. *Wien Med Wochenschr*. 2006;156(19-20):523-6.
23. Wagnerberger S, Schafer C, Schwarz E, et al. Is nutrient intake a gender-specific cause for enhanced susceptibility to alcohol-induced liver disease in women? *Alcohol*. 2008;43(1):9-14.
24. Baraona E, Abittan CS, Dohmen K, et al. Gender differences in pharmacokinetics of alcohol. *Alcohol Clin Exp Res*. 2001;25(4):502-7.
25. Peters MG, Terrault NA. Alcohol use and hepatitis C. *Hepatology*. 2002;36(5 Suppl 1):S220-225.
26. Hezode C, Lonjon I, Roudot-Thoraval F, et al. Impact of moderate alcohol consumption on histological activity and fibrosis in patients with chronic hepatitis C, and specific influence of steatosis: a prospective study. *Aliment Pharmacol Ther*. 2003;17(8):1031-7.
27. Frezza M, di Padova C, Pozzato G, et al. High blood alcohol levels in women. The role of decreased gastric alcohol dehydrogenase activity and first-pass metabolism. *N Engl J Med*. 1990;322(2):95-9.
28. Li TK, Beard JD, Orr WE, et al. Variation in ethanol pharmacokinetics and perceived gender and ethnic differences in alcohol elimination. *Alcohol Clin Exp Res*. 2000;24(4):415-6.
29. Thomasson H. Alcohol elimination: faster in women? *Alcohol Clin Exp Res*. 2000;24(4):419-20.
30. Thurman RG. Sex-related liver injury due to alcohol involves activation of Kupffer cells by endotoxin. *Can J Gastroenterol*. 2000;14 Suppl D:129D-135D.
31. Oshita M, Hayashi N, Kasahara A, et al. Increased serum hepatitis C virus RNA levels among alcoholic patients with chronic hepatitis C. *Hepatology*. 1994;20(5):1115-20.
32. Zhang T, Li Y, Lai JP, et al. Alcohol potentiates hepatitis C virus replicon expression. *Hepatology*. 2003;38(1):57-65.
33. Bellentani S, Tiribelli C, Saccoccio G, et al. Prevalence of chronic liver disease in the general population of northern Italy: the Dionysos Study. *Hepatology*. 1994;20(6):1442-9.
34. Loguercio C, Di Pierro M, Di Marino MP, et al. Drinking habits of subjects with hepatitis C virus-related chronic liver disease: prevalence and effect on clinical, virological and pathological aspects. *Alcohol Alcohol*. 2000;35(3):296-301.
35. Khan KN, Yatsuhashi H. Effect of alcohol consumption on the progression of hepatitis C virus infection and risk of hepatocellular carcinoma

in Japanese patients. *Alcohol Alcohol.* 2000;35(3):286-95.

36. Kumar M, Kumar R, Hissar SS, et al. Risk factors analysis for hepatocellular carcinoma in patients with and without cirrhosis: a case-control study of 213 hepatocellular carcinoma patients from India. *J Gastroenterol Hepatol.* 2007;22(7):1104-11.

37. Okazaki T, Yoshihara H, Suzuki K, et al. Efficacy of interferon therapy in patients with chronic hepatitis C. Comparison between non-drinkers and drinkers. *Scand J Gastroenterol.* 1994;29(11):1039-43.

38. Ohnishi K, Matsuo S, Matsutani K, et al. Interferon therapy for chronic hepatitis C in habitual drinkers: comparison with chronic hepatitis C in infrequent drinkers. *Am J Gastroenterol.* 1996;91(7):1374-9.

39. Tabone M, Sidoli L, Laudi C, et al. Alcohol abstinence does not offset the strong negative effect of lifetime alcohol consumption on the outcome of interferon therapy. *J Viral Hepat.* 2002;9(4):288-94.

40. Morin KH, Stark MA, Searing K. Obesity and nutrition in women throughout adulthood. *J Obstet Gynecol Neonatal Nurs.* 2004;33(6):823-32.

41. Ogden CL, Carroll MD, Curtin LR, et al. Prevalence of overweight and obesity in the United States, 1999-2004. *JAMA.* 2006;295(13):1549-55.

42. McTigue KM, Garrett JM, Popkin BM. The natural history of the development of obesity in a cohort of young U.S. adults between 1981 and 1998. *Ann Intern Med.* 2002;136(12):857-64.

43. Dubnov G, Brzezinski A, Berry EM. Weight control and the management of obesity after menopause: the role of physical activity. *Maturitas.* 2003;44(2):89-101.

44. Pasquali R, Casimirri F, Labate AM, et al. Body weight, fat distribution and the menopausal status in women. The VMH Collaborative Group. *Int J Obes Relat Metab Disord.* 1994;18(9):614-21.

45. Adinolfi LE, Gambardella M, Andreana A, et al. Steatosis accelerates the progression of liver damage of chronic hepatitis C patients and correlates with specific HCV genotype and visceral obesity. *Hepatology.* 2001;33(6):1358-64.

46. Asselah T, Boyer N, Guimont MC, et al. Liver fibrosis is not associated with steatosis but with necroinflammation in French patients with chronic hepatitis C. *Gut.* 2003;52(11):1638-43.

47. Patton HM, Patel K, Behling C, et al. The impact of steatosis on disease progression and early and sustained treatment response in chronic hepatitis C patients. *J Hepatol.* 2004;40(3):484-90.

48. Powell EE, Jonsson JR, Clouston AD. Steatosis: co-factor in other liver diseases. *Hepatology.* 2005;42(1):5-13.

49. Rubbia-Brandt L, Quadri R, Abid K, et al. Hepatocyte steatosis is a cytopathic effect of hepatitis C virus genotype 3. *J Hepatol.* 2000;33(1):106-15.

50. Fartoux L, Chazouilleres O, Wendum D, et al. Impact of steatosis on progression of fibrosis in patients with mild hepatitis C. *Hepatology.* 2005;41(1):82-7.

51. Feldstein AE, Canbay A, Angulo P, et al. Hepatocyte apoptosis and fas expression are prominent features of human nonalcoholic steatohepatitis. *Gastroenterology.* 2003;125(2):437-43.

52. Asselah T, Rubbia-Brandt L, Marcellin P, et al. Steatosis in chronic hepatitis C: why does it really matter? *Gut.* 2006;55(1):123-30.

53. Soresi M, Tripi S, Franco V, et al. Impact of liver steatosis on the antiviral response in the hepatitis C virus-associated chronic hepatitis. *Liver Int.* 2006;26(9):1119-25.

54. Thomopoulos KC, Theocharis GJ, Tsamantas AC, et al. Liver steatosis is an independent risk factor for treatment failure in patients with chronic hepatitis C. *Eur J Gastroenterol Hepatol.* 2005;17(2):149-53.

55. Hickman IJ, Clouston AD, Macdonald GA, et al. Effect of weight reduction on liver histology and biochemistry in patients with chronic hepatitis C. *Gut.* 2002;51(1):89-94.

56. Hadziyannis SJ, Sette H, Jr., Morgan TR, et al. Peginterferon-alpha2a and ribavirin combination therapy in chronic hepatitis C: a randomized study of treatment duration and ribavirin dose. *Ann Intern Med.* 2004;140(5):346-55.

57. Fried MW, Shiffman ML, Reddy KR, et al. Peginterferon alfa-2a plus ribavirin for chronic hepatitis C virus infection. *N Engl J Med.* 2002;347(13):975-82.

58. Akuta N, Suzuki F, Kawamura Y, et al. Predictors of viral kinetics to peginterferon plus ribavirin combination therapy in Japanese patients infected with hepatitis C virus genotype 1b. *J Med Virol.* 2007;79(11):1686-95.

59. Akuta N, Suzuki F, Kawamura Y, et al. Predictive factors of early and sustained responses to peginterferon plus ribavirin combination therapy in Japanese patients infected with hepatitis C virus genotype 1b: amino acid substitutions in the core region and low-density lipoprotein cholesterol levels. *J Hepatol.* 2007;46(3):403-10.

60. Conjeevaram HS, Fried MW, Jeffers LJ, et al. Peginterferon and ribavirin treatment in African American and Caucasian American patients with hepatitis C genotype 1. *Gastroenterology.* 2006;131(2):470-7.

61. Mathew A, Peiffer LP, Rhoades K, et al. Improvement in quality of life measures in patients with refractory hepatitis C, responding to re-treatment with Pegylated interferon alpha -2b and ribavirin. *Health Qual Life Outcomes.* 2006;4:30.

62. Larrey D, Couzigou P, Denis J. [Chronic hepatitis C: management of side effects of treatment]. *Gastroenterol Clin Biol.* 2007;31(8-9 Pt 3):4S20-8.

63. Fried MW. Side effects of therapy of hepatitis C and their management. *Hepatology.* 2002;36(5 Suppl 1):S237-44.

64. Palmer M. Women's Issues With Hepatitis C - Side Effect Management. 2004 [cited 2008 January 10]; Available from: http://www.liverdisease.com/womenhcv.html

65. Bonkovsky HL, Snow KK, Malet PF, et al. Health-related quality of life in patients with chronic hepatitis C and advanced fibrosis. *J Hepatol* 2007;46(3):420-31.

HEPATITIS C IN CHILDREN

Aparna Roy, MD, MPH and Kathleen Schwarz, MD

Introduction

Hepatitis C virus (*HCV*) infection of the liver can occur during childhood and creates many problems and concerns for both the infected children and their families. The purpose of this chapter is to discuss:

- ways that children contract hepatitis C
- the type of liver damage that can occur
- the types of treatment available
- special questions related to hepatitis C in mothers and/or in children such as breastfeeding and school entry

Although there are many challenges for children with hepatitis C infection, families should know that there are a number of pediatric liver disease specialists (pediatric *gastroenterologists*) who are working on solutions to these problems. There are also several sources of information about HCV for families. These are listed in the *Resource Directory*.

Hepatitis C Testing

As with any other area of knowledge in medicine, there is a special vocabulary doctors use in discussing hepatitis C infection. One easy way to screen individuals for hepatitis C is with a blood *antibody* test, usually referred to as *anti-HCV*. A positive antibody test usually indicates that the individual has been infected with the hepatitis C virus and that the person's *immune system* has attempted to get rid of the infection. (See *Chapter 6, Laboratory Tests and Procedures* for more information about hepatitis C antibody testing.) Unfortunately, hepatitis C antibodies are not usually very effective and many people who are anti-HCV positive are still infected with the virus. This is known as viral "persistence."

HCV belongs to a group of viruses called *RNA* viruses (the virus made out of a type of chemical called *ribonucleic acid*). To check for the presence of the hepatitis C virus itself (not the antibody) in the blood, an *HCV RNA* test is used. This test is known by several different names including an HCV molecular test, *HCV PCR*, *HCV TMA*, and HCV *viral load*. (See *Chapter 6, Laboratory Tests and Procedures* for more information about hepatitis C virus testing.)

Hepatitis C Testing in Newborns

Mothers with hepatitis C are usually anti-HCV positive and frequently pass this antibody to their offspring. However, most anti-HCV positive newborns are <u>not</u> actually infected with the hepatitis C virus. The hepatitis C antibodies showing up in the newborn's blood are most often the mother's antibodies that were passed to the baby before birth.

> **Most babies born to mothers with hepatitis C do <u>not</u> have hepatitis C.**
> A baby born to a mother with hepatitis C will probably have antibodies to the virus for the first 12 to 18 months of life. That is, the baby will have a positive hepatitis C antibody test (also known as anti-HCV). But this does <u>not</u> necessarily mean the baby has the hepatitis C virus.

Newborns lose the antibodies from their mothers over time. Most maternal (from the mother) antibodies are no longer detectable in the baby by around 18 months of age. In the case of hepatitis C antibodies, if anti-HCV is still present at 18 months of age, then it is much more likely that the infant is actually infected with the hepatitis C virus. An HCV molecular test is often performed to confirm the presence of HCV in the blood if the anti-HCV test remains positive at 18 months.

Routes of Transmissions and Prevalence of HCV in Children

It is believed that between 68,000 to 100,000 children in the U.S. have *chronic hepatitis* C.[1, 2] However, certain information on hepatitis C virus infection in children is lacking.[3, 4]

The ways in which children become infected with HCV have changed over the past several years. Before 1990, HCV infection in children was mostly due to transfusion of blood or products derived from blood (for example, anti-hemophiliac factor, factor IX, or intravenous *immune globulin*). Screening of blood and its products for the presence of HCV in the last 10 years has drastically decreased this type of transmission. Since 1990 infections in children are primarily caused by transmission from mothers who have chronic hepatitis C.[5]

Mother-to-Child Transmission of HCV

Overall, the risk of HCV transmission from an infected mother to her newborn infant is only about 5%. However, more than one out of every 100 women of childbearing age may be infected with HCV. Therefore, mother-to-child transmission may contribute to a substantial number of cases of new HCV infections in children worldwide.[2]

Overall, the risk of HCV transmission from an infected mother to her newborn infant is only about 5%.

The risk of mother-to-child transmission of HCV also depends on a number of additional maternal, socioeconomic, and geographic factors. The risk of mother-to-child transmission (also called vertical transmission) of HCV depends on the HCV viral load of the mother, and whether she also has HIV. In a recent study among mothers with hepatitis C, the rate of transmission among hepatitis C infected mothers who also had HIV (*human immunodeficiency virus*) was 25.0% [6] compared to 3.8% in mothers who did not have HIV. A high HCV viral load in the mother has also been found to increase the risk of HCV transmission.[7] However, elective Cesarean section is not recommended for women with chronic HCV infection alone.[8]

Natural History of Hepatitis C in Children

Evidence suggests that hepatitis C disease is relatively mild and usually does not cause symptoms in infected children. The rate of liver damage can vary depending on whether the child was infected by the mother or by a blood transfusion. Generally, transfusion-related infection in children with blood disorders such as hemophilia, thalassemia, or leukemia may differ according to the underlying disease. When infection is acquired from the mother, most children only show a signs of mild liver disease for the first one to two decades of life.

There are also many cases of *spontaneous clearance* where an HCV RNA positive infant becomes negative for the virus.[6] The spontaneous clearance of HCV appears to be more common in children than among adults, especially those past the age of 40.

Severe liver disease leading to *cirrhosis*, *liver cancer*, and/or *liver failure* requiring liver transplantation can occur during childhood but is very rare. Children infected with HCV probably do have some risk of developing these serious liver diseases in adulthood, but the exact risks are not known at the present time.

Liver Biopsy in Children

Microscopic characteristics of liver tissue obtained by a biopsy indicate the extent of damage to the liver by the hepatitis C virus as well as the body's immune response to the virus. Changes in the liver cells are typically mild in children. These changes may include swelling (*inflammation*), and death of cells (*necrosis*).

Sometimes permanent replacement of liver cells with scars made of fibrous tissue (*fibrosis*) may be seen. This fibrosis may progress with age and duration of infection. Permanent replacement of the liver cells with fibrous tissue may, in the long run, harm the many functions of the liver, which include the production of proteins related to blood clotting and to processing of medications. [9-12]

Hepatitis C Treatment in Children

There are several factors to consider when discussing treatment of children with chronic HCV infection, including the wide variation of the course of the disease in children as well as lack of definitive information on the safety and effectiveness of drugs in children. Although the issue of who is best treated has not be completely resolved, based on available data, the combination of *interferon* plus *ribavirin* is recommended by the American Association for the Study of Liver Disease for children with HCV who are considered appropriate candidates. The combination of interferon plus ribavirin has been approved by the U.S. Food and Drug Administration (FDA) for use in children 3 to 18 years of age.

Interferon Monotherapy

Alfa-interferon is FDA approved for use in children. How this drug acts is not definitely known, but it stimulates the body's immune response to the hepatitis C virus. Several studies in children have shown that the response rates are better and the side effects are less severe in children compared to adults.[13] The overall sustained viral response (SVR) with standard interferon in children is 36% compared to 10% to 15% in adults. For *genotype* 1, the SVR in children is reported to be 27% compared to 8% to 10% for adults when treated with standard interferon.[13]

Pegylated interferon is a long-acting form of interferon, which only has to be given once per week compared to standard interferon, which has to be given at least 3 times per week. Since treatment with pegylated interferon produces higher SVR's in both adults and children, standard interferon has largely been abandoned as a treatment for HCV in children. Interferon has many side effects including flu-like symptoms, appetite loss, depression, fever, and depression of both white cell and red blood cell counts, all of which are fairly common. More rarely, interferon can cause thyroid disease, *autoimmune* disease, and/or visual problems.

Pegylated Interferon Monotherapy

A small pilot study of *pegylated interferon*-alfa 2a in 14 children (2 to 8 years of age, all but one infected with genotype 1) showed an overall SVR of 43%.[14] The drug was generally well tolerated, but several children developed low white blood cell counts. It is clear that further studies in children with this drug should be done before it can be routinely prescribed. There are two forms of pegylated interferon, and neither of them are FDA-approved for children at the present time (April 2008).

Inteferon Plus Ribavirin

Ribavirin in combination with interferon is more effective for the treatment of HCV in adults compared to each drug when given alone. Interferon plus ribavirin is the FDA approved regimen for treatment of HCV in children aged 3 to 18 years. A recent study found the combination of interferon-alfa 2b in combination with ribavirin in 270 children was effective and safe. The overall SVR was 46%, and SVR for genotype 1 was 36%.[15]

Pegylated Interferon Plus Ribavirin

Pegylated interferon plus ribavirin is the standard of care for adults with chronic HCV infection. To date, only three studies have published the results of pegylated interferon *combination therapy* in children, and all have been performed using pegylated interferon alfa-2b and ribavirin. The largest of these studies (61 children) lends support to the idea that the combination of pegylated interferon plus ribavirin in children will offer the good response rates seen in adults with chronic HCV.[16] "PEDS C" is a multi-center, randomized, controlled trial in 112 children evaluating the safety and effectiveness of 6 to 12 months of pegylated interferon with or without ribavirin.[17] The study should answer whether it is beneficial to add ribavirin to pegylated interferon for the treatment of HCV in children. Because ribavirin can cause birth defects when taken by pregnant females and since children with HCV infection appear to respond better to interferon-based *therapies* than adults do, this question is very important.

To Treat or Not to Treat?

Given present knowledge about the disease, there is enough evidence to treat selected children with chronic HCV infection.

- Children in the 3 to 4 year age group should be considered for treatment before they enter school. The only FDA-approved therapy for this group is the combination of interferon given thrice weekly plus ribavirin (which fortunately is available as a syrup).

- Therapy for children in the 5 to 18 year age group should be individualized. Until the results of PEDS C are available, many authorities would reserve treatment for children with aggressive liver disease.

  - Children 5 to 12 years of age could be treated with the FDA-approved combination of interferon and ribavirin.

  - Off-label use of pegylated interferon could be considered for adolescents, but the treating physician must monitor patients very carefully for side effects such as low white blood cell counts.

There are certain conditions in childhood for which there is little information to guide therapy other than the experience in adults. These conditions include organ or bone marrow transplant, autoimmune diseases including HCV with autoimmune hepatitis, kidney failure, and/or significant disease in another organ system.

Special Pediatric Issues

Pregnancy and HCV Transmission

Pregnant women at risk for HCV infection should be screened for antibodies to HCV (anti-HCV), and HCV RNA testing should be performed if anti-HCV is positive.

Infants born to women with hepatitis C should be tested for anti-HCV at 18 months of age.[18] If the antibody test is positive, HCV RNA testing should be done. If the HCV RNA test is positive, the infant should be referred to a specialist in pediatric liver disease.

Breastfeeding

Currently there is no evidence of mother-to-infant transmission of HCV infection from breastfeeding. According to guidelines from the Centers for Disease Control and Prevention and the American Academy of Pediatrics, maternal HCV infection is not a *contraindication* to breastfeeding. However, the mother should consider not breastfeeding the child if her nipples are cracked and bleeding.[19]

Parenting Issues

Multiple important issues surround parenting with a child with HCV. Women may be particularly concerned about social stigma, sexual transmission, pregnancy, and childcare. These worries may affect their close relationships [20] as well as their ability to take care of their child. Additionally, there might be concerns about the risk of HCV transmission in a household with a chronically infected individual such as a parent or sibling. The HCV infection risk to uninfected children living in the same household of people with chronic hepatitis C is believed to be very low.[4] Blood-to-blood contact should be avoided by <u>not</u> sharing personal hygiene items such as toothbrushes, razors, cuticle scissors, or any other item that may be contaminated with blood. Any blood from an infected person (even dried blood) should be cleaned with a 10% bleach solution (one part bleach to 9 parts water).

> **Hepatitis C is <u>not</u> spread through sharing the same dishes, drinking glasses, silverware, or pots and pans. Hepatitis C is <u>not</u> spread through food.**

HCV in Children With Blood Disorders

HCV infection has been demonstrated in 50% to 98% of children with hemophilia treated with factor concentrates prepared from pooled plasma. Furthermore, there is clear evidence that HCV infection is associated with liver disease in children with hemophilia.[21-24] There is evidence for similar trends in children with thalassemia.[25-27]

Vaccines and HCV

There is currently no *vaccine* to prevent the transmission of HCV. However, children with chronic HCV should be vaccinated against the hepatitis A and *hepatitis B* viruses.[28]

School Issues and Social Stigma

No studies have been performed to date examining the effects of having HCV infection on health-related quality of life or normal childhood development. However, the PEDS C study (currently underway) is examining these issues.

With regard to children's knowledge of hepatitis C, one study conducted in Australia found students' knowledge about HCV to be extremely poor.[29] In the authors' experience, there are significant schooling issues that stem from the infection and the effects of the treatment used. These include missed school days as well as risk of loss of privacy.

In addition to concerns about serious liver disease, children and their families often face the added burden of social stigma, especially when it comes to entry into day care or school. Fortunately, the American Academy of Pediatrics has provided guidelines to ease this burden stating there is <u>no</u> reason to exclude children with HCV from entry into day care and school.[18]

Summary

Hepatitis C (HCV) is an important public health issue that includes both children and adults. An estimated 68,000 to 100,000 children in the U.S. have chronic hepatitis C. Since hepatitis C blood screening procedures have been put in place, children are primarily infected at the time of birth from mothers who have chronic hepatitis C.

Available evidence suggests that chronic hepatitis C is relatively mild and is usually *asymptomatic* in infected children. Rarely, however, severe disease leading to cirrhosis, liver cancer, and liver failure requiring liver transplantation may occur during childhood and adolescence.

Interferon with ribavirin is the FDA-approved regimen for treatment of HCV in children aged 3 to 18 years. It has been found effective and safe in children with chronic hepatitis C virus. Pegylated interferon may, in the future, offer response rates similar to that seen in adults with chronic HCV. However, pegylated interferon is not currently FDA-approved for use in children. Whether it will be necessary to add ribavirin to the treatment regime is not known at present. There is presently no hepatitis C vaccine, but children with HCV should be immunized against the hepatitis A and hepatitis B viruses.

References

1. Alter, MJ. Epidemiology of hepatitis C. *Hepatology*. 1997; 26(3 Suppl 1): 62S-65S.
2. Alter, MJ. D Kruszon-Moran, et al. The prevalence of hepatitis C virus infection in the United States, 1988 through 1994. *N Engl J Med* 1999;341(8):556-62.
3. Gonzalez-Peralta, RP. Hepatitis C virus infection in pediatric patients. *Clin Liver Dis.* 1997;1(3): 691-705, ix.
4. Jonas, M. M. Children with hepatitis C. *Hepatology*. 2002;36(5 Suppl 1):S173-8.
5. Bortolotti, F., M. Resti, et al. Changing epidemiologic pattern of chronic hepatitis C virus infection in Italian children. *J Pediatr.* 1998:133(3): 378-81.
6. Mast EE, Hwang LY, Seto DS, et al. Risk factors for perinatal transmission of hepatitis C virus (HCV) and the natural history of HCV infection acquired in infancy. *J Infect Dis*. 2005:Dec 1;192(11):1880-9 Epub 2005 Oct 28.
7. Newell ML, Pembrey L. Mother-to-child transmission of hepatitis C virus infection. *Drugs Today* (Barc). 2002:May;38(5):321-37.
8. Roberts EA, Yeung L. Maternal-infant transmission of hepatitis C virus infection. *Hepatology*. 2002:Nov;36(5 Supl 1):S106-13.
9. Kage, M., T. Fujisawa, et al. Pathology of chronic hepatitis C in children. Child Liver Study Group of Japan. *Hepatology*. 1997:26(3): 771-5.
10. Badizadegan K, Jonas MM, et al. . Histopathology of the liver in children with chronic hepatitis C viral infection. *Hepatology*. 1998:28(5): 1416-23.
11. Guido, M., F. Bortolotti, et al. Fibrosis in chronic hepatitis C acquired in infancy: is it only a matter of time? *Am J Gastroenterol*. 2003:98(3): 660-3.
12. Guido, M., M. Rugge, et al. Chronic hepatitis C in children: the pathological and clinical spectrum. *Gastroenterology*. 1998:115(6): 1525-9.
13. Jacobson KR, Murray K, Zellos A, et al. An analysis of published trials of interferon monotherapy in children with chronic hepatitis C. *J Pediatr Gastroenterol Nutr*. 2002:Jan;34(1):52-8.
14. Schwarz KB, Mohan P, Narkewicz MR, et al. Safety, efficacy and pharmacokinetics of peginterferon alpha2a (40 kd) in children with chronic hepatitis C. *J Pediatr Gastroenterol Nutr*. 2006;43(4):499-505.
15. Gonzales-Peralta, RP, Kelly DA, Haber B, et al. Interferon Alfa-2b in Combination with Ribavirin for the Treatment of Chronic Hepatitis C in Children: Efficacy, Safety, and Pharmacokinetics. *Hepatology,* 2005;42(5):1010-18.
16. Wirth S, Pieper-Boustani H, Lang T, et al. Peginterferon alfa-2b Plus Ribavirin Treatment in Children and Adolescents with Chronic Hepatitis C. *Hepatology,* May 2005:41(5);1013-18.
17. Maryland Medical Research Institute. PEDS-C: A Clinical Trial for Children with Hepatitis C. Available at: http://www.pedsc.org/. Accessed September 18, 2008.
18. Hepatitis C virus infection. American Academy of Pediatrics. Committee on Infectious Diseases. *Pediatrics* 1998:101(3 Pt 1): 481-5.
19. Mast EE. Mother-to-infant hepatitis C virus transmission and breastfeeding. *Adv Exp Med Biol* 2004:554: 211-6.
20. Teixeira MC, Ribeiro MF, Gayotto LC, et al. Worse quality of life in volunteer blood donors with hepatitis C. *Transfusion*. 2006:Feb;45(2)278-83.
21. Blanchette, V. S., E. Vorstman, et al. Hepatitis C infection in children with hemophilia A and B. *Blood*. 1991:78(2): 285-9.
22. Leslie, D E, Rann S, et al. Prevalence of hepatitis C antibodies in patients with clotting disorders in Victoria. Relationship with other blood borne viruses and liver disease. *Med J Aust*. 1992: 156(11): 789-92.
23. Kanesaki, T., S. Kinoshita, et al. Hepatitis C virus infection in children with hemophilia: characterization of antibody response to four different antigens and relationship of antibody response, viremia, and hepatic dysfunction. *J Pediatr* 1993:123(3): 381-7.
24. Wagner N, and Rotthauwe HW. Hepatitis C contributes to liver disease in children and adolescents with hemophilia. *Klin Padiatr*. 1994:206(1): 40-4.
25. Lai, M. E., S. De Virgilis, et al. Evaluation of antibodies to hepatitis C virus in a long-term prospective study of post transfusion hepatitis among thalassemic children: comparison between first- and second-generation assay. *J Pediatr Gastroenterol Nutr* 1993:16(4): 458-64.
26. Lai, ME, Mazzoleni AP, et al. Hepatitis C virus in multiple episodes of acute hepatitis in polytransfused thalassaemic children. *Lancet* 1994:343(8894): 388-90.
27. Ni YH, Chang MH, et al. Hepatitis C viral infection in thalassemic children: clinical and molecular studies. *Pediatr Res* 1996 39(2): 323-8.
28. Arankvalle, VA, Chadha MS. Who should receive hepatitis A vaccine? *J Viral Hepat*. 2003: May;10(3):157-8.
29. Lindsay J, Smith Am, Rosenthal DA. Uncertain knowledge: a national survey of high school students' knowledge and beliefs about hepatitis C. *Aust N Z J Public Health*. 1999:Apr;23(2):135-9.

HCV / HIV Coinfection

Misha Cohen, OMD, LAc and Tina M. St. John, MD

SECTION

Overview of HIV / HCV Coinfection

Introduction

Both the *human immunodeficiency virus* (*HIV*) and the *hepatitis C virus* (*HCV*) are blood-borne infections. A significant number of people are chronically infected with both HIV and HCV, a condition known as coinfection. The widespread use of increasingly effective *antiviral* therapies for HIV has greatly improved long-term survival among HIV-infected persons. As HIV survival has improved, HCV-related illness and deaths have increased among coinfected persons.[1-3] In recent years, increasing numbers of people coinfected with HIV and HCV are dying from HCV-related complications rather than HIV disease. End-stage liver disease related to HCV is considered by many HIV specialists to be the leading cause of death in HIV-positive people in the United States.[4] Coinfection has a heavier impact on certain communities, including those who are incarcerated and communities of color.[5]

The management of HIV/AIDS and *chronic hepatitis* C is complicated by the presence of the other virus. Researchers are actively studying the most effective approaches for managing coinfection. This section presents an overview of our current knowledge about how HIV and HCV influence one another in people coinfected with both viruses.

Prevalence of HCV, HIV, and HCV/HIV Coinfection

HCV infection is the most common chronic, blood-borne infection in the United States having infected an estimated 4.9 million people.[6] The World Health Organization (WHO) estimates that about 180 million people, some 3% of the world's population, are infected with hepatitis C virus (HCV). WHO further states that 130 million are chronic HCV carriers at risk of developing liver *cirrhosis* and/or *liver cancer*. It is estimated that 3 to 4 million persons are newly infected each year, 70% of whom will develop chronic hepatitis. HCV is responsible for 50% to 76% of all liver cancer cases, and 2/3 of all liver transplants in the developed world.[7]

According to the 2007 AIDS Epidemic Update, global HIV prevalence has leveled off and the number of new infections has fallen in recent years. In 2007, an estimated 33.2 million people worldwide were living with HIV (down from the 40 million estimated in 2003)[8] including an estimated 1.2 million people in the United States.[9]

Although different studies have arrived at varying numbers, most experts now believe that up to 30% of HIV-infected persons in the U.S. are coinfected with HCV.[10-12] An estimated 5% to 10% of Americans living with HCV are also infected with HIV.[12] More than 90% of hemophiliacs treated with blood products during the 1970's and 1980's became infected with HCV.[13] A study in 1998 found more than 80% of hemophiliacs over 18 years of age are infected with HCV.[14] Between 60% to 85% of adult hemophiliacs are coinfected with HIV and HCV.[15] An estimated 50% to 98% of people who acquired HIV though injection drug use are coinfected with HCV.[15] Recent studies at diverse locations and in diverse populations showed a disturbing new trend in increasing sexual transmission among men who have sex with men in HIV-positive populations.[16-18] Prior to these reports, sexual transmission of HCV was considered relatively rare.

Effects of HIV on the Natural History of Chronic Hepatitis C

Immune Response to HCV and Spontaneous Viral Clearance

The *immune system* responds to viral infection with two types of responses, a cellular response and a *humoral immunity* (*antibody*) response (see Figure 1). Cellular responses involve special *white blood cells* called *T cells*. Different kinds of T cells have different actions that help the body fight viral infection.

Humoral responses are antibody responses. Antibodies are proteins produced in response to substances the body sees as foreign such as bacteria and viruses. Antibodies are produced by white blood cells called mature *B cells* or plasma cells. Interestingly, B cells must interact with helper T cells to mature into plasma cells and begin antibody production (see Figure 2). Antibodies tag foreign invaders and cells infected by viruses or bacteria. This alerts the rest of the immune system to the presence of the invader and often leads to the destruction of the viruses, bacteria, or infected cells.

On average, 15% to 30% of people infected with HCV alone spontaneously clear the virus without consequence.[19] However, data suggest that only 5% to 10% of people with HIV spontaneously clear HCV.[20] Further, the likelihood of *spontaneous clearance* of the virus seems to decrease as the number of *T helper cells* decrease.[19-21] T helper cells are the primary target of HIV. They are killed off when HIV infection is untreated or poorly controlled. Therefore, people with well-controlled HIV disease generally have higher T helper (*CD4*) cell counts than those whose disease is poorly controlled.

Normally, people infected with HCV begin producing antibodies to the virus within several weeks after infection. Screening tests for hepatitis C detect *anti-HCV antibodies*. In recent years, researchers have found a very small number of people with apparently normal immune systems who are chronically infected with HCV but do not have any

Figure 1. Types of Immune Responses

Cellular Response	Humoral (Antibody) Response
T lymphocytes (T cells) – there are 3 types	B lymphocytes (B cells)
• T helpers (CD4 cells)	
• T suppressors	B cells interact with T helper cells and mature into
• Killer T cells (NK cells)	plasma cells that produce antibodies.

Figure 2. T and B Cell Interactions Leading to Antibody Production

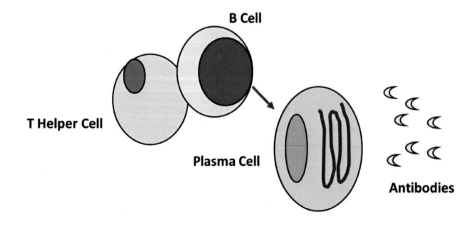

detectable antibodies to the virus.[22-24] This appears to be a very rare situation, and researchers are actively investigating why it occurs.

While the presence of HCV without detectable anti-HCV antibodies is quite rare in people with normal immune systems, it appears to occur in 5% to 19% of people coinfected with HIV.[25, 26] Scientists believe this is probably due to the devastating effects HIV has on the immune system and the loss of CD4 cells. This notion is supported by the fact that generally, people who lack HCV antibodies have lower levels of CD4 immune cells than HIV-infected people who have HCV antibodies.[26] This concept is further supported by recent data that show higher T cell activity improves the chance of spontaneous clearance of HCV among those with HIV.[27]

Effects of HIV on HCV Disease Progression

HCV *viral loads* are significantly higher in the blood and livers of coinfected people compared to people with HCV alone.[28-30] While high HCV viral loads have been correlated with decreased response rates to *interferon-based therapy*, the effect (if any) of viral load on the progression of HCV-related liver disease among coinfected persons is undetermined.[31]

Evidence from multiple studies indicates HIV accelerates the progression of HCV-related liver disease.[32-36] A study of 547 people found the time from infection to cirrhosis was substantially shorter (7 years) in people coinfected with HIV compared to people with HCV alone (23 years).[31] Another 3-year study of 489 people found 8.4% of coinfected persons had *liver failure* (*decompensation*) compared to no cases among those with HCV only.[37] These findings are supported by a separate study that found the rate of *fibrosis* progression (liver scarring) was much faster in HCV/HIV coinfected people than in those with HCV only.[38] A group of eight studies that examined the effects of HIV on HCV-related disease progression were analyzed collectively. Researchers found that compared to people infected with HCV only, coinfected persons had twice the risk for cirrhosis and approximately six times the risk for liver failure (decompensation).[35] As in people infected with HCV alone, several studies have shown that *alcohol* consumption further accelerates the already rapid liver disease progression in those with HCV/HIV coinfection.[39]

People with HCV/HIV coinfection should avoid <u>any</u> alcohol consumption.

Coinfection may also increase the risk of liver cancer.[36] When liver cancer does occur in HCV/HIV patients, it tends to present at a younger age than in those with other causes of underlying cirrhosis.[40, 41]

Effects of HAART on HCV Disease Progression

It is important to note that the studies demonstrating accelerated disease progression associated with HIV coinfection were performed or involved data collected before the widespread use of highly active antiretroviral therapy (HAART) for HIV.

HAART was introduced in 1996 and was a substantial breakthrough in the treatment of HIV infection. For many people, HAART has transformed HIV infection from an imminent life-threatening illness to a condition more akin to a chronic disease. With HAART, HIV is often reduced to an undetectable level and T cell counts generally rebound substantially. Since the introduction of HAART, HIV-related death rates have dropped substantially and survival time has increased dramatically. While serious infections and related deaths have declined steadily in the HIV-infected population since the introduction of HAART, death rates from HCV-related illnesses have been quickly and consistently increasing (see Table 1).[2, 33, 42-46]

Table 1. Mortality Rates Due to End-Stage Liver Disease Among HCV/HIV Coinfected Persons[31]

1987 - 1995	1997 - 2000
1.6 – 13%	7.8 – 50%

In short, the introduction of HAART has enabled HCV/HIV coinfected people to live long enough to experience the effects of chronic hepatitis C. Overall, HAART also slows the progression of HCV disease in coinfected patients (compared to patients with ART or untreated).[47, 48] One study of 182 HCV/HIV coinfected people found the fibrosis stage on *liver biopsy* was lower in people who had been on *combination therapy* with a *protease inhibitor* (one of the drugs used in HAART) compared to people who had never taken a protease inhibitor. The estimated cirrhosis rates at 5, 15, and 25 years post-HVC infection are shown in Table 2.

Table 2. Estimated Cirrhosis Rates in HCV/HIV Coinfected People[49]

Years Since Infection	With Protease Inhibitors	Without Protease Inhibitors
5	2%	5%
15	5%	18%
25	9%	27%

Benhamou Y, Di Martino V, Bochet M *et al.* Factors affecting liver fibrosis in human immunodeficiency virus-and hepatitis C virus-coinfected patients: impact of protease inhibitor therapy. *Hepatology.* 2001;34(2):283-7.

Effects of HAART on HCV Viral Load and Liver Enzymes

Liver enzyme levels increase in approximately 10% of HIV-infected people after beginning HAART therapy.[50] Such increases have been observed in up to 30% of persons coinfected with HCV.[49-61] Some anti-HIV drugs such as nevirapine,[50-52] ritonavir,[52] and stavudine[53, 54] are more likely to cause elevations in liver enzymes than others are.[55] A group of anti-HIV drugs called *nucleoside reverse transcriptase inhibitors* (NRTIs; for example, ddI, ddC and AZT) have also been reported to cause liver enzyme elevations.[56, 57] It appears the increased susceptibility to anti-HIV drug-related liver injury among people coinfected with HCV/HIV is caused by the interplay of many factors. Some of the drugs appear to be directly *hepatotoxic*, meaning they chemically injure liver cells. People with chronic hepatitis may be more susceptible to this type of injury because an inflamed and/or scarred liver may be less capable of processing medications.

Both HCV[58] and some anti-HIV medications have the ability to damage structures called mitochondria inside liver cells. Mitochondria are the "powerhouses" of cells. They provide the energy needed for cells to function properly. When mitochondria are damaged, liver cells do not have the energy to function normally and liver damage occurs. Mitochondrial damage is thought to be one of the mechanisms of liver injury and liver enzyme elevations seen in some HCV/HIV coinfected people on HAART.[59-62] HAART-associated mitochondrial damage appears to be heightened in the presence of underlying hepatitis C.

In 2004, the HCV-HIV International Panel published treatment guidelines entitled, "Care of patients with hepatitis C and HIV coinfection."[63] With regard to the hepatotoxicity of antiretroviral drugs, the panel made this recommendation:

> Liver enzyme elevations after beginning antiretroviral therapy are more frequent in patients with underlying chronic *hepatitis B* and C. Therefore, drugs with more hepatotoxic profiles (i.e., nevirapine, ritonavir) should be used cautiously in coinfected patients. Treatment should be discontinued in patients with symptoms or *grade* 4 increases in *aminotransferase* levels... The close monitoring of these patients during the first weeks may enable them to remain on therapy, because they experience a progressive resolution of liver abnormalities without discontinuing treatment.

Effects of HCV on the Natural History of HIV/AIDS

Research has shown clearly that coinfection with HIV accelerates the natural course of HCV infection. For a number of years, it has been unclear whether the reverse held true as well. New and emerging research now indicates that overall, HCV does not appear to affect HIV disease progression or response to HAART.

A study of 416 people in Italy found patients coinfected with HCV/HIV and those infected with HIV alone progressed to AIDS at a similar rate.[64] A larger study of 1,955 people conducted in Baltimore, Maryland also found no difference in the progression to AIDS or death among coinfected persons compared to people with HIV only.[65] The authors in the large US study of 10,481 patients concluded that coinfection with HCV did not increase the risk of AIDS-defining opportunistic infections or death, and did not affect short-term *immunological* or virological response to first-line HAART.[66] Similarly, a European study of 5,957 patients found HCV did not influence the risk of HIV disease progression, but that coinfection was associated with a markedly increased risk of liver-related death.[67]

Coinfection, Lipid Metabolism, Lipodystrophy, Steatosis and Hyperglycemia

Lipodystrophy is a group of fat *metabolism* disorders commonly seen in people with HIV.[68-70] These disorders can cause several changes in the body including:

- Loss of fat in the arms, legs, buttocks, and/or face is called lipoatrophy. Such fat loss can cause the veins of the arms and legs to protrude and give the face a sunken appearance.

- Lipohypertrophy is a build up of fat stores in the gut, breasts, shoulders, and/or back of the neck. The abdomen often appears bloated and feels hard. The fat around the gut reflects an accumulation of fatty tissue in the abdominal cavity leading to a swollen look.

Some changes in fat metabolism are not visible but are nonetheless abnormal. Levels of fats such as *cholesterol* and *triglycerides* in the blood can become abnormally high with lipodystrophy. High levels of fat may increase the risk for heart disease, stroke, and other disorders.

The exact mechanisms that lead to lipodystrophy in people with HIV are being actively researched. However, it seems clear that several factors are involved including some associated with the virus itself and others associated with anti-HIV therapy. Researchers have found evidence that coinfection with HCV may contribute to the development of lipodystrophy in coinfected persons.[71] HCV damages the powerhouses of liver cells (the mitochondria), thus interrupting normal fat breakdown and storage.[72, 73] One study suggests the incidence of lipoatrophy is higher in people coinfected with HIV and HCV than it is in those infected with HIV only.[74] The redistribution of fat from the arms and legs into the abdomen also causes increased fat in the liver, a situation that can further damage an HCV-infected liver.

HAART-related lipodystrophy has been associated with another condition known as *insulin* resistance (IR).[75] People with insulin resistance have abnormally high *blood sugar* (*glucose*) levels. Some researchers have reported the incidence of IR is higher in HCV/HIV coinfected persons on HAART compared to persons with HIV only.[76] Investigators speculate HAART-related IR may result from anti-HIV medication directly impairing glucose uptake by muscle, effects of HIV per se, or indirect effects such as fat redistribution.[77] *Clinical* scientists hope to soon find effective ways to treat the metabolic abnormalities associated with HAART, HIV, and HCV/HIV coinfection.

Steatosis, or *fatty liver*, is a common finding in people living with HCV. The finding of fatty liver on biopsy can help identify patients at risk for disease progression[78, 79] or those who may respond more poorly to interferon-based therapy.[80] Previous studies have shown associations between the steatosis severity and infection with HCV *genotype* 3[81, 82], obesity[83], and diabetes[84]. However, a recent study of 708 veterans showed that steatosis is highly prevalent and more severe in HCV/HIV coinfection than in HCV infection alone.[85]

The increased prevalence and severity of steatosis in the coinfected population possibly explains the increased rate of fibrosis progression in coinfected persons. Compared to HCV infection alone, HCV/HIV coinfection was associated with a significantly increased odds ratio of steatosis. Among those who were coinfected, the fibrosis progression rate increased in a linear fashion along with the grade of steatosis.

There are several potential pathways by which HIV and HCV may interact to cause steatosis. There are differing opinions on this question. One possibility is that HIV infection itself may lead to development of steatosis by assisting HCV replication. HCV/HIV coinfected people have increased HCV RNA levels inside the liver,[86] and increased HCV viral loads have been associated with increased severity of steatosis in people with HCV alone.[87] HIV may also act in concert with HCV, disrupting *lipid metabolism* and causing steatosis.

According to data from a subset of the APRICOT HCV/HIV coinfection study, the probability of achieving sustained viral response (SVR) was not reduced by steatosis. Also, SVR significantly reduced the prevalence of steatosis in patients infected with HCV genotype 3 but not in those infected with other HCV genotypes.[88]

A recent study of 203 persons with HCV/HIV coinfection demonstrated a strong relationship between *hepatic* steatosis, fibrosis, and *hyperglycemia*. This finding supports efforts to treat HCV and to use ART regimens that have the least associated risk of hyperglycemia in HCV/HIV-co-infected persons.[89]

Harm Reduction

People with HCV/HIV coinfection are at increased risk for other infectious diseases. It is important to take steps to protect yourself from exposure to other infectious diseases.

The simplest and most effective way to protect yourself from food-borne illnesses is hand washing. Although it sounds trivial, hand washing goes a long way toward protecting yourself from many illnesses. A few simple rules to keep in mind include:

- Always wash your hands before eating or preparing food. Be sure everyone in your household does the same.

- Always wash your hands after using the restroom.

- Wash all fresh fruits and vegetables before eating.
  Commercial fruit and vegetable washes are not necessary. Simply rub the fruit or vegetable with your washed hands under running water. Fruits or vegetables with a hard exterior should be scrubbed with a clean vegetable brush. You can clean your vegetable brush in the dishwasher.

Hand washing not only protects you from food-borne illnesses but also helps prevent the spread of cold and flu viruses. Safe sex practices are also essential for coinfected persons. These practices will prevent the spread of HIV and/or HCV to others, and will protect you from being exposed to sexually transmitted infections such as hepatitis B, gonorrhea, syphilis, herpes, chlamydia, and others.

Injection drug use poses many threats to wellness. It is best for coinfected person to avoid all injection drug use and other recreational drug use. However, if you are injecting drugs, be sure to use scrupulously clean injection habits. Avoid reusing needles, and never share needles with others.

People who are coinfected and drink alcohol are at <u>greatly</u> increased risk of developing severe liver disease, cirrhosis, and/or liver cancer. All people infected with HCV should avoid alcohol, but it is even more important for coinfected persons. People coinfected with HCV/HIV should not drink <u>any</u> alcohol. If you have difficulty abstaining from alcohol, you might be addicted to alcohol. Talk with your healthcare providers about the problem. Many resources are available to help you eliminate alcohol from your life. For additional information about the effects of alcohol in HCV and treatment options, see *Chapter 3, Alcohol and Hepatitis C* and *Appendix I, How to Cut Down on Your Drinking*.

Hepatitis A and B

Due to shared routes of transmission, people coinfected with HIV and HCV are at increased risk for also contracting hepatitis B. A recent study conducted in Spain found that among people with HIV, 79% of injection drug users were also infected with both HCV and HBV. Triple infection rates among those with other risk factors ranged from 10% to 20%.[90] Unlike HIV, HCV, and HBV, hepatitis A is a food-borne illness. Hepatitis A causes an acute form of viral hepatitis; there is no chronic form of hepatitis A. Although HAV infection alone is usually a relatively mild disease, it is often a more serious illness in people with HIV, HCV, and/or HBV. Fulminant hepatitis is a rapidly progressive condition characterized by a massive loss of liver cells and liver failure. Fulminant hepatitis is a rare complication of HAV infection (0.3% – 1.8% of cases).[91] Although there have been some conflicting reports,[92] most investigators agree that *acute hepatitis* A in people with chronic hepatitis C is associated with an increased risk for fulminant hepatitis ranging from 0% to 40%.[92-99]

Infections with HBV and HAV among HCV/HIV coinfected persons can be life threatening. All persons with HIV should be tested for HCV and HBV. Most healthcare providers recommend that coinfected persons not already infected or immune to HAV and HBV should be vaccinated against these viruses. The vaccines contain no live viruses, so there is no risk of infection from the vaccines. The two vaccines can be given simultaneously. Hepatitis A and B vaccines are available for little to no cost at public health clinics in the United States and many other countries.

If you have not been previously vaccinated or infected with HAV and are exposed to the virus, treatment with *immune globulin* is recommended.[91] Immune globulin should be given as soon as possible after exposure, but must be given within two weeks of exposure to be effective. Similarly, people who have been exposed to HBV should be treated with hepatitis B immune globulin (HBIG) as soon as possible after exposure, preferably within 24 hours.[100] The effectiveness of HBIG when administered more than seven days after exposure is unknown. The first shot in the hepatitis B vaccine series can be given at the same time as HBIG. If the HBV vaccine is indicated, it too should be given as soon as possible and preferably within 24 hours.

Summary

Overall, up to one-third of people living with HIV in the U.S. are coinfected with HCV. Coinfection with HIV adversely affects hepatitis C disease progression increasing the risk of cirrhosis, liver failure, and liver cancer.

Harm reduction is especially important for people with HCV/HIV coinfection. Vaccination against HAV and HBV is particularly important. Lifestyle choices such as safe sexual practices, avoiding recreational drug use or using clean needles, and abstaining from alcohol can enhance overall wellness and improve quality of life.

References

1. Palella FJ Jr, Delaney KM, Moorman AC, et al. Declining morbidity and mortality among patients with advanced human immunodeficiency virus infection. HIV Outpatient Study Investigators. *N Engl J Med*. 1998;338:853-60.
2. Bica I, McGovern B, Dhar R, et al. Increasing mortality due to end-stage liver disease in patients with human immunodeficiency virus infection. *Clin Infect Dis*.2001;32(3):492-7.
3. Monga HK, Rodriguez-Barradas MC, Breaux K, et al. Hepatitis C virus infection-related morbidity and mortality among patients with human immunodeficiency virus infection. *Clin Infect Dis*. 2001;33:240-7.
4. Martin-Carbonero L, Soriano V, Valencia E, et al. Increasing impact of chronic viral hepatitis on hospital admissions and mortality among HIV infected patients. *AIDS Research and Human Retroviruses*. 2001;17(16):1467-1471
5. CDC IDU HIV Prevention Unit, Hepatitis C Virus and HIV Coinfection, September 2002
6. Armstrong GL, Wasley A, Simard EP, McQuillan GM, Kuhnert WL, Alter MJ. The Prevalence of Hepatitis C Virus Infection in the United States, 1999 through 2002. *Ann Intern Med*. 2006;144:705-714.
7. World Health Organization. Available at http://www.who.int/vaccine_research/diseases/viral_cancers/en/index2.htm. Accessed April 24, 2008.
8. UNAIDS. *2007 AIDS Epidemic Update*. Geneva, Switzerland. 2007. Available at http://www.unaids.org/en/KnowledgeCentre/HIVData/EpiUpdate/EpiUpdArchive/2007/. Accessed April 24, 2008.
9. HIV/AIDS in the United States. CDC HIV/AIDS Facts, March 2008. Available at http://www.cdc.gov/hiv/resources/factsheets/us.htm. Accessed April 24, 2008.
10. Sherman KE, Rouster SD, Chung RT, Rajicic N. Hepatitis C Virus prevalence among patients infected with Human Immunodeficiency Virus: a cross-sectional analysis of the US adult AIDS Clinical Trials Group. *Clin Infect Dis*. 2002;34(6):831-7.
11. Sulkowski M, Benhamou Y. Therapeutic issues in HCV/HIV coinfected patients. *J Viral Hepat*. 2007;14(6):371-386.
12. Sulkowski MS, Thomas DL. Hepatitis C in the HIV-infected person. *Ann Intern Med*. 2003;138:197-207.
13. Ragni MV, Ndimbie OK, Rice EO, Bontempo FA, Nedjar S. The presence of hepatitis C virus (HCV) antibody in human immunodeficiency virus positive hemophilic men undergoing HCV seroreversion. *Blood*. 1993; 82:1010-5.
14. Ewenstein B, Koerper M. Survey of diagnostic and treatment practices of chronic hepatitis C in federally-funded hemophilia treatment centers. Presented at: Medical and Scientific Advisory Council meeting. Orlando, Florida. October 1998.
15. Poles MA, Dieterich DT. Hepatitis C virus/human immunodeficiency virus coinfection: clinical management issues. *Clin Infect Dis*. 2000;31(1):154-161.

16. Danta M, et al. Recent epidemic of acute hepatitis C virus in HIV-positive men who have sex with men linked to high-risk sexual behaviours. *AIDS*. 2007 May 11;21(8):983-91.

17. Gambotti L and the acute hepatitis C collaborating group, Acute hepatitis C infection in HIV positive men who have sex with men in Paris, France, 2001-2004. *Euro Surveill*. 2005; 10(5)

18. van de Laar TJ, et al. Increase in HCV incidence among men who have sex with men in Amsterdam most likely caused by sexual transmission. *J Infect Dis*. 2007 Jul 15;196(2):230-8. Epub 2007 Jun 11.

19. Villano SA, Vlahov D, Nelson KE, Cohn S, Thomas DL. Persistence of viremia and the importance of long-term follow-up after acute hepatitis C infection. Hepatology. 1999;29:908-14.

20. Thomas DL, Astemborski J, Rai RM, et al. The natural history of hepatitis C virus infection: host, viral, and environmental factors. *JAMA*. 2000;284(4):450-6.

21. Alter MJ, Margolis HS, Krawczynski K, et al. The natural history of community-acquired hepatitis C in the United States. The Sentinel Counties Chronic non-A, non-B Hepatitis Study Team. *N Engl J Med*. 1992;327:1899-905.

22. Rossi G, Tucci A, Cariani E, et al. Outbreak of hepatitis C virus infection in patients with hematologic disorders treated with intravenous immunoglobulins: different prognosis according to immune status. *Blood*. 1997;90:1309-14.

23. Durand F, Beauplet A, Marcellin P. Evidence of hepatitis C virus viremia without detectable antibody to hepatitis C virus in a blood donor. *Ann Intern Med*. 2000;133:74-5.

24. Hitzler WE, Runkel S. Routine HCV PCR screening of blood donations to identify early HCV infection in blood donors lacking antibodies to HCV. *Transfusion*. 2001;41:333-7.

25. Bonacini M, Lin HJ, Hollinger FB. Effect of coexisting HIV-1 infection on the diagnosis and evaluation of hepatitis C virus. *J Acquir Immune Defic Syndr*. 2001;26:340-4.

26. George SL, Gebhardt J, Klintzman D, et al. Hepatitis C virus viremia in HIV-infected individuals with negative HCV antibody tests. *J Acquir Immune Defic Syndr*. 2002;31(2):154-162.

27. Falconer K, Gonzalez VD, Reichard O, Sandberg JK, Alaeus A. Spontaneous HCV clearance in HCV/HIV-1 coinfection associated with normalized CD4 counts, low level of chronic immune activation and high level of T cell function. *J Clin Virol*. 2008;41(2):160-163.

28. Cribier B, Rey D, Schmitt C, Lang JM, Kirn A, Stoll-Keller F. High hepatitis C viraemia and impaired antibody response in patients coinfected with HIV. *AIDS*. 1995;9:1131-36.

29. Sherman KE, O'Brien J, Gutierrez AG, et al. Quantitative evaluation of hepatitis C virus RNA in patients with concurrent human immunodeficiency virus infections. *J Clin Microbiol*. 1993;31:2679-82.

30. Bonacini M, Govindarajan S, Blatt LM, Schmid P, Conrad A, Lindsay KL. Patients co-infected with human immunodeficiency virus and hepatitis C virus demonstrate higher levels of hepatic HCV RNA. *J Viral Hepat*. 1999;6:203-8.

31. Verucchi G, Calza R, Manfred R, Chiodo F. Human immunodeficiency virus and hepatitis C virus coinfection: epidemiology, natural history, therapeutic options and clinical management. *Infection*. 2004;33:33-46.

32. Soto B, Sanchez-Quijano A, Rodrigo L, et al. Human immunodeficiency virus infection modifies the natural history of chronic parenterally-acquired hepatitis C with an unusually rapid progression to cirrhosis. *J Hepatol*. 1997;26:1-5.

33. Benhamou Y, Bochet M, Di Martino V, et al. Liver fibrosis progression in human immunodeficiency virus and hepatitis C virus coinfected patients. The Multivirc Group. *Hepatology*. 1999;30:1054-58.

34. Puoti M, Bonacini M, Spinetti A, et al. Liver fibrosis progression is related to CD4 cell depletion in patients coinfected with hepatitis C virus and human immunodeficiency virus. *J Infect Dis*. 2001;183(1):134-7.

35. Bierhoff E, Fischer HP, Willsch E, et al. Liver histopathology in patients with concurrent chronic hepatitis C and HIV infection. *Virchows Arch*. 1997;430(4):271-7.

36. Graham CS, Baden LR, Yu E, et al. Influence of human immunodeficiency virus infection on the course of hepatitis C virus infection: a meta-analysis. *Clin Infect Dis*. 2001;33(4):562-9.

37. Monga HK, Rodriguez-Barradas MC, Breaux K, et al. Hepatitis C virus infection related morbidity and mortality among patients with human immunodeficiency virus infection. *Clin Infect Dis*. 2001;33:240-7.

38. Bedossa P, Poynard T. An algorithm for the grading of activity in chronic hepatitis C. The METAVIR Cooperative Study Group. *Hepatology*. 1996;24(2):289-93.

39. Benhamou Y, Bochet M, Di Martino V, et al. Liver fibrosis progression in human immunodeficiency virus and hepatitis C virus coinfected patients. *Hepatology*. 1999;30:1054-1058.

40. Garcia-Samaniego J, Rodriguez M, Berenguer J, Rodriguez-Rosado R, Carbo J, Asensi V, Soriano V. Hepatocellular carcinoma in HIV-infected patients with chronic hepatitis C. *Am J Gastroenterol*. 2001;96(1):179-83.

41. Bräu N, Fox RK, Xiao P, et al. Presentation and outcome of hepatocellular carcinoma in HIV-infected patients: a U.S.-Canadian multicenter study. *J Hepatol*. 2007;47(4):527-537.

42. Soriano V, Rodriguea-Rosado R, Garcia-Samaniego J. Management of chronic hepatitis C in HIV-infected patients. *AIDS*. 1999;13:539-46.

43. Lesens O, Deschenes M, Steben M, Belanger G, Tsoukas CM. Hepatitis C virus is related to progressive liver disease in human immunodeficiency virus-positive hemophiliacs and should be treated as an opportunistic infection. *J Infect Dis*. 1999;179:1254-8.

44. Cacoub P, Geffray L, Rosenthal E, et al. Mortality among HIV-infected patients with cirrhosis or hepatocellular carcinoma due to hepatitis C virus in French departments of internal medicine/infectious diseases, in 1995 and 1997. *Clin Infect Dis*. 2001;32:1207-14.

45. Soriano V, Martin-Carbonero L, Garcia-Samaniego J, Puoti M. Mortality due to chronic viral liver disease among patients infected with human immunodeficiency virus. *Clin Infect Dis*. 2001;33:1793-4.

46. Puoti M, Spinetti A, Ghezzi A, et al. Mortality for liver disease in patients with HIV infection: a cohort study. *J Acquir Immune Defic Syndr*. 2000;24:211-7.

47. Qurishi N, Kreuzberg C, Luchters G, et al. Effect of antiretroviral therapy on liver-related mortality in patients with HIV and hepatitis C virus coinfection. *Lancet*. 2003;362:1708-1713.

48. Marine-Barjoan E, Saint-Paul MC, Pradier C et al. Impact of antiretroviral treatment on progression of hepatic fibrosis in HIV/hepatitis C virus co-infected patients. *AIDS*. 2004; 18: 2163-2170.

49. Benhamou Y, Di Martino V, Bochet M, Colombet G, Thibault V, Liou A, Katlama C, Poynard T; MultivirC Group. Factors affecting liver fibrosis in human immunodeficiency virus-and hepatitis C virus-coinfected patients: impact of protease inhibitor therapy. *Hepatology*. 2001;34(2):283-7.
50. Sulkowski M, Thomas D, Chaisson R, Moore R. Hepatotoxicity associated with antiretroviral therapy in adults infected with HIV and the role of hepatitis C or B virus infection. *JAMA*. 2000;283:74-80.
51. Martinez E, Blanco J, Arnaiz J, Gatell J. Heptatotoxicity in HIV-infected patients receiving nevirapine-containing antiretroviral therapy. *AIDS*. 2001;15:1261-8.
52. Sulkowski M, Thomas D, Mehta S, Chaisson R, Moore R. Hepatotoxicity associated with nevirapine or efavirenz-containing antiretroviral therapy: role of hepatitis C and B infections. *Hepatology*. 2002;35:182-9.
53. Gisolf EH, Dreezen C, Danner SA, Weel JL, Weverling GJ. Risk factors for hepatotoxicity in HIV-1-infected patients receiving ritonavir and saquinavir with or without stavudine. *Clin Infect Dis*. 200;31:1234-9.
54. Spruance SL, Pavia AT, Mellors JW, et al. Clinical efficacy of monotherapy with stavudine compared with zidovudine in HIV-infected, zidovudine-experienced patients. *Ann Intern Med*. 1997;126:355-63.
55. Sulkowski MS. Hepatotoxicity associated with antiretroviral therapy containing HIV-1 protease inhibitors. *Semin Liver Dis*. 2003;23(2):183-94.
56. Saves M, Raffi F, Clevenbergh, P, et al. Hepatitis B or hepatitis C virus infection is a risk factor for severe hepatic cytolysis after initiation of a protease inhibitor-contained antiretroviral regimen in HIV-infected patients. *Antimicrob Agents Chemother*. 2000;44:3451-5.
57. Brinkman K, ter Hofstede JM, Burger DM. Adverse effects of reverse transcriptase inhibitors: mitochondrial toxicity as common pathway. *AIDS*. 1998;12:1735-44.
58. Okuda M, Li K, Beard MR, Showalter LA, Scholle F, Lemon SM, Weinman SA. Mitochondrial injury, oxidative stress, and antioxidant gene expression are induced by hepatitis C virus core protein. *Gastroenterology*. 2002;122(2):366-75.
59. Moyle G. Hyperlactatemia and lactic acidosis during antiretroviral therapy: causes, management and possible etiologies. *AIDS Rev*. 2001;3:150-6.
60. Lonergan J, Behling C, Pfander H, Hassanein T, Mathews W. Hyperlactatemia and hepatic abnormalities in 10 HIV-infected patients receiving nucleoside analogue combination regimens. *Clin Infect Dis*. 2000;31:162-6.
61. Batisse D, van Huyen J, Piketty C, et al. Severe liver mitochondriopathy with normal liver histology and normal lactate levels in patients receiving nucleoside analogs. *AIDS*. 2002;16:2370-1.
62. Sutinen J, Kakkinen A, Westerbacka J, et al. Increased fat accumulation in the liver in HIV-infected patients with antiretroviral therapy associated lipodystrophy. *AIDS*. 2002;16:2183-93.
63. Soriano V, Puoti M, Sulkowski M, et al. Care of patients with hepatitis C and HIV coinfection. *AIDS*. 2004;18:1-12.
64. Dorrucci M, Pezzotti P, Phillips AN, Lepri AC, Rezza G. Coinfection of hepatitis C virus with human immunodeficiency virus and progression to AIDS. Italian Seroconversion Study. *J Infect Dis*. 1995;172:1503-8.
65. Sulkowski MS, Moore RD, Mehta SH, Chaisson RE, Thomas DL. Hepatitis C and progression of HIV disease. *JAMA*. 2002;288:199-206.
66. Sullivan PS, Hanson DL, Teshale EH, et al. Effect of hepatitis C infection on progression of HIV disease and early response to initial antiretroviral therapy. *AIDS* 20(8): 1171-1179.
67. Rockstroh JK, Mocroft A, Soriano V, et al. Influence of hepatitis C virus infection on HIV-1 disease progression and response to highly active antiretroviral therapy. *J Infect Dis*. 2005;192(6):992-1002.
68. Carr A, Samaras K, Burton S. et al. A syndrome of lipodystrophy, hyperlipidemia and insulin resistance in patients receiving HIV protease inhibitors. *AIDS*. 1998;12:F51-8.
69. Carr A, Samaras K, Chisholm DJ, Cooper DA. Pathogenesis of HIV-1-protease inhibitor-associated peripheral lipodystrophy, hyperlipidaemia, and insulin resistance. *Lancet*. 1998;351:1881-3.
70. Saint-Marc T, Partisani M, Poizot-Martin I. et al. A syndrome of peripheral fat wasting (lipodystrophy) in patients receiving long-term nucleoside analogue therapy. *AIDS*. 1999;13:1659-67.
71. Duong M, Petit JM, Piroth L, et al. Association between insulin resistance and hepatitis C virus chronic infection in HIV-hepatitis C virus-coinfected patients undergoing antiretroviral therapy. *J Acquir Immune Defic Syndr*. 2001;27(3):245-50.
72. Barba G, Harper F, Harada T. et al. Hepatitis C virus core protein shows a cytoplasmic localization and associates to cellular lipid storage droplets. *Proc Natl Acad Sci USA*. 1997;94:1200-5.
73. Barbaro G, Di Lorenzo G, Asti A. et al. Hepatocellular mitochondrial alterations in patients with chronic hepatitis C: ultrastructural and biochemical findings. *Am J Gastroenterol*. 1999;94:2198-2205.
74. Zylberberg H, Nalpas B, Pol S, Bréchot C, Viard JP. Is there a relationship between hepatitis C virus infection and antiretroviral-associated lipoatrophy? *AIDS*. 2000;14(13):2055.
75. Faraj M, Lu HL, Cianflone K. Diabetes, lipids, and adipocyte secretagogues. *Biochem Cell Biol*. 2004;82(1):170-190.
76. Duong M, Petit JM, Piroth L, et al. Association between insulin resistance and hepatitis C virus chronic infection in HIV-hepatitis C virus coinfected patients undergoing antiretroviral therapy. *J Acquir Immune Defic Syndr*. 2001;27(3):245-250.
77. Grinspoon S. Mechanisms and strategies for insulin resistance in acquired immune deficiency syndrome. *Clin Infect Dis*. 2003;37(Suppl 2):S85-90.
78. Castera L, Hezode C, Roudot-Thoraval F., et al., Worsening of steatosis is an independent factor of fibrosis progression in untreated patients with chronic hepatitis C and paired liver biopsies. *Gut*. 2003;52:288–92.
79. Patton HM, Patel K, Behling C, Bylund D, Blatt LM and Vallee M et al. The impact of steatosis on disease progression and early and sustained treatment response in chronic hepatitis C patients. J Hepatol. 2004;40:484–490.
80. Monto A, Alonzo J, Watson JJ, et al, Steatosis in chronic hepatitis C: relative contributions of obesity, diabetes mellitus, and alcohol, *Hepatology*. 2002;36:729–36.
81. Sharma P, Balan V, Hernandez J, et al., Hepatic steatosis in hepatitis C virus genotype 3 infection: does it correlate with body mass index, fibrosis, and HCV risk factors? *Dig Dis Sci. 2004*;49:25–9.
82. Hu KQ, Kyulo NL, Esrailian E, et al., Overweight and obesity, hepatic steatosis, and progression of chronic hepatitis C: a retrospective study on a large cohort of patients in the United States. *J Hepatol.* 40 (2004), pp. 147–154.

83. Sanyal AJ, Contos MJ, Sterling RK, et al., Nonalcoholic fatty liver disease in patients with hepatitis C is associated with features of the metabolic syndrome. *Am J Gastroenterol.* 2003;98:2064–71.

84. Gaslightwala I, Bini E, Impact of human immunodeficiency virus infection on the prevalence and severity of steatosis in patients with chronic hepatitis C virus infection. *J Hepatol.* 44(6):1026-1032.

85. Bonacini M, Govindarajan S, Blatt LM, et al, Patients co-infected with human immunodeficiency virus and hepatitis C virus demonstrate higher levels of hepatic HCV RNA. *J Viral Hepat.* 1999;6:203–8.

86. Rubbia-Brandt L, Quadri R, Abid et al., Hepatocyte steatosis is a cytopathic effect of hepatitis C virus genotype 3. *J Hepatol.* 2000;33:106–115.

87. Bonnet F, Lawson-Ayayi S, Thiebaut R. A cohort study of nevirapine tolerance in clinical practice: French Aquitaine Cohort, 1997-1999. *Clin Infect Dis.* 2002;35:1231-7.

88. Rodríguez-Torres M, et al. Hepatic steatosis in HCV/HIV co-infected patients: correlates, efficacy and outcomes of anti-HCV therapy: a paired liver biopsy study. *J Hepatol.* 2008 May;48(5):756-64. Epub 2008 Feb 7.

89. Mehta S, Thomas D, Torbenson M, Moore R, and Sulkowski M. Liver histology, ART, and hyperglycemia in HCV/HIV coinfected adults. *CROI* 2006. Abstract 165.

90. Rodriguez-Mendez ML, Gonzalez-Quintela A, Aguilera A, Carballo E, Barrio E. Association of HCV and HBV markers in Spanish HIV-seropositive patients in relation to risk practices. *Hepatogastroenterology.* 2003;50(54):2093-7.

91. Centers for Disease Control and Prevention. Prevention of hepatitis A through active or passive immunization: recommendations of the Advisory Committee on Immunization Practices (ACIP). *MMWR.* 1999;48(No. RR-12):1-54.

92. Bianco E, Stroffolini T, Spada E, et al. Case fatality rate of acute viral hepatitis in Italy: 1995-2000. An update. *Dig Liver Dis.* 2003;35(6):404-8.

93. Williams I, Bell B, Kaluba J, Shapiro C. Association between chronic liver disease and death from hepatitis A, United States, 1989–92 [Abstract A39]. IX Triennial International Symposium on Viral Hepatitis and Liver Disease. Rome, Italy, April 1996.

94. Akriviadis EA, Redeker AG. Fulminant hepatitis A in intravenous drug users with chronic liver disease. *Ann Intern Med.* 1989;110:838–9.

95. Willner IR, Uhl MD, Howard SC, Williams EQ, Riely CA, Waters B. Serious hepatitis A: an analysis of patients hospitalized during an urban epidemic in the United States. *Ann Intern Med.* 1998;128:111–4.

96. Vento S, Garofano T, Renzini C, et al. Fulminant hepatitis associated with hepatitis A virus superinfection in patients with chronic hepatitis C. *N Engl J Med.* 1998;338:286–90.

97. Keefe EB. Is hepatitis A more severe in patients with chronic hepatitis B and other chronic liver diseases? *Am J Gastroenterol.* 1995;90:201–5.

98. Vento S. Fulminant hepatitis associated with hepatitis A virus superinfection in patients with chronic hepatitis C. *J Viral Hepat.* 2000;7(Suppl 1):7-8.

99. Reiss G, Keeffe EB. Review article: hepatitis vaccination in patients with chronic liver disease. *Aliment Pharmacol Ther.* 2004;19(7):715-27.

100. Centers for Disease Control and Prevention. Updated U.S. Public Health Service Guidelines for the Management of Occupational Exposures to HBV, HCV, and HIV and Recommendations for Postexposure Prophylaxis. *MMWR.* 2001;50(No. RR-11):1-42.

HCV / HIV COINFECTION

Tina M. St. John, MD and Misha Cohen, OMD, LAc

WESTERN (ALLOPATHIC) TREATMENT OPTIONS

Introduction

The management and treatment of coinfection with the *human immunodeficiency virus* (*HIV*) and the hepatitis C virus (HCV) are complex and challenging. Much progress has been made in recent years, but many unknowns remain. Some of the many questions about HCV/HIV coinfection include:

- Should the infections be treated simultaneously or individually? If the infections are treated individually, which virus should be treated first? If treated simultaneously, what are the best approaches?

- Should all coinfected people be treated for HCV? If not, what subgroup of people should be treated?

- Do the choice of medicines used and their dosages need to be adjusted if both infections are treated simultaneously?

- How can the complications of coinfection be minimized?

- How should liver transplant be managed in the setting of coinfection?

Concerns about treating both HIV and HCV at the same time center on the risk of liver *toxicity* (*hepatotoxicity*) and interactions between *antiviral* drugs. The effects of each virus on the natural disease progression of the other infection are also important issues in treatment decisions.

This section discusses western medicine's current knowledge and approach to HCV/HIV coinfection. Keep in mind, this is a rapidly changing field of study, and all treatment decisions must take into account your unique circumstances and disease status.

Identification of Coinfection

The first issue of coinfection management is accurate diagnosis. Because of the high incidence of HCV/HIV coinfection,[1-8] experts agree that all people with HIV should be screened for coinfection with HCV. HCV screening is accomplished by testing the blood for *anti-HCV antibodies*. While the presence of HCV without detectable anti-HCV antibodies is quite rare in people with normal *immune systems*, it appears to occur in 5% to 19% of people coinfected with HIV.[9, 10] Scientists believe this is probably due to the immunosuppressive effects of HIV and the loss of *CD4 cells*, the immune cells infected by HIV that are also necessary for *antibody* production. Thus, in HIV-infected persons with persistently elevated *liver enzymes* (*ALT* and *AST*) but a negative HCV screening test, most experts recommend testing for the hepatitis C virus (*HCV RNA*).[11]

The Decision to Treat HIV, HCV, or Both

As discussed in *Chapter 20 Section 1, Overview of HCV/HIV Coinfection*, it is clear that HIV infection accelerates HCV disease progression.[12-18] Decompensated cirrhosis is one of the leading causes of death in the coinfected population.[19-21] Further, coinfection appears to increase the risk of liver cancer (*hepatocellular carcinoma*).[16, 22] Thus, the health risks of untreated HCV infection are higher among coinfected persons than in those with HCV alone.

The effects of HCV on HIV disease progression are unclear. Most clinical studies evaluating this topic have failed to show a significant effect of HCV on the progression of HIV disease. However, this was not true in every study.[2, 6, 8, 23 -27] While the possibility still exists that HCV may negatively affect the natural history of HIV, it current appears that this is unlikely.

Both HIV and HCV are potentially life-threatening infections. The stakes involved in treatment decisions are very high and the issues are complex. Therefore, we urge all coinfected persons to consult with healthcare providers who have experience managing coinfection.

The decision to treat HIV, HCV, or both infections simultaneous depends on many factors, including:

- **the timing of diagnosis**
  Were the infections diagnosed at the same time or was one of the infections acquired after the other?

- **immune status**
  What is the CD4 count? What is the HIV *viral load*? Is the client HIV-positive only or has there been disease progression to AIDS? Is the client already on anti-HIV medications? What medications have been prescribed?

- **HCV-related factors**
  Is there evidence of *fibrosis* and/or *cirrhosis*? Is there evidence of liver failure (*decompensation*)? What are the liver enzyme levels? What is the HCV viral load? What is the *genotype*? Has the client received previous treatment for HCV?

- **mental health issues**
  Does the client currently have or have a history of depression or other major mental illness? Is there active substance abuse (drugs or *alcohol*)?

- **overall health status**
  Are there other active illnesses? Are they well controlled?

Depending on the specific circumstances, one of the following choices may be made:

- **Treat the HIV infection first until it can be controlled, then consider treatment for HCV.**
  Low CD4 count has been identified as a factor that may decrease the probability of response to interferon-based therapy for HCV.[28] For this reason, and to prevent the progression of HIV disease to AIDS, many doctors believe treating HIV and gaining control of that infection is the first priority in patients who are coinfected at diagnosis. The partial restoration of immune function that often occurs after beginning highly active antiretroviral therapy (HAART)[29] for HIV may increase the likelihood of response to *interferon-based therapy* for HCV. Further, one preliminary study suggests HAART may actually slow the accelerated HCV disease progression usually observed with coinfection.[30] However, as discussed in *Section 1* of this chapter, liver enzyme levels and HCV viral loads often increase when HAART is initiated.[31- 43] The long-term effects of these spikes in liver enzymes and HCV viral loads are unclear.

- **Treat HCV first, and then begin HIV treatment.**
  In theory, this approach has two potential advantages. It may eliminate the immediate threat of HCV-related liver disease by halting disease progression and allowing for at least partial restoration of liver health. A liver that has been partially or completely restored to normal function is better able to process antiviral drugs when

HIV treatment is initiated. This approach is usually reserved for people who have not received previous therapy for either infection and whose CD4 counts are greater than 350 cells/mm³.[11]

- **Treat both infections simultaneously.**
  This approach addresses both infections at the same time. Caution is required due to potential interactions between anti-HCV and anti-HIV medications.

The decision about which option is most appropriate for your specific circumstances is one that can be made only after a thorough medical evaluation by a healthcare provider experienced in the treatment of coinfection.

Interferon-Based Therapy for HCV in People with HCV/HIV Coinfection

Combination therapy with pegylated interferon plus ribavirin is the treatment of choice for chronic hepatitis C (See *Chapter 8, Sections 1* and *2* for additional information about pegylated interferon plus ribavirin therapy). Pegylated interferon alfa-2a (Pegasys®) in combination with ribavirin was approved by the Food and Drug Administration (FDA) in 2005 for the treatment of chronic hepatitis C in patients with HCV/HIV coinfection. While the manufacturer of pegylated interferon alfa-2b has not sought FDA approval of its drug for this indication (as of this writing), it is also used to treat hepatitis C in coinfected patients.

While overall *sustained response* rates with peginterferon plus ribavirin therapy have been reported to be approximately 50% to 60% in people with HCV only, response rates are lower in coinfected persons. Overall sustained response rates in coinfected persons have been reported to be anywhere from 20% to 44%.[44-53] Recent data indicate that optimal exposure to ribavirin is particularly important for coinfected patients.[54-63] Therefore, the HCV-HIV International Panel issued the following recommendation in 2007:

> The current treatment of chronic HCV infection in HIV-positive persons should be pegylated interferon at standard doses plus weight-based ribavirin (1,000mg/day if <75 kg and 1,200 mg/day if > 75 kg.[64]

Although research is accumulating that suggests duration of therapy may be safely reduced for rapid viral responders (by week 4 of treatment) among monoinfected patients, reduced duration of therapy remains largely unproven for those with HCV-HIV coinfection. There are some data that support the notion that the duration of therapy can be reduced to 24 weeks without significant risk of relapse if the following conditions are met.[65, 66]

- low pretreatment viral load
- HCV genotype 2 or 3
- undetectable HCV viral load by week 4 of treatment
- fibrosis is not advanced
- patient adherence to therapy is good
- weight-based ribavirin dosing is used

Relapses are more frequently observed in the HCV/HIV coinfected population than in those with HCV alone.[45, 50] Researchers speculate the increased relapse rate may be due to the reduced immune function of HIV-infected persons and/or the higher HCV viral loads commonly seen in coinfection. In addition, research suggests that the clearance of HCV after beginning pegylated interferon plus ribavirin therapy is slower in coinfected patients than in those with HCV alone.[67] Recent studies have shown that extending treatment duration (60 to 72 weeks) may be of benefit to coinfected patients with HCV genotype 1 or 4 who have also shown a slow response to treatment (early viral response but not rapid viral response).[68, 69] It is important to note that despite the somewhat slower response seen in HCV/HIV coinfection, early viral response (at least a 100-fold drop in HCV viral load by week 12 of treatment) is predictive of sustained viral response just as it is in patients with HCV alone.[70, 71]

Candidates for Interferon-Based Therapy

All people living with HCV/HIV coinfection should be evaluated for anti-HCV treatment. As noted in *Section 1* of this chapter, response to therapy is partially dependent on the CD4 cell count.[72, 73] Therefore, some doctors prefer treating only patients with CD4 cell counts greater than 350 cells/mm^3.[11] The decision to treat people who have CD4 cell counts between 200 and 350 cells/mm^3 is made on a case-by-case basis. Anti-HCV therapy is uncommon among people with CD4 counts less than 200 cell/mm^3 because of the low response rate.[72, 73]

All factors that may affect response to therapy should be considered before making the decision to begin anti-HCV treatment such as:

- the HCV genotype
- the presence of fibrosis and/or cirrhosis
- current alcohol consumption or drug use
- mental health status

As with people with HCV only, coinfected persons with liver failure are not candidates for interferon-based therapy. Anyone with liver failure should be referred for a liver transplant evaluation. Other relative contraindications to interferon-based therapy are the same in the coinfected population as they are in those with HCV only. They include:

- active substance abuse (alcohol or illicit drugs)
- active mental illness or a history of serious mental illness
- uncontrolled heart disease
- uncontrolled diabetes
- uncontrolled *anemia*

The use of liver biopsy in making treatment decisions in the HCV/HIV coinfected population has become less common in recent years. Many experts share the same opinion expressed in the 2007 updated recommendations of the HCV-HIV International Panel, and that is:

> The higher response to pegylated interferon plus ribavirin compared with that to standard interferon, the faster progression of HCV-related liver disease in the HIV setting, and the chance to assess the virological response at earlier timepoints to identify who will and who will not respond to therapy are all factors that allow the opportunity to prescribe HCV therapy to most patients while avoiding a liver biopsy.[64, 74]

Those experts who believe liver biopsy is unnecessary for most coinfected patients will still generally recommend other noninvasive testing to try to determine the level of liver fibrosis. There are now several noninvasive tests for liver fibrosis available. In general, tests that assess the elasticity of the liver tend to be more accurate in the HCV/HIV coinfected population than those that rely on serum markers.[75-79] It is important to note that among patients with inconclusive or inconsistent results from noninvasive tests for fibrosis, liver biopsy may be necessary.[64]

There are experts who believe anti-HCV therapy should only be initiated in coinfected persons who have evidence of significant fibrosis on liver biopsy. Those who take this approach believe the risk of serious side effects associated with treatment in the coinfected population justifies the requirement for liver biopsy.

Side Effects of HCV Therapy in Coinfected Persons

People with coinfection are subject to the same side effects from combined pegylated interferon plus ribavirin therapy as those with HCV alone (see *Chapter 8, Section 2* for additional information about the side effects of interferon and ribavirin). However, since coinfected people may already have HIV-related symptoms or HAART-related side effects, additional side effects may prove more difficult to tolerate. The high rate of discontinuation of therapy 47-50 in coinfected people may be related to this phenomenon.

White blood cell counts may drop as a side effect of pegylated interferon. In coinfected persons with already reduced CD4 counts, further decreases can be particularly troublesome.[72, 80, 81]

Depression is one of the most common side effects of interferon-based therapy. It is important to report any symptoms of depression to your healthcare provider to prevent this side effect from interfering with completion of therapy. Common symptoms of depression include:

- sleep disturbances – either poor sleep or sleeping too much
- appetite disturbances – eating more or less than usual
- loss of interest in things that used to give you pleasure
- withdrawal from loved ones
- feelings of hopelessness or helplessness
- loss of interest in sex
- suicidal thoughts

Toxic Interactions Between Anti-HIV and Anti-HCV Therapies

Anemia

Anemia is a frequent side effect of ribavirin. Interferon adds to this problem by decreasing the production of both red and *white blood cells*. Overall, significant anemia occurs in approximately 7% to 9% of HCV-infected people treated with combination therapy.[82] A recent study suggests this side effect of pegylated interferon plus ribavirin is more frequent in coinfected persons than in those infected with HCV alone.[83] The anti-HIV drug zidovudine (AZT, ZDV, Retrovir®) is also known to cause anemia.[84] Therefore, most doctors discontinue zidovudine before prescribing ribavirin; it is usually replaced by another drug in the same class.

Mitochondrial Toxicity

As noted in *Section 1* of this chapter, HCV can damage the "powerhouses" of liver cells, the mitochondria.[85] A significant problem in the simultaneous treatment of coinfection is the fact that certain HIV medications may also damage the mitochondria. Anti-HIV drugs that have been implicated in possible mitochondrial damage include.[86-89]

- zidovudine (AZT, ZDV, Retrovir®)
- lamivudine (3TC, Epivir® or combination drugs Combivir®, Epizicom®, and Trizivir®)
- stavudine (D4T, Zerit®)
- didanosine (ddI, Videx®)
- nelfinavir (Viracept®)
- nevirapine (Viramune®)
- zalcitabine (ddC, HIVID®)

Lactic acidosis is a potentially life-threatening condition that may develop with severe mitochondrial toxicity. Lactic acid is a normal byproduct of the energy production process that occurs inside the mitochondria. When the mitochondria are damaged, lactic acid can build up and upset the delicate chemical balances necessary for normal body functions. Symptoms of lactic acidosis include:

- muscular weakness – most noticeable in the arms and legs; the weakness is often severe
- nausea and/or vomiting
- abdominal pain
- breathing difficulty or shortness of breath
- numbness or tingling in the extremities

A blood test is used to confirm the diagnosis of lactic acidosis. If you develop any of the symptoms above, see your doctor immediately. This rare but very serious complication has been specifically linked to didanosine (ddI, Videx®), but has also been linked less frequently with lamivudine (3TC, Epivir®), zidovudine (AZT, Retrovir®), stavudine (D4T, Zerit®), and abacavir (Ziagen®). There have been reports of fatal reactions when didanosine and ribavirin were taken together.[90, 91] These two drugs should not be taken at the same time.

Liver Transplantation in HCV/HIV Coinfection

Chronic HCV infection can eventually lead to end-*stage* liver disease. In end-stage disease, the liver is no longer capable of performing its many vital body functions. Anti-HCV treatment is not useful in such circumstances because the liver has been so severely damaged, and there are potentially life-threatening complications associated with interferon-based therapy when liver failure is present.[92, 93] The primary treatment for patients with HCV/HIV coinfection and liver failure is liver transplantation.[94-97]

Prior to the introduction of HAART, coinfected persons were not eligible for liver transplantation because the likelihood of survival was extremely low.[98] The introduction of HAART, with its ability to suppress HIV replication and the related rebound in immune function, has improved HIV prognosis to the point that coinfection is no longer a contraindication to liver transplantation.

Candidates for liver transplantation typically meet the following criteria:

- no history of opportunistic infections
- CD4 count greater than 100 cells/mm^3
- undetectable HIV-RNA
- no alcohol or illicit drug consumption for at least six months

Although coinfection is not a contraindication to liver transplantation, the potential for complications after transplant are significantly greater for those with both HCV and HIV than for those with HCV alone. A recent analysis of the United Network for Organ Sharing database dating back to 1997 (during the HAART era) found that those with HCV/HIV coinfection had a significantly worse prognosis after liver transplant than those with HCV alone.[99] An earlier, smaller study found that factors associated with poor survival were post-transplant intolerance to HAART, CD4 cell counts <200 cells/mm^3, detectable plasma HIV RNA and HCV infection.[97]

HCV recurrence in transplanted livers occurs in 100% of people with detectable HCV-RNA prior to transplant. Up to 20% of transplanted livers that become reinfected with HCV develop cirrhosis within 5 years. People with genotype 1 HCV appear to be at greater risk for rapid fibrosis progression in transplanted livers compared to other genotypes.[100] Among people with both HCV and HIV, this accelerated rate of liver disease progression is often more pronounced, and makes the long-term viability of the transplanted liver an issue of great concern. Most experts recommend anti-HCV therapy within one to three months post-transplant. A small study of 32 patients found an 18% response rate to pegylated interferon plus ribavirin in liver transplant patients who had been previous non-responders to standard interferon plus ribavirin.[101] Although the response rate is low, it offers some hope to liver transplant recipients. Other strategies to prevent reinfection of transplanted livers are being researched in clinical trials.

Coinfection Treatment Guidelines

The management of HCV/HIV coinfection is an area of active clinical research. Recent developments in the treatment of HCV and emerging research data makes defining ideal treatment much like chasing a moving target. Nonetheless, a group of nine international experts published a series of recommendations for the care of people with hepatitis C and HIV coinfection.[11] A synopsis of the panel's findings and recommendations are shown in Table 1.

Table 1. Issues and Consensus Findings/Recommendations from an International Panel on Care of Patients with Hepatitis C and HIV Coinfection[7, 64]

Treatment Issue	Panel Findings/Recommendations
Influence of hepatitis C virus infection on HIV disease progression and response to antiretroviral therapy	HCV might act as a cofactor for HIV disease progression by several mechanisms.... However, a negative impact of HCV on HIV disease progression has not been recognized in some large clinical-epidemiological studies.
Candidates for anti-hepatitis C virus treatment	All HIV-infected individuals should be screened for HCV antibodies.... Treatment should be provided to patients with repeated elevated *alanine aminotransferase* [ALT] levels, CD4 cell counts greater than 350 cells/mm³, relatively low plasma HIV-RNA levels (i.e., less than 50,000 copies/mL), no active consumption of illegal drugs or high alcohol intake, and no previous severe neuropsychiatric conditions.... Treatment in patients with CD4 cell counts below 350 cells/mm³ should be prescribed cautiously.
Patients with persistently normal aminotransferases (2007 update)	Given that the prevalence of and progression to advanced liver fibrosis in patients with normal ALT is higher in HIV-positive patients, these patients should be considered for anti-HCV therapy. Treatment should be recommended based on patient's motivation, disease duration, fibrosis stage and virological profile regardless of ALT levels.
Management of patients with multiple hepatitis viruses (2007 update)	Multiple viral hepatitis is not uncommon in HIV-positive individuals and worsens liver damage. Complex and dynamic viral interactions occur and making the management of these patients difficult. When possible, treatment of all replicating viruses should be pursued.
Liver fibrosis assessment: when and how? (2007 update)	Information on liver fibrosis staging is important for therapeutic decisions in coinfected patients. However, a liver biopsy is not mandatory for considering the treatment of chronic HCV infection. A combination of non-invasive methods to assess liver fibrosis accurately predicts hepatic fibrosis in most cases.

Treatment Issue	Panel Findings/Recommendations
Treatment of acute hepatitis C (2007 update)	Acute HCV infection in HIV-positive persons should be treated for 24 weeks with a combination of pegIFN plus weight-based ribavirin. However, responses are lower than in HIV-uninfected persons.
Treatment of chronic hepatitis C in HIV-positive patients	The overall response to anti-HCV therapy is lower in patients coinfected with HIV.... Both early virologic responses and relapses are less and more frequent, respectively, in coinfected patients compared with HCV-monoinfected individuals. The benefit of extending therapy... ... in early virological responders should be examined in clinical trials. Moreover, treatment adherence should be considered a critical factor for the attainment of response and must be encouraged actively over the whole treatment period.
Optimal dosages of pegylated interferon and ribavirin (2007 update)	The current treatment of chronic HCV infection in HIV-positive persons should be pegylated interferon at standard doses plus weight-based ribavirin (1000 mg/day if <75 kg and 1200 mg/day if >5 kg).
Optimal duration of therapy (2007 update)	The current treatment of chronic HCV infection in HIV-positive persons should be pegylated interferon plus weight-based ribavirin for 48 weeks. Patients infected with HCV genotype 2–3 and RVR could benefit from shorter (24 weeks) courses of therapy. In contrast, carriers of HCV genotypes 1 and 4 with early virological response (week 12) but not RVR (week 4) might benefit from extended (60–72 weeks) courses of therapy.
Predictors of response to hepatitis C therapy (2007 update)	The achievement of SVR can be predicted on the basis of negative serum HCV RNA at week 4 of therapy. On the other hand, a reduction <2 log IU/ml in HCV RNA at week 12 and/or the presence of detectable viremia at week 24 both predict lack of SVR; accordingly these patients should be advised to stop prematurely anti-HCV therapy.
Monitoring the response to anti-hepatitis C virus therapy in HIV-positive patients	Early virologic response to anti-HCV therapy predicts the chance of sustained response in HIV coinfected patients as it does in HCV-monoinfected individuals. Moreover, the use of an early time point for treatment decision-making seems to be equally appropriate in coinfected patients. Only patients showing a decline in serum HCV-RNA levels greater than 2 logs at 12 weeks on therapy will have a chance of reaching a sustained response. Therefore, treatment might be discontinued in the rest....

Treatment Issue	Panel Findings/Recommendations
Management of adverse effects of anti-hepatitis C virus therapy in HIV-positive patients	Anti-HCV therapy causes fever, malaise, asthenia, depression, etc. in the majority of cases. Patients should be informed in advance about these side effects and how to prevent and manage them... The treatment of depression should be considered as soon as symptoms begin to develop....
Interactions between anti-HIV drugs and those for hepatitis C (2007 update)	While didanosine should never be used with ribavirin, zidovudine should also be avoided when possible.
Treatment of nonresponders and/or relapsers (2007 update)	Non-responders and relapsers to prior courses of HCV therapy are a heterogeneous population and therapeutic interventions in them should be individualized.
Management of end-stage liver disease (2007 update)	HIV infection should no longer be considered a contraindication to orthotopic liver transplantation. However, coinfected patients present unique and highly complex problems post-transplantation, including rapidly progressive recurrent HCV infection and drug interactions (mainly between immunosuppressive agents and protease inhibitors). Accordingly, orthotopic liver transplantation in this population should be limited to transplant centers experienced in the management of such patients, where a multidisciplinary team including surgeons, hepatologists, pharmacologists and infectious diseases physicians can work in concert.
Liver transplantation in HIV coinfected patients	All HIV-infected patients with end-stage liver disease as a result of HCV should be considered candidates for liver transplantation as long as they do not have advanced HIV disease.... HIV-positive candidates should have CD4 cell counts greater than 100 cells/mm^3 and plasma HIV-RNA levels below 200 copies/mL, or the chance of becoming undetectable using optional drugs for successful treatment after transplantation. Moreover, they should have abstained from the consumption of alcohol and illegal drugs for at least 6 months....
Hepatotoxicity of antiretroviral drugs (2007 update)	Patients with chronic HCV infection have an increased risk of liver enzyme elevations following exposure to most antiretroviral drugs. The management of hepatotoxicity should be based on the knowledge of the mechanisms involved for each drug. Treatment of HCV infection may reduce the chances for further development of liver toxicity in these patients.

Adapted from: Soriano V, Puoti M, Sulkowski M, et al. Care of patients with hepatitis C and HIV coinfection. AIDS. 2004;18:1-12.; Soriano V, Puoti M, Sulkowski M, et al. Care of patients with HIV and hepatitis C virus: 2007 updated recommendations from the HCV-HIV International Panel. AIDS. 2007;21:1073-1089.

Summary

Due to common routes of transmission and shared exposures, many people are coinfected with HIV and HCV. Coinfection with HIV is associated with accelerated HCV disease progression and increased risk for liver cancer. Since the introduction of HAART, significant numbers of coinfected persons are experiencing the effects of HCV-related liver disease.

The increased risks associated with coinfection raise the stakes involved in treatment decisions. The management and effective treatment of HCV/HIV coinfection are complex and should be conducted by healthcare providers experienced in this subgroup of clients. All persons being treated for both HIV and HCV must be closely monitored for potentially serious complications.

Many aspects of coinfection are currently being investigated. As these studies are completed, we hope to use the information to develop safer, more effective therapies. The ultimate goal is to reduce the disease burdens currently borne by coinfected persons.

References

1. Thomas, DL. Hepatitis C and human immunodeficiency virus infection. *Hepatology*. 2002;36(Suppl 1):S201-9.
2. Grueb G, Ledergerber B, Battegay M, et al. Clinical progression , survival, and immune recovery during antiretroviral therapy in patients with HIV-1 and hepatitis C virus coinfection: the Swiss HIV Cohort Study. *Lancet*. 2000;356:1800-5.
3. Sherman KE, Rouster SD, Chung RT, Rajicic N. Hepatitis C: prevalence in HIV-infected patients across sectional analysis of the US ACTG. *Antiviral Ther*. 2000;5(Suppl 1):64-5.
4. Waldrep TW, Summers KK, Chiliade PA. Coinfection with HIV and HCV: more questions than answers? *Pharmacotherapy*. 2000;20:1499-1507.
5. Sherman KE, Rouster SD, Chung RT, Rajicic N. Hepatitis C virus prevalence among patients infected with human immunodeficiency virus: a cross-sectional analysis of the US Adult AIDS Clinical Trial Group. *Clin Infect Dis*. 2002;34:831-7.
6. Sulkowski MS, Moore RD, Metha SH, Chaisson RE, Thomas DL. Hepatitis C and progression of HIV disease. *JAMA*. 2002;288:199-206.
7. Soriano V, Sulkowski M, Bergin C, et al. Care of patients with chronic hepatitis C and HIV co-infection: recommendations from the HIV-HCV International Panel. *AIDS*. 2002;16:813-28.
8. De Luca A, Bugarini R, Cozzi Lepri A, et al. Coinfection with hepatitis viruses and outcome of initial antiretroviral regimens in previously naive HIV-infected subjects. *Arch Intern Med*. 2002;162:2125-32.
9. Bonacini M, Lin HJ, Hollinger FB. Effect of coexisting HIV-1 infection on the diagnosis and evaluation of hepatitis C virus. *J Acquir Immune Defic Syndr*. 2001;26:340-4.
10. George SL, Gebhardt J, Klintzman D, et al. Hepatitis C virus viremia in HIV-infected individuals with negative HCV antibody tests. *J Acquir Immune Defic Syndr*. 2002;31(2):154-162.
11. Soriano V, Puoti M, Sulkowski M, et al. Care of patients with hepatitis C and HIV co-infection. *AIDS*. 2004;18:1-12.
12. Verucchi G, Calza R, Manfred R, Chiodo F. Human immunodeficiency virus and hepatitis C virus coinfection: epidemiology, natural history, therapeutic options and clinical management. *Infection*. 2004;33:33-46.
13. Soto B, Sanchez-Quijano A, Rodrigo L, et al. Human immunodeficiency virus infection modifies the natural history of chronic parenterally-acquired hepatitis C with an unusually rapid progression to cirrhosis. *J Hepatol*. 1997;26:1-5.
14. Benhamou Y, Bochet M, Di Martino V, et al. Liver fibrosis progression in human immunodeficiency virus and hepatitis C virus coinfected patients. The Multivirc Group. *Hepatology*. 1999;30:1054-58.
15. Puoti M, Bonacini M, Spinetti A, et al. Liver fibrosis progression is related to CD4 cell depletion in patients coinfected with hepatitis C virus and human immunodeficiency virus. *J Infect Dis*. 2001;183(1):134-7.
16. Bierhoff E, Fischer HP, Willsch E, et al. Liver histopathology in patients with concurrent chronic hepatitis C and HIV infection. *Virchows Arch*. 1997;430(4):271-7.
17. Graham CS, Baden LR, Yu E, et al. Influence of human immunodeficiency virus infection on the course of hepatitis C virus infection: a meta-analysis. *Clin Infect Dis*. 2001;33(4):562-9.
18. Monga HK, Rodriguez-Barradas MC, Breaux K, et al. Hepatitis C virus infection related morbidity and mortality among patients with human immunodeficiency virus infection. *Clin Infect Dis*. 2001;33:240-7.
19. Martin-Carbonero L, Soriano V, Valencia E, Garci´a-Samaniego, J, Lo´pez M, Gonza´lez-Lahoz J. Increasing impact of chronic viral hepatitis on hospital admissions and mortality among HIV-infected patients. *AIDS Res Hum Retroviruses*. 2001; 17:1467–1472.
20. Bica I, McGovern B, Dhar R, McGowan K, Scheib R, Snydman D. Increasing mortality due to end-stage liver disease in patients with HIV infection. *Clin Infect Dis*. 2001; 32:492–497.
21. Rosenthal E, Poiree M, Pradier C, Perronne C, Salmon-Ceron D, Geffray L, et al. Mortality due to hepatitis C-related liver disease in HIV-infected patients in France. *AIDS*. 2003; 17:1803–1809.
22. Garcia-Samaniego J, Rodriguez M, Berenguer J, Rodriguez-Rosado R, Carbo J, Asensi V, Soriano V. Hepatocellular carcinoma in HIV-infected patients with chronic hepatitis C. *Am J Gastroenterol*. 2001;96(1):179-83.
23. Chung RT, Evans SR, Yang Y, et al. Immune recovery is associated with persistent rise in hepatitis C virus RNA, infrequent liver test flares, and is not impaired by hepatitis C virus in coinfected subjects. *AIDS*. 2002;16:1915-23.

24. Dorrucci M, Pezzotti P, Phillips AN, Lepri AC, Rezza G. Coinfection of hepatitis C virus with human immunodeficiency virus and progression to AIDS. Italian Seroconversion Study. *J Infect Dis.* 1995;172:1503-8.

25. Bonacini M, Puoti M. Hepatitis C in patients with human immunodeficiency virus infection: diagnosis, natural history, meta-analysis of sexual and vertical transmission, and therapeutic issues. *Arch Intern Med.* 2000.11-25;160(22):3365-73

26. Sabin CA, Telfer P, Phillips AN, Bhagani S, Lee CA. The association between hepatitis C virus genotype and human immunodeficiency virus disease progression in a cohort of hemophilic men. *J Infect Dis.* 1997;175(1):164-8.

27. Piroth L, Bourgeois C, Dantin S, Waldner A, Grappin M, Portier H, Chavanet P. Hepatitis C virus (HCV) genotype does not appear to be a significant prognostic factor in HIV-HCV-coinfected patients. *AIDS.* 1999 Mar;13(4):523-4

28. Dieterich D, Opravil M, Sasadeusz J, Cooper D, et al. Effect of baseline CD4R % on the efficacy ofpeginterferon alfa-2a plus ribavirin – findings from the APRICOT. 46th Interscience Conference on Antimicrobial Agents and Chemotherapy. San Francisco, September 2006 [abstract H-1888].

29. Mahajan AP, Hogan JW, Snyder B, et al. Changes in Total Lymphocyte Count as a Surrogate for Changes in CD4 Count Following Initiation of HAART: Implications for Monitoring in Resource-Limited Settings. *J Acquir Immune Defic Syndr.* 2004;36(1):567-75.

30. Benhamou Y, Di Martino V, Bochet M, Colombet G, Thibault V, Liou A, Katlama C, Poynard T; MultivirC Group. Factors affecting liver fibrosis in human immunodeficiency virus-and hepatitis C virus-coinfected patients: impact of protease inhibitor therapy. *Hepatology.* 2001;34(2):283-7.

31. Rodriguez-Rosado R, Garcia-Samaniego J, Soriano V. Hepatotoxicity after introduction of highly active antiretroviral therapy. *AIDS.* 1998;12:1256.

32. Saves M, Vandentorren S, Daucourt V. Severe hepatic cytolysis: incidence and risk factors in patients treated by antiretroviral combinations. Aquitaine Cohort, France, 1996-1998. *AIDS.* 1999;13:F115-21.

33. Sulkowski M, Thomas D, Chaisson R, Moore R. Hepatotoxicity associated with antiretroviral therapy in adults infected with HIV and the role of hepatitis C or B virus infection. *JAMA.* 2000;283:74-80.

34. Den Brinker M, Wit F, Wertheim-van Dillen P. Hepatitis B and C virus coinfection and the risk for hepatotoxicity of highly active antiretroviral therapy in HIV-1 infection. *AIDS.* 2000;14:2895-2902.

35. Saves M, Raffi F, Clevenbergh, P, et al. Hepatitis B or hepatitis C virus infection is a risk factor for severe hepatic cytolysis after initiation of a protease inhibitor-contained antiretroviral regimen in HIV-infected patients. *Antimicrob Agents Chemother.* 2000;44:3451-5.

36. Nunez M, Lana R, Mendoza JL, Martin-Carbonero L, Soriano V. Risk factors for severe liver toxicity following the introduction of HAART. *J Acquired Immune Defic Syndr.* 2001;27:426-31.

37. Bonfanti P, Landonio S, Ricci E. Risk factors for hepatotoxicity in patients treated with highly active antiretroviral therapy. *J Acquired Immune Defic Syndr.* 2001;27:316-8.

38. D'Arminio Monforte A, Bugarini R, Pezzotti P. Low frequency of sever hepatotoxicity and association with HCV coinfection in HIV-positive patients treated with HAART. *J Acquired Immune Defic Syndr.* 2001;28:114-23.

39. Aceti A, Pasquazzi C, Zechini B, De Bac C, and the LIVERHAART Group. Hepatotoxicity development during antiretroviral therapy containing protease inhibitors in patients with HIV. The role of hepatitis B and C virus infection. *J Acquired Immune Defic Syndr.* 2002;29:41-8.

40. Wit F, Weverling G, Weel J, Jurrians S, Lange J. Incidence and risk factors for severe hepatotoxicity associated with antiretroviral combination therapy. *J Infect Dis.* 2002;186:23-31.

41. Martinez E, Blanco J, Arnaiz J, Gatell J. Hepatotoxicity in HIV-infected patients receiving nevirapine-containing antiretroviral therapy. *AIDS.* 2001;15:1261-8.

42. Sulkowski M, Thomas D, Mehta S, Chaisson R, Moore R. Hepatotoxicity associated with nevirapine or efavirenz-containing antiretroviral therapy: role of hepatitis C and B infections. *Hepatology.* 2002;35:182-9.

43. Kontorinis N, Dieterich D. Hepatotoxicity of antiretroviral drugs. *AIDS Rev.* 2003;5:36-43.

44. Goelz J, Klausen G, Moll A. Efficacy and tolerance of therapy with IFN-alpha/RIBAVIRIN and pegIFN-alpha/RIBAVIRIN in HCV/HIV coinfected IVDUs. Abstract MoPeB3258. XIV World AIDS Conference. Barcelona, Spain. 2002.

45. Perez-Olmeda M, Nunez M, Romero M, Gonzalez J, Arribas J, Soriano V. Pegylated interferon alpha 2b plus ribavirin as therapy for chronic hepatitis C in HIV-infected patients. *AIDS.* 2003;17:1023-8.

46. Rockstroh J, Schulz C, Mauss S, Klausen G, Voigt E, Gölz J. Pegylated interferon alpha and ribavirin therapy for hepatitis C in HIV-coinfected patients: 24 weeks results. Abstract WePeB6025. XIV World AIDS Conference. Barcelona, Spain. 2002.

47. Perronne C, Carrat F, Bani S. RIBAVIC trial (ANRS HC02): a controlled randomized trial of pegylated interferon alfa-2b plus ribavirin versus interferon alfa2b plus ribavirin for the initial treatment of chronic hepatitis C in HIV coinfected patients: preliminary results. Abstract LbOr16. XIV World AIDS Conference. Barcelona, Spain. 2002.

48. Hopkins S, Lyons F, Brannigan E, Mulcahy F, Bergin C. Tolerability of pegylated interferon and ribavirin in the HCV/HIV coinfected population. Abstract ThPeC7531. XIV World AIDS Conference. Barcelona, Spain. 2002.

49. Chung R, Andersen J, Alston B. A randomized, controlled trial of pegylated interferon alpha 2a with RIBAVIRIN vs. interferon alpha 2a with RIBAVIRIN for the treatment of chronic hepatitis C in HIV coinfection. Abstract LB15. 9th Conference on Retroviruses and Opportunistic Infections. Seattle, Washington. 2002.

50. Cargnel A, Casella A, Angeli E, Gubertini G, Orlando G, De Luca P. Pegylated interferon alfa-2b (PEG-IFN) plus ribavirin for the treatment of HCV/HIV coinfected patients: an open, multicentre, randomized trial. Abstract 115. Digestive Disease Week. San Francisco, California. 2002.

51. Manns M, McHutchison J, Gordon S. Peginterferon alfa-2b plus ribavirin compared with interferon alfa-2b plus ribavirin for initial treatment of chronic hepatitis C: a randomized trial. *Lancet.* 2001;358:958-65.

52. Fried M, Shiffman M, Reddy R. Peginterferon alfa-2a plus ribavirin for chronic hepatitis C virus infection. *N Engl J Med.* 2002;347:975-82.

53. Shire NJ, Welge JA, Sherman KE. Response rates to pegylated interferon and ribavirin in HCV/HIV coinfection: a research synthesis. *J Viral Hepat.* 2007;14(4):239-248.

54. Torriani F, Rodriguez-Torres M, Rockstroh J, Lissen E,Gonzalez- Garcia J, Lazzarin A, et al. Peginterferon alfa-2a plus ribavirin for chronic hepatitis C virus infection in HIV-infected patients. *N Engl J Med.* 2004; 351:438–450.

55. Carrat F, Bani-Sadr F, Pol S, Rosenthal E, Lunel-Fabiani F, Benzekri A, et al. Pegylated interferon alfa-2b vs standard interferon alfa-2b, plus

ribavirin, for chronic hepatitis C in HIV-infected patients: a randomized controlled trial. *JAMA*. 2004; 292:2839–2848.

56. Ballesteros A, Franco S, Fuster D, Planas R, Martinez M, AcostaL, et al. Early HCV dynamics on peg-interferon and ribavirin in HCV/HIV coinfection: indications for the investigation of new treatment approaches. *AIDS*. 2004; 18:59–66.

57. Moreno L, Quereda C, Moreno A, Perez-Elias A, Antela A, Casado JL, et al. Pegylated interferon-a2b R ribavirin for the treatment of chronic hepatitis C in HIV-infected patients. *AIDS*. 2004; 18:67–73.

58. Laguno M, Murillas J, Blanco JL, Martinez E, Miquel R, Sanchez-Tapias JM, et al. Peginterferon alfa-2b plus ribavirin compared with interferon alfa-2b plus ribavirin for treatment of HCV/HIV co-infected patients. *AIDS*. 2004; 18:F27–F36.

59. Chung R, Andersen J, Volberding P, Robbins G, Liu T, Sherman K, et al. Peginterferon Alfa-2a plus ribavirin versus interferon alfa-2a plus ribavirin for chronic hepatitis C in HIV-coinfected persons. *N Engl J Med*. 2004; 351:451–459.

60. Perez-Olmeda M, Nunez M, Romero M, Gonzalez J, Castro A, Arribas J, et al. Pegylated IFN-alpha 2b plus ribavirin as therapy for chronic hepatitis C in HIV-infected patients. *AIDS*. 2003; 17:1023–1028.

61. Voigt E, Schulz C, Klausen G, Goelz J, Mauss S, Schmutz G, et al. Pegylated interferon alpha-2b plus ribavirin for the treatment of chronic hepatitis C in HIV coinfected patients. *J Infect*. 2005; 51:245–249.

62. Cargnel A, Angeli E, Mainini A, Gubertini G, Giorgi R, Schiavini M, et al. Open, randomized, multicentre Italian trial on PEG-IFN plus ribavirin versus PEG-IFN monotherapy for chronic hepatitis C in HIV-coinfected patients on HAART. *Antivir Ther*. 2005; 10:309–317.

63. Santin M, Shaw E, Garcia MJ, Delejido A, De Castro E, Rota R, et al. Efficacy and safety of pegylated interferon alpha-2b plus ribavirin for the treatment of chronic hepatitis C in HIV-infected patients. *AIDS Res Hum Retroviruses*. 2006; 22:315–320.

64. Soriano V, Puoti M, Sulkowski M, et al. Care of patients with HIV and hepatitis C virus: 2007 updated recommendations from the HCV-HIV International Panel. *AIDS*. 2007;21:1073-1089.

65. Crespo M, Esteban J, Ribera E, et al. Utility of the early virological response to individually adjust the duration of treatment for chronic hepatitis C, genotype 2 or 3, in HIV-coinfected patients. 13th Conference on Retroviruses and Opportunistic Infections. Denver, February 2006 [abstract 81].

66. Hopkins S, Lambourne J, Farrell G, et al. Role of individualization of HCV therapy duration in HCV/HIV-coinfected individuals. *HIV Med*. 2006; 7:248–254.

67. Torriani FJ, Ribeiro RM, Gilbert TL, Schrenk UM, Clauson M, Pacheco DM, Perelson AS. Hepatitis C virus (HCV) and human immunodeficiency virus (HIV) dynamics during HCV treatment in HCV/HIV coinfection. *J Infect Dis*. 2003;188(10):1498-507.

68. Berg T, von Wagner M, Nasser S, et al. Extended treatment duration for hepatitis C virus type 1: comparing 48 versus 72 weeks of peginterferonalfa 2a plus ribavirin. *Gastroenterology*. 2006; 130:1086–1097.

69. Sanchez-Tapias JM, Diago M, Escartin P, et al. Peginterferon alfa-2a plus ribavirin for 72 weeks in chronic hepatitis C patients without a response by week 4. *Gastroenterology*. 2006; 131:451–460.

70. Alberti A, Clumeck N, Collins S, et al. Short statement of the first European Consensus Conference on the treatment of chronic hepatitis B and C in HIV co-infected patients. *J Hepatol*. 2005; 42:615–624.

71. Soriano V, Puoti M, Sulkowski M, et al. Care of patients with hepatitis C and HIV co-infection. Updated recommendations from the HIV–HCV International Panel. *AIDS*. 2004; 18:1–12.

72. Soriano V, Garcia-Samaniego J, Bravo R, et al. Interferon alpha for the treatment of chronic hepatitis C in patients infected with HIV. Hepatitis-HIV Spanish Study Group. *Clin Infect Dis*. 1996;23:585-91.

73. Mauss S, Klinker H, Ulmer A, et al. Response to treatment of chronic hepatitis C with interferon alpha in patients infected with HIV-1 is associated with higher CD4+ cell count. *Infection*. 1998;26:16-9.

74. Soriano V, Martı́n-Carbonero L, Garcı́a-Samaniego J. Treatment of chronic hepatitis C virus infection: we must target the virus or liver fibrosis? *AIDS*. 2003; 17:751–753.

75. Saito H, Tada S, Nakamoto N, et al. Efficacy of non-invasive elastometry on staging of hepatic fibrosis. *Hepatol Res*. 2004; 29:97–103.

76. Ziol M, Handra-Luca A, Kettaneh A, et al. Non-invasive assessment of liver fibrosis by measurement of stiffness in patients with chronic hepatitis C. *Hepatology*. 2005; 4:48–54.

77. Castera L, Vergniol J, Foucher J, et al. Prospective comparison of transient elastography Fibrotest, APRI, and liver biopsy for the assessment of fibrosis in chronic hepatitis C. *Gastroenterology*. 2005; 128:343–350.

78. Colletta C, Smirne C, Fabris C, et al. Value of two non-invasive methods to detect progression of fibrosis among HCV carriers with normal aminotransferases. *Hepatology*. 2005; 42:838–845.

79. De Ledinghen V, Douvin C, Kettaneh A, et al. Diagnosis of hepatic fibrosis and cirrhosis by transient elastography in HIV/hepatitis C virus-coinfected patients. *J Acquir Immune Defic Syndr*. 2006; 41:175–179.

80. Vento S, Di Perri G, Cruciani M, Garofano T, Concia E, Bassetti D. Rapid decline of CD4+ cells after interferon treatment in HIV-1 infection. *Lancet*. 1993;341:958-9.

81. Pesce A, Taillan B, Rosenthal E. Opportunistic infections and CD4 lymphcytopenia with interferon treatment in HIV-1 infected patients. *Lancet*. 1993;341:1597.

82. Homma M, Matsuzaki Y, Inoue Y, Shibata M, Mitamura K, Tanaka N, Kohda Y. Marked elevation of erythrocyte ribavirin levels in interferon and ribavirin-induced anemia. *Clin Gastroenterol Hepatol*. 2004;2(4):337-9.

83. Devine EB, Kowdley KV, Veenstra DL, Sullivan SD. Management strategies for ribavirin-induced hemolytic anemia in the treatment of hepatitis C: clinical and economic implications. *Value Health*. 2001;4(5):376-84.

84. Brau N, Rodriguez-Torres M, Prokupek D, et al. Treatment of chronic hepatitis C in HCV/HIV-coinfection with interferon alpha-2b + ribavirin full-course vs 16-week delayed ribavirin. *Hepatology*. 2004; 39:989-998.

85. Okuda M, Li K, Beard MR, Showalter LA, Scholle F, Lemon SM, Weinman SA. Mitochondrial injury, oxidative stress, and antioxidant gene expression are induced by hepatitis C virus core protein. *Gastroenterology*. 2002;122(2):366-75.

86. Lopez S, Miro O, Martinez E, et al. Mitochondrial effects of antiretroviral therapies in asymptomatic patients. *Antivir Ther*. 2004;9(1):47-55.

87. Lafeuillade A, Hittinger G, Chapadaud S. Increased mitochondrial toxicity with ribavirin in HCV/HIV coinfection. *Lancet*. 2001; 357:280-281.

88. Moreno A, Quereda C, Moreno L, et al. High rate of didanosine-related mitochondrial toxicity in HCV/HIV-coinfected patients receiving ribavirin. *Antivir Ther*. 2004; 9:133-138.

89. Garcia-Benayas T, Blanco F, Soriano V. Weight loss in HIV-infected patients. *N Engl J Med.* 2002; 347:1287-1288.
90. Mauss S, Larrey D, Valenti W. Risk factors for hepatic decompensation in cirrhotic patients with HIV-HCV coinfection treated with PEG interferon or interferon and ribavirin or placebo. Abstract PL12.4. Sixth International Congress on Drug Therapy in HIV Infection. Glasgow, Norway. 2002.
91. Perrone C, Carrat F, Banisadr F, et al. ANRS HC02-RIBAVIC: a randomized controlled trial of pegylated interferon alfa-2b plus ribavirin versus interferon alfa-2b plus ribavirin as primary treatment of chronic hepatitis C in HIV coinfected patients. *Hepatology.* 2002;36:283A.
92. Mauss S, Valenti W, Depamphilis J, et al. Risk factors for hepatic decompensation in patients withHCV/HIV coinfection and liver cirrhosis during interferon-based therapy. *AIDS.* 2004;18:F21–F25.
93. Bani-Sadr F, Carrat F, Pol S, et al. Risk factors for symptomatic mitochondrial toxicity in HIV/hepatitis C virus-coinfected patients during interferon plus ribavirin-based therapy. *J Acquir Immune Defic Syndr.* 2005;40:47–52.
94. Miro JM, Laguno M, Moreno A, Rimola A. Management of end stage liver disease: what is the current role of orthotopic liver transplantation? *J Hepatol.* 2006; 44 (suppl):140–145.
95. Neff G, Shire N, Rudich S. Outcomes among patients with end-stage liver disease who are coinfected with HIV and hepatitis C virus. *Clin Infect Dis.* 2005;41 (suppl 1):50–55.
96. Vogel M, Voigt E, Schafer N, Goldmann G, et al. Orthotopic liver transplantation inHIV-positive patients: outcome of 7 patients from the Bonn cohort. *Liver Transpl.* 2005; 11:1515–1521.
97. Ragni MV, Belle SH, Im K, Neff G, Roland M, Stock P, et al. Survival of HIV-infected liver transplant recipients. *J Infect Dis.* 2003; 188:1412–1420.
98. Neff G, Jayaweera D, Tzakis A. Liver transplantation for HIV-infected patients with end-stage liver disease. *Curr Opin Organ Transplant.* 2002;7:114-23.
99. Mindikoglu AL, Regev A, Magder LS. Impact of human immunodeficiency virus on survival after liver transplantation: analysis of United Network for Organ Sharing database. *Transplantation.* 2008 Feb 15;85(3):359-68.
100. Chopra KB, Demetris AJ, Blakolmer K, et al. Progression of liver fibrosis in patients with chronic hepatitis C after orthotopic liver transplantation. *Transplantation.* 2003;76(10):1487-91.
101. Neff GW, et al. Preliminary treatment results of pegylated interferon alpha 2b and ribavirin in liver transplant recipients with recurrent hepatitis C virus nonresponsive to interferon alpha 2b plus ribavirin. Abstract 4447.00. European Association for the Study of the Liver. Geneva, Switzerland. 2003.

HCV / HIV Coinfection

Misha Cohen, OMD, LAc

Alternative Eastern Treatment Options

Traditional Chinese Medicine for HCV/HIV Coinfection

Many people with the *hepatitis C* virus (*HCV*) and/or the *human immunodeficiency virus* (*HIV*) are turning to traditional Chinese medicine (TCM) for treatment. TCM has a long history in the treatment of *chronic hepatitis. Hepatitis B* and C infections are prevalent throughout China, accounting for the increased risk of *liver cancer* (*hepatocellular carcinoma*) in the Chinese population. The Chinese medical system has been dedicated to solving these problems for many years. The Chinese are working to eliminate sources of hepatitis, and to develop treatments for chronic viral hepatitis using both TCM and western medicine.

At the International Symposium on Viral Hepatitis and AIDS held in Beijing, China in April 1991, more than 100 papers on viral hepatitis were presented. Several of these papers documented the positive results of studies involving Chinese herbal medicine. Studies on the use of herbal *antivirals*, and blood cooling and circulating herbs for liver damage repair were presented. These studies corroborated hundreds of years of treatment experience with Chinese herbs for the *symptoms* of hepatitis.[1, 2, 3] A 1995 literature review revealed there are at least 55 herbal formulas that can be used to treat hepatitis.[4] Some recent herbal studies from China and Australia showed positive results in chronic hepatitis C using herbal formulas similar to those widely used in the United States.[5, 6, 7]

In the United States, TCM is a popular *complementary and alternative medicine* (*CAM*) therapy among people with HIV/AIDS and chronic liver diseases. *Anecdotal* reports from one of the largest western medicine hepatology practices in San Francisco suggest that at least 20% to 30% of patients report use of TCM herbs for hepatitis.[8] The rate of use of TCM therapies by HIV positive people is believed to be around 40%.[9] The actual use of TCM may be underestimated because people often choose not to divulge the use of CAM therapies to their western healthcare providers.

TCM uses a variety of healing modalities. *Protocols* have been developed that have successfully helped people infected with HCV and HIV decrease symptoms, normalize or lower *liver enzymes*, and slow the progression of liver disease. A 1995 pilot study conducted among people coinfected with HIV and viral hepatitis (B and C) at the San Francisco's Quan Yin Healing Arts Center indicated acupuncture alone may have an effect in lowering and/or normalizing liver enzymes.[10]

Chinese Medicine Philosophy

The primary goals of TCM are to create wholeness and harmony within a person thereby allowing the mind/body/spirit to self-heal.

Chinese philosophy states there are two opposing principles of life, yin and yang. Imbalances between yin and yang within a person can manifest as illness because the body is considered a microcosm of the world.

TCM defines the *physiological* components of illness using the concepts of *qi* (vital energy), xue (blood), jin-ye (body fluids), jing (essence), shen (spirit), and organ systems. Organ systems are domains within the body that govern particular body tissues, emotional states, and activities.

TCM theory states the key to health is the internal ability of the body to remain strong. According to this theory, people are born with a certain amount of original qi (pronounced "chee"). The qi is easily depleted as energy is used by the body and not replaced. It is difficult to increase the original qi. A person must work hard during life just to retain it. Exercise such as *tai chi* and *qi gong*, healthy eating, and good sleep habits are highly recommended for maintaining the original qi. If a person consistently lacks sleep, does not have a healthy diet, abuses drugs or *alcohol*, and/or has excessive or unsafe sex, he or she becomes qi deficient. When weakened and qi deficient, a person is more susceptible to infection by harmful external elements.[11]

Traditional Chinese Medicine Therapy for HCV/HIV Coinfection

In western medicine, extremely harmful external elements include severe bacterial or viral infections such as HCV and HIV. However, those terms are not used historically in TCM. Instead, Chinese medicine "...recognizes the existence of Pestilences called li qi or yi qi. These are diseases that are not caused by the climatic factors of Heat, Cold, Wind, Dampness, or Summer Heat dryness, but by external infectious agents ... that are severely *toxic* because they strike directly at the interior of the body."[12]

In the case of HIV and/or HCV, the particular pestilence is identified as toxic heat. Toxic heat is considered by TCM to be both an epidemic factor (something that is seen in a number of patients) and its own individual, treatable syndrome. However, HCV and HIV are not identical invasions of toxic heat. They are each characterized by a different set of syndromes involving toxic heat.

Chinese Herbal Medicine for HCV/HIV Coinfection

TCM treatment for HCV/HIV coinfection depends on the *stage* of the disease and the syndromes involved. Herbal medications in conjunction with rest and dietary recommendations can treat the symptoms of *acute hepatitis* fairly rapidly. Chronic hepatitis C is more difficult to treat.

Research and experience both from China and from TCM clinics in the United States suggest that a one-year course of TCM therapy is the minimum needed to alter the progression of hepatitis C. In our clinics, TCM therapy for chronic hepatitis C usually includes combinations of herbal preparations, which are often specifically designed for the disturbed organ system patterns. For example, the combination of Enhance® and Clear Heat® herbal formulas were developed for the treatment of HIV and other chronic viral disease. These formulas were tested in an herbal study at San Francisco General Hospital. Hepatoplex One®, Hepatoplex Two®, and other herbal formulas have been designed specifically for the treatment of chronic hepatitis and related problems

A few Chinese medicine practitioners in the U.S. have developed specific treatments for HCV and HIV infections. Two such practitioners are Dr. Subhuti Dharmananda of Portland, OR and Dr. Qing-Cai Zhang of New York, NY. (See *Chapter 11.2, Modern Chinese Medicine Therapeutics for Hepatitis C* for additional information on Dr. Zhang's protocol.) My own experience treating people with HIV and/or HCV led me to develop the following herbal formulas. The formulas shown in Table 1 can be recommended and prescribed by licensed TCM practitioners who have been trained through the Quan Yin Healing Arts Center's Hepatitis C Professional Training Program.

**Table 1. Examples of Chinese Herbal Formulas Used for HIV and/or HCV
at Chicken Soup Chinese Medicine and Quan Yin Healing Arts Center, San Francisco, CA**

INDICATION	HERBAL FORMULAS
Acute Hepatitis C	Coptis Purge Fire® Clear Heat® Hepatoplex One® Ecliptex®
Chronic Hepatitis C	Hepatoplex One® Hepatoplex Two® Ecliptex®
Immune Disorders	Cordyseng® Enhance® Tremella American Ginseng®
Toxic Heat Related to Chronic Viral *Inflammation*	Clear Heat®
Digestive Problems	Quiet Digestion®
Gallstones or Gallbladder Inflammation	GB6®
Liver Inflammation and Chronic Hepatitis	Milk Thistle 80® Silymarin (Karuna)
Qi Stagnation with Xue Deficiency	Woman's Balance®
Other	Milk Thistle 80® Silymarin (Karuna)

Hepatoplex One® is used for acute and chronic hepatitis symptoms. It may be used when liver enzymes are elevated. It can be used with Clear Heat® to increase the Clear Heat® toxin effect. It is designed to regulate qi, vitalize xue, clear heat, and clean toxin.

While there are herbs to help protect the digestion in Hepatoplex One®, this formula is usually used in conjunction with formulas that protect the spleen and stomach, as there are a number of herbs that are cooling or cold and vitalize xue. For example, to increase the effects of tonifying qi and yin, this formula can be taken with Cordyseng®. If there is spleen dampness and deficiency with loose stools, add Shen Ling®. If there is liver invading spleen, a common scenario in chronic hepatitis patients, you may add Shu Gan®.

To protect the yin in liver disease and specifically in chronic hepatitis, you may use Ecliptex®. For immunodeficiency disorders, you may add Enhance® or Tremella American Ginseng®.
For xue stagnation including liver *fibrosis*, *cirrhosis*, and decreased blood circulation, add Hepatoplex Two®.
For xue deficiency and xue stagnation, or to protect the bone marrow during interferon plus *ribavirin* treatment, add Marrow Plus®.

Hepatoplex Two® is designed to vitalize xue. When used in chronic hepatitis, it should be used in conjunction with other herbal formulas. Its special uses are for liver fibrosis and cirrhosis, and to decrease the size of an enlarged liver. It may also have an effect on splenomegaly (an enlarged spleen). As Hepatoplex Two® is a formula designed to vitalize xue, it should increase circulation of the blood and improve *microcirculation* in the capillaries.

Cordyseng® is used as an adjunct to other herbal formulas to increase the function of qi tonification and increase energy. The formula tonifies both yin and yang. It primarily strengthens the spleen, stomach, kidney, and lung, and helps digestion. It is especially good for the chronic *fatigue* found in chronic hepatitis and AIDS.

Acupuncture Therapies
TCM uses acupuncture extensively in the treatment of chronic hepatitis. Though some of the herbal theories already discussed may apply to acupuncture, the primary goal of acupuncture treatment is to readjust the body's qi in order to enable the body to heal itself. Therefore, acupuncture treatment can be used to treat both specific symptoms and a general epidemic pattern.

After a TCM diagnosis is given for a patient infected with HCV and HIV, an acupuncture treatment plan is developed by considering the epidemic nature of the disease, the individual's complaints, and any underlying constitutional TCM patterns of illness. On a symptomatic level, acupuncture treatments for HCV and HIV infections address digestive functions, appetite, energy level, stress, anxiety, *depression*, pain, and skin complications. Acupuncture has also been used to lower elevated liver enzymes as part of a chronic hepatitis protocol using special acupuncture points.

Moxibustion
An important part of TCM treatment in HCV/HIV coinfection is the use of *moxibustion*. Moxibustion is the burning of the herb mugwort (called moxa in Chinese) over certain points or areas of the body that correspond to acupuncture points. Moxibustion is often used for pain syndromes and areas that appear or feel cold on the body. It is often prescribed for home use in treating both HCV and HIV infections.

Qi Gong
Qi gong *meditation* and exercise is a common practice in China. It is growing in popularity in the United States among people who have HIV and other life-threatening illnesses such as cancer. Many studies from China, Japan, Germany, and the United States show the positive effects of qi gong on immune function. Many locations around the United States offer medical qi gong classes specifically designed for people infected with HCV and HIV.

Dietary Therapy
A healthy diet is considered a key part of maintaining qi and harmony in the body. Most TCM practitioners recommend that their HIV-infected clients eat a cooked, warm diet. Other recommendations are based on the specific organ pattern diagnosis. For example, those suffering from chronic diarrhea may be advised to eat white rice (not brown rice) daily, especially in the form of an easy-to-make rice porridge called congee or jook.

Combining Eastern and Western Therapies

If you decide to use a combination of eastern and western therapies, you must discuss all of your treatment approaches with both your eastern and western practitioners. The use of some herbal therapies in conjunction with *interferon-based therapy* may be inappropriate. However, in my experience, Chinese medicine can be highly effective for the management of side effects from drug therapy. TCM is used as an alternative to western drug therapy in some cases. A list of herbs and drugs that are considered toxic to the liver (*hepatotoxic*) can be found in *Appendix IV*.

Summary

Many people with HCV/HIV coinfection are using TCM as either complementary or alternative treatment. TCM uses a number of therapies for coinfection including acupuncture, moxibustion, Chinese herbs, qi gong, and dietary therapy. While these therapies have not undergone *clinical trials* in the west, many of them have been used for centuries in China for hepatitis and other conditions. The results of modern Chinese research on herbs and other modalities are used in the development of current Chinese medicine treatments for HCV/HIV coinfection.

It is important to discuss all treatment approaches with both your eastern and western practitioners in order to ensure the safety of and to gain the greatest benefit from all of your treatment modalities. For recommended reading on traditional Chinese medicine, please see the *Resource Directory*.

References

1.   Chen Z, et al. Clinical analysis of chronic hepatitis B treated with TCM compositions Fugan No. 33 by two lots. *International Symposium on Viral Hepatitis and AIDS*. Beijing, China. Abstract, p 2. 1991.
2.   Wang C, He J, Zhu C. Research of repair of liver pathologic damage in 63 cases of hepatitis with severe cholestatis by blood-cooling and circulation-invigorating Chinese herbs. *International Symposium on Viral Hepatitis and AIDS*. Beijing China. Abstract, p 5. 1991.
3.   Zhao R, Shen H. Antifibrogenesis with traditional Chinese herbs. *International Symposium on Viral Hepatitis and AIDS. Beijing China*. Abstract, p 20. 1991.
4.   Ergil K. *Fifth Symposium of the Society for Acupuncture Research Conference*. Herbal safety and research panel. Society for Acupuncture Research Conference. Palo Alto, California.1998.
5.   Batey RG, Benssoussen A, Yang Yifan, Hossain MA, Bollipo S. Chinese herbal medicine lowers ALT in hepatitis C. A randomized placebo controlled trial report. Cathay Herbal Laboratories. Sydney Australia. 1998.
6.   Li H, et al. Qingtui fang applied in treating 128 cases of chronic hepatitis C. *Chinese Journal of Integrated Traditional and Western Medicine for Liver Diseases*. 1994;4(2):40.
7.   Wu C, et al. Thirty-three patients with hepatitis C treated by TCM syndrome differentiation. *Chinese Journal of Integrated Traditional and Western Medicine for Liver Diseases*. 1994;4(l):44-45.
8.   Gish R. California Pacific Medical Center, San Francisco. Personal communication. 1996.
9.   Duggan J, Peterson WS, Schutz M, Khuder S, Charkraborty J. Use of complementary and alternative therapies in HIV-infected patients. *AIDS Patient Care STDS*. 2001;15(3):159-167.
10.   Cohen MR, Wilson CJ, Surasky A. Acupuncture treatment in people with HCV and HIV coinfection and elevated transaminases. *XII International Conference on AIDS*. Abstract 60211. Geneva, Switzerland. 1998.
11.   Cohen MR, Donor K. *The Chinese Way to Healing: Many Paths To Wellness*. Universe; 2006
12.   Cohen MR, Doner K. *The HIV Wellness Sourcebook*. New York, New York: Henry Holt & Company; 1998.

HIV / HCV COINFECTION

J. Lyn Patrick, ND

NATUROPATHIC TREATMENT OPTIONS

Introduction

This section discusses the naturopathic treatment options available for people coinfected with the *hepatitis C virus* (*HCV*) and the *human immunodeficiency virus* (*HIV*). See *Chapter 14, Naturopathic Medicine* for more information about the naturopathic approach to treating viral *hepatitis*. See *Chapter 16, Nutritional Supplementation* for additional details on the nutritional supplements mentioned in this section.

Antioxidants

An important similarity between *chronic hepatitis* C and HIV/AIDS is that both infections appear to progress more rapidly in situations of increased oxidative stress. Oxidative stress refers to a state in which there is an overabundance of molecules called *free radicals*. Free radicals can damage cells and are involved in the processes of *inflammation* and scarring. Increased oxidative stress is indicated by low levels of the active form of *glutathione* in the *lymphocytes* and blood of people with HIV and/or HCV. Lack of glutathione can lead to immune suppression, decline of *immune system* function, and an increase in HIV *replication*.[1] While glutathione levels are low in those infected with HCV or HIV alone, they are lowest in those who are coinfected.[2]

Glutathione is produced by the liver. Low levels of glutathione are associated with active liver disease on *liver biopsy* and increased levels of the *liver enzyme ALT*.[2] Several studies have been done in both HCV and HIV to look at the role of *antioxidants* in raising glutathione levels. These studies show the use of antioxidants such as N-acetyl cysteine and *vitamin C* have a positive effect on glutathione levels in the blood and white blood cells of those infected with HIV. Antioxidants have also been shown to significantly lower HIV *viral load*.[3]

N-Acetyl Cysteine

Not all studies of N-acetyl cysteine (NAC) in HIV/AIDS and chronic hepatitis C have shown significant effects.[4] However, studies that showed no effect were generally small and lasted only a few weeks. In studies that have shown NAC has a glutathione elevating effect in people with HIV, this effect was seen only after eight weeks of therapy.[5]

A small study found HCV positive, HIV negative patients who were given 600 mg of NAC three times a day for four weeks experienced normalization of ALT levels. These normalized ALT levels may relate to increased glutathione levels.[6] Two additional randomized studies involving 147 and 77 patients with chronic hepatitis C evaluated the effects of adding NAC to *interferon monotherapy*. The study results were mixed, with one showing significant benefit and the other no evidence of benefit. Additional research with larger study populations and perhaps with higher doses of NAC are needed to determine a definitive role for NAC in the setting of HCV/HIV coinfection.[7, 8]

NAC has been shown to be safe in doses of 1,500 mg to 2,000 mg per day. Researchers in this field suggest this dose is sufficient to affect glutathione levels in people who are HIV infected (personal communication, Lenore A. Herzenberg, PhD,

Stanford University). In a 2007 review article on the topic of NAC, Dr. Herzenberg and her coauthors concluded, "Oral administration of NAC, a safe, well-tolerated drug with no clinically significant adverse effects, has been shown to be beneficial in settings where GSH [glutathione] deficiency occurs, for example, HIV infection..."[9]

Alfa-Lipoic Acid

Alfa-lipoic acid is an antioxidant that exists in small quantities in the food we eat. It has been shown to increase glutathione levels in those with HIV when given at doses of 450 mg per day. This dosage is considered moderate and has been shown to be safe. This dose was also effective at significantly raising the level of *CD4 cells* (a type of immune cell) after 14 days in the same study patients.[10] The findings of a small study published in 2008 showed that daily oral supplementation with alfa-lipoic acid (300 mg three times per day in the study) over a 6-month period resulted in significant elevation of blood glutathione and *CD4 counts*.[11]

Alfa-lipoic acid has positive antioxidant effects in mitochondrial *toxicity*, a common problem inside the cells in coinfected people. In addition, alfa lipoic acid has been shown to prevent damage that results from *free radical* production in both the nervous system and the liver.[12]

Oxidation or production of free radicals occurs in the white blood cells and liver of HCV/HIVcoinfected persons. This can lead to *neuropathy* (nerve damage) and liver damage. Although there have been no large scale studies on the effects of alfa-lipoic acid in HCV/HIVcoinfected individuals, it has been proven to be safe at dosages of up to1,200 mg daily in those who are HIV positive.[13]

Alfa-lipoic acid may be useful in decreasing the risk of kidney stones, a side effect of the protease inhibitor indinavir, an *antiviral* drug used to treat HIV infection.[14]

SAMe

S-adenosylmethionine (SAMe) is a protein made in the liver. It is also available as a nutritional supplement. SAMe has been found to be an effective treatment for certain types of *depression*. A recent study of 20 persons living with HIV and diagnosed with major depression found treatment with SAMe resulted in rapid and progressive decreases in depressive symptoms over the 8-week study period.[15]

SAMe is also used to treat liver disease. SAMe has been shown to be effective in raising glutathione levels in the liver cells of those with *cirrhosis*, and in the nervous systems of HIV positive patients.[16, 17] In addition, a recent animal model study of oxidative liver damage (which is believed to contribute to hepatitis C disease progression), found SAMe supplementation interrupted the experimentally induced liver damage.[18]

Dosages of 1,200 mg daily have been shown to increase liver glutathione levels in people with liver diseases. This dose has been used in other conditions and has been shown to be safe and free of side effects.

Vitamin E

Vitamin E deficiency is common in HIV infection.[19, 20] While vitamin E has not been shown to raise glutathione levels, it does play an important role as an antioxidant in coinfection. Increased intake may be related to slower HIV disease progression. A study of HIV positive men who were followed for over six years showed a decreased risk of disease progression to AIDS in those who took twice the amount of vitamin E as those in the study who did not have HIV.[21] At a moderate dose of 200 IU to 400 IU per day, vitamin E has also been shown to protect against the bone marrow toxicity that is a well-established side effect of the HIV drug zidovudine (AZT).[22,23] As an antioxidant, vitamin E has been shown to protect cell membranes from *lipid* peroxidation, a specific type of free radical damage. This is one of the reasons vitamin E is particularly helpful in preventing liver damage. As explained in *Chapter 16, Nutritional Supplementation*, vitamin E interrupts the biochemical pathways that lead to liver *fibrosis*. However, this does <u>not</u> mean that vitamin E can completely stop the damage caused by HCV, or that it is okay to continue drinking *alcohol* if you take vitamin E.

Research indicates that vitamin E is protective against liver fibrosis and plays a role in preventing the free radical activity that can lead to HIV replication. Vitamin E is nontoxic in doses up to 2,000 IU per day, unless there are blood clotting problems. In this case, vitamin E should only be used with guidance from a doctor. The most beneficial forms of vitamin E are d-alfa-tocopherol, d-alfa tocopherol succinate, and mixed tocopherols.

Selenium

Selenium is probably one of the most important nutrients for HIV positive people. A 1997 research study of HIV-infected people showed that those with the lowest levels of selenium had a 10-fold greater risk of dying from the disease than those with normal levels of selenium. This risk was independent of the *CD4 count* at the time of the study (often an important marker of HIV prognosis), the use of antiviral treatment, and levels of other important nutrients.[24] A more recent 2007 study confirmed the protective effects of selenium supplementation for those with HIV. Investigators found that those receiving daily selenium had decreased HIV viral load, and higher CD4 counts.[25] This held true even for those in the study who were coinfected with HCV.

Studies have found selenium levels in people with HCV/HIVcoinfection are even lower than in those with HIV only, even in people without symptoms.[26] Selenium has been shown to raise blood levels of the active form of glutathione in HIV positive persons.[27]

Clinical trials involving HIV/AIDS patients have shown that 400 mcg of selenium per day resulted in significant increases in blood selenium levels, improved appetite, better digestion, and fewer recurrent infections.[28]

Amino Acids

L-Glutamine

L-glutamine is an *amino acid* found in large quantities in muscle, intestine, and immune cells. L-glutamine and the amino acid cysteine are both required by the body to make glutathione.

L-glutamine is particularly important in people with HIV. L-glutamine is one of the nutrients the body loses because of HIV infection. This loss is compounded by the body's demand for additional L-glutamine resulting from the rapid turnover of immune cells and the stress of infections (including coinfection with HCV and other viruses). This added demand usually results in an L-glutamine deficiency. Glutamine deficiency appears to be one of the causes of wasting (weight loss and muscle loss) that occurs in people with AIDS.[29]

L-glutamine is a primary fuel source for intestinal cells. An L-glutamine deficiency can lead to problems absorbing nutrients from the intestine. About 20% of people with AIDS have abnormal intestinal absorption. This problem has been treated successfully with L-glutamine.[30] Supplemental L-glutamine has been shown to be beneficial in regaining lost muscle and lean body mass (body weight that is not fat) among people with HIV-related wasting. In one study, the daily doses of L-glutamine supplementation ranged from 8 grams to 40 grams. The people who gained the most lean body mass took daily doses of 40 grams per day (divided into four equal doses of 10 grams) for a period of 12 weeks.[30-32] See *Chapter 16, Nutritional Supplementation* for more information.

L-Carnitine

L-carnitine is an amino acid that is particularly important for muscle and immune cells. L-carnitine is another nutrient that can become deficient in certain groups of HIV-infected individuals. One study found carnitine deficiencies in 72% of a group of AIDS patients on AZT.[33] HIV positive patients are at risk for L-carnitine deficiency as a result of *malabsorption*, kidney problems, specific antibiotic and *antiviral* medications, and lipoatrophy (weight loss that is mostly fat tissue).[34] Preliminary studies have shown that people with chronic hepatitis C have a deficiency of acylcarnitine, a specific form of L-carnitine.[35] It is not fully understood why this deficiency occurs; but we know that HCV damages the mitochondria (the powerhouses of cells) in the liver, and that mitochondrial function uses acylcarnitine. Therefore, by causing mitochondrial damage, HCV may cause a need for more L-carnitine in people with chronic hepatitis C. More studies are needed to clarify this issue.

Studies in people with HIV have shown that L-carnitine has a positive effect on the immune system, normalizes high *triglycerides* (blood fats), reduces muscle wasting from AZT, and improves neuropathy symptoms associated with NRTI antiviral medications.[36-41] Carnitine and acetyl-L-carnitine (a specific form used to treat mitochondrial toxicity) are used in Europe to treat the peripheral neuropathy (nerve damage) that often occurs in HIV patients as a side effect of some antiviral drugs. Dosages of 3 grams to 6 grams per day of L-carnitine are used to treat elevated blood fats and muscle wasting in people with HIV. Carnitine is available both as a prescription drug and over-the-counter as a nutritional supplement.

Summary

The biological effects of HIV and HCV on antioxidants in the body make it necessary to restore these nutrients with nutritional supplements. Research has shown that taking N-acetyl cysteine, alfa lipoic acid, SAMe, vitamin E, selenium, L-glutamine, and L-carnitine is safe when appropriate doses are used. These supplements can also be used safely in combination with western therapies and/or traditional Chinese medicine. A healthcare provider who is trained in clinical nutrition and the treatment of coinfection should be consulted for optimal benefit from an antioxidant protocol. It is important to discuss your nutritional supplementation with all of your healthcare providers to make sure your protocol is both safe and effective.

References

1. Muller F, Aukrust P, Svardal AM, et al. The thiols glutathione, cysteine, and homocysteine in human immunodeficiency virus (HIV) infection. In: Watson RR (Ed.). *Nutrients and Foods in AIDS. 1st Edition*. New York, NY: CRC Press; 1998:35-69.
2. Barbaro G, Di Lorenzo G, Soldini M, et al. Hepatic glutathione deficiency in chronic hepatitis C: quantitative evaluation in patients who are HIV positive and HIV negative and correlations with plasmatic and lymphocytic concentrations and with the activity of the liver disease. *Am J Gastroenterol*. 1996;91(12):2569-2573 .
3. Muller F, Aukrust P, Svardal AM, et al. Thiols to treat AIDS. In: Watson RR (Ed.). *Nutrition and AIDS, 2nd Edition*. CRC Press. New York, NY: CRC Press; 2001:84.
4. Treitinger A, Spada C, Masokawa IY, et al. Effect of N-acetyl-L-cysteine on lymphocyte apoptosis, lymphocyte viability, TNF-alpha and IL-8 in HIV-infected patients undergoing anti-retroviral treatment. *Am J Clin Nutr*. 2007;85(5):1335-1343.
5. Herzenberg LA, De Rosa SC, Dubs JG, et al. Glutathione deficiency is associated with impaired survival in HIV disease. *Proc Natl Acad Sci USA*. 1977;94(5):1967-1972.
6. Beloqui O, Prieto J, Suarez M, et al. N-acetyl cysteine enhances the response to interferon-alpha in chronic hepatitis C: a pilot study. *J Interferon Res*. 1993;13(4):279-282.
7. Grant PR, Black A, Garcia N, Prieto J, Garson JA. Combination therapy with interferon-alpha plus N-acetyl cysteine for chronic hepatitis C: a placebo controlled double-blind multicentre study. *J Med Virol*. 2000;61:439–442.
8. Neri S, Ierna D, Antoci S, Campanile E, D'Amico RA, Noto R. Association of alpha-interferon and acetyl cysteine in patients with chronic C hepatitis. *Panminerva Med*. 2000;42:187–192.
9. Atkuri KR, Mantovani JJ, Herzenber LA, Herzenberg LA. N-Acetylcysteine – a safe antidote for cysteine/glutathione deficiency. *Curr Opin Pharmacol*. 2007;7(4):355-359.
10. Fuchs J, Schofer H, Milbradt R, et al. Studies on lipoate effects on blood redox state in human immunodeficiency virus infected patients. *Arzneimittelforschung*. 1993;43(12):1359-1362.
11. Jariwalla RJ, Lalezari J, Cenko D, et al. Restoration of Blood Total Glutathione Status and Lymphocyte Function Following alpha-Lipoic Acid Supplementation in Patients with HIV Infection. *J Altern Complement Med*. 2008;14(2):139-146.
12. Packer L, Witt EH, Tritschler HJ. Alpha-lipoic acid as a biological antioxidant. *Free Rad Biol Med*. 1995;19(2):227-250.
13. Kieburtz K, Schifitto G, McDermott M, et al. A randomized, double-blind, placebo-controlled trial of deprenyl and thioctic acid in human immunodeficiency virus-associated cognitive impairment. Dana Consortium on the Therapy of HIV Dementia and Related Cognitive Disorders. *Neurology*. 1998;50(3):645-651.
14. Jayanthi S, Varalakshmi P. Tissue lipids in experimental calcium oxalate lithiasis and the effect of DL alpha-lipoic acid. *Biochem Int*. 1992;26:913-921.
15. Shippy RA, Mendez D, Jones K, Cergnul I, Karpiak SE. S-adenosylmethionine (SAM-e) for the treatment of depression in people living with HIV/AIDS. *BMC Psychiatry*. 2004;4:38.
16. Vendemiale G, Altomare E, Trisio T, et al. Effects of oral S-adenosyl-L-methionine on hepatic eroxidases in patients with liver disease. *Scand J Gastroenterol*. 1989;24(4):407-415.
17. Castagna A, Le Grazie C, Accordini A, et al. Cerebrospinal fluid S-adenosylmethionine (SAMe) and glutathione concentrations in HIV infection: effect of parenteral treatment with SAMe. *Neurology*. 1995;45(9):1678-1683.
18. Villanueva JA, Esfandiari F, White ME, Devaraj S, French SW, Halsted CH. S-adenosylmethionine attenuates oxidative liver injury in micropigs fed ethanol with a folate-deficient diet. *Alcohol Clin Exp Res*. 2007;31(11):1934-1943.

19. Beach RS, Mantero-Atienza E, Shor-Pozner G. et al. Specific nutrient abnormalities in asymptomatic HIV-1 infection. *AIDS*. 1992;6(7):701-708.
20. Dworkin BD, Wormser GP, Axelrod F, et al. Dietary intake in patients with acquired immunodeficiency syndrome (AIDS), patients with AIDS-related complex, and serologically eroxida human immunodeficiency virus patients: correlations with nutritional status. *JPEN*. 1990;14(6):605-609.
21. Abrams B, Duncan D, Hertz-Picciotto I. A prospective study of dietary intake and acquired immunodeficiency syndrome in HIV-seropositive homosexual men. *J Acquir Immune Defic Syndr*. 1993;6(8):949-958.
22. Ganser A, Greher J, Volkers B, et al. Azidothymidine in the treatment of AIDS. *N Engl J Med*. 1988;318(4):250-251.
23. Geissler RG, Ganser A, Ottmann OG, et al. In vitro improvement of bone marrow-derived hematopoetic colony formation in HIV-positive patients by alpha-D-tocopherol and eroxidasesin. *Eur J Haematol*. 1994;53(4):201-206.
24. Baum MK, Shor-Posner G, Lai S, et al. High risk of HIV-related mortality is associated with selenium deficiency. *J Acquir Immune Defic Syndr Hum Retrovirol*. 1997;15(5):370-374.
25. Hurwitz BE, Klaus JR, Llabre MM, et al. Suppression of human immunodeficiency virus type 1 viral load with selenium supplementation: a randomized controlled trial. *Arch Intern Med*. 2007;167(2):148-154.
26. Look MP, Rockstroh JK, Rao GS, et al. Serum selenium, plasma glutathione (GSH), and erythrocyte glutathione eroxidases (GSH-Px)-levels in asymptomatic versus symptomatic human immunodefiency virus-1 (HIV-1)-infection. *Eur J Clin Nutr*. 1997;51(4):266-272.
27. Delmas-Beauvieux MC, Peuchant E, Couchouron A, et al. The enzymatic antioxidant system in blood and glutathione status in human immunodeficiency virus (HIV)-infected patients: effects of supplementation with selenium or beta-carotene. *Am J Cl Nutr*. 1996;64(1):101-107.
28. Olmstead L, Schrauzer GN, Flores-Arce M, et al. Selenium supplementation of symptomatic human immunodeficiency virus infected patients. *Biol Trace Elem Res*. 1989;29:59-65.
29. Shabert JK, Wilmore DW. Glutamine deficiency as a cause of human immunodeficiency virus wasting. *Med Hypotheses*. 1996;46(3):252-256.
30. Noyer CM, Simon D, Borczuk A, et al. A double-blind placebo-controlled pilot study of glutamine therapy for abnormal intestinal permeability in patients with AIDS. *Am J Gastroenterol*. 1998;93(6):972-975.
31. Clarke RH, Feleke G, Din M, et al. Nutritional treatment for acquired immune deficiency syndrome virus-associated wasting using beta-hydroxy beta-methylbutyrate, glutamine, and arginine: a randomized, placebo-controlled study. *JPEN*. 2000;24:133-139.
32. Shabert J, Winslow C, Lacey JM, Wilmore DW. Glutamine-antioxidant supplementation increases body cell mass in AIDS patients with weight loss: a randomized, double-blind controlled trial. *Nutrition*. 1999;15(11-12):860-864.
33. De Simone C, Tzantzoglou S, Jirillo E, et al. Carnitine deficiency in AIDS patients. *AIDS*. 1992;6(2):203-205.
34. De Simone C, Famularo G, Tzantzoglou S, et al. Carnitine depletion in peripheral blood mononuclear cells from patients with AIDS: effect of oral L-carnitine. *AIDS*. 1994;8(5):655-660.
35. Kuratsune H, Yamaguti K, Lindh G, et al. Low levels of serum acylcarnitine in chronic fatigue syndrome and chronic hepatitis type C, but not seen in other diseases. *Int J Mol Med*. 1998;2(1):51-56.
36. De Simone C, Tzantzoglou S, Famularo G, et al. High-dose L-carnitine improves immunologic and metabolic parameters in AIDS patients. *Immunopharmacol Immunotoxicol*. 1993;15(1):1-12.
37. Campos Y, Huertas R, Lorenzo G, et al. Plasma carnitine insufficiency and effectiveness of L-carnitine therapy in patients with mitochondrial myopathy. *Muscle Nerve*. 1993;16(2):150-153.
38. Dalakas MC, Leon-Monzon ME, Bernardini I, et al. Zidovudine-induced mitochondrial myopathy is associated with muscle carnitine deficiency and lipid storage. *Ann Neurol*. 1994;35(4):482-487.
39. Arnaudo E, Dalakas M, Shanske S, et al. Depletion of muscle mitochondrial DNA in AIDS patients with zidovudine-induced myopathy. *Lancet*. 1991;337(8740):508-510.
40. Davis HJ, Miene LJ, van der Westhuizen N, et al. L-carnitine and magnesium as a supportive supplement with antiviral drugs. Abstract 42384. *Int Conf AIDS*. 1998;12:851
41. Youle M, Osio M. A double-blind, parallel-group, placebo-controlled, multicentre study of acetyl L-carnitine in the symptomatic treatment of antiretroviral toxic neuropathy in patients with HIV-1 infection. *HIV Med*. 2007;8(4):241-250.

MENTAL HEALTH AND HEPATITIS C

Julie Nelligan, PhD, David W. Indest, PsyD, and Peter Hauser, MD

SECTION 1 MENTAL HEALTH AND NEUROCOGNITIVE ISSUES ASSOCIATED WITH HCV INFECTION

Introduction

As with many long-term illnesses, *chronic hepatitis* C infection frequently has associated mental health issues. Because mental health affects every part of life, it is important to understand the many ways mind and body work together in people with the *hepatitis C virus* (*HCV*). We know that mental health conditions such as *depression* may occur along with physical symptoms and difficulties in daily functioning, ability to follow treatment directions, and quality of life. Furthermore, until recently, people with mental illness were discouraged from seeking treatment for HCV for fear of making their mental health problems worse.

This chapter will discuss the link between mental health and HCV, how mental health can affect coping with HCV, and eligibility for HCV treatment. Finally, we will discuss whether HCV can cause problems with thinking and memory.

Mental Health and HCV

Many people with HCV have mental health concerns. A study of Veterans Affairs Medical Centers (VAMCs) in the Northwest United States found that 78% of HCV-infected veterans had at least one psychiatric or substance use disorder.[1] In addition, 54% had a history of both a psychiatric disorder and a substance use disorder.[1] Research at the VAMC in Portland, Oregon found that 93% of HCV-infected veterans said they had a history of at least one psychiatric disorder, and 73% had two or more disorders. *Depression* (81%) was the most common disorder, followed by posttraumatic stress disorder (62%), substance use disorders (58%), bipolar disorder (20%), and other psychotic disorders (17%).[2] Another study at the VAMC in Minneapolis, Minnesota found that 81% of patients being seen in the chronic hepatitis C clinic has at least one positive screening test for psychiatric problems. Among those with a positive screening test, only 38% had an establish mental health provider.[3]

Studies in other settings (not limited veterans) support these findings and suggest that it is not uncommon for people with HCV to have mental health problems.[4-7] Furthermore, it is well established that persons with serious mental health problems and/or substance abuse may be up to 10-times more likely to be infected with HCV than the general population.[8]

Depression

Depression is the most common mental health concern for people with HCV. Stress, loss, loneliness, and certain chemical imbalances in the brain can cause depression. Depression is also a side effect of the medication used to treat HCV (see *Chapter 22.2, Mental Health Issues in the Setting of Interferon-Based Therapy*). One recent study showed that 28% of HCV patients were depressed,[9] compared with 2% to 9% of the general public. Another study found that 35% of HCV patients reported emotional distress. The percentage of patients with depression was similar to patients who reported other long-term medical illnesses such as *HIV* infection and arthritis, and higher than in people without medical illness.[10] Finally, a recent study from the Portland VAMC found that 34% of veterans with HCV admitted to moderate to severe depressive symptoms.[11]

Anxiety

Anxiety is another issue that many patients with HCV experience. One study found that 24% of HCV patients had a current anxiety disorder. It also suggested that many patients do not know they have an anxiety disorder until after they learn they have HCV.[9] Most research about anxiety shows that it is at least as common as depression.[10, 12-14] Despite that, it is common for anxiety disorders to be overlooked by doctors and other medical providers.[9]

Post-Traumatic Stress Disorder (PTSD)

Among veterans, PTSD is particularly common. Early studies showed that between 21% and 43% of veterans with HCV had a diagnosis of PTSD.[14-15] Another study at the Portland VAMC found that among 293 veterans with HCV, 62% screened positive for PTSD suggesting that they had either a diagnosis of PTSD or recent symptoms of PTSD.[2] Studies outside the VA healthcare network have found that PTSD is not nearly as common. For example, a study from 2005 that assessed 90 HCV patients from a university teaching hospital found 22 (24%) patients with an anxiety disorder, 25 (28%) patients with depression, but no patients with PTSD.[9] Community-based studies suggest that PTSD affects about 8% of the general population.[16] Taken together, these studies show that PTSD is common in veterans with HCV, but less common in nonveterans with HCV.

Treatment of Anxiety and Depression

Although patients with HCV have depression and anxiety at higher rates than the general population, medications that are used to treat these disorders are thought to be safe.[17] This is fortunate because providers are often reluctant to give *interferon-based therapy* to patients who have mental health problems.[18] The concern is that *interferon* therapy may make mental health problems worse.

Patients who are being considered for interferon-based therapy will often have a pretreatment psychiatric evaluation. If the evaluation suggests the patient has a mental health problem such as anxiety or depression, then a recommendation for treatment will likely be made that includes medication. Other treatment recommendations may include education about the treatment process (this includes treatment for HCV, as well as depression or anxiety) and regular follow-ups with adjustments as needed.[17]

Severe Mental Illness

Persons with a severe mental illness such as a psychotic disorder (schizophrenia) or bipolar disorder are infected with HCV at much higher rates than the general population. A multi-site study funded by the National Institute of Mental Health found that approximately 20% of adults who have a severe mental illness also have HCV.[19] In contrast, only about 2% of the general population has HCV.

Unfortunately, most people with a severe mental illness do not know they have hepatitis C. Also, they commonly do not have access to or seek medical care as often as people without a severe mental illness. This means they are less likely to be tested for HCV.[19] People with severe mental illness have higher rates of substance use disorders and other behaviors that put them at higher risk of getting HCV. The rate of substance use disorders in people with schizophrenia is almost 5 times higher than the rate in the general population.[20, 21] In addition to injection drug use, crack cocaine is a common problem for this group. Smoking crack cocaine leads to other high-risk behaviors such as unsafe injection practices, unsafe sex, multiple sex partners, and trading sex for drugs. All of these behaviors have been linked with increased risk of HCV infection.[22]

Substance Use Disorders

Many people who have HCV acquired the virus through activities related to injection drug use (IDU).[23] A recent population survey found that of people aged 20 to 59 years, a history of IDU at some point in their lives was the risk factor most strongly associated with HCV.[24] Sixty percent of all HCV infection within the United States is attributed to IDU. It is well-documented that injection drug users often have *clinical* depression.[25, 26] One study recently found that injection drug users who were depressed were more likely to share their "works", increasing their risk of getting HCV.[27] Substance use disorders associated with HCV are not limited to IDU. *Alcohol*, cocaine, methamphetamine, marijuana, and other drugs are also risk factors even if not used intravenously. One study found that 58% of veterans with HCV said they had a history of substance abuse and 51% reported both a psychiatric and substance abuse history.[2] Not only does a history of substance abuse increase a person's risk for acquiring HCV, but often individuals with substance use disorders also have mood or anxiety disorders.

> **Alcohol use in patients with hepatitis C is a dangerous combination. The more alcohol consumed, the greater the increased risk of cirrhosis.**

Alcohol use in patients who have HCV is of particular concern. This is because the combination of heavy alcohol use along with the hepatitis C virus causes more damage to the liver than either alcohol or HCV alone causes.[28] One study found that drinking 75 grams of alcohol per day on average (a little more than a 6-pack of beer) increased the risk of liver *cirrhosis* in people with HCV 26-fold. The more alcohol consumed, the greater the risk of cirrhosis.[28] Heavy alcohol use is usually considered to be more than 4 standard drinks per day for men and more than 3 standard drinks per day for women. A standard drink is one 12-ounce beer, one 4-ounce glass of wine, or one 1.5-ounce shot of hard liquor.

Cognitive Problems

Another common issue that patients with HCV report is problems with thinking and memory, also called cognition. Research looking into the relationship between cognition and hepatitis C has only recently been conducted. There are several factors that may play a role in a link between HCV and cognitive problems. These factors include:

- direct effects of HCV on the brain
- indirect effects of HCV caused by severe liver damage and its consequences
- direct effects of substance use on the brain
- taking the medication that treats HCV (interferon-based therapy)

Direct Effects of HCV

Although HCV primarily affects the liver, it might also affect the brain. Patients with HCV often complain of depression, *fatigue*, and impairments in quality of life. In the hepatitis C community, these symptoms are sometimes called "brain fog." These complaints are not associated with degree of liver disease.[29-32] Many patients also report cognitive changes. Sometimes these are from damage to the brain from substance abuse. But studies have found mild cognitive problems in patients with HCV that are not from substance use.[30, 33] However, one study found that greater liver damage was related to poorer performance on cognitive tests.[34] Overall, individuals with HCV appear to perform below expected levels on tests of attention, concentration, and other functions such as planning and controlling impulses.[32, 34] The reason why is not clear. It could be from liver disease, substance use, the hepatitis C virus, or some combination of these or other factors.

Indirect Effects of HCV

People with HCV are at increased risk of developing cirrhosis of the liver. About 20% of patients will develop cirrhosis within 20 years of being infected.[35] The liver damage caused by HCV may also cause cognitive problems. In advanced stages of liver disease, the liver cannot function properly. As a result, people often experience a condition called *hepatic encephalopathy* that affects their thinking and memory. Hepatic encephalopathy is thought to occur because substances that are toxic to brain cells (neurotoxins), such as *ammonia* and manganese, get into the brain. That makes brain cells not work as well as they normally do.

Symptoms of hepatic encephalopathy depend on the how much damage has been done to the liver. Initially patients have trouble with attention, concentration, coordination, changes in mood (depression or irritability), and mental slowness. As hepatic encephalopathy gets worse, the patient will experience *lethargy*, inappropriate behavior, slurred speech, and drowsiness. In the later more severe stages, patients become disoriented and confused. They may develop amnesia, become incoherent, and fall into a coma.

Direct Effects of Substance Use
It can be hard to tell whether substance abuse or HCV have led to cognitive problems. Many people that have HCV also have a history of substance abuse. That's because substance abuse is the most common way people get HCV. We know that substance abuse can cause permanent cognitive problems. Several studies have documented the negative effects of marijuana, cocaine, opiates, amphetamine, and alcohol use on cognitive function and the brain.[36] In HCV patients with a history of substance abuse, this makes it hard to tell whether substance abuse or the HCV infection caused their cognitive problems. It is likely that both adversely affect cognition and the brain.

Interferon-Based Therapy
Finally, the medication used to treat HCV, interferon, has many side effects. Depression is one of the most common side effects. People with depression often have cognitive problems. The cause of interferon-induced depression may be related to activation of the *immune system*, much like what happens when you have the flu. Common symptoms are irritability, fatigue, slowed movements, and changes in sleep and eating habits.[37] Another possible side effect from taking interferon is cognitive problems. One study[32] found that 1/3 of study participants complained of concentration and memory problems during interferon treatment. As mentioned above, problems with concentration and memory can occur because of depression. However, this study found that cognitive complaints were not related to depression prior to or during interferon treatment.[38] Research into the typical cognitive problems people experience while on interferon is currently being conducted by several researchers. For now, little is known about the potential short- and long-term cognitive effects of interferon.

Coping with HCV

As might be expected, being diagnosed with HCV can seriously affect a person's mental health and quality of life. It is common to have trouble adjusting to a diagnosis of a long-term medical condition. But adjustment is more difficult for some patients than others. How would you know if you were having a hard time adjusting to life with HCV? How would you know if you were becoming depressed or anxious?

Common reactions to being diagnosed with a chronic infectious disease such as hepatitis C include:

- feeling emotionally numb and in shock
- becoming irritable or angry
- crying more than usual
- not spending time with friends and family
- worrying about infecting others
- feeling dirty
- feeling uncertain about your future
- feeling like no one understands
- feeling like life is not worth living

These feelings and reactions are normal, but if they are extreme or continue for more than 3 or 4 weeks, you may be experiencing the first signs of depression. It is important to be aware of changes in any of the following, which may signal depression:

- energy level
- sleeping more or less than normal
- eating more or less than normal
- not spending time with friends and family
- crying for no apparent reason
- feeling hopeless or worthless
- thinking about suicide
- no longer feeling like doing things you normally like doing
- feeling sad or down

A diagnosis of HCV can also cause people to worry more than normal. If you find yourself unable to control how much you are worrying, this may be a sign of an anxiety disorder. If this is the case, it is important to be aware of changes in any of the following, which may signal an anxiety problem:

- feeling restless or on edge
- becoming tired more quickly than normal
- having problems concentrating
- feeling more irritable than normal
- having headaches, cramps, stiffness, and muscle tension
- problems falling or staying asleep

Both of these issues (depression and anxiety) may become serious if they continue for more than a couple of weeks. They can also interfere with your ability to carry out normal activities of living. If this is the case, it is important to talk to someone who can help, such as your healthcare provider.

Summary

Many studies show that patients with chronic HCV infections also have mental health concerns. Concerns such as depression, anxiety, and problems with thinking and memory are common. However, it is unclear how much they are related to the presence of HCV or whether they are related to other factors.

Healthcare providers may not always notice when patients are depressed or anxious, so it may be up to you to tell your healthcare providers if you have any of the symptoms of these disorders (see lists above).

Substance abuse is a significant issue that should be discussed with your healthcare provider. Use of some substances (such as IV drugs) increases a person's risk of acquiring and transmitting HCV. Use of alcohol damages the liver and if a person has HCV, damage to the liver may be increased by continuing to drink alcohol.

Fortunately, patients with depression and anxiety and HCV benefit from treatment for these disorders.[39] Treatment can stabilize mental health conditions, support *abstinence* from drugs and alcohol, and allow for treatment of HCV.

References

1. Loftis JM and Hauser P. Hepatitis C in patients with psychiatric disease and substance abuse: Screening strategies and comanagement models of care. *Current Hepatitis Reports*. 2003;2:93-100.
2. Fireman M, Indest DW, Blackwell A, et al. Addressing tri-morbidity (Hepatitis C Psychiatric and Substance Use Disorders): the importance of routine meantal health screening as a component of a co-management model of care. *Clinical Infectious Diseases*. 2005;40(Suppl 5):S286-91.
3. Knott A, Dieperink E, Willenbring ML, et al. Integrated psychiatric/medical care in a chronic hepatitis C clinic: effect on antiviral treatment evaluation and outcomes. *Am J Gastroenterol*. 2006;101(10):2254-62.
4. Carta MG, Hardoy MC, Garofalo A, et al. Association of chronic hepatitis C with major depressive disorders: irrespective of interferon-alpha therapy. *Clin Pract Epidemol Ment Health*. 2007;3:22.
5. Golden J, O'Dwyer AM, Conroy RM. Depression and anxiety in patients with hepatitis C: prevalence, detection rates and risk factors. *Gen Hosp Psychiatry*. 2005;27(6):431-438.
6. Cruz Neves A, Dickens C, Xavier M. [Comorbidity between hepatitis C and depression. Epidemiological and etiopathogenic aspects. Article in Portuguese.] *Acta Med Port*. 2006;19(1):21-28.
7. Butt AA, Evans R, Skanderson M, Shakil AO. Comorbid medical and psychiatric conditions and substance abuse in HCV infected persons on dialysis. *J Hepatol*. 2006;44(5):864-886.
8. Osher FC, Goldberg RW, McNary SW, et al. Substance Abuse and the Transmission of Hepatitis C Among Persons With Severe Mental Illness. *Psychiatric Services*. 2003;54:842–847.
9. Golden J, O'Dwyer AM, and Conroy RM. Depression and anxiety in patients with hepatitis C: prevalence, detection rates and risk factors. *Gen Hosp Psychiatry*. 2005;27(6):431-8.
10. Fontana RJ, Hussain KB, Schwartz SM, et al. Emotional distress in chronic hepatitis C patients not receiving antiviral therapy. *J Hepatol*. 2002;36(3):401-7.
11. Nelligan J, Loftis JM, Matthews AM, et al. Depression co-morbidity and antidepressant use in veterans with chronic hepatitis C. Submitted.
12. Loftis JM, Matthews AM, and Hauser P. Psychiatric and substance use disorders in individuals with hepatitis C: epidemiology and management. *Drugs*. 2006;66(2):155-74.
13. Yovtcheva SP, Rifai MA, Moles JK, et al. Psychiatric comorbidity among hepatitis C-positive patients. *Psychosomatics*. 2001;42(5):411-5.
14. El-Serag HB, Kunik M, Richardson P, et al. Psychiatric disorders among veterans with hepatitis C infection. *Gastroenterology*. 2002;123(2):476-82.
15. Lehman CL and Cheung RC. Depression, anxiety, post-traumatic stress, and alcohol-related problems among veterans with chronic hepatitis C. *Am J Gastroenterol*. 2002;97(10):2640-6.
16. American Psychiatric Association. Diagnostic and statistical manual of mental disorders. Fourth Edition, Text Revision ed. 2000, Washington, DC: American Psychiatric Association.
17. Rifai MA, Indest D, Loftis J, et al. Psychiatric management of the hepatitis C patient. *Curr Treat Options Gastroenterol*. 2006;9(6):508-19.
18. National Institutes of Health. National Institutes of Health Consensus Development Conference Statement: Management of Hepatitis C. *Hepatology*. 2002. November: p. S3-S20.
19. Rosenberg SD, Goodman LA, Osher FC, et al. Prevalence of HIV, hepatitis B, and hepatitis C in people with severe mental illness. *Am J Public Health*. 2001;91(1):31-7.
20. Mueser K, Bennett M, and Kushner M. Epidemiology of substance use disorders among persons with chronic mental illnesses. In *Double Jeopardy: Chronic Mental Illness and Substance Use Disorder*. A Lehman and L Dixon, Editors. Chur, Switzerland: Harwood Academic; 1995.
21. Regier DA, Farmer ME, Rae DS, et al. Comorbidity of mental disorders with alcohol and other drug abuse. Results from the Epidemiologic Catchment Area (ECA) Study. *JAMA*. 1990;264(19):2511-8.
22. Osher FC, Goldberg RW, McNary SW, et al. Substance abuse and the transmission of hepatitis C among persons with severe mental illness. *Psychiatr Serv*. 2003;54(6):842-7.
23. Alter MJ. Epidemiology of hepatitis C. *Hepatology*. 1997;26(3 Suppl 1):62S-65S.
24. Armstrong GL, Wasley A, Simard EP, et al. The prevalence of hepatitis C virus infection in the United States, 1999 through 2002. *Ann Intern Med*. 2006;144(10):705-14.
25. Golub ET, Latka M, Hagan H, et al. Screening for depressive symptoms among HCV-infected injection drug users: examination of the utility of the CES-D and the Beck Depression Inventory. *J Urban Health*. 2004;81(2):278-90.
26. Sulkowski, M.S. and Thomas, D.L., Epidemiology and natural history of hepatitis C virus infection in injection drug users: implications for treatment. *Clin Infect Dis*. 2005;40 Suppl 5:S263-9.
27. Wild TC, el-Guebaly N, Fischer B, et al. Comorbid depression among untreated illicit opiate users: results from a multisite Canadian study. *Can J Psychiatry*. 2005;50(9):512-8.
28. Corrao G and Arico S. Independent and combined action of hepatitis C virus infection and alcohol consumption on the risk of symptomatic liver cirrhosis. *Hepatology*. 1998;27(4):914-9.
29. Dwight MM, Kowdley KV, Russo JE, et al. Depression, fatigue, and functional disability in patients with chronic hepatitis C. *J Psychosom Res*, 2000;49(5):311-7.
30. Forton DM, Taylor-Robinson SD, and Thomas HC. Cerebral dysfunction in chronic hepatitis C infection. *J Viral Hepat*. 2003;10(2):81-6.
31. Kramer L, Hofer H, Bauer E, et al. Relative impact of fatigue and subclinical cognitive brain dysfunction on health-related quality of life in chronic hepatitis C infection. *AIDS*. 2005;19 Suppl 3:S85-92.
32. Weissenborn K, Krause J, Bokemeyer M, et al. Hepatitis C virus infection affects the brain-evidence from psychometric studies and magnetic resonance spectroscopy. *J Hepatol*. 2004;41(5):845-51.
33. Forton DM, Thomas HC, Murphy CA, et al. Hepatitis C and cognitive impairment in a cohort of patients with mild liver disease. *Hepatology*. 2002;35(2):433-9.

34. Hilsabeck RC, Hassanein TI, Ziegler EA, et al. Effect of interferon-alpha on cognitive functioning in patients with chronic hepatitis C. *J Int Neuropsychol Soc.* 2005;11(1):16-22.
35. Van der Poel CL, Cuypers HT, and Reesink HW. Hepatitis C virus six years on. *Lancet.* 1994;344(8935):1475-9.
36. Verdejo-Garcia A, Rivas-Perez C, Lopez-Torrecillas F, et al. Differential impact of severity of drug use on frontal behavioral symptoms. *Addict Behav.* 2006;31(8):1373-82.
37. Raison CL, Demetrashvili M, Capuron L, et al. Neuropsychiatric adverse effects of interferon-alpha: recognition and management. *CNS Drugs.* 2005;19(2):105-23.
38. Reichenberg A, Gorman JM, and Dieterich DT. Interferon-induced depression and cognitive impairment in hepatitis C virus patients: a 72 week prospective study. *AIDS.* 2005;19 Suppl 3:S174-8.
39. Lang JP, Meyer N, and Doffoel M. [Benefits of a preventive psychiatric accompaniment in patients Hepatitis C Virus seropositive (HCV): prospective study concerning 39 patients]. *Encephale.* 2003;29(4 Pt 1):362-5.

Mental Health and Hepatitis C

Joyce Seiko Kobayashi, MD

Mental Health Issues During Interferon-Based Therapy

Introduction

Most people are aware that the significant benefits of *interferon-based therapy* to treat *chronic hepatitis* C virus (*HCV*) may cause a variety of physical side effects (*see Chapter 8, Western (Allopathic) Medicine*). It is important to be aware that this treatment may also have emotional and mental health side effects.

Approximately 20% to 30% of people undergoing interferon-based therapy for hepatitis C experience *depression*. By being aware of this possibility, you are more likely to recognize the *symptoms* early, request one of the many antidepressant (or mood stabilizing) medications available to treat it, and feel better for the remainder of the treatment period. Although most people do not become depressed during HCV treatment, the depression that does occur is not just a result of adjusting to the changes in your life associated with undergoing treatment. Researchers have recognized for years that interferon-based therapy for HCV can itself cause depression.[1]

While the depressive symptoms caused by interferon-based therapy usually improve as soon as the medication is stopped, this depression also responds well to antidepressant treatment during HCV *antiviral* therapy. Getting help for depression while on interferon-based therapy will prevent early discontinuation of this potentially life-saving course of HCV treatment. This chapter is intended to help you prepare mentally and emotionally for the decision to start HCV treatment. Preexisting mental health or substance use disorders are common among people with HCV and should not be used as reasons for exclusion from treatment.

However, if you have a current psychiatric disorder or are abusing drugs or alcohol, you should consider seeking treatments for these problems — if possible, before you start treatment for HCV. There are many reasons to get clean and sober that are specifically related to HCV infection. Waiting to start HCV treatment can actually serve as an effective motivator to achieve *abstinence* and sobriety, even if that has been difficult for you in the past. In the meantime, continue to discuss the risks and benefits of HCV treatment with your with your healthcare providers.

> **The most important question is not when to start your treatment for HCV, but when you feel ready to make the commitment to complete it once you start.**

Later in this section, you will find some of the ways you can try to prevent, minimize, or treat the mental or emotional side effects of HCV treatment. There is also a discussion of some of the research on the effect of HCV and its treatment on your quality of life, or as researchers call it, "health-related quality of life" (HRQOL).

People tend to tolerate side effects better and can identify them earlier if they know about them in advance, so be sure to discuss these with your healthcare providers until you are sure you understand them.

This chapter will primarily focus on depression and its treatment because it is by far the most common psychiatric side effect of *pegylated interferon* plus ribavirin treatment. Other potential psychiatric side effects will also be discussed.

In the midst of discussing all of these possible side effects of pegylated interferon plus *ribavirin* treatment, it is important not to lose sight of the "goal." The goal is to get the maximum benefit from your pegylated interferon plus ribavirin therapy, that is, achieving a *sustained viral response* (SVR) by clearing the virus from your body, reversing *fibrosis* in your liver, and decreasing the chance of developing *liver failure* and/or *liver cancer*.[2]

My "goal" in this section is to help you do what you can to be mentally prepared so you can do your part by taking the medications as prescribed, following up with appointments, and creating a working partnership with your healthcare providers.

> **Interferon-based therapy can be emotionally and physically challenging.**
> **Remember... Keep your eye on the prize!**

Words of Caution About Drawing Conclusions From Current Research

Anyone with HCV who is trying to understand the mental health aspects of pegylated interferon plus ribavirin treatment should be briefly warned about three different issues that can be confusing when you hear or read about research discussing psychiatric disorders and HCV therapy.

First...

People with HCV have a higher proportion than the general population of preexisting psychiatric disorders and substance abuse disorders, especially if they have a past history of intravenous drug use as a risk factor for HCV. This means that these psychiatric disorders, including mood disorders, predate their treatment for HCV and usually predated their HCV.

During pegylated interferon treatment, however, people who have never had a psychiatric disorder may still experience significant depression directly induced by the pegylated interferon. Further, people with stablized preexisting psychiatric disorders prior to beginning interferon-based therapy may experience a recurrence or worsening of their symptoms, or experience a *relapse* of their substance use disorder during HCV treatment.

If you have had a prior history of depression or another mood disorder (for example, bipolar disorder), studies vary regarding whether you are at higher risk for depression during interferon-based therapy. One study found that half of those with histories of depression had a recurrence during treatment, and half did not.[3] However, if you are depressed or even "subclinically depressed" (meaning the symptoms are severe enough to warrant immediate treatment with antidepressant medication) at the time you start interferon-based treatment, you are still at increased risk for *clinical* depression that may require antidepressant medication during your HCV therapy.[4] In some cases, you may want to consider preventive measures, something discussed later in this section.

Second...

You may hear about results from a variety of research related to interferon or interferon-alfa. But the research that is most pertinent to you is likely to be more recent research about pegylated interferon plus ribavirin, the current standard of care for the treatment of chronic hepatitis C.

And A Final Note of Caution...

Discussions of rates and consequences of depression as a side effect of pegylated interferon plus ribavirin treatment for HCV are based on research that varies significantly in the way "depression" has been measured. Various methods of evaluation can sometimes result in conflicting and often confusing differences in their conclusions. This is a major reason why what you hear about depression and other psychiatric side effects of interferon-based treatment for HCV may not be consistent across studies.

So be cautious in drawing conclusions from studies you may hear about or read because the rates of people experiencing depression that are reported before or during HCV treatment may vary depending on how the depressive symptoms are evaluated.

On the other hand, it usually doesn't help most people to avoid learning about the side effects of HCV treatment. You are likely to feel more in charge of your treatment if you learn more about it. If your healthcare provider gives you a periodic self-rating scale as a means of monitoring you for side effects, be sure to take the time to fill it out accurately. However, if you become aware of feeling more depressed or no longer finding pleasure in anything, you may recognize these symptoms before your healthcare providers because you have learned to monitor them for yourself and you should take an active role in getting treatment or requesting a psychiatric evaluation.

Importance of Knowing About Depression and Other Possible Psychiatric Side Effects of Pegylated Interferon Plus Ribavirin Treatment

Despite the cautions I just gave you about research related to the psychiatric side effects of interferon-based therapy, these potential psychiatric side effects are still important to consider for a number of reasons:

- There is a 20% to 30% chance that you may experience significant depression during interferon-based therapy, even if you have never been diagnosed with depression before.[5]

- Psychiatric side effects are the most common reason for early discontinuation or reduction in medication dosage during HCV treatment.[6]

- Psychiatric side effects of interferon-based therapy such as mania or suicidal thoughts may require emergency intervention, treatment, and possibly psychiatric hospitalization, in addition to immediate discontinuation of HCV treatment.[7]

- Most importantly, most psychiatric side effects of pegylated interferon treatment are treatable. A variety of antidepressant (or mood stabilizing medications) are very effective and can help you feel much better during the entire course of your HCV treatment.

People with severe psychiatric side effects from interferon-based therapy have sometimes unnecessarily discontinued their treatment because they felt so discouraged about their quality of life during treatment, or so depressed as a result of it. Or it may have been discontinued prematurely in the past by their healthcare providers out of concern that they not get worse. Now you and they know that these side effects can be treated, and early discontinuation of HCV treatment or dose reductions are usually not necessary.

You are likely to feel better about your treatment and yourself if you take an active role by:

- learning as much as you can about the treatment before you start it

- knowing what potential side effects to watch out for

- communicating with your healthcare providers about your experiences

Stabilizing Psychiatric and Substance Abuse Disorders Before Starting HCV Treatment

You can begin to prepare yourself mentally and emotionally for HCV treatment by being sure that when you are ready to make the decision to start it, you are also ready to follow through and complete the treatment — so you will get the full benefit from it. If you have a current psychiatric condition, or an alcohol or substance use disorder, consider getting a psychiatric evaluation or enrolling in a substance treatment program to get clean and sober.

For example, if you have a history of one or more episodes of a "major depressive disorder" that has required antidepressant medication in the past, and you are feeling depressed, hopeless, tearful or not finding pleasure in anything, you should consider consulting with a psychiatrist or asking your healthcare provider to restart antidepressant medication.

In the meantime, you should discuss your individual risks and benefits of HCV treatment with your healthcare providers in order to be a full participant in the important decision about when you are ready to start the treatment. You will likely consider your liver enzymes, your genotype, and the *stage* of disease in your liver in light of your past treatment history. (See *Chapter 8, Western (Allopathic) Medicine* for additional information.)

Prior to the 2002 Consensus Statement on the Treatment of HCV from the National Institutes of Health[8], HCV-infected individuals with associated psychiatric and substance use disorders were often unnecessarily excluded from HCV treatment, and there have been discussions about whether this was ethical.[9] While it is advantageous for these disorders to be evaluated and stabilized before HCV treatment, they should not prevent anyone from being eligible for *antiviral* treatment on the basis of that history alone.

Excluding individuals with psychiatric and substance use disorders from HCV treatment has been justified historically because of the assumption of decreased adherence and follow-up with treatment.[10] But research suggests this is not a valid assumption. This is an important question for a large segment of the HCV-infected population. For example, up to 85% of HCV-infected veterans also have psychiatric and substance use disorders.

While there are few large studies separating preexisting from current psychiatric and substance use disorders among HCV-infected individuals, one review of the medical records of 1.9 million veterans between 1992 and 1999 found that 1.77% were HCV-infected. Among those with HCV, 85% had a past history of psychiatric or substance use disorders, 31% had an active psychiatric or substance use disorder, most frequently cocaine (69%) and opiates (48%). Among those with comorbid disorders (that is, both psychiatric and substance use disorders), 85% had depression, 71% had anxiety disorders, 43% had posttraumatic stress disorder, 42% had psychotic disorders, and 30% had bipolar disorders.[11]

A recent review of the records of 294 HCV-infected veterans with psychiatric and substance use disorders compared to 353 controls found that the former group was more often considered ineligible for treatment for HCV, and were treated less frequently despite comparable viral and liver characteristics.[12] These researchers found that rates of HCV therapy completion rates and SVR were similar between the groups.

Most clinicians now recommend a case-by-case, individualized risk-benefit assessment between you and your healthcare providers to make the decision about when to start HCV treatment. You should not accept being told you are ineligible simply because you have a preexisting psychiatric or substance use disorder. But it is likely to be to your advantage to seek treatment before starting HCV therapy.

If you feel ready not just to start, but to complete the treatment, be sure to let your healthcare providers know, even if they have not yet started that discussion with you.

Intravenous Drug Use and HCV

The most common exposure to the hepatitis C virus is through intravenous drug use. The figures that are often cited are alarmingly high: 50% to 80% of intravenous drug users become HCV-infected after one year of drug use, and nearly all become infected after eight years of use.[13] However, a more recent study in New York[14] suggests that HCV prevalence declined from 80% to 59% among HIV-negative individuals and from 90% to 63% overall between 1990 and 2001. The authors felt this was attributable to the availability of needle exchange programs. Their estimated HCV incidence in 2000 to 2001 among new injectors was 18 per 1,000 person-years at risk.

The 1997 NIH Consensus statement[15] recommended that people who use illicit drugs not be offered HCV treatment until they had been abstinent for at least six months. One academic group[16] has argued that the four reasons used to justify this guideline - expectations of decreased adherence, increased side effects of treatment, risk of reinfection, and the fact that the timing of treatment should allow for a period of abstinence before starting HCV treatment - are not valid in routinely denying treatment to illicit drug users. They also argue that treatment decisions should be individualized on the basis of evidence-based risk-benefit considerations, and augmented by substance treatment programs (including needle exchange programs), establishing increased trust in the doctor-patient relationship, and providing close monitoring of side effects of HCV treatment and relapse behavior.

There have been a number of studies of people who use intravenous drugs (IDUs) and the impact of depressive symptoms or a period of abstinence prior to HCV treatment on their completion of treatment. One Italian study[17] found that the presence of depressive symptoms among IDUs before or during pegylated interferon plus ribavirin treatment did not affect their virologic response or predict early treatment discontinuation. However, the presence of other physical side effects did increase the likelihood of early treatment discontinuation, and they encouraged healthcare providers to address these physical side effects as soon as they were identified in order to promote higher rates of treatment completion, rather than making a large group ineligible for treatment or allowing early discontinuation.

Another study from San Francisco[18] found that among 76 recovering heroin users on methadone, 28% had a sustained viral response and 24% discontinued treatment early. Neither drug use during HCV treatment nor a short duration of pretreatment drug abstinence diminished the virologic outcomes.

So people should not be excluded from HCV treatment because of their substance abuse. But there are many reasons to get clean and stay clean before HCV treatment. For example, there have been important questions raised about whether ongoing opiate dependence may negatively affect the outcome of HCV treatment by enhancing viral replication, liver injury, and hepatic fibrosis.[19] These authors suggest that being on methadone is not a contraindication to HCV treatment, but should be further studied in this regard.

The two substitution therapies for opiate dependence, methadone and buprenorphine, promote harm reduction and may help HCV-infected individuals stabilize their abstinence before HCV treatment (see *Chapter 20, Interferon-Based Therapy in Recovery*). Patients on methadone may continue on their usual doses with stable chronic liver disease, including advanced *cirrhosis*. Buprenorphine is another substitution therapy that may be administered directly by physicians who have received training and certification, in contrast to the highly regulated methadone maintenance treatment programs. However, patients should be warned that attempts to abuse it can cause liver dysfunction after sublingual and especially after intravenous administration.[20]

Despite the fact that people who are using intravenous drugs often feel that they have "many strikes against them," being able to start interferon-based therapy may be a great motivator. The possibility of clearing HCV from their body, and especially, helping them feel better on a daily basis, can be a powerful force for major changes in their lives. Many people find that they can start a new chapter in their life book. If you are using intravenous drugs, you are likely to do better with an organized treatment program, but the hepatitis C virus may give you the challenge you need not only to make the decision to stop using, but to stay clean.

Alcohol Dependence and HCV

People with histories of alcohol abuse and alcohol dependence have a rate of HCV infection that is double that of the general population, even when individuals with other HCV risk factors are excluded.[21] It is possible that intranasal cocaine use and sharing of cocaine "straws", or tattooing by friends are additional risk factors for HCV among these individuals who have never used intravenous drugs.

There are many reasons to get sober and stay sober before starting HCV treatment. Median daily alcohol use of more than 30 grams is associated with failure to respond to interferon-based treatment for HCV, despite a period of abstinence before starting treatment.[22] Individuals with chronic hepatitis C who continue to use alcohol are two to three times more likely to develop cirrhosis and associated complications, and HCV-infected patients admitted to the hospital with alcohol-related diagnoses have longer hospital stays and are more likely to die in the hospital.[23]

Alcohol decreases the cellular effects of interferon, increases HCV *viral load*, reduces the virologic response to HCV treatment, and accelerates the progression of fibrosis in the liver. For all these reasons, some authors suggest that the potential liver *toxicity* from disulfiram (Antabuse®) is likely to be lower in people with HCV than the toxicity from alcohol, despite the fact that this has not been studied directly. Disulfiram (Antabuse®), monitored Antabuse®, or acamprosate

(Campral®) can be effective in helping you maintain sobriety. A 12-step program such as Alcoholics Anonymous is often successful in helping people stop drinking. (See *Chapter 3, Alcohol and Hepatitis C* for additional information.)

In one 28-day substance treatment program for alcohol and other substance dependence (without IDUs), 23.1% were HCV-infected, and those who completed the substance treatment program were more likely to receive HCV treatment than HCV-positive individuals who had never been in a substance treatment program. These authors[24] report that as part of their treatment program, they educated people about HCV and its treatment, tested them for HCV, and told people at the beginning of the treatment program that they would only be eligible for treatment if they remained abstinent. Almost 90% of the HCV-positive participants completed the program and had a planned discharge versus 67% of the HCV-negative group. Forty-nine percent of HCV-positive participants were abstinent six months after program completion compared to 31% of the HCV-negative individuals. The association between HCV positive status, program completion, and sobriety at six months was statistically significant. HCV-infected participants were more likely to complete the substance treatment program and remain abstinent for 6 months after program completion than the other program participants who were not HCV-infected.

This suggests that a desire to get HCV treatment can be a powerful motivator for remaining clean and sober when people are educated about HCV and its major risks to health over a lifetime. It is also a reminder that you will probably have a better chance of getting clean and sober with the support and structure a formal substance treatment program. But you will know what works best for you.

Severe Mental Illness and HCV

Five percent to 7% of adults in the United States have a severe mental illness. Half of all people with a severe mental illness also have a substance use disorder and are at increased risk for HCV and HIV. From 1997 to 1998, one group studied coinfection with HIV, hepatitis B and HCV in a multisite sample of 755 patients with severe mental illness. They found that 14.4% were positive for HCV, 3% were positive for HIV, and 1.7% were coinfected with both HIV and HCV. Coinfection in this very vulnerable population was associated with psychiatric illness severity, ongoing drug abuse, poverty, homelessness, incarceration, urban residence and minority status.[25]

Of note, HCV monoinfected individuals continued to engage in behaviors that are high risk for HIV. Studies suggest that while people with severe mental illness tend (on average) to be less sexually active, those who are sexually active tend to engage in more behaviors that are high risk for HIV[26], and possibly HCV. It is likely that HCV treatment programs for the most severely mentally ill populations will need to incorporate concrete services such as help with access to housing, public assistance programs, and education about high risk behaviors.

People who are HIV-positive and are coinfected with HCV are another undertreated population. Success rates with pegylated interferon plus ribavirin treatment are for HCV/HIV coinfection are more modest than seen with HCV infection alone. In one study of HCV/HIV coinfected individuals, 90% had access to primary medical care, but only 21% were referred to a specialist for evaluation of their HCV, and less than 4% were treated with interferon-based therapy.[27] Compared with HCV uninfected individuals, HCV co-infected patients were more likely to be using injection drugs, to be homeless for more than one year, and to be actively depressed.

In summary, there is generally little to lose and a lot to be gained by waiting to start HCV treatment until you have sought treatment to stabilize any psychiatric disorders and to get clean and sober. You will not be able to clear HCV from your body if you relapse with drugs, alcohol, or psychiatric symptoms and have to stop therapy. You can maximize the chance of a good treatment outcome by remaining clean and sober during treatment.

However, if you do relapse or have a recurrence of psychiatric symptoms during HCV treatment, let your healthcare providers know so you can get treatment as soon as possible. If the HCV treatment needs to be discontinued, it should be possible to restart once your symptoms have been stabilized. However, remember that whenever you do make the decision to start HCV treatment, make the decision to finish it as well.

Health-Related Quality of Life and Physical Side Effects of Interferon-Based Therapy

Historically, chronic hepatitis C had been considered an asymptomatic illness (meaning without significant symptoms).[28] However, there have been a number of studies[29-31] that focus on measures of "health related quality of life" (HRQOL), and it has been demonstrated that people living with chronic hepatitis C have a lower HRQOL than others without it, independent of the present of cirrhosis.[32] While these studies were largely done during the era of standard interferon plus ribavirin treatment, they suggest significant reductions in physical function[33] that impact the HRQOL for HCV-infected individuals even before starting interferon-based therapy.

Researchers use several standardized measurements to compare the effects of different illnesses on the quality of life of people living with them.[34] For example, there is a greater effect in lowering the HRQOL in individuals with chronic hepatitis C than among people with chronic hepatitis B.[35] The magnitude of decrease in HRQOL is at least as large as other chronic diseases such as diabetes mellitus and chronic arthritis.

While the once weekly schedule of pegylated interferon has reduced the intrusion of this treatment in the course of people's lives, the physical side effects during a lengthy treatment course on pegylated interferon may make some people feel worse before they feel better. Reflecting this experience, researchers have found that the HRQOL for people on pegylated interferon tends to decline after 12 to 24 weeks of treatment, but then generally returns to baseline.[36] Both fatigue and depression tend to improve at the conclusion of pegylated interferon treatment.

The following are the percentages of some of the physical side effects of pegylated interferon alfa-2a plus ribavirin treatment that were reported from one of the major pegylated interferon treatment studies, involving 1,121 patients at multiple sites.[37] The side effects listed are common and are among those that can particularly affect your quality of life. Decreased interest in sex can also occur with pegylated interferon treatment, perhaps as a result of a combination of the other side effects. It is included here, although it was not originally reported in this study.

- fatigue 54%

- headache 47%

- insomnia 37%

- nausea 29%

- decreased appetite 21%

- decreased interest in sex

Remember that no one experiences all the side effects of any medication, and some people don't experience any. Many of these can also be decreased or improved by other treatments. For a more detailed discussion of the potential side effects of pegylated interferon treatment, refer to *Chapter 8, Western (Allopathic) Medicine.*

One study of fatigue and HRQOL found that scores were not as impaired on pegylated interferon as with standard interferon in the realms of physical or emotional role limitation, general health, vitality, and social function.[38] But it will take more studies to know if the effects of pegylated interferon are different from standard interferon on the quality of peoples' daily lives. More reassuring, while not surprising, is the finding that HRQOL measures improve among patients even before they knew they had achieved an SVR.[39]

As with any medical illness, people differ in the way they respond to the demands of the treatment they require for that illness. Some experience the treatment itself - such as the need for multiple medical appointments, getting blood tests, taking or self-administering medications, and medication side effects - as an additional burden of the illness. Others look to the treatment as a possible salvation from their illness and consider the demands of that treatment a passing phase on the way to recovery or cure.

Symptoms that are considered "reactive" or in response to the demands of treatment or the symptoms of the illness are considered "adjustment" issues and usually do not require treatment with psychiatric medications. Often, psychotherapy or counseling can be very beneficial for reactive symptoms. For example, someone who experiences fatigue and decreased interest in sex may benefit more from a few couples sessions with a therapist (who can facilitate communication about the effects of the illness on both the patient and the partner) than from a course of antidepressant medications.

While ribavirin may have a role in side effects such as insomnia (37% on pegylated interferon with ribavirin and 23% without ribavirin) and decreased appetite (21% on pegylated interferon with ribavirin and 11% without ribavirin)[40], one well known side effect of ribavirin affecting HRQOL is anemia. Many people on pegylated interferon plus ribavirin experience significant fatigue because they are anemic from the ribavirin.

In a Swedish study[41], patients who had a fall of more than 20% of their hemoglobin levels were significantly lower in measures of HRQOL than those who had decreases in hemoglobin of less than 10%. While treatment-related anemia is often taken care of by decreasing the ribavirin dose, people who experience fatigue related to anemia will often experience more energy and a higher quality of life after treatment with erythropoietin. This may be an option to explore with your healthcare provider.[42]

One study found that while fatigue and depression both negatively affect the HRQOL of people on combination therapy, the effect of depression far outweighed the effect of fatigue or any other side effect on the HRQOL in the experience of most patients.[43] Another study of 271 patients found that although both anemia and depression were associated with impairment in HRQOL, but depression was the "most consistent predictor."

Some studies suggest that patients who take on physical symptoms and the experience of illness as a "challenge" (as opposed to another unfortunate effect of the illness that must be accepted, or even as a punishment) tend to cope better overall.[44] Not only do many patients feel they just "need to be strong" and accept difficult side effects, many healthcare providers feel that it is "understandable" and "natural" that people with HCV might feel depressed. This can cause both patients and providers not think as actively as they could about using treatments to intervene when side effects occur to help people feel better.[45] You may need to be the one to activate such interventions.

You can have an active role in decreasing the impact of these side effects on the quality of your life by learning about them. In learning about possible side effects, you will be prepared to tell your healthcare providers if they occur. You can request the treatments to minimize any side effects you may experience instead of just trying to accept them as another burden of the illness. In addition, by learning as much as you can about this illness, its treatment, and possible side effects, you may experience improved self-esteem by feeling "empowered" and advocating for yourself. Knowing more about your situation may make it more likely that you will find ways to feel better!

Psychiatric Side Effects and Interferon-Based Therapy

Psychiatric side effects of interferon-based therapies for HCV include depression, mania, psychosis, suicidal thoughts, and anxiety. There are no consistent predictors of who will develop these disorders as side effects of interferon-based therapy, even among those with clear histories of preexisting psychiatric disorders.

In a study of people receiving interferon-based therapy who had preexisting psychiatric disorders (but were not in psychiatric care at the beginning of interferon-based treatment), ½ did not require any psychiatric intervention or develop significant psychiatric symptoms during the treatment. The only two factors that seemed to be associated with progression to frank psychiatric symptoms during interferon-based therapy were a family history of psychiatric disorders and having more than one psychiatric disorder at baseline.[46]

Depression on Interferon-Based Therapy

Many studies have documented the occurrence of depression during standard interferon and standard interferon plus ribavirin treatment for HCV.[47-49] Depression occurred in 20% to 30 % of patients in these studies.[50] There have been fewer studies investigating the effects of pegylated interferon on mood.

The previously cited study of 1,121 subjects from 81 sites[51] found lower rates of depression (20% and 22%) among patients treated with pegylated interferon compared to those treated with standard interferon (30%). This is a particularly significant percentage since the baseline rate of both a history of depression and active depression was very low for this sample (less than 5%). Notably, psychiatric side effects (mostly events related to depression) were still the most common reasons for early discontinuation of treatment.

However, not all studies have noted this difference between standard interferon and pegylated interferon. A study conducted in Germany[52] compared psychiatric side effects in 48 patients who were treated with standard interferon and 50 patients who were treated with pegylated interferon. They found the rates of depression between the two groups were not statistically different. Furthermore, measures of HRQOL (primarily depression and anger/hostility) were similar in the two groups.

Notably, while major depressive disorders are consistently found to be twice as common in women as in men in the general population, most studies have found that men and women are equally at risk for becoming depressed as a result of the pegylated interferon plus ribavirin treatment.

Finally, one study stressed the importance of identifying and treating depressive symptoms because their results suggested that people who experience significant depressive symptoms on interferon-based therapy may be less likely to clear HCV.

> **Fortunately, depressive symptoms related to interferon-based therapy respond well to antidepressant medication so be sure to consider asking for it — and feel better.**

Mania and Irritability on Interferon-Based Therapy

A French study[53] of 93 patients treated with pegylated interferon-alfa 2b plus ribavirin reported "psychiatric events" or side effects in 32% of their sample. The mood disorders were diagnosed as follows: mania (10%), irritable hypomania (50%) and depressive mixed states (40%). Three patients in that study exhibited classic euphoric manic symptoms and there is another extensive case report of mania that arose during pegylated interferon plus ribavirin treatment.[54] In a study of 943 patients on standard interferon, one of the 43 patients who developed psychiatric symptoms was manic.[55]

The development of frank manic symptoms (such racing thoughts, grandiose thoughts, extreme irritability, hypersexuality, hyperactivity, and decreased need for sleep) with or without psychotic symptoms requires emergency intervention, discontinuation of interferon treatment, and the immediate initiation of psychiatric treatment.

The French study highlights the question of how to consider irritability, anger, and hostility in the diagnosis of depression versus bipolar depression. This is important for several reasons. Irritability is very common during the course of HCV treatment. Many patients with irritability on interferon-based therapy reportedly show improvement with antidepressant medication. However, patients with significant irritability and depression who are diagnosed with a bipolar disorder are usually treated with a mood stabilizer, and are considered at risk for deterioration if incorrectly treated with antidepressants. Several papers have discussed these issues in detail.[56, 57] In general, a psychiatrist should be consulted if there is a question about diagnosis or treatment.

People who are manic or especially "hypomanic" (where manic symptoms are not as fully symptomatic) may, understandably, not want to let go of those feelings as they are experienced as positive and/or pleasant. But the problem is that these feelings and thoughts always "spin out of control" and result in impaired judgment that can end up being highly self-destructive. As illogical as it may seem, if you feel "on top of the world" and it is "too good to be true," it probably is. You may be manic and need psychiatric treatment.

Suicidal Thoughts on Interferon-Based Therapy

A survey of 15 hospitals from 10 countries estimated one patient in 5[15] on standard interferon treatment developed suicidal thoughts, and these were not preceded by prior histories of suicide attempts.[58]

While very few suicides have been reported among HCV patients on alfa interferon therapy[59, 60], it is critical to identify anyone with suicidal thoughts or feelings. People with a sense of hopelessness beyond depression, and those actively making plans to take their own lives are at highest risk for actual suicide attempts. Suicidal thoughts with active intent are always an emergency and require immediate psychiatric intervention and discontinuation of the pegylated interferon treatment until the risk of suicide has passed.

"Suicidal ideation" is the term psychiatrists use to refer to suicidal thoughts. The response to "passive suicidal ideation" (those suicidal thoughts that are not driven by active intent nor accompanied by plans to act on them) is different than for people with "active suicidal ideation." In contrast to active suicidal ideation that requires an emergency response, passive suicidal ideation is not uncommon among people with HCV even when they are not on interferon-based therapy. Passive suicidal ideation requires careful monitoring and assessment for antidepressant medication, but does not necessarily require discontinuation of pegylated interferon treatment or psychiatric hospitalization.

One study found that 27% (15/55) of HCV-infected persons who were not on interferon-based treatment reported suicidal ideation compared to 43% (18/42) among those on treatment.[11] Individuals with passive suicidal ideation can benefit from increased support, clinical assessment, and management. However, passive suicidal ideation is often related to passing moments of sadness, or may reflect some instinctual effort to reestablish a sense of control at a time when illness and treatments can leave people feeling powerless and out of control.

Passive suicidal ideation is not related to an actual wish to die, and is not accompanied by a readiness to put thoughts into action. In fact, in the study mentioned above, 94% (17/18) of those HCV-infected individuals in the study who expressed suicidal ideation were able to complete a course of at least six months of interferon-based therapy. On the other hand, psychiatric evaluation should be considered if there is a question of active suicidal ideation.

> **If you find yourself having even passing thoughts of "ending it all" or "feeling better off dead," talk to your healthcare providers and ask to see a psychiatrist.**

Psychosis on Interferon-Based Therapy

A study of 43 out of 943 patients who experienced psychiatric symptoms on standard interferon included four patients with a psychotic disorder (delusions and hallucinations).[61] There have also been a few case reports of individuals who experienced psychotic symptoms on standard interferon[62] and one series of four such patients.[63] While there have been few reports of psychotic symptoms on pegylated interferon, it is likely that some patients will also experience psychotic symptoms on pegylated interferon therapy as well.

The term "psychotic" refers to auditory hallucinations (hearing voices others don't hear), visual hallucinations (seeing things other people don't see), grandiose or paranoid delusions (extreme thoughts of fictional power or feelings that strangers on the street are talking about you or knowing your thoughts).

If you experience or have experienced any of these symptoms, be sure to let your healthcare providers know. You may be afraid or even ashamed to admit to your healthcare providers that you are experiencing these symptoms (or have previously experienced them while on or off drugs). Your fear may be because you have never experienced anything like this before and you don't want anyone to think you are "crazy." Or you may have had these experience before but are afraid because you have never told anyone about them before. You are not crazy, but you may be having side effects or symptoms that are very treatable. Remember, your healthcare providers can only help you with things they know you are experiencing.

Anxiety on Interferon-Based Therapy

Very few studies have focused on the symptoms of anxiety with inteferon-based therapy. The previously mentioned study found that 13 patients of the 43 patients who experienced psychiatric side effects on standard interferon therapy for HCV (total study involved 943 patients) were diagnosed with anxiety disorders.[61] Another found that 2 out of 60 patients required treatment for anxiety disorders while on standard interferon-based therapy.[64] While there are higher baseline rates of anxiety among patients with HCV prior to treatment[65], this seems to be a relatively uncommon side effect of standard interferon treatment, and is relatively unstudied with pegylated interferon.

Anxiety is more common among people with HCV before they start treatment. If you have experienced more severe anxiety than others on a chronic basis, or have ever been treated with psychiatric medications for anxiety or panic attacks, be sure to let your healthcare providers know. Together, you can consider restarting treatment for your anxiety before you begin your pegylated interferon plus ribavirin therapy.

Mood Changes Related to The Effects of Interferon-Based Therapy on Thyroid Function

Both hypothyroidism (low *thyroid* hormone levels) and hyperthyroidism (high thyroid hormone levels) have been associated with interferon-based therapy for HCV infection. Hypothyroidism is a well-known, reversible cause of depression that is associated with weight gain, decreased energy, sleepiness, and physical and mental slowness. Hypothyroidism often subsides once interferon treatment is completed. If the condition persists, it can be treated with thyroid hormonal supplements.

Severe hyperthyroidism (Grave's disease or destructive thyrotoxicosis), can cause symptoms that appear similar to mania with racing thoughts, physical agitation, excess energy, and rapid speech. If symptoms are severe and do not respond to medication to control the hyperthyroidism, interferon therapy may need to be discontinued.[65]

Prevention and Treatment of Psychiatric Side Effects of Interferon-Based Treatment

There are a number of important decisions you can make for yourself, even before you discuss whether to start pegylated interferon plus ribavirin treatment with your healthcare providers. If you start your treatment feeling in charge of yourself and with a commitment to complete therapy, you may feel more hope and pride as you complete each day of treatment - closer to reaping the full benefits of these powerful medications.

> While there is no guarantee that any measure will prevent the occurrence of depression or other psychiatric side effects of interferon-based therapy, there are many things you can do to decrease the likelihood you will need to stop HCV treatment because of these side effects.

One of the most important things you can do is to be sure to seek treatment for preexisting psychiatric and substance use disorders, and to be sure that you are not in a state of depression before you start treatment for your HCV infection. Optimally, try to achieve a stable state of abstinence and sobriety — especially sobriety.

Stopping alcohol as soon as you can after you have been diagnosed with HCV is one of the most important steps you can take on behalf of your own health. If you drink alcohol before you start HCV treatment, you are in a sense, increasing the activity of HCV in your liver while thinking about starting a year-long treatment whose major goal is to decrease its activity. If there were a pill you could take that would eliminate the effects HCV on your liver that stopping all alcohol actually does, you would want to take it.

Seek out both formal treatment programs as well as 12-step programs such as Alcoholics Anonymous, Cocaine and Narcotics Anonymous. Consider taking disulfiram (Antabuse®) or acamprosate (Campral®), even in a monitored program if that would give you more support in your goal of sobriety. Consider methadone or buprenorphine as substitution therapy for opiate addiction. Set up both formal and informal sponsors you can call when you need to talk with someone about impulses to relapse.

Consolidate your natural support networks by letting others who are close to you know what you are going through. Make your healthcare providers feel part of "your team" by talking with them and establishing a relationship of trust and collaboration.

And do all those things you already know are good for you - and that your primary care providers have been telling you - such as paying attention to healthy nutrition, good sleep hygiene with regular hours, and some exercise. There is never a better time to start to pay more attention to these than now.

Preventive (Prophylactic) Antidepressant Medication

In addition to treating a current major depressive disorder, some people have recommended that antidepressant medications be started before interferon-based therapy begins in people who have a prior history of major depressive episodes. One trial using citalopram (Celexa®) pretreatment in patients on pegylated interferon plus ribavirin with a psychiatric history found lower rates of depression in pretreated patients than in those who did not receive citalopram.[67]

However, another study already discussed[11] indicated that only half of those with a prior history of psychiatric disorder at baseline required antidepressant treatment during pegylated interferon plus ribavirin treatment. Preventive (prophylactic) use of antidepressant medications would be exposing half of the treatment population to medications (and their side effects) that they didn't actually need.

If you have had a course of antidepressant medication and then relapsed with depression and required another course of antidepressants, you are at higher risk of relapse during interferon-based therapy. You should consider discussing going back on antidepressant medication with your psychiatrist before beginning interferon-based therapy. Or you may feel, as many people do, that you are already taking enough medication and because pegylated interferon plus ribavirin induced depression usually responds well to treatment, you may choose to wait and see how you feel during the treatment. This is likely a workable solution as long as you are closely monitoring for depressive symptoms, or are seeing a psychiatrist regularly during your HCV treatment.

Antidepressant and Mood Stabilizing Medication

If you experience a major depressive disorder during pegylated interferon plus ribavirin treatment, almost all antidepressants have been reported to be effective and tolerated as treatment. The choice of one antidepressant over the other is usually based on their side effect profile, as it routinely is for non-HCV patients.

One study specifically assessed citalopram (Celexa®) in the treatment of depression among patients with chronic hepatitis C. It was found that in patients with liver enzymes less than 2.5 times above the normal range, citalopram blood levels were not significantly different in depressed patients with and without liver disease[67] and that it was an effective, well-tolerated antidepressant.

There are many case reports of antidepressants that have been successfully used in the treatment of major depressive disorders during interferon-based therapy. These are extensively reviewed in papers[57, 68] that also discuss side effects, drug-drug interactions (such as the caution regarding bleeding problems when using the combination of interferon, non-steroidal anti-inflammatory agents and selective serotonin reuptake inhibitor [SSRI] antidepressants), metabolism, dose and duration of treatment, and choice of agent that are beyond the scope of this chapter.

Antidepressant agents showing efficacy and tolerability for HCV patients on interferon-based therapies are shown in Table 1.

**Table 1. Antidepressant Medications Showing Efficacy and Tolerability
for HCV Patients on Interferon-Based Therapy**

Drug Class	Specific Medications
selective serotonin reuptake inhibitors (SSRIs)	citalopram (Celexa®) fluoxetine (Prozac®) paroxetine (Paxil®) sertraline (Zoloft®)
noradrenergic/serotonergic antidepressants	duloxetine (Cymbalta®) mirtazapine (Remeron®) venlafaxine (Effexor®)
noradrenergic/dopaminergic agents	buproprion (Wellbutrin®)

These papers also discuss the possible role of psychostimulants such as methylphenidate (Ritalin®) or modafinil (Provigil®) for interferon-induced fatigue.

Similarly, most mood stabilizing agents have been reported to be safe and effective in the treatment of bipolar disorders among patients with HCV and those on interferon-based therapy. Valproic acid (Depakote®), of particular concern because of an occasional association with elevated liver enzymes, was not shown to elevate liver enzymes more in patients with chronic hepatitis C than other psychiatric medications, specifically antidepressants, lithium, and gabapentin.[69] However, many doctors are still cautious about the use of valproic acid in patients with HCV and significantly elevated liver enzymes. Often other medications are substituted instead of using valproic acid to control psychiatric symptoms in such situations. Another study[70] reviews a number of competing concerns with mood stabilizers such as the lithium and carbamazepine (Tegretol®). Olanzapine (Zyprexa®) has been used safely to help with mood stabilization in chronic hepatitis C patients with bipolar disorder.

There are also many antianxiety agents such as lorazepam (Ativan®), and medications to help you sleep such as trazadone (Desyrel®) or zolpidem (Ambien®) that have been used by people with HCV safely and with good result.

The biggest barrier to getting treatment for depression and bipolar mood disorders is likely to be not recognizing their symptoms early and not acknowledging these symptoms need treatment. In general, there are as many psychiatric medications available to people with HCV (with a few exceptions that your healthcare provider will know about) as there are to the general population.

Summary

Combination therapy with pegylated interferon plus ribavirin has significantly improved response rates across all genotypes compared to standard interferon. But this therapy is still associated with depression and physical side effects that can negatively affect quality of life.

Depression and other mood disorders are effectively treated with standard antidepressant and mood stabilizing medications. If you have a prior history of psychiatric, alcohol or substance use disorders, you should consider getting psychiatric and/or substance treatment for stabilization before starting pegylated interferon plus ribavirin treatment.

On the other hand, patients with psychiatric and substance used disorders should not automatically be considered ineligible for pegylated interferon plus ribavirin treatment. Similarly, psychiatric disorders induced by pegylated interferon plus ribavirin treatment should be treated directly and not by reduction of dosage or early discontinuation of HCV treatment unless necessary.

You are likely feel better about yourself and your treatment if you learn as much as you can about them, and continue to discuss your experiences and concerns with your healthcare providers and your support system. Despite a potentially challenging course of treatment over 6 to 12 months, many people with HCV completely clear the virus and achieve a sustained virologic response with normalization of their mood and resolution of physical side effects as soon as they complete their treatment.

References

1. Asnis GM, De La Garza R II. Interferon-induced depression: strategies in treatment. *Prog Neuropsychopharmacol Biol Psychiatry*. 2005;29(5):808-18. Review.
2. Bonkovsky HL, Woolley JM, The Consensus Interferon Study Group. Reduction of health-related quality of life in chronic hepatitis C and improvement with interferon therapy. *Hepatology*. 1999;29:264-70.
3. Braitstein P, Montessori V, Chan K, et al. Quality of life, depression and fatigue among persons co-infected with HIV and hepatitis C: outcomes from a population-based cohort. *AIDS Care*. 2005;17(4):505-15.
4. Chang A, Skole K, Gautam, M, et al. The impact of past alcohol use on treatment response rates in patients with chronic hepatitis C. *Aliment Pharmacol Ther*. 2005;22(8):701-6.
5. Constant A, Castera L, Dantzer R, et al. Mood alterations during interferon-alfa therapy in patients with chronic hepatitis C: evidence for an overlap between manic/hypomanic and depressive symptoms. *J Clin Psychiatry*. 2005;66(8):1050-7.
6. Córdoba J, Flavià M, Jacas C, et al. Quality of life and cognitive function in hepatitis C at different stages of liver disease. *J Hepatol*. 2003;39(2):231-38.
7. Dan AA, Martin LM, Crone C, et al. Depression, anemia and health-related quality of life in chronic hepatitis C. *J Hepatol*. 2006;44(3):491-8.
8. Davis GL, Rodrigue JR. Treatment of chronic hepatitis C in active drug users. *N Engl J Med*. 2001;345(3):215-7. Erratum in N Engl J Med. 2001;345(23):1716.
9. Des Jarlais DC, Perlis T, Arasteh K, et al. Reductions in hepatitis C virus and HIV infections among injecting drug users in New York City, 1990-2001. *AIDS*. 2005;19(Suppl 3):S20-5.
10. Dieperink E, Ho SB, Tetrick L, et al. Suicidal ideation during intefereon-α2b and ribavirin treatment of patients with chronic hepatitis C. *Gen Hosp Psychiatry*. 2004;26:237-40.
11. Dieperink E, Ho SB, Thuras P, et al. A prospective study of neuropsychiatric symptoms associated with interfereon-α-2b and ribavirin therapy for patients with chronic hepatitis C. *Psychosomatics*. 2003;44(2):104-12.
12. Dieperink E, Willenbring M, Ho SB. Neuropsychiatric symptoms associated with hepatitis C and interferon alfa: a review. *Am J Psychiatry*. 2000;157(6):867-76.
13. Dominguez S., Ghosn J, Valantin MA, et al. Efficacy of early treatment of acute hepatitis C infection with pegylated interferon and ribavirin in HIV-infected patients. *AIDS*. 2006;20:1157-61.
14. Edlin BR, Seal KH, Lorvick J, et al. Is it justifiable to withhold treatment for hepatitis C from illicit-drug users? *N Engl J Med*. 2001;345(3):211-5.
15. Foster GR, Goldin RD, Thomas HC. Chronic hepatitis C virus infection causes a significant reduction in quality of life in the absence of cirrhosis. *Hepatology*. 1998;27:209-12.
16. Fraenkel L, McGraw S, Wongcharatrawee S, et al. What do patients consider when making decisions about treatment for hepatitis C? *Am J Med*. 2005;118(12):1387-91.
17. Fried MW, Shiffman ML, Reddy KR, et al. Peginterferon Alfa-2a plus ribavirin for chronic hepatitis C virus infection. *N Engl J Med*. 2002;347(13):975-82.
18. Geppert CMA, Dettmer E, Jakiche A. Ethical Challenges in the Care of persons with hepatitis C infection: a pilot study to enhance informed consent with veterans. *Psychosomatics*. 2005;46(5):392-401.
19. Gleason OC, Yates WR. Five cases of interferon-alfa-induced depression treated with antidepressant therapy. *Psychosomatics*. 1999;40(6):510-12.
20. Gochee PA, Powell EE, Purdie DM, et al. Association between apolipoprotein E ε4 and neuropsychiatric symptoms during interferon α treatment for chronic hepatitis C. *Psychosomatics*. 2004;45(1):49-57.
21. Golden J, O'Dwyer AM, Conroy RM. Depression and anxiety in patients with hepatitis C: prevalence, detection rates and risk factors. *Gen Hosp Psychiatry*. 2005;27(6):431-38.
22. Guadagnino V, Trotta MP, Carioti J, et al. Does depression symptomatology affect medication compliance during the first weeks of anti-HCV therapy in intravenous drug users? *Dig Liver Dis*. 2006;38(2):119-24.
23. Hauser P. Neuropsychiatric side effects of HCV therapy and their treatment: focus on IFNα-induced depression. Gastroenterol Clin North Am. 2004; 33(Suppl 1):S35-50.
24. Hauser P, Khosla J, Aurora H, et al. A prospective study of the incidence and open-label treatment of interferon-induced major depressive disorder in patients with hepatitis C. *Mol Psychiatry*. 2002;7:942-47.
25. Hoffman RG, Cohen MA, Alfonso CA, et al. Treatment of interferon-induced psychosis in patients with comorbid hepatitis C and HIV. *Psychosomatics*. 2003;44:417-20.
26. Hollander A, Foster GR, Weiland O. Health-related quality of life before, during and after combination therapy with interferon and ribavirin in unselected Swedish patients with chronic hepatitis C. *Scand J Gastroenterol*. 2006;41:577-585.
27. Hosoda S, Takimura H, Shibayama M, et al. Psychiatric symptoms related to interferon therapy for chronic hepatitis C: clinical features and prognosis. *Psychiatry Clin Neurosci*. 2000;54(5):565-72.
28. Inciardi JA, Surratt HL, Kurtz SP. HIV, HBV, and HCV infections among drug-involved, inner-city, street sex workers in Miami, Florida. *AIDS Behav*. 2006;10(2):139-47.
29. Joseph J, Stoff DM, Van der Horst C. HIV/hepatitis C virus co-infection: basic, behavioral and clinical research in mental health and drug abuse. *AIDS*. 2005;19(Supple 3):S3-7.
30. Kalyoncu OA, Tan D, Pektas O, et al. Major depressive disorder with psychotic features induced by interferon-alfa treatment for hepatitis C in a polydrug abuser. *J. Psychopharmacol*. 2005 Jan;19(1):102-5.
31. Kang SC, Hwang SJ, Lee SH, et al. Health-related quality of life and impact of antiviral treatment in Chinese patients with chronic hepatitis C in Taiwan. *World J Gastroenterol*. 2005;11(47):7494-8.
32. Kramer L, Hofer H, Bauer E., et al. Relative impact of fatigue and subclinical cognitive brain dysfunction on health-related quality of life in chronic hepatitis C infection. *AIDS*. 2005;19(Suppl 3):S85-92.

33. Kraus MR, Schäfer A, Csef H, et al. Psychiatric side effects of pegylated interferon alfa-2b as compared to conventional interferon alfa-2b in patients with chronic hepatitis C. *World J Gastroenterol*. 2005;11(12):1769-74.

34. Kraus MR, Schäfer A, Faller H, et al. Psychiatric symptoms in patients with chronic hepatitis C receiving interferon alfa-2b therapy. *J Clin Psychiatry*. 2003;64(6):708-14.

35. Kresina TF, Bruce RD, Cargill VA, et al. Integrating care for hepatitis C virus (HCV) and primary care for HIV for injection drug users coinfected with HIV and HCV. *Clin Infect Dis*. 2005;41(Suppl 1):S83-88.

36. Lieb K, Engelbrecht MA, Gut O, et al. Cognitive impairment in patients with chronic hepatitis treated with interferon alfa (IFNα): results from a prospective study. *Eur Psychiatry*. 2006;21:204-10.

37. Maddock C, Baita A, Orrù MG, et al. Psychopharmacological treatment of depression, anxiety, irritability and insomnia in patients receiving interferon-α: a prospective case series and a discussion of biological mechanisms. *J Psychopharmacol*. 2004;18(1):41-6.

38. Malek-Ahmadi P, Ghandour E. Bupropion for treatment of interferon-induced depression. *Ann Pharmacother*. 2004;38(7):1202-5.

39. Mauss S. Treatment of viral hepatitis in HIV-coinfected patients-adverse events and their management. *J Hepatol*. 2006;44(Suppl):S114-8.

40. Moore K, Dusheiko G. Opiate abuse and viral replication in hepatitis C. *Am J Pathol*. 2005;167(5):1189-91.

41. Moriguchi H, Sato C. Treatment of chronic hepatitis C in blacks and non-Hispanic whites. *N Engl J Med*. 2004;351(8):831-2. Letter.

42. Olson SH, Iyer S, Scott J, et al. Cancer history and other personal factors affect quality of life in patients with hepatitis C. *Health Qual Life Outcome*. 2005;3:39-46.

43. Onyike CU, Bonner JO, Lyketsos CG, et al. Mania during treatment of chronic hepatitis C with pegylated interferon and ribavirin. *Am J Psychiatry*. 2004;161(3):429-35.

44. Reichenberg A, Gorman JM, Dieterich DT. Interferon-induced depression and cognitive impairment in hepatitis C virus patients: a 72 week prospective study. *AIDS*. 2005;19(Suppl 3):S174-8).

45. Rifai MA, Moles JK, Lehman LP, et al. Hepatitis C screening and treatment outcomes in patients with substance use/dependence disorders. *Psychosomatics*. 2006;47(2):112-21.

46. Rosenberg SD, Drake RE, Brunette, MF, et al. Hepatitis C virus and HIV co-infection in people with severe mental illness and substance use disorders. *AIDS*. 2005;19(Suppl 3):S26-33.

47. Sepkowitz, KA. One disease, two epidemics – AIDS at 25. *N Engl J Med*. 2006;354(23):2411-14.

48. Sockalingam S, Balderson K. Major depressive episode with psychotic features induced by pegylated interferon-alfa-2b and ribavirin treatment. *Int Clin Psychopharmacol*. 2005;20(5):289-90.

49. Sulkowski MS, Thomas DL. Perspectives on HIV/hepatitis C virus co-infection, illicit drug use and mental illness. *AIDS*. 2005;19(Suppl 3):S8-12.

50. Teoh NC, Farrell GC. Management of chronic hepatitis C virus infection: a new era of disease control. *Intern Med J*. 2004;34(6):324-37.

51. Torriani FJ, Rodriguez-Torres M, Rockstroh JK, et al. Peginterferon alfa-2a plus ribavirin for chronic hepatitis C virus infections in HIV-infected patients. *N Engl J Med*. 2004;351(5):438-50.

52. Trask PC, Esper P, Riba M, et al. Psychiatric side effects of interferon therapy: prevalence, proposed mechanisms, and future directions. *J Clin Oncol*. 2000;18(11):2316-26. Review.

53. Ware JE, Bayliss MS, Mannocchia M, et al. Health-related quality of life in chronic hepatitis C: impact of disease and treatment response. *Hepatology*. 1999;30:550-5.

54. Onyike CU, Bonner JO, Lyketsos CG, Treisman GJ. Mania during treatment of chronic hepatitis C with pegylated interferon and ribavirin. *Am J Psychiatry*. 2004;161(3):429-435.

55. Willenbring ML. Integrating care for patients with infectious, psychiatric, and substance use disorders: concepts and approaches. *AIDS*. 2005;19(Suppl 3):S227-37.

56. Wilson MS 2nd. Interferon for Hepatitis C patients with psychiatric disorders. *Am J Psychiatry*. 2004;161(12):2331-2.

57. Raison CL, Demetrashvili M, Capuron L, and Miller AH. Neuropsychiatric Adverse Effects of Interferon-α: Recognition and Management. *CNS Drugs*. 2005;19(2):105–123.

58. Janssen HL, Brouwer JT, van der Mast RC, Schalm SW. Suicide associated with alfa-interferon therapy for chronic viral hepatitis. *J Hepatol*. 1994 Aug;21(2):241-3.

59. Rifflet H, Vuillemin E, Oberti F, et al. [Suicidal impulses in patients with chronic viral hepatitis C during or after therapy with interferon alfa]. *Gastroenterol Clin Biol*. 1998;22(3):353-7.

60. Janssen HL, Brouwer JT, van der Mast RC, Schalm SW. Suicide associated with alfa-interferon therapy for chronic viral hepatitis. *J Hepatol*. 1994;21(2):241-3.

61. Hosoda S, Takimura H, Shibayama M, Kanamura H, Ikeda K, Kumada H. Psychiatric symptoms related to interferon therapy for chronic hepatitis C: clinical features and prognosis. *Psychiatry Clin Neurosci*. 2000 Oct;54(5):565-72.

62. Banerjee A, Jain G, Grover S, Singh J. Mania associated with interferon. *J Postgrad Med*. 2007;53:150.

63. Rosalind G, et al. Treatment of Interferon-Induced Psychosis in Patients With Comorbid Hepatitis C and HIV. *Psychosomatics*. 44:417-420, October 2003.

64. Maddock C, et al. Psychopharmacological treatment of depression, anxiety, irritability and insomnia in patients receiving interferon-alfa: a prospective case series and a discussion of biological mechanisms. *J Psychopharmacol*. 2004 Mar;18(1):41.

65. Dieperink E, Willenbring M, Ho SB: Neuropsychiatric Symptoms Associated with Hepatitis C and Interferon Alfa: A Review. *Am J Psychiatry* 2000; 157:6: 867-876.

66. Davies TF. *A Case-Based Guide to Clinical Endocrinology*. Totowa, NJ: Humana Press;2008:53-55.

67. Kraus MR, Schäfer A, Schöttker K, Keicher C, Weissbrich B, Hofbauer I, Scheurlen M. Therapy of interferon-induced depression in chronic hepatitis C with citalopram: a randomised, double-blind, placebo-controlled study. *Gut*. 2008 Apr;57(4):531-6.

68. Fontana RJ. Neuropsychiatric toxicity of antiviral treatment in chronic hepatitis C. *Dig Dis*. 2000;18(3):107-16.

69. Felker B., et al The Safety of Valproic Acid Use for Patients With Hepatitis C Infection. *Am J Psychiatry* 2003; 160:174–178

70. Catherine C. Managing the neuropsychiatric side effects of interferon-based therapy for hepatitis. *Clinic Journal of Medicine volume*. 2004;71 supplement 3.

Mental Health and Hepatitis C

Amy E. Smith, PAC and Diana L. Sylvestre, MD

3

Interferon-Based Therapy in Recovery

Introduction

So-called special populations, that is, persons with a history of addiction, mental illness, homelessness, and the like, represent the majority of patients with *hepatitis C (HCV)*.[1] It is sometimes assumed that these people are less-than-ideal *interferon-based treatment* candidates, incapable of completing HCV therapy. This misconception is driven by unfamiliarity, disinterest, or lack of knowledge.[2] The result? Many needy patients cannot access medical services for HCV. Fortunately, a growing body of evidence suggests that special populations can be successfully tested and treated for HCV in a setting that addresses their special needs.[3-5]

O.A.S.I.S. (Organization to Achieve Solutions in Substance Abuse) is a nonprofit organization located in Oakland, California dedicated to providing state-of-the-art medical care to drug users and other marginalized populations, the majority of whom have HCV. O.A.S.I.S. has developed a unique peer-based model of HCV intervention that combines contemporaneous education, peer support, and medical care. Using this strategy, even the most challenging patients can be successfully treated for HCV. More importantly, this success can carry over into many other aspects of their lives. The O.A.S.I.S. model serves as one example of how to successfully deliver interferon-based treatment for HCV in the setting of recovery, and will the be model discussed throughout this section.

> **Evidence suggests that special populations can be successfully tested and treated for HCV in a setting that addresses their special needs.**

About the Disease of Addiction

The disease of addiction is far more lethal than hepatitis C. According to the Centers for Disease Control and Prevention (CDC), 5% to 20% of people with chronic hepatitis C will develop *cirrhosis* over a 20 to 30 year period, and approximately 3% die of complications of HCV.[6] In contrast, the 33-year mortality of active heroin users is approximately 50%.[7] Despite this, it is common for a patient with both addiction and hepatitis C to focus on the less important viral illness instead of the much more important problem of drug or *alcohol* use. It is not hard to understand why: dealing with one's addiction is vastly more difficult than dealing with hepatitis C.

It is important to understand that addiction is different from drug use.[8] Addiction is a brain disease. People with addictive disorders have well-defined *neurochemical* abnormalities that are slow to resolve and, in some cases, are irreversible. These abnormalities lead to characteristic behaviors such as lack of control over drug use and a lifelong tendency toward relapse. Short-term strategies (such as "detox" or detoxification) are rarely successful because they fail to address the neurochemical underpinnings of addiction. Detoxes are a lot like crash diets — possibly effective for the short term, but rarely of long-term benefit. Just as losing weight is a lot easier than keeping it off, the hard part of sobriety isn't getting there, it's staying that way.

Addiction shares features with other chronic conditions such as diabetes, *hypertension*, and asthma in which weight loss, dietary restraint, and smoking cessation do not eliminate the predisposition the condition but help minimize the consequences. Similar to these conditions, addiction is highly genetically determined. And as with other chronic conditions, retention (sticking with one's recovery program) is the key to a successful outcome in a patient with addiction. Over time and with continued treatment, alcohol and substance use relapse become less frequent and severe.

Relapse is part of the definition of addiction. It is not a personal failing. Just as you would not consider a doughnut-eating diabetic hopeless, understanding that drug relapse is a normal and treatable characteristic of addiction is an important aspect of understanding the disease of addiction itself. In order to achieve maximal benefit, a person with an addiction should be guided toward long-term strategies to deal with his/her problem.

For opiate users, maintenance with methadone or buprenorphine is a highly effective strategy to stabilize behaviors and should be encouraged. Twelve-step programs such as Alcoholics Anonymous (AA) and Narcotics Anonymous (NA) are at least as effective as many fancier treatment modalities and are often much more accessible. In some instances, long-term residential treatment may be the only option, especially if less intensive outpatient strategies are repetitively failing. The bottom line? Any treatment for addiction is better than no treatment. Whatever works to maintain sobriety is good, good, good.

The O.A.S.I.S. HCV Model

The O.A.S.I.S. model of HCV intervention is called Educate-Motivate-Facilitate (see Figure 1). Each component is integral to the model's success. If this model is not available in your area, we hope that the information provided here will help you organize and prioritize information about hepatitis C and the treatment possibilities.

Figure 1. Components of the O.A.S.I.S. Model of HCV Intervention

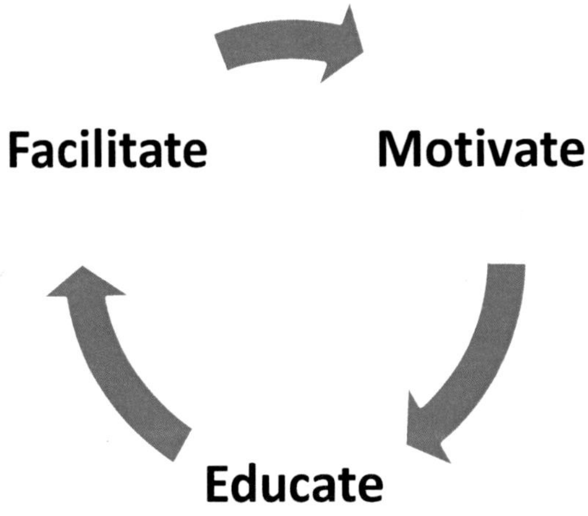

Get Educated

Hepatitis C is a complicated disease that affects each individual differently. Some people need interferon-based treatment, but many others do not. Among those who elect interferon-based treatment, there are a number of possible side effects and treatment-related problems. Add to this the bigger issue of addiction and recovery, and there is a lot of ground to cover in becoming educated about hepatitis C and its treatment.

The O.A.S.I.S. model uses peer-based support groups to teach everything from the fundamentals of hepatitis C, anatomy and *physiology* of the liver, and treatment-related issues. These groups also address how all of these other topics relate to addiction and recovery. We want patients to be active participants in the decisions made about their healthcare. It is not the provider's choice whether to treat. It is a decision to make together. And the more educated you are, the better your treatment-related decisions will be.

Get Motivated

It is not enough just to know things. The knowledge must be translated into action. If you know that alcohol is a big problem with hepatitis C but continue to drink, then how far have you really gotten? It is easy to get bogged down in your own self pity. Remember, hepatitis C is a treatable and often curable disease — and that is much more than can be said about many other serious conditions.

It is hard to stay motivated without a good support system. In the O.A.S.I.S. program, groups provide not only education but motivation by creating a nurturing environment. People are there to cheer you on, give you a shoulder to cry on, lift your spirits with a phone call at the right time, offer honest and constructive dialog and the occasional dose of tough love that only someone who has "been there and done that" can give. A positive mental attitude and being motivated to take care of your health and well-being will go a long way in making the right choices regarding this and all aspects of your health.

Get Help/Facilitate

This is often the most challenging aspect of HCV intervention: once motivated, how do you access the services you need? At O.A.S.I.S., we are in the unique position of being able to provide all HCV services on-site. But we know this is the exception rather than the rule. Use all available resources. You may need to assist your provider in finding and accessing the necessary services, which include HCV screening tests, viral tests, and doctors that offer biopsy and HCV treatment.

Mental health services and programs for substance users are important, especially during HCV treatment. Do not forget 12-step programs such as AA and NA. Research has shown that 12-step programs are just as effective as many other types of recovery programs, and they are free.

County clinics are often overwhelmed. Getting an appointment may take weeks to months. It is easy to get impatient, but fortunately, most people with hepatitis C have plenty of time. Please try to remember this important bit of information. It is common to get motivated to address hepatitis C but lose interest when your needs are not met quickly enough to suit you. Hepatitis C tends to progress slowly over a long period of time. Take a deep breath and do not become needlessly frustrated by the process.

Addiction: Understanding the Stages of Change

Drug users can and do care about their health. You may have awoken from the era of *HIV* with relief that you did not contract it, only to find that you have been infected with another potentially life-threatening medical condition, hepatitis C. This belief can be very destabilizing and contribute to continued use of drugs as well as conscious avoidance of medical care.

Addiction is a chronic illness. Understanding the "Stages of Change" model of substance use behaviors can be useful when seeking help for yourself or someone you care about. The Stages of Change model, which grew out of work in the area of smoking cessation, is now a widely-used approach to substance use.[9] By understanding the stage, we can help create an environment more conducive to a positive change in behaviors.

The Stages of Change is a five-stage model originally developed at the University of Rhode Island by James Prochaska and Carlo DiClemente (see Table 1). All people faced with a behavioral change fit somewhere along a continuum of motivation to accept advice. This applies to all behavioral changes, be it eliminating ongoing drug use, excessive caloric intake, dietary indiscretions, or poor medication adherence. The key to success is recognizing where you are along the continuum, and pursuing an intervention that will help you move though the motivational steps and closer to the goal.

Table 1. Stages of Change

Stage	Characteristics
Precontemplation	Not yet acknowledging that there is a problem behavior that needs to be changed
Contemplation	Acknowledging that there is a problem but not yet ready or sure of wanting to make a change
Preparation/Determination	Getting ready to change
Action/Willpower	Changing behavior
Maintenance	Maintaining the behavior change
Relapse	Returning to older behaviors and abandoning the new changes

People in the precontemplation stage are unaware or underaware that their substance use behaviors are a problem or might be contributing to other problems. Obviously, without an understanding of the need for sobriety, a message to stop using drugs at this stage is destined for failure. The key to this stage is being open to information that can help you consider making a behavior change, such as alcohol use makes hepatitis C more dangerous or that drug use may increase the risk of infections.

In the contemplation stage, you may be aware that your behavior is a problem but are not yet ready or sure about making changes. You may be torn between the difficulties created by the drug use and the challenges required to stay sober. Interventions in this stage should target some of these challenges as a means of facilitating progress to the next stage. At this stage, you are not yet mentally or physically prepared for sobriety. You will need further education and encouragement to achieve this goal.

Once a decision has been made in favor of change, you have entered the preparation stage. Goals are being set even though drug use continues. Typically, this is a stage at which the quantity or frequency of drug use is reduced, and information about treatment options will be more welcome. A quit date can usually be set.

When the action stage is reached, an attempt to stop using drugs is made. At this stage, your healthcare provider may need to help with withdrawal symptoms. The consequences of sobriety, such as the emergence of an unrecognized anxiety or panic disorder, may also need to be addressed. During this stage, an honest and open partnership is critical. It must be safe and comfortable to discuss problematic behaviors or sobriety will be brief and unsuccessful.

Once you have successfully negotiated the action stage, you enter the maintenance stage. In this stage, new coping patterns for emotions and relationships are developed and the foundations are laid for long-term sobriety. Relapse at this stage is common and often a product of success. People in this stage feel dramatically better after a sustained period of *abstinence*. You may begin to believe you can return to occasional use and maintain other gains. Although it often causes feelings of remorse and shame, relapse is normal and offers an opportunity to learn more about addiction and recovery.

Treating HCV in Substance Users

There are surprisingly few data about how best to treat HCV in substance users. Perhaps the most important piece of information would be to foster a climate of honesty. Patients need to be honest with providers. And providers need to understand addiction and be willing to work closely with patients dealing with addiction.

If a relapse occurs, you must be able to discuss it with your healthcare providers without fear of retribution. Catching a relapse early and making the proper referrals to treatment programs can allow treatment to continue and further the recovery process.

Frequently Asked Questions

HOW LONG DO I HAVE TO BE DRUG FREE BEFORE I CAN START HCV TREATMENT?

A period of six months is generally considered to be a reasonable period of time for patients to be drug-free prior to starting HCV treatment. That is probably not a bad starting point, but there is nothing magical about the six month period. Indeed, some patients with more limited sobriety can do better than those who have been drug free for years. The bottom line is that this decision should be individualized. [10]

IS METHADONE A PROBLEM?

Overall, patients maintained on methadone do well and should not be detoxed prior to HCV treatment. In fact, it may be easier for patients to be treated while taking methadone because it helps stabilize the craving and drug use behaviors that can potentially be destructive. A recent review of published research found that methadone-maintained patients have virologic response rates no different from nonsubstance users. [11]

IF I HAVE A HISTORY OF MENTAL ILLNESS, CAN I BE TREATED FOR HCV?

While a history of mental illness necessitates extra planning and monitoring, many people with stable mental health issues can be successfully treated with interferon-based therapy. It can be a challenge for both the healthcare provider and the patient, but in many cases, it can be done successfully. Please see section 2 of this chapter for additional information.

WHAT IF I RELAPSE?

If you relapse during HCV treatment, you may find it hard to take the medicines as directed. In addition, the drugs or alcohol may affect your *immune system* and lessen your body's response to the HCV medicines. You can also become reinfected during a relapse. Any or all of these circumstances may decrease your chance of getting rid of the hepatitis C virus. It is always best to get help quickly should a relapse occur to help you get the situation under control and to prevent an interruption in your HCV treatment.

ARE THE INTERFERON INJECTIONS GOING TO MAKE ME CRAVE DRUGS?

Some people are concerned about this potential problem, but fortunately, it appears to be uncommon. If you feel that the syringe might be a trigger for you, please discuss this with your healthcare provider. See if you can have the interferon shots administered at the doctor's office.

Interferon-based treatment can cause *fatigue*, nausea, headache and a general feeling a low energy. These side effects can be a trigger for some people and should be discussed prior to beginning HCV treatment.

Summary

Addiction and hepatitis C are closely intertwined. Both are chronic medical conditions and both be successfully treated. Although patients with alcohol or drug addictions may have additional challenges when undergoing treatment for HCV, the data show that HCV treatment outcomes in addicted patients are similar to those without a history addiction.

The trick is to find a place where you can be honest about your conditions and that has the expertise to guide you through any barriers that may present themselves. Remember that hepatitis C is almost never a medical emergency; protecting your sobriety is the most important thing that you can do for yourself.

Because of misunderstandings and misconceptions, you may need to learn to be an *advocate* for your own healthcare. The best road to successful advocacy is information. The more you understand about HCV and addiction, the more you will be able to work with your medical provider to make the best decisions for you.

References

1. Alter MJ, Moyer LA. The importance of preventing hepatitis C virus infection among injection drug users in the United States. *J Acquir Immune Defic Syndr Hum Retrovirol*. 1998;18 Suppl 1:S6-10.
2. Davis GL, Rodrigue JR. Treatment of chronic hepatitis C in active drug users. *N Engl J Med*. 2001;345(3):215-7.
3. Backmund M, Meyer K, Von Zielonka M, Eichenlaub D. Treatment of hepatitis C infection in injection drug users. *Hepatology*. 2001;34(1):188-93.
4. Sylvestre DL, Litwin AH, Clements BJ, Gourevitch MN. The impact of barriers to hepatitis C virus treatment in recovering heroin users maintained on methadone. *Journal of Substance Abuse Treatment*. 2005;29(3):159-65.
5. Van Thiel DH, Anantharaju A, Creech S. Response to treatment of hepatitis C in individuals with a recent history of intravenous drug abuse. *Am J Gastroenterol*. 2003;98(10):2281-8.
6. Centers for Disease Control and Prevention. Recommendations for prevention and control of hepatitis C virus (HCV) infection and HCV-related chronic disease. *MMWR*. 1998;47(No. RR-19):12-13.
7. Hser YI, Hoffman V, Grella CE, Anglin MD. A 33-year follow-up of narcotics addicts. *Arch Gen Psychiatry*. 2001;58(5):503-8.
8. Leshner AI. The disease of addiction. *Lippincotts Prim Care Pract*. 2000;4(3):249-53.
9. Prochaska JO, DiClemente CC, Norcross JC. In search of how people change. Applications to addictive behaviors. *Am Psychol*. 1992;47(9):1102-14.
10. Strader DB, Wright T, Thomas DL, Seeff LB; American Association for the Study of Liver Diseases. Diagnosis, management, and treatment of hepatitis C. *Hepatology*. 2004;39(4):1147-71.
11. Novick DM, Kreek MJ. Critical issues in the treatment of hepatitis C virus infection in methadone maintenance patients. *Addiction*. 2008 Jun;103(6):905-18.

Mental Health and Hepatitis C

Susan L. Zickmund, PhD

Psychosocial Issues and HCV

Introduction

Having the *hepatitis C virus* (*HCV*) raises many questions and concerns. With the diagnosis comes information about a chronic and often progressive disease that may lead to significant complications. Treatment is indeed possible and increasingly successful, but it can be cumbersome and may lead to significant side effects.

Yet, concerns about HCV go beyond medical questions about the disease and its treatment. Hepatitis C is a liver disease caused by a virus that is typically transmitted parenterally, meaning through blood products or contaminated needles or surgical instruments. All these seemingly simple facts affect the lives of many patients infected with HCV. There is guilt by association. Suffering from a blood-borne illness, an illness affecting the liver, carries a stigma.

There is the concern about passing the virus to others. Patients themselves or others may shy away from personal contact, fearing that the disease might spread. And then there is the experience of a disease and its treatment that drains energy as if invisible forces were at work, not allowing patients to meet expectations.

Such problems can cause patients to feel alone, isolated, and rejected from their much-needed social support system. Several recent studies have focused on the social implications of HCV. This section will present an overview of the effects HCV can have on patients' social support systems. It is our hope that:

- Recognizing these problems will function as the first step toward solving them.

- Reading about such difficulties may help some patients prepare for future challenges or to see that they are not alone in their experiences.

Problems in Close Personal Relationships

The social implications of HCV can be very important to patients. The significance was effectively shown in a study by Coughlin and her team where they found that the level of social functioning for female patients with HCV was the best predictor of patients' psychological well-being and overall mental health.[1] Yet what remains more elusive in the published literature are the specific social challenges that patients with the HCV diagnosis face. Given the lack of available information to provide these details, we will draw on our own investigations on social issues affecting patients with HCV and place these in the larger context of the medical literature. We will especially focus on the voice of the patients themselves and the concerns they express.

We conducted a large study interviewing several hundred patients with HCV seen in a university-based *hepatology* clinic.[2-4] We asked about the effects of their disease on their interactions with others. Nearly half of these patients noted that having HCV had resulted in a significant strain or actual loss of at least one relationship.[4] They reported problems with sexual partners (17%), family members (16%), and friends (12%).[4] Nearly 1 in 10 of the patients had lost contact with more than one person in their lives due to the disease.[4] As one man expressed, "When I got here [to the clinic] they told me I had hep C and then, when I was honest about it and told a girlfriend. I no longer had a girlfriend."

Patients often used powerful language to describe their isolation after the diagnosis, employing terms such as "lepers" and "hermits."[2] "When I first found out, I always felt dirty, like someone who had leprosy or something." Interestingly, it was not just the people around those with HCV who shied away from close contacts. A small number of patients saw themselves as a potential cause of harm, with 7% noting that they themselves had limited their social interactions.[4] One man mentioned that he was too concerned to interact with others. "I'm constantly aware of being around people in my surroundings, because you don't want to give it to anybody else. So it kind of plays with your mind a little bit. I was really depressed at first because it felt like you were just unclean or you [could] contaminate them. I got isolated from society and kind of stayed by myself."

Stress and Concern, and the Erosion of Social Support

In discussing the loss of social support, patients explained various reasons for the toll HCV had taken on their relations. Surprisingly often, it was the physical symptoms and consequences of the disease itself and its treatment that had caused the difficulties. About one-quarter of patients described stressful situations where family members worried about their health, or where they themselves worried about being able to stay healthy for their loved ones.[4] One woman noted that, "my relationship with my daughter has changed as well, because, after I found out, she got pretty angry with me. I think it's just because I was so sick."

A professor of nursing shared a similar experience in her narrative account of her infection and successful treatment for HCV.[5] Dr. Jana C. Saunders wrote that, "my HCV illness was very difficult for both of my daughters. While they never told me about all their concerns until after I had completed the treatment, they now tell me they were afraid I would not survive the treatment or the disease. I could tell by their physical and emotional distancing from me, they also had a hard time coping with my new disease."[5] Such accounts exemplify the extent to which HCV and the side effects of treatment can affect patients' lives.

Fatigue and Misunderstanding can Affect Social Networks

One of the major physical symptoms affecting relationships was *fatigue*. Unfortunately, fatigue is a prevalent symptom of HCV infection and a common side effect of antiviral treatment. In a study of patients who had never been treated, 86% described fatigue as a symptom.[6] In our study, participants described the effect fatigue had had on their lives. Whether caused by the HCV disease or its treatment, this symptom had become a real burden on relationships for 14% of patients.[4] In addition to having strained relations with his wife and children, one man explained, "The relationships with friends have pretty much died out, too. I have a few friends that I keep in contact with...Basically I do not have any good relationships with anyone."

Patients associated fatigue with lower social support. In our study it was associated with many symptoms, both mental (*depression*, anxiety) and physical (mobility, ambulation, body care and movement).[4] Similarly, Hilsabeck and colleagues reported that poor social functioning was the biggest predictor of fatigue.[7] This study raises the interesting question of whether there can be a two-way association between fatigue and social support where poor support worsens physical symptoms or their perceived effects on patients, which in turn, further reduces social support.

In addition to the physical manifestations of hepatitis C disease, the public comprehension of the disease posed a source of relationship problems. Patients encountered individuals who demonstrated a complete lack of understanding of HCV. This in turn affected their social interactions.[4] For example, when asked about changes in relationships, one man noted, "Don't have any. Lot of stress. Extreme amount of stress. Because they don't want to take time to read. They don't want to take time to listen to what you got to say.....I didn't know nothing about this until I started reading on it." Other patients noted that family and friends did not believe they were physically limited by HCV as they did not appear classically "sick." This led to accusations that HCV was not a "real" disease, like cancer or heart failure, and that instead the patient must be pretending to be ill.[4]

Employment and Financial Issues and the Straining of Social Support

The diagnosis of HCV and its effects on physical and psychological health also negatively affected patients' ability to meet professional expectations. In our own treatment study, nearly a third of our patient sample had experienced difficulties in the work environment.[8] Such problems at work, especially when it resulted in a demotion or even the frank loss of work, resulted in turmoil for patients and their social lives. One man and his wife described the emotional and social impact of losing a job due to HCV. "I used to be able to work and do things on my own and I don't feel like it. I'm not able to do anything like that anymore. So I feel kind of low, more than I'm use to. And this female [turning to wife] would go to work every day and bring home a paycheck. It's kind of a drag on me and makes it even tougher on her...and the little ones feel it also."

Although our studies have found employment to be an area of major stress for patients with HCV and their families,[2, 4, 8] little in the published literature has helped to shed light on this phenomenon.[9] Minuk in his study of expressed concerns of HCV patients reported this problem,[10] as did Hopwood and Treloar in their qualitative study of patients' experiences in undergoing antiviral treatment.[11] However, more work is needed to clarify the stressors that HCV patients face in the work force and the effect it has on their social lives and health.

A related concern emerges from the financial problems patients experience, which can add to their already significant emotional stress.[4] Patients stated they were often supporting treatment costs out-of-pocket, and the rising level of debt from treatment helped to further strain familial relationships. Such experiences became especially difficult when patients faced a job loss caused by their HCV. One woman explained that she had been fired for absences incurred due to her disease. When asked to describe what the effect of the disease had been, she explained, "Tremendous! I had to quit my job. I am a single parent raising four kids, two of which are teenagers. It's hard. I cannot work full-time and parent. I had probably the best job I ever had. I had to give it up in March because it was either work full-time or parent. And I am not about to give my kids up." These findings are supported by Zacks and colleagues who found that 66% of HCV-positive participants expressed concern over their financial security.[12]

Fear of Transmitting the Virus and the Effect on Social Support

Another common concern voiced by 25% of our study participants was the fear of potentially transmitting HCV.[4] Although the current literature indicates that the likelihood of spreading HCV through casual or sexual contact is low, patients and their family, friends, and coworkers remained concerned.[13] In one study, patients indicated a substantial change in sexual behavior due to the disease, with 20% of participants saying that they kissed less frequently and 27% noting that they engaged in less sexual intercourse.[12] In our own study, 20% of patients spontaneously stated that they worried about possibly infecting sexual partners and family members.[4] A patient shared the stress he experienced in his relationship: "From the very get-go of knowing I had this, the changes were that my wife was more scared...All of a sudden she wanted to use protection and I was like, why, we have been married twenty years and you don't have it. I do."

Another isolating aspect of the disease came when patients chose to limit contacts in order to avoid any potential spread of disease.[4] In our interviews, patients agonized over the hope of ever finding a partner if they were not currently in a stable relationship. This concern was reflected in the statement by one young man, "[HCV] is hard on friends. It's hard on families, and extremely hard on relationships. That's one of my major concerns right now. Suppose I meet somebody and we hit it off pretty well. It's like, well, do I tell them I have hep C? I feel you should tell them right away instead of going on with something and getting along and saying `I have hep C' and `oh, oh,' you know? Because whenever you mention a blood virus the first thing that comes to people's mind is *HIV*." These findings are consistent with results published by Zacks, with 19% of participants reporting that they were less likely to date due to HCV disease.

Perhaps more surprising, 1 in 6 patients mentioned fears related to transmission through casual contacts with friends and/or children.[4] "My family's aware of [the HCV] and I've become super protective of them. Not a total quarantine, of course, but we practice very strict hygiene rules."

Our results have been corroborated by others. In a study by Minuk and colleagues, patients listed transmitting the virus to family members and to others as two of the biggest stressors related to their HCV diagnosis.[10] Additionally, in a study of HCV and attitudes toward blood donation by Waldby and colleagues, patients with HCV were described as viewing their blood as a danger that they needed to protect others from.[14] Finally, the study by Zacks also found that participants changed behavior by especially limiting exposures to their body fluid, by not sharing a drinking glasses (45 %), towels (35 %), and not preparing food for others (14 %).[12]

Lifestyle & Emotional Difficulties and Social Support

Having a liver disease and adhering to treatment recommendations often requires significant lifestyle modifications. *Abstinence* from drug and *alcohol* often changed interaction patterns with friends and acquaintances. In our study of patients undergoing antiviral therapy, 22% of the participants admitted having difficulties in eliminating all alcohol or illegal substances from their daily routine.[8] To remain compliant with treatment recommendations, patients felt the need to restrict their contact with family and friends in social situations that traditionally involved alcohol, such as going out to a bar or restaurant. One man shared his experience saying, "I don't go out as much. Since this is a liver disease, I hardly drink. I do slip occasionally because, hey, it is a good time. I have got friends that are social and relationships are built around hitting the bars and talking and having a good time, maybe seeing some music. So, while I still go out, I don't drink as much and, frankly, it is not as exciting as when you don't have a few drinks. So those relationships have changed." Others who had lived a life involving alcohol or drugs also experienced difficult challenges as they felt compelled to change their social circle. One man described the progress he had made but also the struggles he experienced in re-orienting his social life. "My friends have really changed to where I used to have a bunch of drinking buddies.... A lot of those buddies are gone."

The emotional problems caused by HCV and/or its treatment also worsened interpersonal relations. A study by Lang and her colleagues found that for patients who had never experienced treatment, irritability was the second most prominent symptom (behind fatigue).[6] One in five patients in our study felt their temper had led to deteriorating relations with friends and family members.[8] "My wife said that I've been moodier. There's been swings towards raising my voice to the children and to her maybe." The isolating impact of the emotional irritability was revealed by one man who noted, "I think I've withdrawn a lot more. I've been a little testier, harder to get along with those I've maintained contact with. The close ones have gotten the worst of it, unfortunately."

The Isolating Effect of Social Stigmatization

Having a liver disease, a disease most likely caused by contaminated blood or instruments, is often also associated with a value judgment. The links between alcohol, intravenous drug use, and liver disease frequently trigger reactions in others that the disease may well be a consequence of inappropriate behavior, thus casting the shadow of stigmatization over patients.

Several patient groups have been found to experience such negative stereotyping, especially those with active intravenous drug habits or mental disorders. Crockett and Gifford found that female drug users in Australia have experienced widespread and extensive stigmatization.[15] This phenomenon extends beyond actual drug users and can affect individuals regardless of how HCV was contracted. In the study by Zacks, 51% of participants noted that they experienced social rejection due to their disease.[12] In our own study, 57% of participants had experienced some type of stigmatization related to HCV.[2]

Patients described three major reasons for feeling stigmatized.[2] First, they felt others confused or associated HCV with HIV/AIDS.[2] Some mentioned that the acronym "HCV" led to confusion. One man shared the story of being informed of the diagnosis via a letter from the blood bank where he had donated blood. "When I first found out about it from the blood bank saying I had HCV – `wait a minute HIV!?' I confused it and said 'oh no!' and worried how to tell my wife I had this."

Second, given the commonly perceived link between blood-borne diseases such as HIV/AIDS and sexual transmission, patients were frequently viewed as sexually promiscuous.[2] One woman noted, "You know, my doctor was telling me, it's almost like AIDS. You can catch it from kissing or having sex, or using the same container, drinking out of the same milk jug. So, it kind of scares your friends away."

Finally, many patients were automatically seen as drug users.[2] One woman explained, "People don't understand what [HCV] is about. When they hear hepatitis, they think of IV drug users. That's what I always thought when I heard of it years ago."

The experience of stigmatization is not trivial. It may disrupt important and close ties with family members and friends. Nearly 1 in 5 patients reported that HCV-related stigmatization had negatively affected relations with family and/or friends.[2, 4] One patient noted that she had been denied the right to see a family member. "We have to file for grandparent visitation rights. They tried to hold my disease against us, so I could not see my grandson." Another man shared the experience of losing contact with family members. "My real daughter from a previous marriage really got farther away quick; won't have anything to do with me any more. . . I have no idea what that was all about. She had a couple of babies there and I don't know if she thought that I was going to contaminate the kids or what, but she hasn't called for about two years since she found out."

Based in part on such experiences, 18% of the persons interviewed had decided that they would not tell others about their disease in order to decrease the chance of receiving a negative reactions.[4] However, such a lack of disclosure could ultimately result in a lessening of social support as well. One woman responded to the question of what effect her disease had had on relationships, "I don't have any...I avoid them. In fact, I'm really cold with people. I don't let no one warm up to me, to get close, because I don't want nobody to know."

As noted above, suffering from a viral infection of the liver affects the work environment. In addition to physical problems, 26% of patients shared examples of being stigmatized in the work environment due to their disease.[2] One woman wrote, "When I first found out and they phoned at work, it was like I had leprosy because everyone stayed away and did not talk to me...That was pretty bad." Others noted that they had directly lost work due to prejudice and stigmatization. One man stated that he had lost multiple jobs due to stigmatization. "The next job I was terminated from I told my supervisor, because I was working handling bread trays that were 13 feet off the floor, I told my supervisor if I ever got knocked unconscious, don't touch my blood. Less than a week later, I was in the unemployment line. The third job I got fired from I was working at [Blank] Foods and I cut my hand and they out and out told me point blank...the reason they fired me is that I have hepatitis C and I pose a direct threat."

Stigmatization Within the Provider-Patient Relationship

Some patients with HCV have experienced stigmatization in the medical environment. Often the healthcare provider is the first person the patient learns the diagnosis from. The healthcare provider is also the person the patient needs to turn to in order for management and treatment of the disease. Therefore, feeling stigmatized by doctors, nurses, or other healthcare workers can have significant implications.

We studied patient perception of communication with doctors taking care of their HCV and found that 41% of the HCV patients had some type of communication difficulties with their doctors.[3] This included 9% feeling directly stigmatized by their doctors, with 16% feeling that they had been abandoned by their healthcare provider either in the context of a misdiagnosis or as a result of poor care.[3] Such an experience can cause frustration, as described in a comment a patient made to his wife during an interview. "Remember when we went into the emergency room? You said I have hepatitis C, and I just inhaled some *ammonia*, and they thought we were drug dealers? I was farming this fall and I took a big dose of anhydrous ammonia. Four hours of waiting because the first thing they think of is `he's a meth dealer', you know?"

Our findings do not stand alone. Grundy and his colleagues found that female HCV patients experiencing stigmatization within the medical environment held negative feelings toward their healthcare providers.[16] Day, Ross and Dolan reported stigmatizing experiences among heroin users infected with HCV.[17] Banwell and her group revealed similar experiences of medical discrimination amongst HCV infected lesbians and bisexual women.[18] Schaefer and colleagues noted that 39% of patients in their study had experienced stigmatization and other difficulties communicating with their healthcare providers.[19] Perhaps as a result, 55% of patients in the study stated that they had not told at least some of their medical providers of their HCV diagnosis, thereby limiting the medical insight into their disease.[19]

Two large studies conducted by Gifford and his group determined that nearly half of the HCV infected patients rated their treatment by medical professionals as poor and attributed this to their HCV status.[20, 21] Finally, Paterson and her team described abandonment and frustration by patients, noting that those who were ineligible for treatment or who had experienced treatment failure felt they had nowhere left to turn.[22]

As the doctor-patient relationship is so important to helping those with HCV adjust to and live with their disease, the question arises of why such problems exist. While no study definitively answers this important question, some data suggest that poor knowledge of HCV may contribute. Previous studies have demonstrated that primary care providers, medical residents, and other healthcare providers are often not sufficiently trained or comfortable in diagnosing and treating HCV infection. Nicklin and colleagues found widely varying recommendations for HCV-infected patients among primary care providers.[23] Similarly, Shehab and his group reported that 25% of primary care providers did not know what treatment to recommend for HCV, thereby delivering suboptimal care.[24] Negative attitudes that providers may hold toward *interferon-based therapy* itself (given its early low success rates and of the array of possible side effects) may further complicate this situation.[25, 26]

Studies suggest that healthcare providers may also have an aversion toward HCV-infected patients themselves.[11] The reasons for this stigmatizing treatment are not clearly known.[27] Negative attitudes may further exacerbate knowledge deficits, which can be caused by rapidly changing medical recommendations, and the complexities of managing patients with multiple psychiatric and medical conditions.[27] Fear of exposure to the hepatitis C virus may also lead to potentially stigmatizing behavior.[28]

Regardless of why some healthcare providers may hold such beliefs, the ultimate result is that patients with HCV can experience problems in developing the relationships they need in order to effectively face and manage their condition.

Summary

In conclusion, this section has described some of the challenges that people living with hepatitis C may face. Hopefully, an improved understanding of the disease will lessen the likelihood of negative social stereotyping. While educational efforts should emphasize and explain appropriate precautions, they need to more specifically address unnecessary concerns about endangering others through the spread of the hepatitis C virus.[29-31] Such information should be easily available for healthcare professionals, patients, relatives, friends and/or others interacting with individuals living with hepatitis C.

As the powerful narratives of patients who experience the physical, emotional, and social effects of their hepatitis C disease show, educational campaigns should devote some efforts toward dispelling myths that may underlie some of the stereotyping or unwarranted anxieties patients or other have.

References

1. Coughlan B, Sheehan J, Hickey A, Crowe J. Psychological well-being and quality of life in women with an iatrogenic hepatitis C virus infection. *Br J Health Psychol.* 2002; 7(Pt 1):105-116.
2. Zickmund S, Ho EY, Masuda M, Ippolito L, LaBrecque DR. "They treated me like a leper". Stigmatization and the quality of life of patients with hepatitis C. *J Gen Intern Med.* 2003; 18(10):835-844.
3. Zickmund S, Hillis SL, Barnett MJ, Ippolito L, LaBrecque DR. Hepatitis C virus-infected patients report communication problems with physicians. *Hepatology.* 2004; 39(4):999-1007.
4. Blasiole JA, Shinkunas L, LaBrecque DR, Arnold RM, Zickmund SL. Mental and physical symptoms associated with lower social support for patients with hepatitis c. *World J Gastroenterol.* 2006;12(29):4665-4672.
5. Saunders JC. Living with hepatitis C: a nurse's story. *Gastroenterol Nurs.* 2004; 27(5):239-241.
6. Lang CA, Conrad S, Garrett L, Battistutta D, Cooksley WG, Dunne MP et al. Symptom prevalence and clustering of symptoms in people living with chronic hepatitis C infection. *J Pain Symptom Manage.* 2006; 31(4):335-344.
7. Hilsabeck RC, Hassanein TI, Perry W. Biopsychosocial predictors of fatigue in chronic hepatitis C. *J Psychosom Res.* 2005; 58(2):173-178.
8. Zickmund SL, Bryce CL, Blasiole JA, Shinkunas L, LaBrecque DR, Arnold RM. Majority of patients with hepatitis C express physical, mental, and social difficulties with antiviral treatment. *Eur J Gastroenterol Hepatol.* 2006; 18(4):381-388.

9. Crofts N, Louie R, Loff B. The Next Plague: Stigmatization and Discrimination Related to Hepatitis C Virus Infection in Australia. *Health Hum Rights*. 1997; 2(2):86-97.
10. Minuk GY, Gutkin A, Wong SG, Kaita KD. Patient concerns regarding chronic hepatitis C infections. *J Viral Hepat*. 2005; 12(1):51-57.
11. Hopwood M, Treloar C. Receiving a hepatitis C-positive diagnosis. *Intern Med J*. 2004; 34(9-10):526-531.
12. Zacks S, Beavers K, Theodore D, Dougherty K, Batey B, Shumaker J et al. Social stigmatization and hepatitis C virus infection. *J Clin Gastroenterol*. 2006; 40(3):220-224.
13. Brusaferro S, Barbone F, Andrian P, Brianti G, Ciccone L, Furlan A et al. A study on the role of the family and other risk factors in HCV transmission. *Eur J Epidemiol*. 1999; 15(2):125-132.
14. Waldby C, Rosengarten M, Treloar C, Fraser S. Blood and bioidentity: ideas about self, boundaries and risk among blood donors and people living with hepatitis C. *Soc Sci Med*. 2004; 59(7):1461-1471.
15. Crockett B, Gifford SM. "Eyes Wide Shut": narratives of women living with hepatitis C in Australia. Women Health 2004; 39(4):117-137.
16. Grundy G, Beeching N. Understanding social stigma in women with hepatitis C. *Nurs Stand*. 2004; 19(4):35-39.
17. Day C, Ross J, Dolan K. Hepatitis C-related discrimination among heroin users in Sydney: drug user or hepatitis C discrimination? *Drug Alcohol Rev*. 2003; 22(3):317-321.
18. Banwell C, Bammer G, Gifford SM, O'Brien ML. Australian lesbian and bisexual women's health and social experiences of living with hepatitis C. *Health Care Women Int*. 2005; 26(4):340-354.
19. Schafer A, Scheurlen M, Felten M, Kraus MR. Physician-patient relationship and disclosure behaviour in chronic hepatitis C in a group of German outpatients. *Eur J Gastroenterol Hepatol*. 2005; 17(12):1387-1394.
20. Gifford SM, O'Brien ML, Bammer G, Banwell C, Stoove M. Australian women's experiences of living with hepatitis C virus: results from a cross-sectional survey. *J Gastroenterol Hepatol*. 2003; 18(7):841-850.
21. Gifford SM, O'Brien ML, Smith A, Temple-Smith M, Stoove M, Mitchell D et al. Australian men's experiences of living with hepatitis C virus: results from a cross-sectional survey. *J Gastroenterol Hepatol*. 2005; 20(1):79-86.
22. Paterson BL, Butt G, McGuinness L, Moffat B. The construction of hepatitis C as a chronic illness. *Clin Nurs Res*. 2006; 15(3):209-224.
23. Nicklin DE, Schultz C, Brensinger CM, Wilson JP. Current care of hepatitis C-positive patients by primary care physicians in an integrated delivery system. *J Am Board Fam Pract*. 1999; 12(6):427-435.
24. Shehab TM, Sonnad SS, Lok AS. Management of hepatitis C patients by primary care physicians in the USA: results of a national survey. *J Viral Hepat*. 2001; 8(5):377-383.
25. Patil R, Cotler SJ, Banaad-Omiotek G, McNutt RA, Brown MD, Cotler S et al. Physicians' preference values for hepatitis C health states and antiviral therapy: a survey. *BMC Gastroenterol*. 2001; 1(1):6.
26. Cotler SJ, Patil R, McNutt RA, Speroff T, Banaad-Omiotek G, Ganger DR et al. Patients' values for health states associated with hepatitis C and physicians' estimates of those values. *Am J Gastroenterol*. 2001; 96(9):2730-2736.
27. Fontana RJ, Kronfol Z. The patient's perspective in hepatitis C. *Hepatology*. 2004; 39(4):903-905.
28. Dement JM, Epling C, Ostbye T, Pompeii LA, Hunt DL. Blood and body fluid exposure risks among health care workers: results from the Duke Health and Safety Surveillance System. *Am J Ind Med*. 2004; 46(6):637-648.
29. Kerbleski M. Hepatitis C: are you confused?: Issues related to patient education. *Gastroenterol Nurs*. 2005; 28(3 Suppl):S19-S23.
30. Cormier M. The role of hepatitis C support groups. *Gastroenterol Nurs*. 2005; 28(3 Suppl):S4-S9.
31. Fraenkel L, McGraw S, Wongcharatrawee S, Garcia-Tsao G. Patients' experiences related to anti-viral treatment for hepatitis C. *Patient Educ Couns*. 2006; 62(1):148-155.

Military Veterans and Hepatitis C

Terry Baker

Introduction

America's military veterans have been plagued with many health issues since the founding of this country. *Hepatitis* has long been associated with U.S. military service. Military training and combat present many opportunities for transmission of viral hepatitis through blood-to-blood contact. Field bleeding, surgery, transfusions, and exposure to blood by military medics and surgeons all constitute high risks.

Since the identification of the *hepatitis C virus* (*HCV*) in 1989, physicians and Veterans Administration (VA) officials have seen large numbers of infection among veterans. Veterans appear to have unusually high rates of hepatitis C. While the prevalence of hepatitis C in the general population is approximately 1.6%, various studies in VA facilities have shown hepatitis C prevalence rates between 5% to 22% among veterans.[1-4] Veterans of foreign combat appear to be at the highest risk for infectious hepatitis. All major engagements of the last 70 years - World War II, the Korean War, and the Vietnam War - were associated with high rates of infectious hepatitis. Viral hepatitis was viewed as a single disease in the early years, and most treatment and documentation of it were for the acute forms of the disease. Table 1 shows a timeline of major developments in the history of the U.S. military and the current hepatitis C epidemic.

Table 1. Military Veterans and the Hepatitis C Timeline

1941-1953	Many World War II and Korean War veterans were diagnosed with non-A, non-B hepatitis.
1967-1969	Field hospitals performed 364,900 blood transfusions on American personnel in Vietnam. Soldiers, medics, and nurses were exposed to blood while caring for the wounded.[5]
1989	Researchers identified the hepatitis C virus, 48 years after the start of World War II.
1992	Researchers developed an accurate blood test for hepatitis C.[6]
1998	The number of hepatitis C cases at U.S. Department of Veterans Affairs facilities rose to 22,000 in 1998, up from 6,600 in 1991.[1,7]
1999	The VA established two HCV research and education centers and issued HCV treatment guidelines.
	VA leaders argued that investing in early treatment would save public dollars by reducing future hospital stays and liver transplants.
	Legislation was introduced to ensure wider coverage for hepatitis C treatment through VA facilities.
	Veterans Aimed Toward Awareness (VATA) launched a nationwide campaign to alert U.S. veterans they may be at risk for hepatitis C.
	A national survey about hepatitis C was conducted with 504 veterans.
2000	The National Hepatitis C Program was created.
2001	Four Hepatitis C Resource Centers (HCRC) were established and funded.
2003	113,927 veterans in the VA's care diagnosed with HCV, up from 22,000 in 1998.[8]
2008	250,000 veterans in the VA's care diagnosed with HCV.[9]

Military Veterans' Hepatitis C Survey

Bruskin-Goldring Research conducted a national survey commissioned by Veterans Aimed Toward Awareness (VATA) of 504 veterans in 1999. Veterans age 40 to 60 years were surveyed. Some findings from that survey include:

- 74.8% were "not very" or "not at all" concerned about their risk for HCV.
  - 67.5% were "not very" or "not at all" familiar with the disease.
- 60.1% had not been tested for HCV.
  - 58.3% were "not very" or "not at all" likely to be tested for HCV.
- 63.3% recognized flu-like symptoms, and 57.7% recognized yellow skin as possible symptoms of liver disease.
  - 1.6% knew that hepatitis C often has no symptoms.
- 9% initially acknowledged they might be at risk for hepatitis C.
  - 45% acknowledged they might be at risk after being informed of risk factors.
  - 65.1% stated their greatest fear about HCV is the possibility of infecting a loved one.
  - 62.9% stated their next greatest fear was the possibility of having a serious illness or dying from a serious illness.

There is clearly a need for HCV education. Veterans must be informed of their risk for hepatitis C, and about the seriousness of the disease.

The Prevalence of Hepatitis C Among U.S. Military Veterans

Veterans' *advocates* are concerned about the prevalence of hepatitis C among military veterans. Several studies have shown that veterans have a higher prevalence of HCV than the general public.[2-4] Studies at the VA Medical Centers (VAMC) in Washington, D.C. and San Francisco found the prevalence of HCV positive inpatients was 20% and 10%, respectively.[1] One of these studies also found 52% of patients requiring liver transplant were HCV positive.[1]

In 1998, a national tracking system analyzed the findings from 95,000 hepatitis C screening tests.[7] Of those who tested positive:

- 64% were Vietnam veterans
- 18.5% were post-Vietnam veterans
- 4.5% were Korean War veterans
- 4.2% were post-Korean War veterans
- 9.1% were veterans from other periods of service

Of the 8.1 million surviving veterans of the Vietnam War, 3.2 million had active duty in Asia between 1964 and 1973.[10] It is conservatively estimated that 10% of these Asian theater veterans are now infected with HCV.[1]

Transmission of HCV in the Asian Theater of the Vietnam War

There are a number of HCV risk factors for veterans who were in Asia during the Vietnam War, many related to the high prevalence of HCV in Southeast Asian countries. It is estimated that 5% to 8% of the Vietnamese population is infected with HCV.[11]

TRANSFUSIONS

Transfusion of blood or blood products before 1992 is a known risk factor for HCV infection. Prior to 1992, there were no accurate HCV screening tests to ensure the safety of the blood supply with respect to HCV.[6] Three hundred thousand

Americans were wounded and 153,329 were hospitalized during the Vietnam War. Between March 1967 and June 1969, 364,900 Americans in Vietnam received blood transfusions.[5] It is estimated that a minimum of 10% of those transfused received HCV-infected blood.[12]

MEDICAL CONTACT
Surgeons, nurses, medics, helicopter crews, and others involved in the evacuation and treatment of the wounded from Vietnam were also placed at risk for HCV infection because of their blood exposure. An estimated 41.1% of all soldiers deployed to Vietnam, approximately 2.1 million veterans, were involved in combat. Many soldiers assisted the more than 300,000 wounded. Medical personnel on hospital ships were also placed at risk via their exposure to wounded soldiers from the Vietnam theater.[13]

TATTOOS
Unclean needles that pierce the skin can transmit HCV. Tattoos have now been recognized as a significant route of transmission for HCV.[14, 15] An estimated 34% of active-duty military personnel have tattoos (personal communication, Capt. John Mateczun, Principal Director, Clinical Affairs, Office of Health Affairs, Department of Defense). Many of these tattoos were and continue to be acquired in countries where sanitation is often substandard.

SEXUAL CONTACT
Although sexual transmission of HCV occurs, it is believed to be relatively uncommon. Nevertheless, a portion of those infected with HCV during the Vietnam War were probably infected through sexual contact with Vietnamese nationals.

RECREATIONAL DRUG USE
Sharing drug paraphernalia is currently the most common cause of newly acquired HCV infections. This was also a risk factor during the Vietnam War. A study from the Centers for Disease Control and Prevention on the health status of Vietnam veterans found 3% had used "hard drugs," including amphetamines, barbiturates, cocaine, heroin, psychedelics, phencyclidine, and methaqualone.[16]

Veterans Affairs Response to Hepatitis C

The Department of Veterans Affairs has noted a decided increase in the number of HCV cases diagnosed over the past several years.[9, 17, 18]

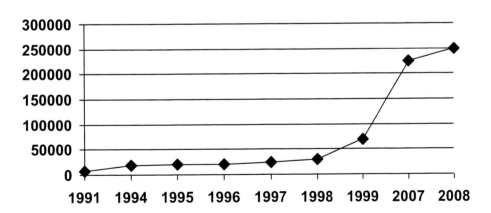

Veterans Diagnosed with HCV, 1991 to 2008

Testing of veterans outside the VA medical system has confirmed the high HCV prevalence in this population. A 1998 screening program that tested 200 apparently healthy leaders of the Vietnam Veterans of America found 9% of those tested were infected with HCV.[19] A more recent screening at a Vietnam Veterans' Standdown in New Orleans found 36% of those screened tested positive for HCV (unpublished data). These data all support the reality that veterans have consistently and markedly higher rates of HCV infection than the general population.

In June 1998, the VA issued HCV screening guidelines for veterans entering VA facilities. In December 1999, the VA adopted treatment guidelines for HCV infection. The guidelines recommend that eligible veterans be given the very best medical care, including the most recently approved treatment. Of course, only veterans who are income eligible or service connected for HCV can receive treatment through a VA medical center. Despite the treatment guidelines, veterans report problems obtaining care due to constraints put on HCV healthcare at the Veterans Integrated Service Network (VISN) level.

In 2001, the VA established four Hepatitis C Resources Centers (see Table 2).[18] These centers coordinate HCV treatment and research efforts, and develop educational programs for patients and their families. Healthcare providers who specialize in HCV and patient counselors are also located at these centers. The Hepatitis C Resource Centers build on the success of the previous Centers of Excellence in Hepatitis C program, established by VA in 1999. In 2007, the funding for these centers was renewed through September 30, 2011.

Table 2. Veterans Affairs Hepatitis C Resource Centers

Veterans Administration Medical Center, San Francisco, California www.hepatitis.va.gov/vahep?page=prin-con-hcrc-sf
Veterans Affairs Medical Center, Minneapolis, Minnesota www.hepatitis.va.gov/vahep?page=prin-con-hcrc-mn
Veterans Affairs Connecticut Healthcare System, West Haven, Connecticut www.hepatitis.va.gov/vahep?page=prin-con-hcrc-ct
VA Northwest Hepatitis C Resource Center at the VA Puget Sound Healthcare System, Seattle, Washington in collaboration with the VA Portland Medical Center, Portland, Oregon www.hepatitis.va.gov/vahep?page=prin-con-hcrc-nw

Projects of the Hepatitis C Resource Centers include:
- Improved screening and testing methods
- Assessment and treatment of patients traditionally excluded from hepatitis C treatment (including those with mental illness, substance abuse, or concurrent *HIV* infection)
- Development and dissemination of models of interdisciplinary care to optimize treatment outcomes
- Development and dissemination of *clinical* standards for treating patients with all stages of hepatitis C infection.

The National Hepatitis C Program, which includes the Hepatitis C Resource Centers (HCRC), falls under the VA National Clinical Public Health Program. The goals of the National Hepatitis C Program through 2012 are shown below.[18]

- Improvements in the management and treatment of the growing patient population with advanced liver disease and its complications

- The evaluation of the implementation and application of the knowledge, products, and clinical practices developed by the HCRC program across the entire VA system

- The preparation of the healthcare system for meeting the demand that will occur when new and better HCV treatment becomes available, which is likely in the next five years;

- A cross-cutting component of the previous three goals is the management of comorbidities in patients with hepatitis C such as mental illness, HIV infection and substance abuse

Each VA Medical Center Director must designate a Hepatitis C Lead Clinician to be the principal point of contact for all clinical hepatitis C program information and reporting between the facility, the Clinical Public Health Program office, and other facility program offices.

The Need For a Service Connection to HCV to Receive Treatment Through a VA Facility

As a result of the reorganization of the VA Medical Center system, all veterans have been put into one of seven categories according to his or her medical priority. Currently, all veterans, regardless of their category, receive medical treatment when they come to a VA Medical Center. Unless a veteran is 100% service connected, a copayment is required for all services and medicines.

It is critically important for veterans with HCV to be granted presumptive service connection to the disease so they can be treated. However, veterans infected with HCV during their military service are generally unable to establish the necessary service connection. A lack of knowledge about hepatitis C and how it is contracted, a historic lack of a reliable screening test, and the prolonged, often *asymptomatic* course of disease progression all conspire to make it extremely difficult to prove that infection was acquired during military service. Without a service connection to HCV, most veterans are unable to meet the standard of proof necessary to show that they contracted HCV during their military service. As the VA's budget continues to shrink, veterans without a service-connected injury, or veterans not enrolled in the VA healthcare system, including veterans with HCV, will be turned away from VAMCs.

Currently, Vietnam veterans are the military group most significantly affected by hepatitis C. Many veterans who contracted HCV in Vietnam 25 to 30 years ago are only now exhibiting symptoms of liver disease. When they were first infected, HCV had not been distinguished from other forms of hepatitis. In 85% of the cases, there would have been no acute symptoms at the time of infection.

Detecting HCV infection at the time of discharge was also impossible. Many of today's HCV-infected veterans were discharged from the military before tests for hepatitis C existed. Even today, when there are reliable tests for hepatitis C, the military does not conduct HCV testing as part of the routine discharge physical.

HCV-infected veterans who were treated for *acute hepatitis* during their military service and who now appear before the Board of Veterans' Appeals (BVA) to establish service connection are most often denied because they cannot prove their current HCV infection is related to their prior acute hepatitis. The Board often rejects a claim for service-connection because the veteran's medical record does not show the presence of HCV at the time of discharge. In fact, in the review of all 1,599 cases of *chronic hepatitis* brought before the BVA between 1994 and 1996, only 37 resulted in approval of a service-related disability rating for hepatitis.[20] Making a service connection to HCV enables those veterans who desire treatment to obtain it through the VA system. It also enables veterans who progress to advanced liver disease to get adequate healthcare through the VA.

Establishing a Service Connection to Hepatitis C

To establish a successful claim for military service connected disability from hepatitis C, you must meet the following requirements.

- You must show that you currently have hepatitis C. The VA is obligated to test you for hepatitis C, but it is suggested that you also get a diagnosis from a private doctor.

- You must show that hepatitis C was caused by or aggravated by military service. Because hepatitis C is blood-borne, you must show that while you were in the military you had:

  - a blood transfusion

  - hemodialysis

  - blood-to-blood contact

  - tattoo(s) in service, if your doctor states that this is the risk factor

  - shared a razor, tooth brush, or any other item that could carry infected blood.

Successful claims often include a private physician's (often a *gastroenterologist* or *hepatologist*) letter indicating that, in his or her opinion, your hepatitis C is a direct result of your military service.

You should be aware that activities that show "willful misconduct" could disqualify you from compensation. These activities include body piercing, tattoos, and/or use of injected recreational drugs, snorted cocaine, and other drug use. If you are a veteran diagnosed with hepatitis C, the first thing you should do is to find a qualified Veterans Service Officer to assist you in filing a claim for a service connection to hepatitis C. Most Service Officers work for a county or state veteran's service. To find a Veterans Service Officer in your area, visit the National Association of County Veterans Service Officers Internet site at www.nacvso.org and click on "Find a Service Officer." All VFW's, A.L.'s, and VVA chapters, have service officers.

Summary

Veterans' advocates have made it a priority to see that service men and women are tested for hepatitis C. We are working to ensure that treatment is affordable, and that information will be available for those who need it. It is my heartfelt commitment to work to see these goals accomplished.

References

1. Kizer KW. Hepatitis C standards for provider evaluation and testing. Under Secretary for Health information letter (IL 10-98-013). Department of Veterans Affairs. Veterans Health Administration. Washington, D.C. 1998.
2. Briggs ME, Baker C, Hall R, et al. Prevalence and risk factors for hepatitis C virus infection at an urban Veterans Administration medical center. *Hepatology.* 2001;34(6):1200-1205.
3. Dominitz JA, Boyko EJ, Koepsell TD, et al. Elevated prevalence of hepatitis C infection in users of United States Veterans Medical Centers. *Hepatology.* 2005;41(1):88-96.
4. Sloan KL, et al. Hepatitis C tested prevalence and comorbidities among veterans in the US Northwest. *J Clin Gastroenterol.* 2004;38:279-284.
5. Neel S. Medical support of the US army in Vietnam 1965-1970. Department of the Army. CMH Pub. No. 90-16. US Government Printing Office. Washington, DC. 1991.
6. Centers for Disease Control and Prevention. Recommendations for prevention and control of hepatitis C virus (HCV) infection and HCV-related chronic disease. *MMWR.* 1998;47(RR19):1-39. [Note: At the time of publication, this document was available at: http://www.cdc.gov/mmwr/preview/mmwrhtml/00055154.htm.]
7. Kralovic S, Roselle GA, Simbartl L, et al. Hepatitis C virus antibody (HCAb) positivity in Department of Veterans Affairs (VA) facilities. Presented at the Ninth Annual Scientific Meeting of the Society for Healthcare Epidemiology of America (SHEA). San Francisco, California. 1999.
8. Butt AA, Justice AC, Skanderson M, Rigsby MO, Good CB, Kwoh CK. Rate and predictors of treatment prescription for hepatitis C. *Gut.* 2007;56(3):385-389.
9. United States Department of Veterans Affairs. VA Hepatitis C Prevalence Study Results and VA Hepatitis C Program Actions: Summary.

Available a www.hepatitis.va.gov/vahep?page=prtop01-rs-01. Accessed April 26, 2008.

10. Projected veteran population as of July 1,1998. Office of the Deputy Assistant Secretary for Policy, Department of Veterans Affairs Document. [Note: The referenced text from this document is also contained in The Maimes Report on Hepatitis C Infection in New Hampshire by Steven Maimes. 2002. This text was available at the time of publication for non-commercial purposes at: http://www.cc-info.net/hepatitis/Hepatitis_C_Report.pdf.]

11. Song P, Duc DD, Hien B, et al. Markers of hepatitis C and B virus infections among blood donors in Ho Chi Minh City and Hanoi, Vietman. *Clin Diag Lab Immunol*. 1994:1(4):413-418.

12. National Institutes of Health, Department of Transfusion Medicine. A controlled prospective study of transfusion-associated hepatitis (TAH). Intramural Research Project Z01 CL-02005-28 DTM. Bethesda, Maryland. 1997.

13. National Center for Veteran Analysis and Statistics. National Survey of Veterans. US Government Printing Office. Washington, D.C. Pub. No. NSV9503. 1995.

14. Bini EJ, Dhalia CT, Tenner T, et al. Strong association between tattoos and hepatitis C virus infection: a multicenter study of 3,871 patients. American Association for the Study of Liver Diseases Annual Meeting 2007. Boston, Massachusetts. Abstract 136.

15. Pavli P, Bayliss J, Dent O, Lunzer M. The prevalence of serological markers for hepatitis B virus infection in Australian naval personnel. *Med J Aust*. 1989;151(2):71-75.

16. Health status of Vietnam veterans. II. Physical health. The Centers for Disease Control Vietnam Experience Study. *JAMA* 1988;259(18):2708-2714.

17. Roselle GA, Danko LH, Mendenhall CH. A four-year review of patients with hepatitis C antibody in Department of Veterans Affairs facilities. *Mil Med*. 1997;162(11):711-714.

18. Department of Veterans Affairs, Veterans Health Administration. VHA Directive 2007-022, National Hepatitis C Program. July 2007. Available at www1.va.gov/vhapublications/ViewPublication.asp?pub_ID=1586. Accessed April 26, 2008

19. Spolarich AW, Russo B. Hepatitis C and veterans. December 1998/January 1999. The VVA Veteran®.

20. United States Department of Veterans Affairs, Board of Veterans' Appeals. Board of Veterans' Appeals Decisions 1994-1996. Pub. No. 98-09166 (CD-ROM). US Government Printing Office. Washington, DC. 1998.

Choosing: My Journey, My Choices

Randy Dietrich

> **The key to your universe is that you can choose.**
> ~ Carl Frederick

January 1999

My sister and I have come to the medical library at the Cleveland Clinic—partly to seek information, but mostly to fill time as our mother recovers from heart surgery. We launch an Internet search for *hepatitis C*. That's the term my doctor used when ordering additional tests after routine blood work indicated elevated *liver enzymes*. Except for suggesting that I avoid *alcohol* while waiting for the test results—a recommendation I took only half to heart—he had not indicated the problem was serious.

I'm 42. Energetic. About to be named president of my company.

And I am totally unprepared for what I see on the computer screen.

Article after article paints a grim picture. Studies project more people will die of hepatitis C than from AIDS. There are treatments, but the side effects are serious. "*Cure*" isn't a word I can find anywhere.

Later, I will realize that I have just taken the first steps on an amazing physical, emotional, and spiritual journey. One that, for me, would be a journey of health. But for now, all I know is that my life is about to change radically.

And I am frightened.

That was more than nine years ago.

The fact you're reading this chapter of *Hepatitis C Choices* tells me you, or someone you love, has been diagnosed with the virus. While my experience navigating hepatitis C certainly hasn't made me an expert on the subject, I think my story may prove helpful as you move forward on your own journey. It details the health decisions one man has made and where they've led. And it reinforces what may be the most important lesson I've learned along the way — that the very act of choosing can bring us to a place of greater wellness.

Each of us facing hepatitis C does so with a unique set of health factors, genetics, support, and financial resources. Yours will play a role in setting your course just as mine did. But regardless of your circumstances, I sincerely hope you'll remember one thing: **This is your journey. These are *your* choices.**

Beginning

> **To choose is also to begin.**
> ~ Starhawk

Countless questions

Needless to say, the night after my medical library introduction to hepatitis C was a long one. I read. I cried. I wondered how I might have contracted the virus, as I'd had no blood transfusions and had never used drugs intravenously. I worried that I might have infected my wife or children. And I kept thinking there had been some mistake. After all, I'd had a physical shortly before and it had shown nothing like this.

The next morning, I called my doctor's office for my test results. Not only was I positive for the virus, I had a viral load of 799,000. For about 20 minutes, the tears came again, accompanied by a flood of concerns. What should I do? How much time did I have? What were my odds of beating it?

Then the thought hit me: *Did you really think you would escape having to deal with any major problems?* I had always encouraged others with serious health challenges to become experts in their disease. I had given out copies of Dr. Bernie Siegel's book *Love, Medicine and Miracles* to friends fighting cancer. I had "talked the talk." Now I was going to have to "walk the walk."

With my sister's help, I searched the articles we'd printed for names of expert resources I might contact. My first call was to Hep C Connection, a national organization for people affected by hepatitis C. A very helpful gentleman there began answering my questions. I learned some basic facts, such as the meaning of the term *viral load*, and that my level was not high. My liver enzymes were clearly above normal, but not off the chart. Still, I wasn't clear about what the disease might mean to me. What was my prognosis? How fast or slow would liver damage occur? Would I require a liver transplant?

The evening I returned home to Denver, I told my wife about my diagnosis. We vowed we would fight it together—even though we had no idea what that meant or where it would take us in the future. In the near term, however, we had a 12-day trip to Australia slated that same week. We went, accompanied by a small library of books and journals discussing hepatitis C and its treatment.

I read every one. And before long, a better picture of the disease emerged. For most people, hepatitis C is not a death sentence. The term *"chronic hepatitis C"* simply means the virus persists in the liver—not that I would develop all the symptoms, that my liver would become cirrhotic, or that I would need a liver transplant. I would, however, be wise to avoid substances that negatively affect the liver, starting with alcohol. Fried foods, coffee, red meat and many of my favorite foods would also need to go.

Flying home from Australia, I drew the diagram shown in Figure 1 and began playing a little game.

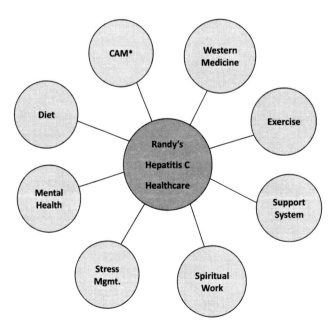

*Complementary and Alternative Medicine
Figure 1. Components of Health and Wellness

I would cover up each of the outer circles in succession, asking myself, "Can I ignore this aspect of my healthcare?" What I realized was that each category of care was important to maintaining my health. I would need to investigate all the various disciplines to figure out what I needed to do now and what to do next.

Taking a Team Approach

> "When opportunity knocks on your door, it is not always a friendly or welcome sound.
> Sometimes the opportunity is hidden in the very concerning and frightening sound
> of a doctor telling you that you have a serious, perhaps even life-threatening illness.
> Often there can be a positive outcome, and there are ways
> to turn these words into a positive life experience."
> ~ Jim Possehl, Founder
> Republic Financial Corporation

There's an old proverb that says, "If you want to make God laugh, tell Him your plans." Hepatitis C definitely was not in my plans. I'm guessing it wasn't in yours, either.

It's like the barnacled sailor's response in *Pirates of the Caribbean* when the heroine told him she didn't believe in ghost stories: "Well, you better start believing, because you're in one now."

It took some time for the initial shock of my diagnosis to fade. But it did. At that point, I met with Jim Possehl, the founder and CEO of my company, Republic Financial Corporation.

I told him of my test results, the *liver biopsy,* and that my doctor recommended immediate *interferon-based therapy.* When Jim asked what course I would take, I replied that I had some research to do before making any decisions — *a lot of research.* We discussed hiring a medical professional to assist me in investigating options, or possibly even a physician, but decided any one person would be biased by his/her own training and experience. What was needed, we agreed, was a true team approach.

At our company, we make decisions by convening many different business disciplines in the same room—sales, legal, operations, financial, and management. Each discipline challenges the other. It's a process we call *teamstorming,* and it's proven quite effective in yielding more creative solutions that benefit all involved. What if we were to employ the teamstorming process in this arena? Could we break down some of the preconceptions and prejudices that keep various healing disciplines from respecting and integrating best practices and outcomes?

It was worth a try.

At the end of our discussion, Jim and I concurred that I would postpone becoming president of the company until I had a better feel for what having hepatitis C would mean. We also agreed that I would take a 3- to 5-month sabbatical to assemble a team of healthcare professionals to brainstorm possible common solutions for people affected by chronic hepatitis C.

The four-and-a-half months I took marked the beginning of the Caring Ambassadors Hepatitis C Program. With Republic Financial Corporation's underwriting and understanding, I now had the opportunity to gather nearly a dozen medical experts and hear their theories on clearing the virus or living with it. What we learned through this process of communication and challenge could then help energize the current hepatitis C knowledge base.

For knowledge *is* power. And information *empowers.*

Securing Support

I noted earlier that each of us comes to this challenge with our own unique set of resources. One of my most powerful assets was and is my support system. From the beginning, it has been *great*.

- **My sister Lorren**, who had been with me in the medical library the day I first learned of the virus, agreed to work with me to establish the Caring Ambassadors Hepatitis C Program. She was instrumental in researching the virus and its treatment, separating truth from fiction, and assembling the brainstorming team. Personally, she wanted me to pursue interferon-based treatment at the start. But she supported my choices at every step.

- **Kim, my wife**, offered love and support without bounds. She became a wizard with the juicer and a gourmet where healthy foods are concerned. It's really not hard to eat well when someone else does all the work.

- **My kids** were amazing and their confidence strengthened my resolve. My then 12-year-old daughter wrote on the Caring Ambassadors Internet site, "My dad is very strong and when he gets better, it will be the happiest day of my life." She didn't say *if*. She said *when*.

- **My team** of healthcare providers gave me love and support along with their skill and knowledge. They were willing to engage in intellectual arguments, consider other input, and always keep my best interests at heart.

- **My company** gave me five months to start an organization focused on hepatitis C. My colleagues offered encouragement and understanding. Together, they made it possible for me to take the time necessary to maintain and improve my health.

- **My friends, neighbors, and parents of the kids I coach**. Having hepatitis C was never a secret. Why be ashamed? The result was a lot of people telling me I inspired them — which inspired *me.* Our openness also allowed additional help to flow in from many different sources.

It's as my colleague and friend Jim Possehl says, "When opportunity knocks on your door, it is not always a friendly or welcome sound." Hepatitis C was my gift—my opportunity to explore some dynamic health changes. I truly believed, within a year of my diagnosis, that I would live longer because of the choices I have made.

Determining Priorities

Because I do not know *how* I became infected with the *hepatitis C virus*, I do not know *when* the infection occurred. That made it more difficult to determine my disease progression. But the fact that I was diagnosed prior to developing any significant symptoms figured heavily into my decision-making.

I decided early on—being symptom-free—that my treatment goals were two-fold:

- to have good health as long as possible
- to rid my body of the hepatitis C virus

It has always important to me, however, that I never sacrifice the first goal for the second. It's a cornerstone of care that I encourage everyone encountering hepatitis C to consider building into his or her foundation. The other six suggestions I readily share:

- Gather all the information you can.
- Talk to and use the services of healthcare professionals from many different disciplines.
- Rely on your support network—and develop one if you need to.
- Make the choices that work best for you.
- Focus on your larger life—not just the illness.
- This journey is yours. Enjoy the moments and the meaning.

Exploring

> **"Whether you think you can or you think you can't, you're right."**
> ~Henry Ford

An Integrated Approach to Healing: The Best of Everything

At the time I began my journey through hepatitis C, I wasn't familiar with the term *integrative medicine*. It refers to a multidimensional way of looking at health and healing that brings together Western medicine's scientific model and Eastern approaches to health. Where western medicine has traditionally focused on the physical, an integrative approach emphasizes that we're also emotional, spiritual, and mental beings. If we are to have true health, all these components must be considered, along with our cultural experiences, our environment, and the fact that our lives are forever changing.

Though I may not have known the term, that was the model I chose for myself. I simply thought of it as the power of the best of everything. It fit well with my personal philosophy of "navigating life" —a philosophy wrapped up in one of my favorite jokes.

> *A man was caught in a flood. The water was up to his waist when a boat came by.*
> *The people in the boat yelled, "Get in!" "No," said the man. "I have lived my life as God desires. God will save me. Go help someone else."*
>
> *The water was up to his shoulders when a second boat came by. Once again, the people yelled, "Get in!" "No," said the man. "I have lived my life as God desires. God will save me. Go help someone else."*
>
> *After a while, the water rose over the man's head. Just then, a helicopter appeared and dropped a rope down to him. "No," yelled the man over the rotors' roar, "I have lived my life as God desires. God will save me. Go help someone else."*
>
> *A short time later, the man drowned. He arrived in Heaven, thoroughly confused and asking God, "What happened? I lived my entire life just the way I thought you wanted me to. Why didn't you save me?" To which God replied, "Well, I tried! I sent two boats and a helicopter."*

So I started a journey using boats and helicopters, common sense, intuition, and the best advice experts had to offer. I integrated all the things we've been told are "optimal" but never wanted to consider: diet, exercise, stress management, supplements, positive menal attitude, juicing, yoga, *meditation*, and support. It didn't take long for the answer to become obvious. *Live a health-centered lifestyle over an extended period of time and the effect is tremendously powerful.* Being an analyst at heart, I saw it like this (Figure 2).

Figure 2. Progression of Hepatitis C in an Individual Patient

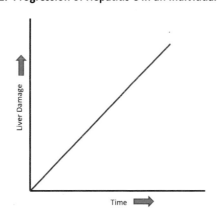

We know that, over time, the hepatitis C virus causes progressive liver damage. How quickly the disease progresses is variable. A person's general well-being, health habits, genetics, and many other factors come into play — which means that while the life span of someone with hepatitis C may well be affected, it is not with a precise calibration.

I know people who have lived with the hepatitis C virus for more than four decades and are still considered to be in phase I of the disease process. They may die with hepatitis C, but is unlikely the virus will be the primary cause of their demise. The reverse is true, as well. I have met people for whom the disease has progressed rapidly. I do not presume to know the factors involved in that process nor the outcome.

As to my own treatment for hepatitis C, I did not have a data baseline for tracking disease progression because I did not know when I became infected. Moreover, I had received divergent opinions from the doctors who read my liver biopsies, a frustration I'll expand upon later. Suffice it so say that the same biopsy garnered a stage 2 from one professional, and a stage 3 from another.

Since I didn't have certainty about where I was in terms of disease progression and I wasn't ready for interferon-based treatment, I focused my full attention on making those "optimal lifestyle changes." I wanted to find a natural way to rid my body of the virus. And I saw the opportunity to alter the course of the disease (Figure 3).

Figure 3. Altering the Progression of Hepatitis C With Lifestyle Changes

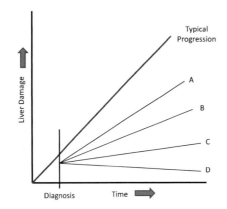

Knowing alcohol's negative effect on liver function, I could stop drinking (A). Knowing nutrition's positive effect on cellular restoration, I could improve my diet (B). And knowing how stress compromises natural *immunity*, I could exercise, practice relaxation, meditate, take supplements, have regular bodywork sessions, and more (C+D). Even if each of these changes improved my odds only a few percentage points, I reasoned that the cumulative effect could prove significant.

That was my theory going in.

The accuracy of my theory has been borne out in my experience.

I could sense my health was improving. And I was learning more all the time about how wellness works:

- The better you eat, the fewer supplements you need to take.

- All stress is not the same. Getting rid of the stress that comes from monotony and constant pressure—what I call "production line stress"—is good. Staying challenged and motivated can also create stress, but it's a positive force and can be balanced with relaxation, meditation, and exercise.

- There's no magic pill. Your system didn't get out of sync overnight, and it won't heal with a day or week of healthy living. It takes time, patience, and discipline to bring your body back into balance. But it's so worth it!

One of my doctors asked me why such a "normal guy" who studies all the data with such intensity "would try so many things on the outer edges of medicine?" My answer is simple: I follow what I call results-based medicine. When exploring options, I would ask about success rates (even if *anecdotal*), side effects, and the medical theory of why it works. Then I would make a decision to try it or not. If I did try it, I would track the results to see if my experience was congruent with the information I had received in advance. Since there is so much we don't know, this was my way of navigating the journey.

Integrated Professional Care

Throughout my journey through hepatitis C, I have made decisions based on the best data I could get. It's been my practice to correlate the results of my Western medicine tests with the findings of my acupuncturist, medical intuitive, chiropractor, and BioScan™ practitioner. When results have been similar, I felt confident in proceeding along that path. When they have conflicted, I took it as a "boat and helicopter" to keep investigating.

Western medicine has and continues to be an essential part of my treatment. It provided my diagnosis, which gave me the opportunity to make lifestyle changes, such as stopping alcohol. It has given me information—through successive liver biopsies and regular enzyme blood tests—of the damage done to my liver by the virus. And, as I'll detail later, it offered the interferon-based treatment I elected eight years after my diagnosis.

In my opinion, Western medicine does the best job of gathering data regarding disease progression, how a person is affected by the disease, and the length of time between various disease stages. All of this information was and continues to be important to me as I monitor my health. This data/decision-making relationship is reflected in the appendix of this chapter, where I have shared my liver enzymes (*ALT* and *AST*) and viral load tests over time. My hope is that, in sharing this information, others will become more inclined to, as well.

My primary care doctor is an allopathic doctor (an MD) who practices integrative medicine. He has not only been very supportive of my treatment choices, but works with me actively to find alternative treatment options and to determine the efficacy of various treatments. The treatment approach I chose integrated Western, Chinese, homeopathic and naturopathic medicine, and various forms of bodywork. All of these have been supported and encouraged by my primary care physician.

As to the downside...

It's sometimes difficult to determine whether a problem lies in the service or the system—and that's certainly the case with Western medicine. I deeply disliked the fact that I could not obtain answers in a timely manner following my initial diagnosis. The first incident occurred immediately after learning I had the hepatitis C virus, when I was leaving the country for two weeks and wanted to speak with the specialist. After numerous calls to and promises from his office, he simply left a message with my wife to not worry and he'd see me when I returned. Once I was back, it took three weeks before he could see me, whereupon he told me my only real option was interferon-based therapy. He told me diet did not matter, despite everything I had read indicating the contrary. Ultimately, he agreed to *genotype* testing and I agreed to a liver biopsy.

The genotype test was not ordered. When I inquired why, his nurse replied that they had 50 people going through treatment they had only ordered one genotype test before. Today, it's standard of care. But it points out how diligent you must be to make sure you're getting the best of Western medicine.

The biopsy— described as a "routine" 15-minute procedure—resulted in internal bleeding requiring an overnight hospital stay. (Two subsequent biopsies, I must interject, went well.) Currently, a biopsy is the best way to measure your status and despite my complications, I would encourage everyone to get a biopsy if your doctor recommends it.

When the specialist called to discuss biopsy findings, he stated I should begin interferon-based treatment immediately. My response that I was still researching the best decision was met with his response that it was fine if I wanted to consider some "witchcraft remedies" but he wanted to see me and my plan in a month. Since the only "remedies" I'd mentioned had been diet and supplements, I was furious. But the anger was motivating, and for that I'm grateful.

I'm also frustrated by Western medicine's "missed opportunities." This is a discipline that relies on scientific evidence from *clinical trials*, surveys, case studies, and other research methods. The results and observations gathered determine which health practices and products are promoted or rejected. While there are numerous clinical trials involving medications to treat hepatitis C, these trials often fail to collect detailed information about participants' medical histories and lifestyles (diet, exercise, smoking history, nutritional supplements, etc.) that may well influence the course of the disease.

The fact is, we only know about 10 percent of what we need to know about hepatitis C, despite the fact that some tremendous people are working to fill the knowledge gaps. Currently, ALT levels are an indicator we have on which to gauge inflammatory activity—but they don't predict the degree of liver damage. Biopsies are the best procedure we have for gathering facts on disease staging—but I've had seven experts look at the same biopsy data and render very divergent opinions.

We simply do not have a perfect path.

In fact, the more one deals with and explores a long-term illness, the clearer it becomes that "errors and omissions" not only occur in treatment, but can reduce the number of options one sees. Physicians provide the best information they have based upon research conducted. But only a certain number of variables can be considered in the typical research effort. Whether drug Y was more effective because of study participants' nutritional differences or meditation practices is not information that's captured. But just because something hasn't been tested doesn't mean it doesn't work.

Western medicines are often studied against the *placebo* effect. As you're probably aware, the placebo effect is the actuality that a particular treatment works because you believe it will work, and therefore, contributes to your healing. Well, if what we want to do is heal ourselves of the hepatitis C virus, it only makes sense we would do whatever we can to enhance this placebo effect and make it more powerful. We can tell ourselves that a pill or herb will be effective and visualize it working in our bodies. Many times, I've had people tell me that a particular treatment was beneficial because of my mind. My response, "So what? It's about healing!"

I believe strongly these are calls we have to make, and actions we have to take, for ourselves.

Western medicine has been a constant of my care equation over the nine-plus years I've dealt with hepatitis C. I have worked with skilled and sensitive practitioners who understood my choice of merging allopathic and alternative treatments and offered guidance within that framework. I have encountered physicians who could not support my course of action and were not interested in the potential I saw. And I have met a few medical professionals whose manner left me feeling depersonalized and devalued.

How I choose to process those experiences is up to me.

I happen to believe in what I call the "95/5 rule." According to this rule, 95 percent of people are good and do their best to live life in a positive, supportive way. The remaining 5 percent do not. When we pay inordinate attention to the minority, we diminish the good of the majority and disempower ourselves.

The same holds true for practitioners caring for persons with hepatitis C. Although there are great differences of opinion on the optimal course of treatment, most are trying very hard to do their best for their patients; a small portion is not. While we can learn from each others' experiences, it's up to each of us to deal with the caregivers we encounter on our respective journeys.

I would urge you to be realistic about the time the typical Western medicine physician can allocate to you and your condition. Being a numbers guy, I did the math. On average, most internists have about 2,000 patient contact hours annually to spend with about 2,500 patients. That's about 45 minutes per patient per year for diagnosing and managing some 100-plus diseases. So, what is the likelihood that this individual can do so and be up to speed on all the latest and greatest treatments for hepatitis C?

If you are referred to a hepatitis specialist, you will get more answers. But there is much Western medicine does not yet know about the effects this virus has, given individual variations.

We are all learning together.

Complementary and Alternative Medicine

When I was first diagnosed with hepatitis C, I mentally grouped all *complementary and alternative medicine* (*CAM*) treatments together. The truth is, each is a distinct discipline in its own right (see Figure 4). If you are interested in the specific treatment modalities and my experiences with each, please visit www.hepcchallenge.org/randy.htm.

CAM was an essential part of my healing plan; I used CAM healing techniques every day in my journey. Because these methods focus on getting and keeping the body healthy and balanced, I advise every person dealing with hepatitis C to start his or her journey by exploring CAM options and choosing those that fit. Whether you are preparing to begin interferon-based treatment to rid your body of the virus or are simply working to maintain your health, CAM provides are variety of beneficial options from which to choose.

Figure 4. Complementary and Alternative Healing Options

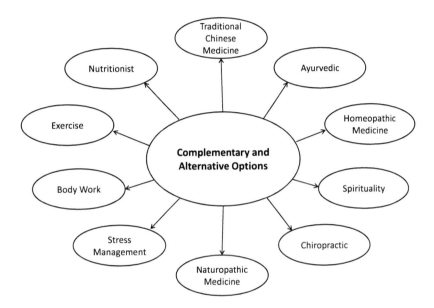

All of the options shown in this diagram contribute to healing from a holistic perspective. Most practitioners strongly encourage those of us with hepatitis C to focus on all aspects of our lives. While we may be looking and hoping for a "magic" pill or herb, they know that ignoring other health factors will prove detrimental to our overall well-being. This can sometimes make us very uncomfortable.

The health plan I chose looked like this:

NUTRITION

EAT	AVOID	SUPPLEMENTS

A balanced diet of:
  fruits
  vegetables
  fish
  turkey/chicken
  whole grains
  dairy (limited)
	Foods and substances that tax
	liver function:
	  red meat (beef/pork)
	  fried foods
	  refined sugar
	  shellfish
	  preservatives
	  additives
	  artificial sweeteners
		As advised:
		  multiple vitamin (no iron)
		  omega-3 oils
		  acidophilus
		  vitamin C
		  various other supplements
		    from time to time

BODYWORK AND EXERCISE

Type	Frequency
acupuncture	weekly
energy work	weekly
chiropractic	bi-weekly
massage	monthly
running	daily
basketball	weekly

I reasoned then—and affirm now—that anything that enhances my ability to manage disease and gives me greater energy is a positive. The other aspect that I appreciate is that these forms of healing require me to deal with all aspects of my health, not just hepatitis C.

The downside of CAM approaches is that there is little scientific testing or documentation about the effects of the various prescribed treatments. There are few clinical trials, and some CAM practitioners do not keep statistics on their patients. This lack of scientific data makes it difficult for many Western doctors to believe in or recommend CAM treatments, regardless of how beneficial they may be.

Over the past nine years, I've had countless calls and encounters relating to CAM success stories for curing hepatitis C. I always ask that the "cured" individual contact me and share their medical records. To date, I've had no response. Some of these *anecdotes* have come from CAM practitioners promoting a particular course of treatment. When I suggested we survey their patients and medical records to document these outcomes, their interest evaporated. Many CAM practitioners judge the efficacy of a given therapy according to how the person is feeling. Depending on the situation, this may or may not be an accurate reflection of disease progression.

Spiritual Practice

If there is an ultimate gift of my journey through hepatitis C, it is my spiritual development. I have never been a religious man, but I have always believed there is a universal spiritual power. Ironically, I had begun a prayer practice just prior to being diagnosed with hepatitis C, primarily to help someone I cared about who was sick.

After my diagnosis, I found many of the books I read and most of the healthcare practitioners I saw spoke of developing a spiritual practice. I did so, but not because I was afraid of dying. For within a month or so of my diagnosis, I began to understand I could live with this disease for a long time. My choice came more from a desire to heal, and once I got started, it took on a life of its own.

My spiritual practice includes a range of approaches, all of which integrate mind, body, and soul. I practice various forms of qi gong, a Chinese movement method that develops one spiritual sense. I also practice two forms of yoga. Ashtanga yoga is a rather strenuous form that is intended to realign and detoxify the physical body. The poses require a focused concentration that brings the mind and body into sync. Bikram yoga is practiced in a heated room to facilitate profuse sweating. The heat is used to bring about deeper stretching, prevent injuries, and reduce stress and tension. Bikram yoga is designed to build strength, flexibility, balance, and mental focus. In addition to these forms, I also meditate at times, using either an "aah" or "ohm" sound.

Spirituality has opened my eyes to a world I barely knew existed before. I believe each person has his or her own spiritual journey. I also believe that the type of spirituality one practices is less important than the fact that it works for you and allows you to continue growing.

When you open up to spirituality, things happen that do not seem logical or rational— especially to the "normal guy, normal job, normal life" type of person I am. I'm choosing to share some here specifically because I think there are many of us who may discount the importance of these messages. And I really believe paying attention to them helps us to tune into our lives and our healing.

The first experience that shook me up was a dream. In it, another person and I are digging up a man who died of liver disease. He had been buried in the 1950s. As we reach the part of the grave that holds the casket, I see a piece of paper on top. As I reach for it, a ghost comes out of the casket, grabs me by the ankles, carries me across a room, and dumps me on a couch. I turn to the ghost and ask, "Are you mad at me?" The ghost says, "No." I then ask if it's trying to help me, and get an affirmative answer. Then the ghost says, "Take this." When I ask what it is, the spirit responds, "Bee propolis."

I knew when I woke this was no ordinary dream. So clear...so vivid...and I was so freaked out. I was up in mountains at the time, but checked the Internet for information on bee propolis when I returned. The first article explained it is the substance bees use to fight off viruses. I immediately knew this was no accident.

So I went to the natural foods store and purchased every kind of bee propolis I could find. I took them to my medical intuitive/naturopath and my BioScan™ practitioner. Both confirmed that I should be taking it. Other than vitamin C, it is the only substance that is always part of their recommended protocol.

My sense is that the dream has more to tell me. But I'm waiting.

This was one of the first synchronicities I link directly to developing my spiritual nature. Another happened during a meditation. I'd been told that if you pray with emotion, it has a greater effect, and I decided to give it a try. I began praying with deep emotion, and my body began shaking all over. I could stop the shaking by stopping my meditation... but when I resumed, so did the shaking.

It was clear to me that this, too, was no accident. I have incorporated this shaking meditation into my spiritual work. I can now begin it simply by breathing deeply.

Treating

> **"Things turn out best for people who make the best of the way things turn out."**
> **~John Wooden**

When summarizing my experience for the 2005 edition of Hepatitis C Choices, I wrote, "For now, I have chosen to hold off on interferon-based therapy. This may be a mistake, but the decision is very clear to me at this time."

The following year, I made a different choice. Why? Because I started getting new boats and helicopters.

Practitioners began sharing new information. Fellow hepatitis C patients started telling me new experiences. Where all my indicators had pointed to not treating before, they now shifted to "yes."

Pre-Treatment

As I actively considered interferon-based treatment, I saw what an advantage I had gained. For eight years, I had been living an extremely healthy lifestyle. Actively integrating the best of Western and CAM approaches had brought me to a point where my body felt strong and my mind ready.

I want to note, this advance preparation was the key point of consensus reached by the multidisciplinary medical brainstorming group assembled by the Caring Ambassadors Hepatitis C Program. The team now referred to it as "setting the table" and acknowledged that this practical prescription could benefit virtually every patient with a long-term disease considering treatment intervention.

Getting ready for interferon-based treated, I kicked it up a notch:

- Thirty days before beginning treatment, I adjusted my work schedule to my "new normal" of 9 a.m. to 5 p.m.— two to three hours shorter than typical.

- I focused on keeping my *immune system* in great shape through excellent nutrition and took key vitamins and supplements (i.e., omega-3 oils, acidophilus, vitamins C and E).

- I exercised regularly and maintained my body weight.

- I received regular body and energy work treatments.

- I worked on making sure my mind wanted the treatment to succeed.

In short, I did everything possible to connect my mind, body, and spirit. My intention was to have nothing in my life that did not support the medicinces working for the optimal outcome. Some actions were symbolic—such as writing "PURE LOVE" on the syringes I used to inject the interferon. It was my way of intentionally working to enhance the placebo effect. Others were relational — assuring my family members and colleagues that this was simply the next step in my journey and all would be well.

And I knew in my heart it would.

Treatment

I received combination interferon plus *ribavirin* treatment for 42 weeks—from September 2006 through June 2007. My physician advised me to continue the therapy for six additional weeks, but I chose to end it at the nine-month mark. By then, it had been 36 weeks since my viral load had become undetectable. For me, it was time to stop.

As with so many of my hepatitis C decisions, this one was multifactorial. I could tell my toxicity levels were rising and that my body needed relief. My internal guidance system told me the objective had been achieved, something my medical intuitive confirmed. Moreover, I had a running tally of viral-load report levels — western Medicine's best indicator of treatment efficacy — for visual proof.

Wanting to make my results and experience part of the knowledge base for hepatitis C study, I had viral-load measurements at 24 hours after the first treatment and each week, thereafter. Ideally, one would like to see a 100-fold drop after four weeks and undetectable virus at 12 weeks. My viral loads through treatment are shown in Figure 5.

Figure 5. Randy's Viral Load Results Through the First 6 Weeks of Treatment

Timing with Treatment	Viral Load: (IU/mL)
(started treatment)	6,315.680
(+ 16 hrs)	2,069,030
(+ 1 week)	63,930
(+ 2 weeks)	3,640
(+ 3 weeks)	310
(+ 4 weeks)	60
(+ 5 weeks)	10
(+ 6 weeks)	undetectable
(+ 42 weeks) (treatment stopped)	undetectable
(+ 66 weeks)	undetectable
(+ 92 weeks)	undetectable

I experienced what is referred to as a rapid viral response, or RVR. Whether my RVR was because of genetics, "setting the table," spirituality, prayer, using the power of the mind (enhancing the placebo effect), or a combination of all of these — we may never know. However, I would highly encourage anyone going on treatment to employ each of these and others they discover on their journey.

Those who choose interferon-based therapy report a wide range of side effects from the treatment. I would classify mine as moderate, with some days being very difficult and all requiring management. Specifically, I:

- *Chose Thursdays for my injections*, knowing I could use weekend time to regain energy for the following week.

- *Remained active* but adjusted whatever I was doing to the appropriate level. Basketball is my sport, and I played regularly. However, I could only stay in the game for approximately three minutes at a time. At the beginning of treatment, my goal was to still run 10 miles a week; that ultimately changed to walking.

- *Focused on getting sufficient sleep* and became a sofa-lounging sitcom watcher for the first and only time in my life.

- *Ate an extremely healthy diet*—no alcohol or preservatives; fresh foods, whenever possible; primarily vegetables, fruits, whole grains, lean meats, and key supplements.

- *Forced myself to go to work*. I love what I do. I work with great people in an exciting company. But there were days when getting there at 9 and staying until 5 was tough. But I can't overemphasize how important it was to have a reason to get up and stay active.

- *Connected with friends and family*. My wife and kids were amazing, and their support gave me an unbelievable amount of energy. I continued coaching youth sports throughout treatment and engaging socially as much as possible.

- *Acknowledged the toxic effects of treatment on my emotions*. I'm generally quite laid-back, and I found myself getting angry more often and easily. Relaxation and spirituality helped immensely in this regard.

- *Avoided the "downward spiral."* It's easy for any of us to let things slide when we're not feeling well. I worked hard to maintain my structure—work, family, service, relaxation, spirituality. I encourage you to keep life in balance as best you can during this time. The more you help yourself, the more powerful you become to help others.

Post-Treatment

I would love to say everything returned to normal the moment I stopped taking my treatment medications. Not true. In fact, the post-treatment period of my hepatitis C journey brought some new and unexpected challenges.

- **I felt worse.** My *metabolism* was affected and I had lost muscle tone—both of which affected my performance. I maintained the same diet as before treatment, but my appetite was affected.

- **I had to adjust my exercise program.** I started training using the Jeff Galloway method of beginning slowly and increasing one's pace/distance on a weekly schedule. Instead of running, I began walking. Interestingly, each time I upped my activity level, I could feel the "detox effect." It was like a delayed drug response as the toxins were released.

- **Naturally ridding my body of toxins took more time than I anticipated.** My healthcare practitioners urged me to not rush this process.

- **Some things were better.** I was far less emotional. I could feel my energy growing. And at six months, tests showed no virus.

I was also extremely fortunate to not have some of the long-term side effects some have with interferon-based treatment. My thyroid function remains normal by Western medicine standards but is a little slow according to my complementary medicine practitioners. No other systems have been negatively affected.

Living

> **"Luck is what you have left over after you give 100 percent."**
> ~Langston Coleman

My Life Now

Today, I am 52 and healthy. Western medical tests nine months post-treatment showed my body had cleared the hepatitis C virus and my CAM practitioners concurred. Now, the only "souvenir" I have is the fact that my life and the way I live it will never be the same.

My lifestyle choices remain much the same as during my journey to health. More than 80 percent of the time, I follow the same nutrition plan I outlined earlier. I did, however, recently enjoy my first glass of wine in nine years and now drink alcohol in moderation.

I am not big on giving unsolicited advice. But when someone with hepatitis C asks me for my best thinking on charting their journey, here's my response:

- If you want to get rid of the virus, get as healthy as possible. Set the table. This is the foremost finding of the Caring Ambassadors Hepatitis C Program team of western and eastern healthcare practitioners.

- Understand the effect the virus is having on your body.

- If you can't stop drinking, focus there first.

- Get your body weight to a healthy level. Even modest weight loss will help.

- Don't use marijuana to reduce side effects. To take into the body something we know compromises immunity defies logic.

- Do the things that make common sense and you know will make you healthier.

- Use your intuition. Listen and watch for your own "boats and helicopters."

10 Truths

For all we now understand about hepatitis C, there is much we do not. I personally believe that each journey shared strengthens the collective knowledge base and makes the path slightly smoother for those affected, and their families and friends. My attempt to distill the essential lessons I've learned over the past nine-plus years since my diagnosis has yielded the following "top 10" list.

To borrow from the words of Thomas Jefferson in the Declaration of Independence, I hold these truths about living with hepatitis C to be self-evident:

1. It's all about the immune system! We know the immune system is the body's defense against viruses. We also know that much of the liver damage occurring with chronic hepatitis C is mediated by the immune system. It follows, therefore, that anything we can do to enhance the function of this system is potentially helpful and anything that impairs its function is potentially harmful. A note of caution: It's easy to fall into the pattern of thinking that if a little immune enhancement is good, a lot must be better. Not true. Excessive vitamins, supplements, herbs and even exercise can have a negative impact. Best bet? Moderation.

2. You are what you eat. This is a fact of life. With the help of our liver, our bodies transform what we eat and drink into the very substance of our physical selves. While we may want to think that what we ingest doesn't matter, logic and basic biology say otherwise.

3. Stress management is crucial. Scientists have known for decades that stress depresses immune function. And, to revisit #1, anything that interferes with that function is potentially detrimental to people with hepatitis C. Recognizing and managing your stressors is an important way to influence your course and condition.

4. Protect your liver. The liver processes virtually every substance that enters the human body. Every step you take to decrease the demands on that vital organ while it is under siege from the hepatitis C virus is potentially helpful. You can protect your liver by eating a healthy diet, eliminating alcohol, limiting your intake of complex chemicals (such as medications and supplements), and avoiding toxins such as smoke, pollutants and chemicals.

5. Time is on your side. For the vast majority of people, chronic hepatitis C is a disease that progresses very slowly. With the exception of those diagnosed with advanced *cirrhosis*, it is not an immediate threat to one's life, nor will it become one. In no way am I minimizing the challenges of living with hepatitis C. I do, however, want to emphasize the most people with the virus have time to make choices about how to manage their disease and change their lifestyle.

6. You are as you think. As with all life experiences, your outlook, perceptions and attitudes influence your journey through hepatitis C. No one wants this virus. But if you have been diagnosed, you are now free to choose how you will react to it. Don't be surprised if your emotions range widely in the beginning—from anger and fear to helplessness and shame. But over time, staying in the negative can make living more difficult. Keep in mind there's no "good" or "bad" feeling. What's important is now they add to or detract from your sense of well-being.

7. Body and mind work in tandem. The more I worked with the CAM modalities, the better I understood how healing takes everything we are and have. We cannot separate how we think, act and feel. If you have not read Bill Moyers' book *Healing and the Mind,* the transcripts of his PBS interview series on the subject, I strongly encourage you to.

8. Information can be healing. Knowledge is power. In fact, I've learned since my diagnosis that information is a very real antidote to fear. So search fearlessly. Do be wise, however, that there are many unsubstantiated claims about so-called cures. Make sure the information you gather—whether from the Internet, library or your own contacts—is reliable. With that said, don't let your quest for facts and findings take over your life. Moderation...there's that word again.

9. Support helps. My journey has been made much easier because my wife, kids, extended family, friends, and colleagues have been there for me. I can count on these people, and they can count on me. Some people draw the same strength from hepatitis C support groups. My own support group experience — which I admit was very

limited—left me feeling less supported and more singled out because of the collective mood. Knowing myself, I knew I could not afford to spend a minute in the victim role. I understand some groups can be very helpful. For me, in the sessions I attended, the victim mentality promoted was not healthy. You will need to figure out what works best for you.

10. There is no magic bullet. When first diagnosed, I was certain I could find a medicine or treatment that would clear the virus from my body with no pain and no interruption to my life. It doesn't work that way...at least for now. Like most of the long-term illnesses affecting millions of individuals worldwide, living with hepatitis C requires us to make some difficult choices and changes. The good news is, when you accept your responsibilities with this condition, you are rewarded with a renewed sense of control and self-determination.

Sharing

> "We make a living by what we get,
> but we make a life by what we give."
> ~Winston Churchill

There was a time when I very much wanted hepatitis C to be something I was a victim of, not something I was responsible for. That's changed. And along with a shifting sense of responsibility came an awareness that I was on this path for a reason.

And that I was supposed to share what I found along the way.

It's why I've made my ALT, AST and viral load test results public and why the CAM treatments I explored are detailed on the Caring Ambassadors Hepatitis C Program Internet site (www.HepCChallenge.org).

I strongly encourage you to do the same.

No other journey will be like yours.

The world needs to hear your story.

Recommended Reading

Love, Medicine and Miracles, Siegel, Bernie, MD., HarperCollins Publishers. New York, NY. 1986.
Why People Don't Heal and How they Can, Myss, Caroline, Ph.D., Three Rivers Press, New York, NY. 1997.
Healing and The Mind, Moyers, Bill, Doubleday, New York, NY. 1993.

A Look Into the Future

Lorren Sandt

Introduction

Hepatitis C is a major global health problem. More than 180 million people worldwide are infected with the *hepatitis C virus* (*HCV*). An estimated 3 to 4 million people are newly infected each year.[1] Yet hepatitis C is largely a preventable disease. Prevention requires multilevel education programs, rigorous efforts to protect the blood supply, and intervention programs for at-risk populations.

Despite significant advances in hepatitis C diagnosis and treatment, there is still much to be learned. Research is being conducted on several fronts in the race to gain control over the virus. *Advocates* are working diligently to raise public awareness and provide information to the millions of people infected with HCV. Healthcare providers from all healing disciplines are looking for better ways to treat people living with hepatitis C.

So, where do we go from here?

Information and Awareness

Despite the fact that most new cases of hepatitis C are preventable, the disease continues to spread globally. Many consider the worldwide HCV prevalence rate to be grossly underestimated. For example, current estimates for the United States do not include incarcerated, homeless persons, and others who do not participate in the mainstream healthcare system.

> The number of people living with HCV demands the attention and intervention
> of public health professionals and advocates worldwide.

Multilevel education, public awareness, and effective, affordable testing are essential for disease prevention. When prevention fails, effective treatment is imperative.

The federal government is responsible for educating citizens of the United States about communicable diseases such as hepatitis C. The Centers for Disease Control and Prevention (CDC) is the principal agency managing this task. However, much of the HCV education and awareness efforts in the U.S. continues to be conducted by grassroots hepatitis C organizations and support groups throughout the country. Why is this the case?

Hepatitis C is largely an unfunded epidemic, meaning neither the federal government nor the private sector has earmarked funds for combating this public health problem. Remarkably, many decision makers are still unaware of the magnitude and severity of the hepatitis C epidemic currently threatening the health of hundreds of thousands of Americans. The seriousness of the HCV epidemic and the widespread suffering it is causing must become common knowledge if adequate funding to address this disease is to be obtained.

Both government and private funding are desperately needed to support HCV public awareness campaigns. Many grassroots organizations that conduct the majority of hepatitis C education and awareness programs are funded solely by monies from pharmaceutical companies that manufacture drugs used to treat hepatitis C. While this had caused some people to mistrust the provided information, public awareness about hepatitis C would be even less than it currently is without this funding.

HCV Research

Remarkable advances in medical research have been made during the past six decades. Each decade seems to bring advances even more rapidly than the one before. Computer technology has been an incredible boon to the advancement of medical research, especially with respect to viral illnesses. Computer modeling of viral *genomes* has allowed scientists to carefully target and attack specific patterns of viruses. As our knowledge increases and pieces of the puzzle are put in place, a more complete picture is revealed.

We have learned much about HCV since it was first identified in 1989. But we are far from having a thorough and complete understanding of the virus. The factors that lead to persistent HCV infection are still poorly understood as are many of the mechanisms that contribute to disease progression, treatment response, and the relationship of HCV to liver cancer. Until additional information is available, we must do the best with what we have.

Treatment is available that is a cure for some (but not all) people with HCV. Some *antiviral* therapies offer the possibility of *viral clearance*, but may cause significant discomfort during treatment. Other therapies may improve quality of life, but offer no potential for viral clearance.

A few short years ago, people treated with interferon-based therapy had only a 12% chance of achieving a *sustained viral response*. Today, approximately 50% of people treated with *pegylated interferon* plus *ribavirin* are sustained responders. With long-term follow up data now in hand, the medical community is now using the word "cure" for those who experience a sustained viral response. This has been a significant cause for hope for many. Response rates may be as high as 80% for patients with specific *genotypes* using pegylated interferon-based therapy.

Chapter 8.4, Future of Allopathic Hepatitis C Treatment outlines many new drugs in development. As we look to the future, we hope for continued progress in HCV prevention, treatment, and access to care.

HCV and the Immune System: Is It the Virus or the Host?

Every day, HCV researchers around the world ponder the same questions.

- Why do some people infected with HCV develop *acute hepatitis* that quickly resolves while others develop *chronic hepatitis*?

- How does HCV infect the cell?

- Why do some people develop *cirrhosis* and/or *liver cancer* as a result of chronic HCV infection while others do not?

- Why do some chronically infected patients have only mild disease with few *symptoms* while others experience severe symptoms and disability as a result of the disease?

The ability of the hepatitis C virus to reproduce itself (a process called *replication*) is staggering. In a **single** day, in **one** HCV-infected person, there may be more copies of the virus produced than there have been humans on Earth since civilization began! Considered another way, an HCV viral particle can replicate roughly 600 to 900 generations each year. By comparison, it is estimated there have been only 300 generations of humans on Earth since civilization began. The numbers are so large, it is almost impossible to comprehend them.

Virologists (scientists who study viruses) generally believe characteristics of the hepatitis C virus are primarily responsible for the harm caused by chronic infection. However, many immunologists (scientists who study the immune system) conducting HCV research have a different thought. They believe limitations of the host's *immune system* are primarily responsible for the severe consequences some people experience in response to HCV infection. Western researchers are studying people who spontaneously clear HCV to identify regions of the virus particle that may be involved in triggering a specific and successful immune response. This work is providing potential targets for the development of *vaccines* that may be used to prevent or treat HCV infections.

In the end, most HCV researchers agree that **both** the virus and the host's immunological capabilities play a role in the natural history of the disease in any given person.

Research Frontiers

To address the burden of liver diseases in the United States, the National Institutes of Health (NIH) developed the Action Plan for Liver Disease Research. The plan, originally launched in 2004, calls for coordination between the NIH and industry to avoid overlap and maximize results. The primary goals for research are to develop practical, safe, and effective means of prevention, treatment, and control of viral hepatitis. Areas of HCV research in the plan include:

Short Term (0 to 3 years)	• develop a cell culture system that is fully permissive for HCV replication • fully define the pathways of interferon induction and effector action against HCV in vitro and in vivo • define basis for interferon resistance of HCV in humans • to better define the optimal dose and duration, rates of response, early predictors of response, and safety and tolerance of current regimens of therapy for hepatitis C in special populations, such as children, patients with solid organ transplants, renal failure, HIV-coinfected individuals, and persons with problems of substance abuse and psychiatric illness
Intermediate Term (4 to 6 years)	• develop small animal models of HCV replication and liver disease • identify new targets in viral replication and the host for development of small molecule therapeutics • fully define early events during HCV infection • define whether longterm interferon therapy is beneficial in nonresponders with HCV
Long Term (7-10 years)	• develop HCV vaccine • develop ways to prevent reinfection after liver transplant for HCV • achieve sustained response rate of over 90 percent in chronic hepatitis C • evaluate new approaches to therapy in hepatitis C

The complete plan is available online at: www2.niddk.nih.gov/AboutNIDDK/ResearchAndPlanning/Liver_Disease/Action_Plan_For_Liver_Disease_Intro.htm. An in-depth progress report was released in 2006 (see Figure 1). The complete progress report can be viewed at: http://www2.niddk.nih.gov/NR/rdonlyres/A5CD343D-6E5D-49D1-8CB3-6BB903D1DCA0/0/EntireDoc_3282007.pdf

Figure 1. Estimated Progress on Viral Hepatitis Research Goals, 2006 (Year 2)
[Crosshatching indicates recent year's progress.]

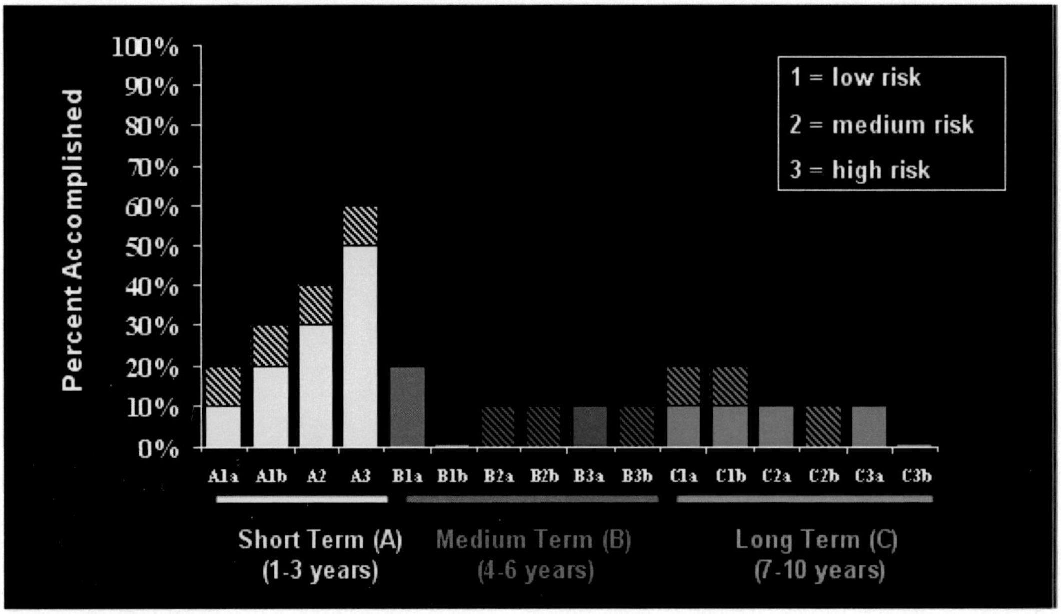

Complementary and Alternative Medicine (CAM) Research

The use of *complementary and alternative medicine (CAM)* treatment approaches is common in many countries of the world. CAM use is increasingly popular in western countries as well. This is particularly true among people with hepatitis C. Much of upsurge in interest in these therapies has been facilitated by easy access to information via the Internet. However, there are concerns about the use of CAM therapies among people with chronic hepatitis C. The National Center for Complementary and Alternative Medicine (NCCAM) was established by the National Institutes of Health (NIH) in 1998. The mission of NCCAM is to:

- Explore complementary and alternative healing practices in the context of rigorous science.
- Train complementary and alternative medicine researchers.
- Disseminate authoritative information to the public and professionals.

NCCAM has four primary areas of focus:

Advancing scientific research	NCCAM has funded more than 1,200 research projects at scientific institutions across the United States and around the world.
Training CAM researchers	We support training for new researchers as well as encourage experienced researchers to study CAM.
Sharing news and information	We provide timely and accurate information about CAM research in many ways, such as through our Web site, our information clearinghouse, fact sheets, Distinguished Lecture Series, continuing medical education programs, and publication databases.
Supporting integration of proven CAM therapies	Our research helps the public and health professionals understand which CAM therapies have been proven to be safe and effective.

Research to establish the safety and efficacy of various CAM therapies for a variety of ailments is a priority for NCCAM. *Clinical trials* are needed to establish the actions of herbs and nutritional supplements in the body. While NCCAM is conducting research on some herbal therapies and other CAM practices, they cannot possibly look into all of the thousands of products currently available.

NCCAM currently states, "No CAM treatment has yet been proven safe and effective for treating hepatitis C. There are many CAM treatments for which benefits for health are claimed. Clinical trials are needed of CAM therapies that may show some potential for benefit for hepatitis C, such as milk thistle." For this reason, NCCAM is currently sponsoring a clinical trial of milk thistle.

Product manufacturers and other proponents of CAM must get involved in funding clinical trials that will allow for more careful definition of the risks and benefits of these products and services. While it is important that medical research be scientifically sound, many people question the need for randomized, double-blind, *controlled clinical trials* for complementary therapies to establish reliable *clinical* information. Randomized, controlled trials are very costly and time-consuming. While it is true that research on CAM therapy can be a compromise, the same is also true of western research. The best information will come when there is true collaboration between CAM and western practitioners. Until research data are available on the efficacy and safety of CAM approaches, few western doctors are willing to recommend them out of concern for potential harm. Often, people interested in using CAM therapies must seek information on their own. Unfortunately, a significant amount of the information available on the Internet and from other sources is unreliable, inaccurate, and sometimes, deliberately misleading. The lack of easily accessible and reliable information was one of the primary reasons *Hepatitis C Choices* was written — to give people accurate information upon which to base their treatment decisions.

If you are considering using CAM products, you should use the same precautions you would with a prescription medicine. Just because a product is "natural" does not mean it cannot harm you. If you intend to use CAM in your hepatitis C management approach, gather information from someone who is trained and knowledgeable about CAM therapy.

> **Always be sure to let all your healthcare practitioners know about each and every product, supplement, medication, and practice you are using.**

The Future Of Medicine – An Integrated Approach

Can, should, or must we explore combining CAM and western treatments? Would this provide potentially less expensive and more effective treatments with better quality of life, not only for people in the U.S., but for the rest of the world's population as well?

As we move forward in the 21st century, the general public, CAM practitioners, and western doctors are increasingly accepting the idea of *integrative medicine*. As CAM therapies and interventions are incorporated into western medical education and practice, the exclusionary term "complementary and alternative medicine" will hopefully be replaced with the more inclusive term "integrative medicine."

A number of respected healthcare institutions, medical schools, and teaching hospitals are setting up or have already set up integrative medicine clinics. Some doctors-in-training are being taught not only about western medical treatments, but also about the many herbs, supplements, and other forms of treatment their patients are using and/or requesting. Respected professionals from all healing disciplines are talking, listening, and working together as colleagues, much like the authors of this book. We hope that in the not too distant future, integrative medicine will be seen as providing novel insights and tools for whole body health.

The Role of the Patient Advocacy Community

Patient advocates play a major role in the hepatitis C community. HCV advocates have been largely responsible for the hepatitis C public awareness and information programs that currently exist. They work in communities and in prisons. They work with military veterans. They work with police and firefighters, and with IV drug users. They speak before Congress and state legislatures, appear on television, and reach out to other media outlets. They have been responsible for setting up testing sites where people can be screened for HCV free of charge. They are encouraging states to develop their own testing plans to help prevent the continued spread of this disease. They are organizing the development of community-based HCV task forces.

Advocates are clearly a necessary and vital component in the fight against HCV. But HCV is a huge problem. Many people are needed if we are going to continue to make strides for the good of all those living with HCV.

We encourage you to get involved with one or more of your local HCV groups. Volunteer your time if you can. Just a few hours a week can make a big difference. If you do not have time to volunteer, you can still help by writing your state and local representatives. Tell them you want hepatitis C moved to the top of their healthcare agenda.

Financial support is also needed. Public awareness campaigns, offering free or low-cost testing, conducting educational programs, and all of the many other activities advocates perform daily require funding. If you can help the HCV advocacy community do its work through a financial contribution, we encourage you to pick up the phone or get online today to make your donation.

Giving Hepatitis C a Face and a Voice

Each and every day, HCV advocates hear stories from the community of people living with hepatitis C about the negative stigma associated with the disease. Stigmatization and prejudice are often based on two factors: ignorance and impersonalization or "facelessness." While people may have heard of HCV, many have little knowledge about the disease, or worse yet, have mistaken notions about the disease.

Ignorance often leads to fear, which is expressed as prejudice. For example, a commonly held misconception is that you can catch hepatitis C through casual, day-to-day contact with someone who has HCV. Of course, this is not true. But someone who holds this mistaken notion may develop a prejudice toward people with HCV as a result of his or her unwarranted fears. This is just one example of how lack of knowledge can contribute to stigmatization.

Impersonalization is also a factor in stigmatization and prejudice. It is often easy to hold on to judgmental thoughts about others when we think of them as a group, separate and distinct from ourselves. We often use phrases such as "those people" or "what they're like" when describing groups of people with whom we feel no sense of connection. Lacking a sense of connection, we are just a step away from forgetting the humanity we share with "those people."

This type of "facelessness" can contribute to the stigmatization of people with hepatitis C. But such stigmatization often quickly fades when one realizes that "those people" are not separate, but are one's friends, neighbors, and loved ones. Understandably, the stigmatization associated with hepatitis C has caused many people living with the disease to remain silent. However, we've all heard the old adage and have certainly experienced its truth at some point: "The squeaky wheel gets the grease."

Becoming Involved in the Hepatitis C Community by Working With an HCV Advocacy Organization has Many Potential Benefits:

- You will be contributing to the process of raising public awareness and knowledge about hepatitis C. Increased public awareness and knowledge will help contain the spread of HCV, and will decrease the stigmatization associated with ignorance and misconceptions about the disease.

- Involvement with the community is likely to expand your own support system while at the same time providing help for others facing similar challenges.

- Giving a face to hepatitis C will help others see that those living with HCV are people just like their friends, neighbors, and loved ones. This is often a powerful antidote to stigmatization and prejudice.

- There is strength in numbers!
  In an ideal world, facts and need should speak for themselves. In the real world with many competing interests vying for a limited number of funding dollars, it is often those who are most vocal and have the support of the largest numbers of people who are heard. As noted earlier in the chapter, the success of future HCV prevention, research, and treatment are dependent upon an infusion of governmental and private funds to support these efforts. We need to join our voices together so that decision makers can gain an understanding of the problems at hand. We must also let them know the hepatitis C community is **strong**, and we will not settle for insufficient resources to meet the needs of those who require our help.

> You are an important part of the hepatitis C community, and we need your help!
> *C* the Problem and Become Part of the Solution.

The National Hepatitis C Advocacy Council

The Caring Ambassadors Hepatitis C Program mission statement addresses the need to motivate HCV advocacy organizations to work together. In the summer of 2000, all the existing HCV advocacy groups were invited to participate in a meeting to determine if a collaborative approach would benefit people living with HCV. The meeting resulted in the formation of The National Hepatitis C Advocacy Council (NHCAC).

Since NHCAC was formed, it has grown into a 27-member, national organization with three additional advisory organizations. NHCAC is a forum for discussing common goals and developing strategies to become a formidable national force to advance the issues of importance to all people affected by hepatitis C.

NHCAC has established ethical guidelines for all participating groups. The guidelines promote a better quality of life for people living with hepatitis C, and stress that all member organizations must act responsibly and provide accurate, unbiased information.

NHCAC is working on a variety of issues. Currently, the primary focus is to increase the capacity of member organizations to deliver HCV prevention, education, and patient care services to all persons affected by hepatitis C.

For more information on the National Hepatitis C Advocacy Council, visit www.hepcnetwork.org. The *Resource Directory* lists the members of NHCAC as well as many other educational resources.

Summary

Much has been learned about hepatitis C, but there is still much yet to discover.

For the vast majority of people, infection with HCV is not fatal. In fact, most people with HCV will not die **from** the virus, but **with** the virus. Given enough time and financial support from the government and private sectors, researchers will undoubtedly answer many of the questions nagging scientists today.

Even if all the scientific questions were answered tomorrow and effective treatments were available for everyone infected with HCV, there would still be hundreds of thousands of people worldwide who already have the disease, and hundreds of thousands more to whom it could be spread. Prevention is crucial if we want to control the spread of hepatitis C. A critical need for information exists and will continue to exist for a long time to come.

We, as individuals and as organizations, have the opportunity to play a pivotal role in putting the spotlight on this slowly progressive, insidious, and potentially devastating disease. It will take a concerted effort on the part of everyone involved — researchers, government agencies, the private sector, patient advocates, and the public at large — if we are to overcome hepatitis C.

> So many of our dreams at first seem impossible,
> then they seem improbable,
> and then, when we summon the will,
> they soon become inevitable.
> ~ Christopher Reeve

References

1. World Health Organization. Hepatitis C Fact Sheet, No. 164, Revised October 2000. [At the time of publication, this fact sheet was available at: www.who.int/mediacentre/factsheets/fs164/en.]
2. National Institues of Health, National Center for Complementary and Alternative Medicine (NCCAM). Expanding horizons of healthcare, five-year strategic plan, 09/25/00. [At the time of publication, this report was available at: nccam.nih.gov/about/plans/fiveyear/fiveyear.pdf.]
3. National Institutes of Health, National Center for Complementary and Alternative Medicine (NCCAM). Hepatitis C and Complementary and Alternative Medicines: 2003 Update. NCCAM Pub. No. D004. Reviewed May 2004 . [At the time of publication, this report was available at nccam.nih.gov/health/hepatitisc.]

Appendix I: How to Cut Down on Your Drinking

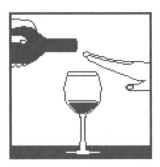

NATIONAL INSTITUTE ON ALCOHOL ABUSE AND ALCOHOLISM
NATIONAL INSTITUTES OF HEALTH

How to Cut Down on Your Drinking

If you are drinking too much, you can improve your life and health by cutting down. How do you know if you drink too much? Read these questions and answer "yes" or "no":

- Do you drink alone when you feel angry or sad?
- Does your drinking ever make you late for work?
- Does your drinking worry your family?
- Do you ever drink after telling yourself you won't?
- Do you ever forget what you did while you were drinking?
- Do you get headaches or have a hang-over after you have been drinking?

If you answered "yes" to any of these questions, you may have a drinking problem. Check with your doctor to be sure. Your doctor will be able to tell you whether you should cut down or abstain. **If you are an alcoholic or have other medical problems, you should not just cut down on your drinking - you should stop drinking completely. Your doctor will advise you about what is right for you.**

If your doctor tells you to cut down on your drinking, these steps can help you:

1. Write your reasons for cutting down or stopping.

Why do you want to drink less? There are many reasons why you may want to cut down or stop drinking. You may want to improve your health, sleep better, or get along better with your family or friends. Make a list of the reasons you want to drink less.

2. Set a drinking goal.

Choose a limit for how much you will drink. You may choose to cut down or not to drink at all. If you are cutting down, keep below these limits:

Women: No more than one drink a day
Men: No more than two drinks a day

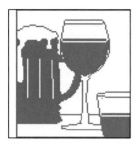

A drink is:
- a 12-ounce bottle of beer;
- a 5-ounce glass of wine; or
- a 1 1/2-ounce shot of liquor.

These limits may be too high for some people who have certain medical problems or who are older. Talk with your doctor about the limit that is right for you.

Now--write your drinking goal on a piece of paper. Put it where you can see it, such as on your refrigerator or bathroom mirror. Your paper might look like this:

My drinking goal
- I will start on this day _____.
- I will not drink more than _____ drinks in 1 day.
- I will not drink more than _____ drinks in 1 week.
  or
- I will stop drinking alcohol.

---

3. Keep a "diary" of your drinking.
To help you reach your goal, keep a "diary" of your drinking. For example, write down every time you have a drink for 1 week. Try to keep your diary for 3 or 4 weeks. This will show you how much you drink and when. You may be surprised. How different is your goal from the amount you drink now? Use the "drinking diary" below to write down when you drink.

Week:			
	# of drinks	type of drinks	place consumed
Mon.			
Tues.			
Wed.			
Thurs.			
Fri.			
Sat.			
Sun.			

Week:

	# of drinks	type of drinks	place consumed
Mon.			
Tues.			
Wed.			
Thurs.			
Fri.			
Sat.			
Sun.			

Week:

	# of drinks	type of drinks	place consumed
Mon.			
Tues.			
Wed.			
Thurs.			
Fri.			
Sat.			
Sun.			

Week:

	# of drinks	type of drinks	place consumed
Mon.			
Tues.			
Wed.			
Thurs.			
Fri.			
Sat.			
Sun.			

Now you know why you want to drink less and you have a goal. There are many ways you can help yourself to cut down. Try these tips:

Watch it at home.
Keep a small amount or no alcohol at home. Do not keep temptations around.

Drink slowly.
When you drink, sip your drink slowly. Take a break of 1 hour between drinks. Drink soda, water, or juice after a drink with alcohol. Do not drink on an empty stomach! Eat food when you are drinking.

Take a break from alcohol.
Pick a day or two each week when you will not drink at all. Then, try to stop drinking for 1 week. Think about how you feel physically and emotionally on these days. When you succeed and feel better, you may find it easier to cut down for good.

Learn how to say NO.
You do not have to drink when other people drink. You do not have to take a drink that is given to you. Practice ways to say no politely. For example, you can tell people you feel better when you drink less. Stay away from people who give you a hard time about not drinking.

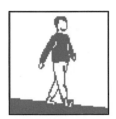

Stay active.
What would you like to do instead of drinking? Use the time and money spent on drinking to do something fun with your family or friends. Go out to eat, see a movie, or play sports or a game.

Get support.
Cutting down on your drinking may be difficult at times. Ask your family and friends for support to help you reach your goal. Talk to your doctor if you are having trouble cutting down. Get the help you need to reach your goal.

Watch out for temptations.
Watch out for people, places, or times that make you drink, even if you do not want to. Stay away from people who drink a lot or bars where you used to go. Plan ahead of time what you will do to avoid drinking when you are tempted.
Do not drink when you are angry or upset or have a bad day. These are habits you need to break if you want to drink less.

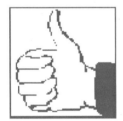

DO NOT GIVE UP!
Most people do not cut down or give up drinking all at once. Just like a diet, it is not easy to change. That is okay. If you do not reach your goal the first time, try again. Remember, get support from people who care about you and want to help. Do not give up!

NIH Pub No. 96-3770
Printed 1996
Updated: May 28, 2001

This information was provided by the National Institute on Alcohol Abuse and Alcoholism (NIAAA).
If you would like additional copies of this pamphlet, visit their website at:
http://pubs.niaaa.nih.gov/publications/handout.htm

The most important herbs used in the formulas described in *Chapter 10, Ayurvedic Medicine* for the treatment of liver disorders are provided below. Their botanical names, distribution, parts used, and medicinal uses are described. In addition, information on the dosage forms and side effects are provided.[1-10]

Bhringaraj

Botanical Name:	*Eclipta alba, Eclipta erecta*
	The name means "ruler of the hair."
Family:	Compositae
Distribution:	This herb is found throughout India as well as the southwestern part of the United States.
Parts Used:	Herb, roots, and leaves
Actions:	Roots and leaves stimulate the flow of bile into the intestine. The root is used as an emetic and purgative. The leaf juice is used as a liver tonic. This is the main herb for the hair, and cirrhosis. It is believed to prevent aging, maintain and rejuvenate hair, teeth, bones, memory, sight, and hearing. It is a rejuvenative for pitta, kidneys, and liver. The root powder is used in Ayurvedic medicine for hepatitis, enlarged spleen, and skin disorders.
Dosage:	Infusions, *decoction*, powder, medicated oil, and ghee (clarified butter)
Safety Caution:	This herb can cause severe chills. <u>Do not use this herb without the supervision of a qualified health care provider.</u>

Bhuamalaki

Botanical Name:	*Phyllanthus niruri, Phyllanthus urinaria, Phyllanthus amarus*
Family:	Euphorbiaceae
Distribution:	This perennial herb is found from central and southern India to Sri Lanka. *Phyllanthus* species are also found in other countries including China (e.g., *Phyllanthus urinaria*), the Philippines, Cuba, Nigeria, and Guam.
Parts Used:	Leaves, roots, and whole plant
Active Compounds:	*Phyllanthus* primarily contains lignans (phyllanthine and hypophyllanthine), alkaloids, and *flavonoids* (quercetin). While it remains unknown which of these ingredients has an *antiviral* effect, research shows that this herb acts primarily on the liver. This action in the liver confirms its historical use as a remedy for jaundice.
Actions:	*Phyllanthus* has been used in Ayurvedic medicine for over 2,000 years and has a wide number of traditional uses. It is the main herb for treating liver disorders. Other uses include using the whole plant for jaundice, gonorrhea, frequent menstruation, and diabetes. It is also used topically as a poultice for skin ulcers, sores, swelling, and itchiness. The young shoots of the plant are administered in the form of an infusion for the treatment of chronic dysentery.

Dosage:	Infusion, juice, poultice, powder, or pill
Safety:	No side effects have been reported using *Phyllanthus* as recommended. Researchers have used the powdered form of *Phyllanthus* in amounts ranging from 900-2,700 mg per day for three months.

Guduchi

Botanical Name:	*Tinosporia cordifolia, Menisper mum cordifolium, Cocculuc cordifolia*
Family:	Menispermaceae
Distribution:	This herb is found in the Himalayas and in many parts of southern India.
Parts Used:	Whole plant, roots, and stems
Actions:	This herb is used to treat HIV/AIDS, other immune diseases, and pitta diseases. It is used as a blood purifier, to treat fever, and to aid recovery from fevers. It is also used for jaundice, digestion, constipation, hemorrhoids, dysentery, and cancer (strengthens persons before and after chemotherapy).
Dosage:	Extract, powder, concoctions for serious illnesses like cancer. Use one or more ounces daily.
Safety:	No information available.

Haridra (Turmeric)

Botanical Name:	*Curcuma longa*
Family:	Zingeberacae
Description:	This herb is found throughout India especially in Bengal, Mumbai and Chennai.
Parts Used:	Rhizome
Actions:	The active ingredient is curcumin. This herb is dry and light. The plant is bitter, astringent, and heating. It is used as a anti-inflammatory, anti-oxidant, and hepato-protective agent. It is useful in gastrointestinal colic, flatulence, hemorrhage, hematuria, menstrual difficulties, jaundice, hepatomegaly, skin disorders, fever, and wounds.
Dosage:	Juice extract 10-20 mL, powder 1-3 gm
Safety Caution:	No information about the safety of this plant is available.

Haritaki (Myrobalan)

Botanical Name:	*Terminalia chebula, Terminalia reticulata*
Family:	Combretaceae
Description:	This tree grows in many parts of India.
Parts Used:	Fruit

Actions:	This fruit is a blood purifier and is used to treat jaundice, colic, anemia, cough, asthma, hoarse voice, hiccups, vomiting, hemorrhoids, diarrhea, malabsorption, abdominal distention, gas, fevers, parasitic infections, tumors, and spleen and liver disorders. Small doses are good for constipation and diarrhea. It also improves digestion.
Dosage:	Decoction, powder, paste, and gargle
Safety Caution:	<u>Do not take this fruit if you are pregnant or are suffering from dehydration, severe exhaustion, and/or emaciation.</u> No other information about the safety of this plant is available.

Kalmegha (King of Bitters)

Botanical Name:	*Andrographis paniculata*
Family:	Acanthaceae
Distribution:	This herb is found throughout India and southeast Asia.
Part used:	Leaves
Active ingredient:	Andrographolide
Actions:	This herb is reported to possess astringent, anodyne, and tonic properties. The plant is bitter, acrid, and cooling. It is used as a laxative, anti-inflammatory, expectorant, and digestive. It is useful in treating dysentery, cholera, diabetes, influenza, bronchitis, hemorrhoids, gonorrhea, *hepatomegaly*, skin disorders, fever, worm infestations, burning sensations, wounds, ulcers, leprosy, itching, flatulence, colitis, and diarrhea.
Dosage:	Powder, decoction, and extract
Safety:	No information about the safety of this plant is available.

Katuka or Kutki

Botanical Name:	*Picrorrhiza kurroa*
Description:	This plant is found in the western Himalayas from Kashmir to Sikkim.
Parts Used:	Dried rhizome
Actions:	This herb is used with equal parts of licorice and raisins to treat constipation. It is also used with neem bark for bilious fever, and with aromatics to treat fevers, malaria, and worms in children.
Dosage:	Tincture, extract, powder, or pills
Safety:	No information about the safety of this plant is available

Musta (Nutgrass)

Botanical Name:	*Cyperus rotundus*
Family	Cyperaceae

Description:	This plant is found in southern India.
Parts Used:	Rhizome
Actions:	This plant is used to treat poor appetite, diarrhea, dysentery, fevers, gastritis, indigestion, and sluggish liver. It is also used to harmonize the liver, spleen, and pancreas and to treat malabsorption.
Dosage:	Decoction or powder
Safety Caution:	Prolonged use of this herb may cause constipation and excess flatulence or gas. No further information about the safety of this plant is available.

Pippali (Long Pepper)

Botanical Name:	*Piper longum*
Distribution:	This plant is indigenous to northeastern and southern India and Sri Lanka. It is cultivated in eastern Bengal.
Family:	Piperaceae
Parts Used:	Fruit
Actions:	*Piper longum* is used to treat abdominal tumors and distention, and to improve the digestive fire. It is used to treat flatulence, gout, laryngitis, paralysis, rheumatic pain, sciatica, and worms. It is also used to enhance the *immune system*.
Dosage:	Infusion, powder, and oil
Safety Caution:	This herb causes high pitta. No information about the safety of this plant is available.

Punarnava (Red Hogweed)

Botanical Name:	*Boerrhavia diffusa*
Family:	Nyctaginae
Description:	This herb is found throughout India. It can be white or red.
Parts Used:	Herb or root
Actions:	White and red species are used to treat *edema*, *anemia*, heart disease, cough, intestinal colic, jaundice, *ascites*, peritoneal concerns such as urethritis, and kidney disorders.
	Other uses of red plant include hemorrhoids, skin diseases, rat and snake bites, alcoholism, wasting diseases, insomnia, rheumatism, eye diseases, and asthma (moderate doses). It induces vomiting in large doses. Leaf juice is used to treat jaundice. Root decoction or infusion is used to treat constipation, gonorrhea, and internal *inflammations*. It is used externally to treat *edema*, and rat and snake bites.
Dosage:	Juice, decoction, infusion, powder, paste, oil, sugar water or honey paste
Safety Caution:	No information about the safety of this herb is available. However, large doses are known to cause vomiting.

Current Ayurvedic Research on Plants for the Treatment of Liver Disorders

Research regarding plants traditionally used in Ayurveda for the treatment of liver disease has advanced significantly in the past 15 years. Much of what has been discovered supports traditional knowledge.

The following descriptions of some of these research studies are technical and may be somewhat difficult to understand. They are provided here for reference only. If you choose to incorporate Ayurvedic medicine into your treatment *protocol*, you should give this information to your non-Ayurvedic health care providers. It will help them understand what you are taking and how it may or may not affect any other treatments you are using.

The *hepatoprotective* effect of the ethanol to water (1:1) extract of *Eclipta alba* (Ea) has been studied at subcellular levels in rats against carbon tetrachloride-induced *hepatotoxicity*. Its hepatoprotective action is created by regulating the levels of hepatic microsomal drug metabolizing *enzymes*.[11]

Studies on *Phyllanthus niruri* have revealed that it blocks *DNA polymerase*, the enzyme needed for the *hepatitis B* virus (*HBV*) to *replicate*. Fifty-nine percent of those infected with chronic viral hepatitis B lost one of the major blood markers of HBV infection (hepatitis B surface antigen) after using Phyllanthus for 30 days. While *clinical studies* on the outcome of *Phyllanthus* and HBV have been mixed, the species *P. urinaria* and *P. niruri* seem to work far better than *P. amarus*. Many previous studies on the hepatoprotective effects of *P. niruri* corroborated traditional knowledge of its role in liver disorders.[12]

Turmeric has shown evidence of hepatoprotective effects in laboratory and animal studies. However, there are no human clinical studies. Like silymarin, turmeric has been found to protect animal livers from a variety of hepatotoxic substances including carbon tetrachloride, galactosamine, pentobarbitol, 1-chloro-2,4-dinitrobenzene[7], 4-hydroxy-nonenal, and *acetaminophen*. Giving curcumin along with piperine (long pepper) can enhance its absorption when taken orally. The hepatoprotective effects of turmeric may stem from its potent *antioxidant* effects. Turmeric contains several water and fat soluble antioxidant compounds. Curcumin was found to be the most active of these compounds. The antioxidant effects of other components of turmeric are also significant. A heat-stable *protein* isolated from the aqueous extract of turmeric was found to be more effective against superoxide than was curcumin, and more effective in inhibiting oxidative damage to DNA. In addition to its antioxidant effects, curcumin has also been shown to enhance liver detoxification by increasing the activity of *glutathione* S-transferase.[10,20] Glutathione S-transferase is an enzyme that joins glutathione with a wide variety of *toxins* to facilitate their removal from the body.[13-15]

Glycyrrhiza (licorice) has been shown to have a direct hepatoprotective effect. Glycyrrhiza flavonoids provide protection to *hepatocytes* exposed to carbon tetrachloride and galactosamine. Research points to the antilipid peroxidation effect of glycyrrhiza as the central mechanism contributing to its protective action against carbon tetrachloride-induced hepatotoxicity. Glycyrrhiza has also been shown to significantly quench *free radicals*. Recent studies have shown glycyrrhiza to enhance the detoxification of medications and toxins. Several mechanisms seem to be involved, one of which is increased liver glucuronidation. Glycyrrhiza exerts *antiviral* activity *in vitro* toward a number of viruses, including *hepatitis A*, varicella zoster, *HIV*, herpes simplex type 1, Newcastle disease, and vesicular stomatitis viruses. Intravenous glycyrrhizin has been shown to be effective in a double blind study against viral hepatitis, chronic viral hepatitis in particular. Administered in a physiologic saline solution in combination with cysteine and glycine (a product called Stronger Neo Minophagen-C, or SNMC), glycyrrhiza has been shown to stimulate *endogenous interferon* production in addition to its antioxidant and detoxifying effects.[16-18]

Picroliv, the active constituent isolated from the plant *Picrorhiza kurroa*, was evaluated as a hepatoprotective agent against ethanol-induced *hepatic* injury in rats. Alcohol feeding (3.75 g/kg x45 days) produced 20-114% alteration in selected *serum* (AST, ALT and ALP) and liver markers (lipid, glycogen and protein). Further, it reduced the viability (44-48%) of isolated hepatocytes ex vivo as assessed by Trypan blue exclusion and rate of oxygen uptake. Its effect was also seen on specific alcohol-metabolizing enzymes (aldehyde dehydrogenase, 41%; acetaldehyde dehydrogenase, 52%) in rat hepatocytes. The levels of these enzymes were reduced in the cells following alcohol intoxication. Ethyl alcohol also produced cholestasis (41-53%), as indicated by reduction in bile volume, bile salts, and bile acids. Picroliv treatment (3-12 mg/kg p.o. x45 days) restored the altered parameters in a dose-dependent manner (36-100%).[19, 20]

Andrographolide, a chief constituent of A. paniculata, exhibits protective effects in galactosamine and paracetamol induced toxicity in rats. Andrographolide was demonstrated to possess antihepatotoxic effects in carbon tetrachloride-induced hepatotoxicity in albino rats. The LD50 of aqueous ethanolic extract of whole plant was determined to be >215 mg/kg, i.p. in mice. Andrographic paniculata (Kalamegh) was used in an uncontrolled study at Kaya Chikitsa Dept. BHU Varanasi, India. Average duration of treatment was 23 days. In 90% of patients, clinical as well as liver function parameters improved significantly.[21]

Sample Panchkarma and Rasayana Therapy for Treatment of Liver Disease

As noted in *Chapter 10, Ayurvedic Medicine*, panchakarma and rasayana are two treatments commonly used to treat chronic liver disorders. Following are sample protocols for each of these Ayurvedic treatments. However, keep in mind that Ayurvedic treatments are customized for each individual, and these are just sample protocols. Further, these treatments can only be done under the supervision of a qualified Ayurvedic practitioner.

If you are interested in adding Ayurvedic therapy to your hepatitis C treatment plan, you will need to see a qualified Ayurvedic practitioner. He or she can evaluate you, and then decide on the treatments that are appropriate for your unique situation.

Panchakarma Therapy (Body Cleansing)

Panchakarma is used in Ayurveda to eliminate excess doshas from the body. This therapy is widely used throughout India and the United States. It is used to balance humors and eliminate toxins from the body, thus treating various physical and psychiatric disorders.

Most liver disorders are typically aggravated conditions of pitta, which is also the predominant humor for the liver.

Panchakarma consists of three parts: *poorva karma*, *pradhana karma*, and *paschat karma*.

Poorva Karma (Pre-Purification Measures)

This procedure helps prepare the body for the main purification process. This treatment includes *abhyanga* (massage) and *pinda svedana* (warm massage with a small cotton bag containing the warmed herbs).

<u>Abhyanga</u>: The term abhyanga is used as a synonym for oil bath. Oil is anointed all over the body, especially on the head and feet.

<u>Pinda Sveda (fomentation)</u>: This treatment is very efficacious wherever sweating is advised. The subject is massaged with warm oil all over the body. Then the subject is massaged with small bags containing cooked old rice that is warmed in a milk decoction mixture. The heat of the bags is maintained by re-warming them whenever necessary.

Medicaments for Panchakarma

<u>For abhyanga</u>:	*Balaguduchyadi taila*
Main Ingredients:	*Sida cordifolia (bala), Tinospora cordifolia (guduchi), Santalum album (candana), Pluchea lanceolata (rasna), Valeriana wallichii (nata), Withania somnifera (ashwagandha)*
<u>For pinda sveda</u>:	Old rice/rice powder cooked with milk and *Sida cordifolia* (bala) decoction.

Pradhan Karma (Main Purification Measures)

Pradhan karma includes *virechana* (purgation), *pizhichil*, and *yapana vasti*.

VIRECHANA (PURGATION)

This treatment is advised for the pitta disorders to eliminate aggravated pitta. Pitta disorders include liver disorders. The subject's physical constitution (prakruti) and strength will determine the dosage of the purgative herbs. Subjects are advised to consume purgative herbs in the early morning.

PIZHICHIL (MEDICATED WARM LIQUID OIL MASSAGE)

This is a modified form of sarvangadhara. Warm liquid is poured from a certain height all over the body of the patient with unctuous liquids. After anointing the head with *ksheerabala* oil, warm *trivrit* oil is applied all over the body. The patient is then laid in a wooden compartment and again smeared with the warm unctuous fluid all over the body.

YAPANA VASTI

This treatment is in the form of an enema. It helps improve strength and builds up muscle and tissue. It is intended to improve quality of life by alleviating ailments. This treatment is used only in subjects who can tolerate the procedure.

Medicaments for Pradhan Karma

For Virechana: Based on the subject's physical constitution and strength either Avipattikara choorna (a mild powder laxative) or triphala churna powder (a combination of Terminalia chebula, Terminalia bellirica, and Emblica officinals) is administered.

For Yapana Vasti: An herbal concoction is used along with milk and honey. The herbs used are Glycyrrhiza glabra (yasti madhu), Tinospora cordifolia (guduchi), Picrorrhiza kurroa (katuki), Hemidesmus indicus (sariva), and Rubia cordifolia (manjista). The dose of each herb is 500 mg for a total treatment dose of 2.5 grams.

Paschat Karma

This treatment includes diet and lifestyle guidelines to bring about balance in the tridoshas after the subject has undergone the main purification procedure. Subjects are advised to follow the diet and lifestyle that will reestablish the balance of pitta. Paschat karma should be practiced during the entire treatment process.

Lifestyle: Patients should avoid sleeping in the afternoon, exposure to hot sun, exertion, anxiety, alcohol abuse, smoking, and irregular eating habits.

Diet: Vegetarianism is best for liver disorders. After mild purgation, subjects will be managed with a wholesome diet including non-spicy food, barley, wheat, basmati rice (old rice), and soup of lentils and mung bean. The consistency of food should be gradually increased from a thin consistency on the first meal to thicker one on seventh meal. A drink of warm water should follow each meal.

Rasayana Therapy (Rejuvenation Therapy)

Rasayana therapy is advised after the subject has undergone panchakarma therapy. Rasayana is a clinical specialty in Ayurveda wherein a specialized rejuvenating diet, herbs, and lifestyle are advised. Rasayana promotes tissue repair and the formation of healthy tissues. It alleviates exertion, lassitude, exhaustion, and debility. In other words, it builds up all the body tissues, improves immunity against diseases, and enhances the mental competence.

By its immunomodulatory and antioxidant effects, rasayana helps enhance the immune system, and prevent diseases and premature aging. The diet, herbs and lifestyle also help alleviate already existing ailments and restore health. Therapy ensures proper transportation and absorption of nutrients, and builds normal tissues. Through rasayana, one attains longevity, memory, intelligence, youthful age, optimum strength of physique, and optimum sensory ability.

There are two types of rasayana treatments, kutipravesika (indoor) and vataatapika (outdoor). In this sample protocol, we discuss an outdoor rasayana.

People with liver disorders are prescribed rasayana therapy that is both hepatoprotective and immune enhancing. The therapy includes rejuvenation of the liver with herbs (mainly Piper longum in a powder formula, in a graded dose) and diet.

PIPPALI RASAYANA

Mainly indicated for fever, fatigue, inflammation, liver and spleen enlargements, cough, and/or *dyspnea*.
Main Ingredient: *Pippali*
Dose: 1 tablespoon twice a day with warm water

ASHWAGANDHA RASAYANA

Mainly indicated in fatigue and immunodeficiency. It is an immune enhancer and a rejuvenator. Used when antioxidants are needed. Therapy is intended to decrease viral load.

Main Ingredients: *Withania somnifera (ashwagandha), Hemidesmus indicus (sariva), Cuminum cyminum (jiraka), Vitis vinifera (draksha)*

Dose: 1 tablespoon twice a day with warm water or milk

TRIPHALA RASAYANA

Mainly indicated in immunodeficiency and chronic illness.

Main Ingredients: *Terminalia chebula (haritaki), Terminalia bellirica (bibhitaki), Emblica officinals (amalaki), Madhuca indica (madhuka), Piper longum (pippali)*

Dose: 1 tablespoon at night with warm water

References

1. Mishra ,Shri K. Recent advances in liver diseases in Ayurvedic medicine in complementary and alternative medicine in chronic liver disease. National Institutes of Health Conference on Complementary and Alternative Medicine in Chronic Liver Diseases. Bethesda, Maryland. 1999.
2. www.Holistic-online.com/yoga
3. Nadkarni KM, Nadkarni KA. *Indian Materia Medica, Vols. I and II*. Bombay, India: Popular Prakashan; 1993.
4. Luper S. A review of plants used in the treatment of liver disease: part two. *Altern Med Rev*. 1999;4(3):178-188.
5. Madhava Nidanam. *Kaamala roga*. Madras, India: Vavilla Ramaswamy Sastrulu & Sons; 1975.
6. Sharma PV, Ed. *Charaka Samhita*. Varanasi, India: Chaukambha Orientalia; 1981.
7. Vagbhata, D. *Ashtanga Hridayam*. Varanasi, India: Chaukambha Orientalia; 1980.
8. Madhava Nidanam. *Kaamala roga*. Madras, India: Vavilla Ramaswamy Sastrulu & Sons; 1975.
9. Frawley, D. *Ayurvedic Healing*. New Delhi, India: Motilal Banarasi Das Publishers; 1992.
10. Susruta Samhita. *Sutrasthanam*. New Delhi, India: Motilal Banarasidas Publishers; 1983.
11. Saxena AK, Singh B, Anand KK. Hepatoprotective effects of Eclipta alba on subcellular levels in rats. *J Ethnopharmacol*. 1993;40(3):155-61.
12. Wang M, Cheng H, Li Y, Meng L, Zhao G, Mai K. Herbs of the genus phyllantus in the treatment of chronic heptatitis B: observations with three preparations from different geographic sites. *J Lab Clin Med*. 1995;126(4):350-352.
13. Adithan C, Sivaperuman A, Shashindran CH. *Indian Journal of Pharmacology*. 1999;31(1): 71.
14. Xiang ZX, He XQ, Zhou GF, et al. Protective effects of an ethanolic extract and essential oil of Curcuma kwangsinensis s. against experimental liver lesions in mice. *Chung Kuo Chung Yao Tsa Chih*. 1989;14(5):303-305, 320.
15. Piper JT, Singhal SS, Salameh MS, et al. Mechanisms of anticarcinogenic properties of curcumin: the effect of curcumin on glutathione linked detoxification enzymes in rat liver. *Int J Bioch Cell Biol*. 1998;30(4):445-456.
16. Wang BE. Treatment of chronic liver diseases with traditional Chinese medicine. J Gastroenterol Hepatol. 2000;15(May 15 Suppl):E67-70.
17. Kiso Y, Suzuki Y, Watanabe N, et al. *Planta Medica*. 1983;49:185-187.
18. Piper JT, Singhal SS, Salameh MS, et al. *International Journal of Biochemistry and Cell Biology*. 1998;30:445-456.
19. Visen PKS, Saraswat B, Patnaik GK, Agarwal DP, Dhawan BN. Protective activity of picroliv isolated from Picrorhiza kurrooa against ethanol toxicity in isolated rat hepatocytes. *Indian J Pharmacol*. 1996;28:98-101.
20. Saraswat B, Visen PK, Patnaik GK, Dhawan BN. Ex vivo and in vivo investigations of picroliv from Picrorhiza kurroa in an alcohol intoxication model in rats. *J Ethnopharmacol*. 1999;66(3):263-269.
21. Deshpande UR, Gadre SG, Raste AS, Pillai D, Bhide SV, Samuel AM. Protective effect of turmeric (Curcuma longa L.) extract on carbon tetrachloride-induced liver damage in rats. *Indian J Exp Biol*. 1998;36(6):573-77.
22. Subramoniam, P. Pushpangadan development of phytomedicines for liver diseases. *Indian Journal of Pharmacology*. 1999;31:166-175.

Appendix III: Chinese Medicine Herbs and Formulas

Composition of Herbal Therapies

Capillaris Combination (plus blood cooling and toxin resolving herbs)

- Artemisiae capillaris, Gardeniae fructus, Rhei rhizoma, Desmodii herba, Paeoniae rubra radix, Polygoni cuspidati, Plantaginis herba, Polyporus umbellatus, Scutellariae radix, Turmeric radix, Glycyrrhiza uralensis fisch

Modified Formulas of Bupleurum and Tang-kuei Formula, and Bupleurum and Peony and Six Major Herb Combination

- Bupleuri radix polyporus, Poria (Hoelen), Atractylodes rhizoma, Paeoniae alba radix, Urantii fructus, Fructus oryzae germinatus, Fructus hordei germinatus, Endothelium corneum gigeriae galli, Fructus citri sarcodactylis, Glycyrrhiza uralensis fisch

Modified Glehnia and Rehmannia Formula

- Paeoniae alba radix, Aurantii fructus, Angelicae radix, Rehmanniae radix, Ophiopogonis radix, Fructus lycii, Glehniae radix, Cortex moutan radicis, Fructus meliae toosendan, Ligustri fructus, Polygoni multiflori radix, Zizyphi spinosi semen

Modified Aconite, Ginseng, and Ginger Combination, and Gardenia and Hoelen Formula (Four Major Herb Combination and Rehmannia Eight Formula)

- Aconiti praeparata raix, Cinnamomi ramulus, Zingiberis rhizoma, Atractylodes rhizoma, Dioscoreae batatis rhizoma, Polyporus, Poria (Hoelen), Polyporus umbellatus, Alismatis rhizoma, Arecae pericarpium, Glycyrrhiza uralensis fisch

Modified Persica and Achyranthes Combination, and Persica and Cinidium Combination (Persica and Eupolyphaga Combination)

- Carthami flos, Persicae semen, Cortex moutan radicis, Aurantii fructus, Leonuri herba, Cyperi rhizoma, Turmeric radix, Rhei rhizoma, Angelicae radix, Cnidii rhizoma, Rehmanniae radix, Paeoniae rubra radix, Achyranthis radix, Citri aurantii fructus, Bupleuri radix, Glycyrrhizae radix, Platycodi radix

AI #3 Capsule

- Mucunae caulis, Sargentodoxae caulis, Paederiae caulis

Allicin Capsule

- Allii sativum bulbus (garlic)

BM Capsule

- Momordica charantia, Fagophyrum tatarium

Capillaris Combination

- Artemisiae capillaris herba, Gardeniae fructus, Rhei rhizoma

Circulation No. 1 Capsule

- Carthami flos, Persicae semen, Angelicae radix, Cnidii rhizoma, Rehmanniae radix, Paeoniae rubra radix, Achyranthis radix, Citri aurantii fructus, Bupleuri radix, Glycyrrhizae radix, Platycodi radix

Coptin Capsule

- Coptis chinensis franch

Cordyceps Capsule

- Cordyceps sinensis

Gall No. 1 Capsule

- Bupleuri radix, Artemisiae capillaris herba, Desmodii herba, Taraxaci herba, Gardeniae fructus, Saussureae radix, Citri pericarpium, Citri immaturi pericarpium, Salviae miltiorrhziae radix, Angelica radix, Scutellariae radix, Gentianae radix

Ginseng and Atractylodes Formula

- Ginseng radix, Dioscoreae rhizoma, Dolichoris album semen, Coicis semen, Nelumbinis semen, Atractylodis macrocephalae rhizoma, Poriae alba, Glycyrrhizae radix, Amomi fructus, Platycodi radix, and Zizipi jujubae fructus

Glycyrrihzin Capsule

- Glycyrrhiza uralensis fisch (licorice root)

Hepa Formula No. 2 Capsule

- Schizandrae fructus, Artemisiae capillaris herba, Alismatis rhizoma, Polyporus, Poria (Hoelen), Atractylodes rhizoma, Cinnamomi ramulus, Citri pericarpium, Magnoliae cortex, Zingiberis rhizoma (ginger), Glycyrrhizae radix (licorice)

HerbSom Capsule

- Corydalis yanhusao rhizoma, Zizyphus spinosi semen, Schizandrae fructus

Ligustrin Capsule

- Ligustrum lucidum ait

Red Poeny Combination

- Paeoniae rubra radix, Puerariae radix, Salviae miltiorrhziae radix, Persicae semen, Artemisiae capillaris herba, Aristolochiae fangchi radix

Rhubarbin Capsule

- Rhei rhizoma

Tiao Ying Yin

- Angelicae radix, Cnidii rhizoma, Paeoniae rubra radix, Rhei rhzoma, Polyporus, Porie (Hoelen), Corydalis yanhusao rhizoma, Dianthi herba, Zedoariae rhizoma, Mori radicis cortex, Leonuri fructus, Arecae pericarpipum

Pharmacology of Herbs and Formulas

The following list of the pharmacology of the major herbal remedies is for reference only. If you choose to take any of these herbal remedies, it may be helpful to provide your western healthcare provider with this information. It will help your doctor better understand what you are taking and how it may interact with other treatments he or she is prescribing.

Herbs

ALLICIN
- Allicin has a wide spectrum of anti-infectious capabilities.
- It acts against bacteria, mycobacteria, fungi, protozoa, and certain viruses.

- It is potent enough to be used in many common infections such as bacillary dysentery, amebic dysentery, deep fungal infections, whooping cough, endobronchial tuberculosis, oxyuriasis (pinworms), trichomonas vaginitis, and others.
- It has been used in China for more than 20 years.
- It is virtually nontoxic. Its LD50 is 134.9 times higher than the therapeutic dose.

ARTEMISIAE CAPILLARIS THUNB HERBA
- This is the main herb used to treat jaundice in TCM.
- It fosters bile secretion in both healthy and carbon tetrachloride liver damaged animals.
- It has liver protective effects.
- It reduces carbon tetrachloride-induced liver damage and ALT elevation. It also helps recover liver glycogen and RNA.
- It lowers blood lipids and has fibrolytic effects.

ASTRAGALI RADIX
- Astragalosides is the main active ingredient of Astragali Radix.
- It has extensive pharmacological actions and beneficial effects on regulating immunity, antiviral effects, cardiovascular system protection, anti-neoplastic actions, and anti-inflammatory effects.
- Its liver protective and antifibrosis actions can be used for treating fibrosis in chronic liver disease. An experimental study found it can suppress hepatic stellate cell proliferation and the synthesis of collagens.[1, 2]

BUPLEURI RADIX
- Bupleuri radix has liver-protective and biliary effects.
- It can protect the liver from toxic damage caused by galactosalmine, Penicillium notatum, and carbon tetrachloride.
- It can increase bile secretion and the amount of bile salt in the bile.
- Its anti-inflammatory effect can be used to treat inflammation of the liver and gall bladder.

COPTIS CHINENSIS FRANCH
- Coptis chinensis franch has antimicrobial properties.
- It can strongly suppress Staphylococcus aureus, Streptococcus, pneumococcus, Vibrio comma, anthrax bacillus, Bacillus dysenteriae, hay bacillus, pneumobacillus, Bacillus diphtheriae, Bordetella pertussis, Brucellaceae, and Mycobacterium tuberculosis.
- It can suppress influenza viruses and Newcastle disease virus in vitro.
- It can act against ameoba, Chlamydia trachomatis, trichomonas, and Leptospira.
- It is virtually nontoxic. The LD50 is 205mg/kg.

CORDYCEPS CAPSULE (CORDYCEPS SINESIS)
- The various actions ascribed to Cordyceps sinesis are lung and kidney nourishment, vital essence and energy tonification, hemostasis, and phlegm resolution.
- It is used in general debility after sickness, and for elderly persons.
- Its therapeutic effects have been confirmed in many controlled, well-designed studies carried out by medical schools in China including Beijing, Shanghai, and Nanjing.

- It is virtually nontoxic.

- The effects of this herb have been studied in chronic viral hepatitis. The efficacy rate was reportedly above 80% in a 256 patient clinical study. Cordyceps sinesis can lower ALT, improve liver function, relieve liver related symptoms, and increase albumin. It has also been used for cirrhosis caused by chronic viral hepatitis. In the previously mentioned study, 17 out of 22 patients had increased albumin levels after three months of treatment. Twelve of 17 patients with ascites experienced complete resolution while the other five had a reduction in ascites.[3]

- This herb is helpful for immunodeficiency caused by viral infection, chemotherapy, radiotherapy, major illnesses, or surgery.

- Cordyceps sinesis is used to treat impotence, premature ejaculation, low libido, low sperm counts and/or activity, irregular menstruation, and leukorrhea.

- Observed in a rat CCl4 fibrotic model, Cordyceps sinensis treatment led to less inflammation, fatty degeneration, and liver cell damage. From clinical observations, Cordyceps sinensis appears to improve regeneration of hepatocytes and suppression of fibroblast activities.[4, 5]

- This substance is the main ingredient of the Cordyceps Capsule.

CURCUMA LONGA LINN

- Curcumin is an active ingredient extracted from Chinese herb Curcuma longa Linn.

- It has strong antioxidant effects. An animal study found it inhibits hepatic stellate cell proliferation without cytotoxicity, and also inhibits the formation of type I collagen, HA, and LN to different degrees.[6]

DANSHENSUAN A

- Danshensuan A is a water soluble ingredient of Salvia miltiorrhiza with antioxidant effects.

- Animal experiments found it suppresses the proliferation of fibroblastic cells and the synthesis of intracellular collagen.[7]

- Extract IH764-3 of Salvia miltiorrhiza has been shown to markedly reduce fibrosis in rat fibrotic models and reduce the content of hydrooxyproline (Hyp), type I and III collagen, HA, and LN. It can also improve liver function and liver histology.[8]

- These substances are the main ingredients of the Circulation P Capsule.

DESMODII STYRACIFOLIUM HER

- This herb can facilitate bile secretion and help expel sandy gall stones.

- It can relax the sphincter of Oddi, helping to abate biliary obstruction and pain.

- It prevents the precipitation of gallstone-forming elements.

GLYCYRRHIZIN (GL)

- GL, the active ingredient in licorice root, has various pharmacological actions that can be used in treating hepatitis C.

- GL has antiviral effects. It can induce production of interferon-gamma in test animals and humans. It can prolong the survival of mice after being injected with mouse hepatitis virus (MHV). In rabbits, it can inhibit Vaccinia virus proliferation.

- GL protects liver cells from chemical injuries. It can alleviate histological changes due to carbon tetrachloride intoxication, and lower ALT. It can reduce liver cell degeneration and necrosis, and help recover glycogen and RNA. Experimental hepatitis and cirrhosis studies in rats found GL can promote regeneration of liver cells and inhibit fibrosis.[9] It can also reduce gamma globulin and interstitial inflammation in the liver.

- It has antiallergic, antiinflammatory, and detoxifying activities that resemble those of glucocorticoid. GL also inhibits the release of histamine from mast cells.

- Although licorice root is a nontoxic herb, long-term use of GL can cause adverse reactions in about 20% of patients. Adverse reactions include edema, rise in blood pressure, low blood potassium, dizziness, muscle fatigue, and others. People with hypertension should not take GL.

LIGUSTICUM CHUANZIONG

- The active ingredient of Ligusticum chuanziong is chuanxionyzine, also known as pyrazine.

- In the rat CCl4 -induced fibrotic model, it can reduce ALT, HA, type III pre-collagen, and reduce fibrosis. It is an antioxidant and can increase superoxide dismutase activities and reduce the level of methylene dioxyamphetamine.[10]

- It can improve microcirculation, promote regeneration and repair of the liver cells, and eliminate free radicals. Its liver-protective and antifibrosis effects are realized by its anti-oxidant mechanism.[11]

- This substance is an ingredient of the Circulation P Capsule.

LIGUSTRUM LUCIDUM AIT

- Ligustrum is a highly purified extract of Ligustrum lucidum fructus. Its active chemical component is oleanolic acid. It can protect the liver from chemical and biological injuries.

- Ligustrum can lower ALT levels. In experimental cirrhosis studies, it has been found to inhibit degeneration and reduce liver cell death.[12] It can increase the glycogen in the liver, and accelerate the regeneration of liver cells. It can also inhibit inflammation and collagen formation.

- It can raise the white blood cell count, and is used to treat leukopenia caused by chemotherapy and radiotherapy.

- In clinical trials for hepatitis, ligustrum reduced ALT, AST, and jaundice.

- It promotes lymphoblast cell transformation and macrophage phagocytosis.

- Ligustrum can increase coronary blood flow.

- Acute and chronic toxicity tests have shown ligustrum has very low toxicity.

MARMODICA CHARNATIA (BITTER MELON)

- A 1981 clinical trial in England found that bitter melon (BM) can significantly improve glucose tolerance in type II diabetes.[13] A water-soluble extract of BM can significantly reduce blood glucose concentrations during oral glucose tolerance tests.

- Animal studies with normal and diabetic rats and rabbits have shown BM has a hypoglycemic effect.[14] Insulin-like molecules in the extract of BM have physiological effects similar to those of insulin. The extract of BM can also stimulate the pancreas to secret insulin. Some of the ingredients of BM can also prolong the effects of insulin. Comparative studies conducted in China found that BM's blood sugar reducing effects were similar to those of tolbutamide.[15]

- In China and southeast Asia, BM is a commonly consumed vegetable, which indicates that it is very safe.

NOTOGINSENG

- Notoginseng's active ingredient can suppress fibrotic rat expression of TGF-β1, type I and III collagen, and reduce fibrosis.[16]

- This substance is a main ingredient of the Circulation P Capsule.

PAEDERIAE CAULIS

- This herb has antirheumatic, digestant, antitussive, mucolytic, analgesic, hypotensive, and corticosteroid-like effects. It also has sedative actions and can elevate the pain threshold.

- Paederiae caulis inhibited spontaneous activity in mice experiments, and prolonged pentobarbital-induced sleep.[15]

- The total alkaloids of this herb inhibit the contraction of the isolated intestine, and antagonize spasm due to acetylcholine and histamine.

- Paederiae caulis has been used for many skin diseases such as eczema, neurodermatitis, and leprosy. This herb is also used to treat respiratory diseases such as bronchitis and whooping cough.

- It has a high LD50 with virtually no toxicity.

EXTRACTS OF PERSICAE SEMEN

- Studies done at Shanghai TCM University found that Persicae Semencan promote the action of collagenase to reduce type III pre-collagen synthesis and increase the degradation of collagen, and cause the hydroxyproline level to increase in the blood.

- This herbal extract has been successfully used to treat cirrhosis caused by viral hepatitis and parasitic hepatitis.[17]

- It is one of major ingredients of the Circulation P Capsule.

POLYGONI CUSPIDATI RHIZOMA

- The 10% decoction of Polygoni cuspidati rhizoma inhibited Asian influenza virus type A, Jingke 68-1 strain, ECHO 11, and herpes simplex viruses.[18] A stronger inhibitory action was exhibited by a 2% decoction against adenovirus type III, poliomyelitis virus type II, Coxsackie virus group A and B, ECHO 11 group, encephalitis B virus, and herpes simplex I strain.

- A 20% solution showed significant inhibitory action against the hepatitis B surface antigen (HBsAg). Active principles I and II of the herb were able to decrease the HBsAg titer eight-fold.

- This herb has been used for chronic viral hepatitis, acute inflammatory diseases, neonatal jaundice, and leukopenia.

RHEI RHIZOMA (RHUBARB ROOT)

- Alcohol extracts of this herb contain aloe-emodin, rhein, and chrysophanol.

- Pharmacological studies have found it has a wide antimicrobial spectrum. It can effectively suppress Staphylococcus, anthrax bacillus, Bacillus dysenteriae, Streptococcus, and E. coli.[19] It is especially effective for Staphylococcus and Streptococcus.

- This herb also has antiviral effects. The herb decoction has been shown to strongly inhibit the influenza virus.[20]

- Clinically, rhubarb root has been used for indigestion, constipation, acute inflammatory diseases, infectious and parasitic diseases, hemorrhage, and thrombocytopenia (low platelets). Its strong purgative and laxative effects can be used to treat constipation.

- Chrysophanol has hemostatic effects (stopping bleeding), and is often used for bleeding in the gastrointestinal system.

- The LD50 of rhubarb root is 250-500mg/kg. The LD50 of chrysophanol is 10grams/kg and is very safe.

- Emodin is an active compound of Rhei Rhizoma. It antagonizes fibrosis and has been used as an effective treatment for cirrhosis and other organ fibrosis. Its antifibrosis effects are based on its actions to protect against cell damage from inflammation and reducing necrosis, and regulating the synthesis and decomposition of the ECM.[21-23]

SALVIAE MILTIORRHZIAE RADIX (SALVIA)

- Salvia improves the microcirculation in the liver. It markedly increases liver blood flow in acute and chronic carbon tetrachloride (CCl4) toxic models.[24] The fibrosis preventive effects of Salvia are mainly the result of its microcirculation improving effects.

- In the CCl4 toxic rat model, Salvia can quickly lower ALT, and reduce inflammation, necrosis, and steatosis (fatty liver degeneration). In the control group, CCl4 caused liver collagen and globulin to increase and every rat in the control group developed cirrhosis. In the Salvia treated group, not a single rat developed cirrhosis, and the collagen and globulin did not increase.[25]

SCHIZANDRAE FRUCTUS

- Animal studies have shown the alcohol extract of the kernel of the fruit of schizandra (AEKFS) has many pharmacological activities such as:

  - lowering ALT caused by CCl4-induced liver damage

  - reducing fat deposits in liver cells caused by CCl4 intake

  - reducing the histological damage of the liver cells caused by CCl4

  - promoting glycogen and serum protein synthesis in the liver

  - promoting liver regeneration after partial removal of the liver, and

  - increasing metabolic enzymes in the liver.

- Clinical trials using tablets made from the whole AEKFS conducted in three hospitals in China found that of 107 chronic viral hepatitis cases, ALT was normalized for 73 with an associated improvement in clinical symptoms. There were no serious side effects reported.[26]

SOPHORAE SUBPROSTRATAE RADIX

- The active ingredient of Sophorae subprostratae radix is oxymatrine. In three commonly used liver damage models, oxymatrine prevented liver cell damage. Compared with the control group, the oxymatine treated group had much lower ALT levels, less liver cell necrosis, and less inflammation.[27]

- Oxymatrine can increase cytochrome P-450 content and activity, and increase the amount of smooth surfaced endoplasmic reticulum of the liver cell. Thus, it can strengthen the detoxification capability of the liver.

- It also has viral suppressive, anti-inflammatory, immunoregulatory, anticancer, and leukogenic (raising the white blood cell count) effects.

- Recent studies have shown oxymatrine at a concentration of 62.5 ng/ml, suppresses fibroblastic cell activities and suppresses the expression of mRNA of type III precollagen. The potency of these effects is dose dependent. Clinical studies found that the treated group showed lower levels of ALT, collagen IV, HA, and TNF-β, and less inflammatory activities and fibrosis than that of the control group.[28, 29]

- This substance is one of the main ingredients of Hepa F #2 and Hepa F #1a Capsules.

TAURINE

- Taurine is an active ingredient of Nature Calculus Bovis.

- In TCM, the gallstone of Bos Taurus demesticus is used to remove heat from the heart, induce resuscitation, eliminate phlegm, relieve convulsion and remove heat and toxic substances.

- Recent studies found that taurine can suppress hyaluronic acid (HA) and the expression of mRNA of type I and III precollagens. In rat fibrotic models, it was found that treatment with this substance was associated with reduction in collagen deposition in the liver tissue and reduced hydrooxyproline (Hyp) in the liver. In rat CCl4 fibrotic model, it reduced the content of Hyp, type I and III precollagen, HA, LN, and improved liver function and liver histology.[30]

TETRANDRINE

- Tetrandrine is the active ingredient of Stephania tetrandra S. Moore.

- This substance can affect the calcium channel and calcium distribution in cells. It also exhibits antiinflammatory, antiallergic, analgesic, and antibacterial effects. It can suppress the collagen and DNA synthesis in the HSC. The suppression is dose dependent. After being treated with this substance, the serum HA, P-II-P, and the collagen deposit levels decreased significantly. At the same time, inflammation, cell necrosis, and inflammatory cell infiltration decreased. This substance has been used in treating lung fibrosis with successful clinical outcomes.[31, 32]

Herbal Formulas

CAPILLARIS COMBINATION

- This is a very old and famous formula was originated by the Chinese medical sage Zhang Zhongjing 2,000 years ago.

- Clinical Pharmacology

  - Clears dampness-heat type jaundice that manifests as bright yellowish coloration of the eyes and skin, oliguria with dark yellow urine, yellow and greasy fur on the tongue, a smooth and rapid pulse, and other signs and symptoms.

  - The whole formula has cholegogic and choleretic (facilitating bile secretion) effects. Intraduodenal administration of the alcohol extracts of this formula in rats markedly increased the bile collected by up to 51.28%, and increased the solid composition of the bile by 85%.[33] Its choleretic effects are mainly due to increasing the secretion of the bile in the micro bile ducts.

  - It has liver protective effects and can reduce the liver damage caused by α-naphthylisothiocyanate (ANIT). While using this formula, the ALP, total bilirubin, ALT, and AST elevations caused by ANIT all improved dramatically.[34]

  - Histological examination revealed that hypertrophy of the micro bile duct cells, necrosis of liver cells, and inflammatory cell infiltration were much milder in treated animals compared with the untreated control group. The liver glycogen and RNA content were normalized, and the ALT activity was markedly reduced.[35]

CIRCULATION NO.1 CAPSULE

- This is a modified formula based on Persica and Achyranthes Combination and Persica and Cnidium Combination. Traditionally, these formulas were used for blood stagnancy or stasis that manifests with symptoms such as dark or purplish tongue, cold hands and feet, dark rings around the eyes, liver palm, spider moles, dry and itchy skin, rashes, lumps, and upper abdominal discomfort.

- Clinical Pharmacology

  - This formula can noticeably ameliorate the acute microcirculation disorder induced by macromolecular dextran in rats.[36] It dilates the microcapillaries, accelerates blood flow, and opens more micro-capillary networks. The result is to increase blood infusion to the tissues and stop the pathology caused by the microcirculation disorder. It can promote the phagocytosis by macrophages (Kupffer cells) in the liver. It can also clear the clotting factors in DIC (disseminated intravascular coagulation) and stop the progress of DIC.[37]

  - It will not prolong the PTT or prothrombin time. It can suppress the clustering of platelets.

  - It can improve phagocytosis by macrophages. It can also regulate cellular and humoral immunity.

  - It can noticeably suppress granuloma formation (a fibrotic activity).[38]

GINSENG AND ATRACTYLODES FORMULA

- This formula was first created by the National Medical Bureau of the Song Dynasty 1,000 years ago.
- Clinical Pharmacology
  - This formula is used for strengthening digestion and vital energy. It is helpful for treating diarrhea, poor appetite, emaciation, and white and greasy fur on the tongue.
  - This formula can improve absorption in the intestinal tract. Giving the decoction of the formula increased water and chloride absorption in the intestine of rabbits under anesthesia.[39] It is an antagonist to the spastic effects of acetylcholine on the intestine.

HERSOM CAPSULE

- Clinical Pharmacology
  - This formula has been studied in teaching hospitals in China. Randomized, controlled clinical trials have shown that this formula has sleep-inducing effects and improves the quality of sleep. In a study of 374 patients, improvement in sleep was found to be statistically equivalent to that of methaqualone.[40] HerbSom formula is not habit forming and has no hangover effect.
  - The pharmacological data of these herbs show that they may also have many beneficial effects on the cardiovascular and neurological systems of the body.
  - These herbs have no harmful effects on the liver.
- **CAUTION**: Keep this formula out of reach of children. This product should not be taken while driving a car or operating heavy machinery.

YUNNAN PAIYAO CAPSULE

- This is a very famous traditional herbal medicine.
- Clinical Pharmacology
  - This formula can quickly stop bleeding in rat and rabbit liver injury models, and rabbit large artery injury models.[41] It has been shown to dramatically reduce clotting time in human and rabbit experiments.[42] The hemostatic effects begin 30 minutes after administration, and peaks 2-3 hours after administration. These effects can last for more than four hours. The hemostatic effect is due to a permeability change in the cell membranes of platelets. This causes the release of clotting factors from platelets that promote clotting.
  - This formula can suppress inflammation in various animal models.[43] The strength of its antiinflammatory effect is similar to that of corticosteroids.
  - It also has analgesic and antineoplastic (antitumor) effects.

References

1. Zheng B, et al. Astragalus' anti- liver fibrosis effect and its relationship with TGF-β1 and γ-interferon. *J Clinical Military Medicine*. 2000, 28(3):22-23.
2. Wang YJ, et al. The immunohischemical study of astragalus's effect on the expression of ICAM-I in experimental liver fibrosis. *Chin J Clinical Pharmacology and Therapeutics*. 2000, 5(1):49-51.
3. Zheng FR. The current clinical applications of cultured Cordyceps. *Chinese Journal of Hospital Pharmacy*. 1992;12:84.
4. Liu C. et al. Observation of treating post-hepatitis cirrhosis with extracts of Persicae Semen and Cordyceps. *J of Chinese Medicine*. 1991 (7):20.
5. Zhu JL. Et al. The immune regulatory effects of extracts of Persicae Semen and Cordyceps on post hepatitis cirrhosis patients. *Chinese J of Integrative Chinese and Western Medicine*. 1992, 12(4):207.
6. Yang WF, et al. Effect of curcumin on proliferation and extra-cellular matrix secretion of rat hepatic stellate cells in vitro. *Chin J Hepatol*. 20(3):142-143.

7. Zheng YY, et al. The studies on the mechanism of antifibrosis effects of Salvia miltiorrhiza. *Chinese J of Liver Diseases*. 2003, 11(5):288-290.
8. Liu C, et al. Danshensuan A's anti-oxidation action and its effects on the hypertrophy of HSC. *CJITWM on Digestion*. 2001, 9(1):15-16.
9. Cai Y, et al. Glycyrrhizin's effects on the gene expression during the rat liver fibrosis. *Chinese J of Medicine*. 2003, 83(13):1122-1125.
10. Wang H, et al. Chuanxionyzine's effects on liver fibrosis and fat over oxidation. *Chin J of Liver Diseases*. 2000, 8(2):98.
11. Chen ZZ, et al. The experimentally study on Chuanxionyzine's antifibrosis effects. *CJITWM on Liver Diseases*. 1997, 7(3):156-158.
12. Jie YB. Pharmacological Action and Application of Available Composition of Chinese Materia Medica. Harbin, China: Helongjian Science and Technology Press; 1992.
13. Leatherdale BA, Panesar RK, Singh G, et al. Improvement in glucose tolerance due to Momordica charantia (karela). *British Medical Journal*. 1981;282(6279):1823-24.
14. Day C, Cartwright T, Provost J, Bailey CJ. Hypoglycaemic effect of Momordica charantia extracts. *Planta Medica*. 1990;56(5):426-29.
15. *The Great Dictionary of Chinese Materia Medica*. Shanghai, China: Shanghai Science and Technology Press; 1985.
16. Xio JZ, Shi XF, et al. Effect of the total glycocide of Noto ginseng on liver fibrosis in rats type I, III collagen and TGF-β1. *Pharmacol Clin Chin Materia Med*. 2001, 17(2):7-8.
17. Wang YS. The studies on the antifibrosis effects of extracts of persicae semen. The Symposium of International Conference on TCM. Beijing, China's Academic Press; 1987.
18. Ying J, et al. *Modern Studies and Clinical Applications of Chinese Materia Medica, Vol. 1*. Beijing, China: Xue Huan Press; 1994:1214-1215.
19. Chen ZB. The anti-microbial effects of Rhei rhizoma. *Academic Journal of Chinese University of Pharmacy*. 1990;21(6):373.
20. Chen JH, et al. Anti-viral effects of Rhei rhizoma. *Journal of New Medicine*. 1974;(5):34.
21. Gao ZQ, et al. Emodin and Organ Fibrosis. *CJITWM*. 2005, 25(11):1030-1032.
22. Zhan YT, et al. Effect of emodin on development of hepatic fibrosis in rats. *CJITWM*. 2000, 20(4):276-278.
23. Zhan YT, et al. Mechanism of emodin's anti- liver fibrosis effects. *Chin J Hepatol*. 2004, 12(4)245-246.
24. Wang BJ, et al. Blood activating and stasis expelling herbs for chronic hepatitis: Salvia miltiorrhiza. *TCM Hepatology*. Beijing, China; Chinese Medical Technology Press: 1993:96-97.
25. Ma XH, et al. The liver-protective effects of Salvia miltiorrhiza. *Chinese Journal Integrated Traditional and Western Medicine*. 1983;3:180.
26. Bao TT, et al. *Modern Studies of Chinese Materia Medica, Vol. 1*. Beijing, China: Beijing Medical University and Union Medical University Press; 1995:371.
27. Sa JM. Treating chronic viral hepatitis with Sophorae subprostratae radix. *Pharmaceutical Bulletin*. 1983;18(10):37.
28. Yang WZ, et al. Experimental study on preventing and treating fibrosis with Oxymatrine in rats. *Chin J on Digestion*. 2003, 23(3):165-168.
29. Wang GX, et al. The pharmacology and clinical applications of Oxymatrine and matrine. *The Liver*. 2000, 5(6):116-117
30. Liang J, et al. The studies on taurine's antifibrosis effects on CCl4 induced liver fibrosis and its mechanism. *World Oversea-Chinese J of Digestion*. 2003, 11((9):1392-1395.
31. Wang ZR et al. The suppression of ECM expression in fibrotic rats by combined treatment with tetrandrine and glycyrrhizin. *World Oversea-Chinese J of Digestion*. 2003, 11((7):970-974.
32. He YS, et al. The suppressive effects of tetrandrine on collagen protein synthesis of rats fibrosis model. *Chinese J Materia Medica*. 1996, 21(3):177-179.
33. Kimura M. The choleretic effects of Capillaris combination. *Proc Symp WAKAN-YAKU*. 1977;(10):121.
34. Bai G, et al. The Basic Studies and Clinical Applications of TCM Formulas. Beijing, China: Chinese Science and Technology Press; 745.
35. Zheng SX. The study of treating acute jaundice in rat model with Capillaris combination. *Chinese Journal of Integrated Traditional and Western Medicine*. 1985;(6):356.
36. Fan QL. The effects of Persica and Achyranthes combination on microcirculation. *TCM Patent Medicine*. 1988;(7):29.
37. Tianjin First Central Hospital. Treating DIC with Persica and Achyranthes combination. *Chinese Journal of Internal Medicine*. 1977;2(2):79.
38. Liang YJ. Treating nodular vasculitis with Persica and Achyranthes combination. *Journal of TCM*. 1984;(4):44.
39. Liu WX. The effects of Ginseng and Atractylodes combination on intestinal functions on experimental rabbits model. *The Study of TCM Patent Medicine*. 1982;(8):25.
40. Ma YD, et al. Observation on efficacy and experimental study with compound Suanzaoren Ansen capsules for insomnia. *Chinese Journal of Integrated Traditional and Western Medicine*. 1989;9(2):85.
41. Zhou JM. Observation of Yunan paiyao's bleeding-stopping effects. *The Study of TCM Patent Medicine*. 1980;(2):43.
42. Ogle CW, Dai S, Ma JC. The haemostatic effects of the Chinese herbal drug Yunnan Bai Yao: a pilot study. *American Journal Chinese Medicine*. 1976;4(2):147-152.
43. He GM. Yunan pai yao's anti-inflammatory effects. Proceedings of First National Conference of the Association of TCM Materia Medica of China. Beijing, China. 987:949.

Appendix IV: Liver-Toxic Medications and Herbs

The following information is based on an appendix found in The Hepatitis C Help Book and is reprinted with the permission of the publisher, St. Martin's Griffin.

There is a great deal of research still to be done to identify those prescription medications, over-the-counter drugs, herbs and chemicals that are liver toxic. Some substances affect everyone negatively, some are dangerous for people who have liver disease. Others are hazardous when taken in too large a quantity, in combination with other substances or by people who have unusual immune responses.

The following list of suspected or confirmed liver-toxic medications and herbs should help guide anyone with hepatitis. It is not comprehensive, however, and any time a person with liver disease contemplates taking a drug or herb, even when prescribed by a health care practitioner, he or she should be on the lookout for negative reactions. Combining herbs with interferon and/or ribavirin demands particular care. Anyone with HCV should discuss potential reactions and drug interactions with both western and Chinese medicine practitioners before taking any medication or herbal remedy. Although liver-toxic substances are identifiable in the laboratory, liver hypersensitivity problems are not predictable. In some cases, hypersensitivity may result in organ failure. Although hypersensitivity is hard to anticipate, some indicators offer clues as to who may be vulnerable. Indicators of possible negative reactions to medical substances include:

- having multiple allergies and having had previous adverse reactions to drugs or herbs
- a history of chronic skin rashes
- current liver disease

Important! You should discontinue taking any drug or herb if you experience a skin rash, substantial nausea, bloating, fatigue and/or aching in the area of the liver, yellowing of the skin, or pale feces.

Dr. Gish has contributed information on liver-toxic drugs.

David L. Diehl, MD, FACP, an associate clinical professor of medicine at UCLA School of Medicine, focuses on herbal toxicity. He, Ken Flora, MD, formerly of the University of Oregon Health Sciences Center, and Misha Cohen are currently undertaking an extensive survey of the literature concerning the liver toxicity of herbal medicines.

Prescription and Over-The-Counter Drugs

Patients who take the following medications regularly should undergo monthly laboratory testing for the first three months and then every three to six months to check on changes in liver function. Sample brand names are listed after the pharmaceutical name. Other products in addition to those mentioned may contain these drugs. Talk with your doctor and read all package inserts carefully.

- acetaminophen or APAP (Tylenol®), particularly hazardous when taken with alcohol or anti-seizure medications
- alpha-methyldopa (Aldomet®)
- amiodarone (Cordarone®)
- azathioprine (Imuran®, 6-mecaptopurine [6MP])
- carbamazapine (Tegretol®, Epitol®, Mazepine®, Atretol®, Carbatrol®)
- chlorzoxazone (Parfon Forte DSC®, Paraflex®, Chlorzone Forte®, Algisin®)
- dantrolene (Dantrium®)
- diclofenac (Voltaren®, Cataflam®)
- fluconazole or ketoconazole (Diflucan®, Nizoral®)

- flutamide (Drogenil®, Euflex®, Eulexin®)

- hydralazine (Apresolin®, Novo-Hylazin®)

- ibuprofen (Advil®, Motrin®, Nuprin®)

- isoniazid (INH) (Laniazid®, Nydrazid®)

- long-acting nicotinic acid

- leukotriene synthase inhibitors (Zafirlukast®, Accolate® and Zileuton®, Zyflo®)

- methotrexate (Maxtrex®)

- nitrofurantoin (Macrodantin®)

- perihexilene maleate

- phenylbutazone (Mapap®, Marnal®, Lanatuss®)

- phenytoin (Ethotoin®, Mephenytoin®, Dilantin®)

- pravastatin, fluvastatin, simavastatin, lovastatin

- quinidine (Cardoquin®, Cin-Quin®, Duraquin®)

- rifampin (Rifampicin®, Rifadin®, Rimactane®)

- sulfa medications (especially Septra® or Bactrim®)

- tacrine (Cognex®)

- ticlopidine (Ticlid®)

- tolcapone (Tasmar®)

- troglitzone (Rezulin®)

- vitamin A (in doses greater than 5,000 units a day; beta-carotene is safe at all doses)

According to an article published in the April 1996 New England Journal of Medicine, the most common cause of acute liver failure in the United States is the negative interaction between acetaminophen (Tylenol) and alcohol. In addition, there are interactions that are less common but equally as serious. Research suggests individual genetic variations in liver enzymes may be the cause.

Chinese Herbal Perparations

Herbal patent medicines, tonics, elixirs and prepackaged solutions are particularly risky for anyone, whether they have liver disease or not. Ingredient labels may be incomplete or mistranslated. Herbs may be mistakenly used in the concoctions that are dangerous or inappropriate in combination with other herbs. Toxic herbs may be substituted for beneficial ones. The best bet is to avoid self-prescribed premixed preparations. Rely on the best-trained and most experienced herbalist available to individualize your herbal therapy and monitor your reactions.

Some reportedly hazardous herbs and herb formulas:

- **Shosaikoto** – a Japanese preparation used for improving hepatic dysfunction in chronic hepatitis. Its Chinese name is Xiao Chai Hu Tang. It may trigger interstitial pneumonia in people with chronic HCV who also are taking interferon, according to Precautions from the Pharmaceutical Affairs Bureau.

- **Jin Bu Huan** – for insomnia and pain. This formula caused some liver problems but the exact trigger was never identified.

- **Aristolochia** – used to treat fluid retention and rheumatic symptoms; has been banned in England after it was confused with an herb from the clematis plant that has the same name in Chinese as aristolochia: Mu Tong. The Mu Tong used was in fact the toxic species aristolochia rather than the other harmless herb. Aristolochia was part of a formula implicated in seventy cases of kidney failure in Belgium in 1993.

In addition, some Chinese patent medicines may contain heavy metals, poisons, and other potentially liver-toxic substances. In other cases, patent medicines contain western pharmaceutical agents that are not listed on the label.

Common Toxic Ingredients Found in Asian Patent Medicines

Be on guard for these ingredients:

- aconite or aconitum: causes paralysis and death if not highly processed before use
- acorus: causes convulsions and death
- borax: triggers severe kidney damage
- borneol: triggers internal bleeding and death
- cinnabar or calomel: a mercury compound
- litharge and minium: contain lead oxide
- myiabris: can trigger convulsions, vomiting and death
- orpiment or realgar: contains arsenic
- scorpion or buthus: causes paralysis of the heart and death
- strychnos nux vomica or semen strychni: strychnine-containing seeds cause respiratory failure and death
- toad secretion or bufonis: can paralyze heart muscle and lungs

Toxic Individual Herbs

Dr. Diehl writes: "Herbal medicine is generally safe – safer than western pharmaceuticals. There are certain plants that are highly toxic. The most common examples are those that contain pyrolizidine alkaloids." Those that contain alkaloids or that reportedly have triggered toxic reactions include the following.

- Chaparral (creosote bush, greasewood)
- Comfrey (if taken internally)
- Crotalaria (Ye Bai He)
- Eupatorium
- Germander (This toxic herb is often substituted for skullcap, and skullcap is not toxic in well-formulated herbal remedies. However, always insist that any ingredient identified as skullcap be the genuine article and not germander.)
- Groundsel (senecio longilobus)
- Heliotropium
- Mentha pulegium
- Mistletoe
- Pennyroyal (squawmint) oil or Hedeoma pulegoides
- Sassafras
- Senicio species

Special Cases

Licorice: a mainstay of Chinese formulas, licorice is used in very small quantities to balance herbal action and often appears as glycyrrhizin (licorice root). However, licorice produces well-documented side effects such as hyperaldosteronism (an increase in levels of the adrenal hormone aldosterone, triggering imbalance of electrolytes) when taken in doses of more than 50 grams a day or for six weeks or longer. However, no side effects have been seen in smaller doses over thirty days or in higher doses for a very short period of time.

Skullcap: also called scutelleria or scute, this herbv is used in many formulas to good effect. However, it appears that the toxic substance germander often is substituted for skullcap in formulas without being properly identified. As a result skullcap looks like the offending substance. Dr. Diehl found several mentions of skullcap toxicity in the literature, but those mentions may in fact refer to unidentified substitutions of germander. Further research is needed to clarify this. Until then, whenever skullcap appears in a formula, make sure that it, not germander, is in fact being used. If you cannot be sure, do not take the formula or herb.

Dr. Diehl has found one mention of toxicity in the literature for the following herbs. Further documentation of toxicity is needed.

- Calliepsis laureola
- Atractylis gunnifera
- margosa oil
- valerian (Valerian officinalis)

For more detailed information on substances toxic to the liver, please see:
The HIV Wellness Sourcebook, Henry Holt & Misha Cohen, 1998 and *The Hepatitis C Help Book, Revised Edition*, Misha Cohen & Robert Gish, St. Martin's Griffin, 2007.

Disclaimer

The information contained in this Resource Directory is intended as reference material only. The Caring Ambassadors Hepatitis C Program makes no representation nor implies endorsement of any product or service, nor does it accept any responsibility for any claims made by any resources listed.

ORGANIZATIONS AND SUPPORT GROUPS

National Hepatitis C Advocacy Council

P.O. Box 1748

Oregon City, OR 97045

Phone: 503-632-9032

Fax: 503-632-9030

Internet address: www.hepcnetwork.org

The organizations listed below with an asterisk (*) are members of the National Hepatitis C Advocacy Council. The National Hepatitis C Advocacy Council is an association of organizations that creates a unified voice, promotes ethical guidelines, and improves quality of services for people affected by hepatitis C. From this Internet address, you can reach all member sites.

African American Council on Liver Awareness (AACLA)

10515 Blue Ridge Blvd. Suite 207

Kansas City, Missouri 64134

Phone: 1.888.436.HEPC (8472)

Office: 1.816.767.8472

Fax: 1.816.442.8089

Internet address: www.aacla-national.org

The African American Council on Liver Awareness (AACLA) is a national organization promoting viral hepatitis prevention, treatment and research in order to optimize the health of the African American community. Hepatitis C Multicultural Outreach and Strengthened by Grace Ministries are two outreach programs of the AACLA, offer free screening, testing and referral services to underserved communities.

AIDS Community Research Consortium (ACRC)

1048 El Camino Real, Suite B

Redwood City, CA 94063-1633

Phone: 650-364-6563

Fax: 650-364-9001

Internet address: www.acrc.org

ACRC's mission is to improve health and quality of life through compassionate programs that address prominent and emerging public health concerns.

AIDS Treatment Data Network (The Network)

611 Broadway, Suite 613

New York, NY 10012

Phone: 212-260-8868 or (800)734-7104, ext. 16 (toll free in New York)

Fax: 212-260-8869

Internet address: www.atdn.org

The Network provides local and national services to people with HIV and coinfected with HCV/HIV. The Access Project (TheAccessProject@aol.com) is the agency's national treatment advocacy and access program. They advocate for patients and assist providers in obtaining treatments for hepatitis, HIV, and AIDS related conditions.

Alert Health*
660 Northeast 125th Street
North Miami, FL 33161
Phone: 877-HELP-4-HEP
Fax: 305-893-7998
Internet address: www.hep-c-alert.org
Founded as Hep-C ALERT, the organization was a pioneer in the hepatitis C field. ALERT Health's mission is to improve the health and quality of life for people at risk for chronic disease, by providing accessible, integrated preventive health services.   ALERT's clients are offered a variety of counseling and screening options during a single encounter. Services include counseling and testing for hepatitis A, B and C, HIV, and STDs; on-site treatment for bacterial STDs; and vaccination to prevent liver and cervical cancers.

American Liver Foundation*
75 Maiden Lane, Suite 603
New York, NY 10038-4810
Phone: 212-668-1000 or 800-676-9340
Fax: 212-483-8179
Internet address: www.liverfoundation.org
The American Liver Foundation is a national, voluntary, nonprofit health agency dedicated to preventing, treating, and curing hepatitis and all liver diseases.

California Hepatitis Alliance*
Center for Health Improvement
1330 21 Street, Suite 100
Sacramento, California 95811
Phone: 916-930-9200
Internet address: www.calhep.org
The California Hepatitis Alliance (CalHEP) seeks to reduce the scope and consequences of the hepatitis B and C epidemics, which disproportionately affect California's ethnic communities and the socioeconomically underserved. Committed to culturally competent public education and awareness, CalHep focuses on sound public health policy and advocacy to improve California's public health approach to liver wellness.

Caring Ambassadors Hepatitis C Program*
604 East 16th Street, Suite 201
Vancouver, WA 98663
Phone: 360-816-4186
Internet address: www.HepCChallenge.org
The Caring Ambassadors Hepatitis C Program is a national nonprofit organization devoted exclusively to meeting the needs of the hepatitis C community. The mission is to improve the lives of people living with hepatitis C through information and awareness.

HCV Support*
P.O. Box 1077
South Dennis, MA 02660
Internet address: www.hcvsupport.org
HCV Support offers an informational forum and chat room for persons with Hepatitis C. They provide a place to post questions and share personal experiences regarding hepatitis C.

Hep C Advocate Network (HepCAN)*

2023 Seabiscuit Trc. A
Longview, TX 75604
Phone: 903-291-9700
Internet address: www.hepcan.org
HepCAN is devoted to legislative changes for more testing and treatment of HCV infected individuals on the state and national level. They also work to increase professional education about hepatitis C.

Hep C Aware

P.O. Box 3122
North Hollywood, CA 91609
Phone: 818-769-2701
Internet address: www.hepcaware.org
Hep C Aware's mission is to raise public awareness about hepatitis C through community events such as concerts, promotional materials, postcards, and other means.

Hep C Connection*

1325 S. Colorado Boulevard, B-302
Denver, CO 80222
Phone: 303-860-0800 or 800-522-4372
Fax: 303-860-7481
Internet address: www.hepc-connection.org
Hep C Connection provides a hepatitis C network and support system to assist hepatitis C-challenged individuals and their families.

Hepatitis C Association*

1351 Cooper Road
Scotch Plains, NJ 07076
Phone: 866-437-4377
Fax: 908-561-4575
Internet address: www.hepcassoc.org
The Hepatitis C Association focuses on educating the public, creating awareness, promoting organ donation, and offering support to hepatitis patients. They do this through publications, an Internet site, a 24-hour toll-free support line, awareness pins, and educational programs.

Hepatitis C Support Project*

P.O. Box 427037
San Francisco, CA 94142-7037
Phone: 415-587-8908
Internet address: www.hcvadvocate.org
The Hepatitis Support Project offers support to those who are affected by the hepatitis C virus (HCV). Support is provided through information and education, and access to support groups. The Project seeks to serve the HCV community and the general public.

H.E.A.L.S of the South*
PO Box 180813
Tallahassee, FL 32318
Phone: 850-443-8029
Internet address: www.HEALSoftheSouth.org
The goal at HEALS is to expand awareness about liver health through educational programs, literature, and public speaking. Young people, veterans, minorities, and prison populations are some of the groups targeted by HEALS. By educating the public, they hope to aid in the prevention of hepatitis in all its forms.

Hepatitis Education Project*
The Maritime Building
911 Western Ave #302
Seattle WA 98104
Phone: 206-732-0311
Internet address: www.hepeducation.org
The Hepatitis Education Project works to raise awareness about the facts concerning hepatitis patients and the resources available to help those who live with the disease..

Hepatitis Foundation International
504 Blick Drive
Silver Spring, MD 20904-2901
Phone: 301-622 4200
Internet address: www.hepfi.org
Hepatitis Foundation International works to increase awareness of the worldwide problem of viral hepatitis, and to educate the public and health care providers about its prevention, diagnosis, and treatment.

Help & Education for Liver Patients (HELP!)
P.O. Box 2028
Santa Cruz, CA 95063-2028
Phone: 831-462-2979
Internet address: www.myspace.com/help4hcv
HELP! provides support, education, and advocacy for anyone affected by liver disease, especially hepatitis C. The Gordon's have experienced the progression of hepatitis C from having no symptoms to receiving a liver transplant. They provide patient support, community education, and public awareness through meetings, presentations, counseling, e-mail news (available upon request), and other services.

Hepatitis Prevention, Education, Treatment and Support Network of Hawaii (HEPTS)*
3254 Olu Street
Honolulu, HI 96816
Phone: 808-221-6204
Fax: 808-758-5797
E-mail: KenAkinaka@aol.com
HEPTS is the only hepatitis B and C advocacy organization in Hawaii. It offers educational presentations and training opportunities for people with hepatitis and health care professionals.

Hepatitis Research Foundation*
RR 2 Box 12
Verbank, NY 12585
Internet address: www.heprf.org
The Hepatitis Research Foundation's mission is to raise money for research into new treatments for hepatitis.

Latino Organization for Liver Awareness (LOLA)
1560 Mayflower Avenue
Bronx, NY 10461
Phone: 718-892-8967
Internet address: www.lola-national.org
LOLA is a bilingual, bicultural, volunteer organization dedicated to raising awareness of liver disease through prevention, education, and treatment-referral services.

Liver Health Today*
523 N. Sam Houston Parkway East, Suite 300
Houston, TX 77060
Phone: 281-272-2744
Fax: 281-847-5440
Internet address: www.liverhealthtoday.org
Liver Health Today is the only national magazine dedicated to people with hepatitis B and C. The magazine is a bimonthly resource guide to assist hepatitis patients and their families in taking control of their health care by providing current, comprehensive information in one source.

LiverHope*
16807 Canterbury Drive
Minnetonka, MN 55345
Phone: 952-933-0932
Internet address: www.liverhope.com
LiverHope provides support, promotes education, generates awareness, and advocates for quality medical care for all people with hepatitis in the metropolitan Minneapolis and St. Paul area of Minnesota.

MO Hepatitis C Alliance
601 Bus Loop 70 W., Suite 106
Columbia, Mo 65203
Phone: 866-434-1975
Internet address: www.mo-hepc-alliance.org/2/2.htm
The MO Hepatitis C Alliance mission is to provide education, testing, and follow-up care to all people affected by HCV in rural and Mid Missouri. They work to increase awareness of HCV to the general public, healthcare providers, and the corporate community.

National Alliance of State and Territorial AIDS Directors (NASTAD)
444 North Capitol Street, NW, Suite 339
Washington D.C. 20001
Phone: 202-434-8090
Internet address: www.nastad.org
NASTAD strengthens state and territory-based leadership, expertise, and advocacy and brings them to bear in reducing the incidence of HIV infection and on providing care and support to all who live with HIV/AIDS. NASTAD's vision is a world free of HIV/AIDS.

National Viral Hepatitis Roundtable
Internet address: www.nvhr.org
The National Viral Hepatitis Roundtable is a coalition of public, private, and voluntary organizations dedicated to reducing the incidence of infection, morbidity, and mortality from viral hepatitis in the United States through strategic planning, leadership, coordination, advocacy, and research.

New Mexico Hepatitis C Alliance*
PO Box 1106
Albuquerque, NM 87048-1106
Phone: 505-314-6555
Internet address: www.nmhepcalliance.org
The New Mexico Hepatitis C Alliance advocates for equal access to quality hepatitis C treatment, information, education, prevention, and support services for all individuals.

Nor-Cal Hepatitis C Task Force*
P.O. Box 3307
Yuba City, CA 95992
(530) 713-0090
(530) 671-7441 Support Line
Internet address: www.norcalhepc.org
Nor-Cal Hepatitis C Task Force serves Northern California providing awareness, education and support to the medical community, the general public and those affected by the hepatitis C virus.

San Louis Obispo Co. Hepatitis C Project*
P.O. Box 15130
San Luis Obispo, Ca 93406
Phone: 805-543-4372
Internet address: www.slohepc.org
The San Luis Obispo County Hepatitis C Task Force is dedicated to educational outreach, public awareness, and the on-going study of community needs regarding the impact of Hepatitis C in San Luis Obispo county.

The Spears Foundation*
4208 Old Hillsboro Road Suite 8
Franklin, TN 37064
Phone: 888-773-2779
Internet address: www.helpwithhepc.org
The Spears Foundation works to provide current and accurate information about the potentially dangerous liver disease, hepatitis C by enabling people to identify whether they may be at risk and encourage testing.

Status C Unknown*
P.O. Box 735
Medford, NY 11763
Phone: 631-776-8095
Toll-Free 866-466-5086
Internet address: www.statusCunknown.org
Status C Unknown is an awareness organization that is dedicated to dispelling myths regarding hepatitis C. They provide support and education to all communities.

Treatment Action Group
611 Broadway, Ste. 308
New York, NY 10012-2608
Phone: 212-253-7922
Internet address: www.aidsinfonyc.org/tag/index.html
The Treatment Action Group's Hepatitis/HIV Project collaborates with activists, community members, scientists, government, and drug companies to make life-saving information, prevention, and safer, more tolerable, and more effective treatment for viral hepatitis and HIV available to all people who need it. It forges coalitions with activists worldwide to demand universal access to prevention, care and treatment for viral hepatitis and HIV.

Veterans Aimed Toward Awareness (VATA)*
111 West Main St.
Middletown, DE 19709
Phone: 302-378-1415
VATA is a member-run organization of veterans. Their outreach and advocacy is by and for the men and women who served in the nation's military services and their families. VATA seeks political and social change within the veteran's health system, the community, our state, and our country.

GENERAL MEDICAL INFORMATION INTERNET SITES THAT INCLUDE INFORMATION ABOUT HEPATITIS C

Aetna Intelihealth
Internet address: www.intelihealth.com
This site is sponsored by the Aetna, Inc., an insurance company that is part of a larger international conglomerate. This site features Harvard Medical School's Consumer Health Information.

The Alternative Health News On-Line
Internet address: www.altmedicine.com
The Alternative Health News On-Line site provides information on alternative and conventional medicine as it relates to various health issues including hepatitis.

The American Association of Naturopathic Physicians
Internet address: www.naturopathic.org
This official site of the American Association of Naturopathic Physicians offers a variety of resources on naturopathic medicine including a message board, library, and a naturopathic physician finder.

The American College for Advancement in Medicine (ACAM)
Internet address: www.acam.org
The American College for Advancement in Medicine (ACAM) is a nonprofit medical society dedicated to educating physicians and other health care professionals on the latest findings and emerging procedures in preventive/nutritional medicine. ACAM's goals are to improve skills, knowledge, and diagnostic procedures as they relate to complementary and alternative medicine, to support research, and to develop awareness of alternative methods of medical treatment.

The American Board of Medical Specialties (ABMS)
Internet address: www.certifieddoctor.org
The American Board of Medical Specialties (ABMS) site has a public education program, a physician locator, and information services. The board certification status, location by city and state, and specialty of any physician certified by one or more of 24 member boards of the ABMS can be checked through this site. This service is free to consumers. Listed physicians have subscribed to be included in this service.

The American Medical Association (AMA)
Internet address: www.ama-assn.org
The American Medical Association (AMA) site has a consumer health section that includes links to general health issues, specific conditions, your body, your family's health, Kids Health Club, Doctor Finder, Hospital Finder, and a Medical Group Practice Finder. The nutrition section has information on such things as vitamins and fitness. It also has a medical glossary. There is a link to recipes, and new ones are posted every two weeks. This link also has information on health-oriented cookbooks and nutritional resources.

Benson-Henry Institute for Mind Body Medicine
Internet address: www.mbmi.org
The Benson-Henry Institute for Mind Body Medicine at Massachusetts General Hospital is a world leader in the study, advancement, and clinical practice of mind/body medicine. The BHI provides outpatient medical services, training for health professionals, corporate and school-based programs, women's health services, and affiliation for national and international health care systems.

The British Medical Journal
Internet address: www.bmj.com
The British Medical Journal is a free publication with up-to-date information about hepatitis C, among many other topics.

Center for Mindfulness in Medicine, Health Care, and Society (CFM)
Internet address: www.umassmed.edu/cfm
The Center for Mindfulness is an innovative leader in mind-body medicine and mindfulness-based treatment and research investigations, pioneering the integration of meditation and mindfulness into mainstream medicine and health care. They offer a number of pathways for people to cultivate a sense of well-being, confidence, and creativity.

CenterWatch
Internet address: www.centerwatch.com
CenterWatch is a clinical trials listing service of industry and government sponsored trials including recently FDA approved drug therapies.

ClinicalTrials.gov
Internet address: www.clinicaltrials.gov
This site is sponsored by the National Cancer Institute. It provides current information on many clinical trials.

ConsumerLab.com
Vitamins, herbs, and other supplements are not regularly tested by any government organization. ConsumerLab.com continually evaluates nutritional supplements in a laboratory environment. It also investigates problems with drugs.

Doc Misha's Chicken Soup Chinese Medicine
Internet address: www.docmisha.com
This site has general information about Chinese medicine. There is specific information about HIV/AIDS and hepatitis C.

Dr. Koop.com
Internet address: www.drkoop.com
Dr. Koop is a former United States Surgeon General. This site provides up-to-date information on hepatitis C and available treatments.

Dr. Weil.com
Internet address: www.drweil.com
Dr. Andrew Weil is a leader in the integration of western medicine and the exploding field of alternative medicine. This site has extensive information about integrated medicine.

Dr. Zhang.com
Internet address: www.dr-zhang.com
This site provides information on modern Chinese medicine specifically related to hepatitis C. There is also information about some other diseases such as Lyme disease and inflammatory bowel syndrome.

eBioCare.com
Internet address: www.eBioCare.com
This site provides information on risk factors, lifestyle, diet, and treatment options for people living with hepatitis C.

The Glycemic Index
Internet address: www.glycemicindex.com/
Not all carbohydrate foods are created equal, in fact they behave quite differently in our bodies. The glycemic index or GI describes this difference by ranking carbohydrates according to their effect on our blood glucose levels.

Harvard School of Public Health Nutrition Source
Internet address: www.hsph.harvard.edu/nutritionsource/index.html
Harvard School of Public Health Nutrition Source is to provide timely information on diet and nutrition for clinicians, allied health professionals, and the public.

Healthfinder
Internet address: www.healthfinder.gov
The Healthfinder site is easy to navigate and has a tremendous amount of information. There is a lot of good information on hepatitis C and non-western medicine under the "Hot Topics" section. The non-western medicine information includes links for general information, therapies, nutrition and lifestyle information, quackery and fraud, training and associations, and other topics.

Health World On-line
Internet address: www.healthy.net
This comprehensive site provides access to information on a variety of therapies including acupuncture, Ayurveda, Chinese medicine, chiropractic medicine, homeopathy, and others. There are links to finding a health care provider in several different disciplines. This site has links to information on several diseases and conditions including hepatitis.

The Hepatitis B Foundation
Internet address: www.hepb.org
The Hepatitis B Foundation is a national nonprofit organization dedicated to finding a cure for hepatitis B and improving the quality of life of people affected by the illness. There are Chinese, Korean, and Vietnamese language versions of this site.

Hepatitis C Advocacy
Internet address: www.hepcadvocacy.org
This site is dedicated to providing up-to-date information on hepatitis C, HIV, and HCV/HIV co-infection as it relates to federal and state lobbying efforts, and HIV and HCV public policies and funding programs.

Hepatitis C Meditations
Internet address: www.HepCMeditations.org
Hepatitis C Meditations offers a meditation CD to help meet the challenges that hepatitis C brings.

Hepatitis Central
Internet address: www.hepatitis-central.com
Hepatitis Central offers extensive information about all forms of hepatitis including hepatitis A, B, C, D, E, G, autoimmune hepatitis, and more.

Hepatology
Internet address: www.hepatology.org
This site provides access to Hepatology, the official journal of the American Association for the Study of Liver Diseases.

HIVandHepatitis.com
Internet address: www.HIVandHepatitis.com
The staff of HIV and Hepatitis.com state their common objective is to create a quality online publication that provides accurate, timely and cutting-edge information about treatment for HIV/AIDS, chronic hepatitis B and hepatitis C, and co-infection with HIV/HCV and HIV/HBV. This site has an extensive list of consulting editors who review all materials before posting.

ITM On-line (Institute for Traditional Medicine)
Internet address: www.itmonline.org
This is the site of the Institute for Traditional Medicine. The Articles section has a Disorders Index that will take you to articles on hepatitis C. The START Index has good basic information on a wide variety of topics including acupuncture, the best time of day to take herbs, qi gong, the immune system, pregnancy, and Chinese herbs.

The Lancet
Internet address: www.thelancet.com
The Lancet is a peer-reviewed medical journal. You are able to search for articles on hepatitis C and are able to view the abstracts free of charge; full text articles can be viewed for a fee.

Lab Tests Online
Internet address: www.labtestsonline.org/understanding/index.html
Lab Tests Online is designed to help patients and caregivers better understand the many clinical lab tests that are part of routine care as well as diagnosis and treatment of a broad range of conditions and diseases.

National Association of County Veteran Service Officers
Internet address: www.nacvso.org
The National Association of County Veterans Service Officers is an organization made up of local government employees. Their members are tasked with assisting veterans in developing and processing their claims.

National AIDS Treatment Advocacy Project (NATAP)
Internet address: www.natap.org
The NATAP mission is to educate individuals about HIV and hepatitis treatments and to advocate on the behalf of all people living with HIV/AIDS and HCV. The information on the site is scientifically oriented, abundant, and comprehensive in its coverage of both HIV and hepatitis. The site is regularly updated with new articles, studies, and highlights from various major conferences.

National Center for Complementary and Alternative Medicine (NCCAM)
Internet address: www.nccam.nih.gov
The National Center for Complementary and Alternative Medicine (NCCAM) at the National Institutes of Health (NIH) conducts and supports basic and applied research and training and disseminates information on complementary and alternative medicine to practitioners and the public. There are sections on health information, current and completed research, news and events, and alerts and advisories.

The New England Journal of Medicine
Internet address: www.nejm.org
This is the site of the well-respected medical journal, The New England Journal of Medicine. It provides access to the PubMed database from which you can search for and order medical journal articles on hepatitis C.

Net Wellness

Internet address: www.netwellness.com

This site is sponsored by the University of Cincinnati but is a joint project of Case Western Reserve University, Ohio State University, and the University of Cincinnati. The site is a consumer health information site and has sections on current health news, health topics, clinical trials and more.

Oasis, Inc.

Internet address: www.oasisclinic.org

The Organization to Achieve Solutions in Substance Abuse (O.A.S.I.S.) is a nonprofit organization. The primary mission of Oasis is to provide low-cost, subsidized medical care, clinical research studies, and provision of and/or access to social and vocational rehabilitation services for medically marginalized former or current drug and alcohol users.

United Network for Organ Sharing

Internet address: www.unos.org

This is the site of the United Network for Organ Sharing whose mission is to advance organ availability and transplantation. The site has news articles related to organ transplantation.

U.S. Pharmocopeia (USP)

Internet address: www.usp.org

In pursuit of its mission to promote public health, U.S. Pharmocopeia establishes state-of-the-art standards to ensure the quality of medicines for human and veterinary use. USP also develops authoritative information about the appropriate use of medicines. The site has prescription drug information and information about supplements.

The VA National Hepatitis Program

Internet address: www.hepatitis.va.gov

The Veterans Affairs National Hepatitis C Web site provides information about viral hepatitis for health care providers inside and outside the VA system, veterans, and the general public. The "Patient's Corner" area of the site has basic information on hepatitis C for patients, their families, and the general public.

WebMD

Internet address: www.webmd.com

This site is owned by WebMD Corporation. This is a comprehensive on-line resource committed to providing general health information and support. The site is extensive.

Wholistic Healing Research

Internet address: www.WholisticHealingResearch.com

Wholistic approaches empower patients to participate in their own health care. The WHR site is a gateway for you to connect with many wholistic healing approaches through more than 900 pages of references and gateways to experiential learning.

INTERNET SITES ON HARM REDUCTION AND SUBSTANCE ABUSE RESOURCES AND TREATMENT

American Association for the Treatment of Opioid Dependence (AATOD)

Internet address: www.aatod.org

AATOD was founded to enhance the quality of patient care in treatment programs by promoting the growth and development of comprehensive methadone treatment services throughout the United States. AATOD works with federal agencies and state substance abuse authorities concerning opioid treatment policy. The organization offers a program for providers entitled, the Hepatitis Education Training for Opioid Treatment Providers.

Centers for Disease Control and Prevention/Injection Drug Users

Internet address: www.cdc.gov/ncidod/diseases/hepatitis/c/index.htm#idu

This location on the CDC site has links to sources of information about viral hepatitis and its prevention in the setting of injection drug use.

Chicago Recovery Alliance (CRA)

Internet address: www.anypositivechange.org/menu.html

CRA is a racially and ethnically diverse group composed of people living with HIV and drug use, working in addiction treatment, health care, education, law and assorted other areas. See also CRA's better vein care/safer injection guide at www.anypositivechange.org/bvcsi.htm.

Florida Hepatitis and Liver Failure Prevention and Control Program

Internet address: www.doh.state.fl.us/disease_ctrl/aids/hep/index.html

Operated by the Florida Department of Health, this site provides viral hepatitis information, and hepatitis vaccine and testing availability. The Florida Hepatitis C Hotline is toll free at 1-866-FLA-HEPC. The hotline provides hepatitis C education and describes testing options.

Harm Reduction Coalition (HRC)

Internet address: www.harmreduction.org

The Harm Reduction Coalition is committed to reducing drug-related harm among individuals and communities by initiating and promoting local, regional, and national harm reduction education, interventions, and community organizing. HRC fosters alternative models to conventional health and human services and drug treatment; challenges traditional client/provider relationships; and provides resources, educational materials, and support to health professionals and drug users in their communities to address drug-related harm.

Immunization Action Coalition, Model Programs for Hepatitis A, B, and C Prevention

Internet address: www.hepprograms.org/drug/index.asp

This location on the Immunization Action Coalition Internet site provides links to harm reduction programs and resources.

Lifeguard Harm Reduction Services

Internet address: www.lifeguardonline.org

Lifeguard Harm Reduction Services is part of the Partnership for Increasing Harm Reduction Services (PIHRS). This collaborative effort is designed to provide comprehensive harm reduction services for persons who inject drugs.

National Development and Research Institutes, Center for Drug Use and HIV Research

Internet address: cduhr.ndri.org

CDUHR is funded by the National Institute on Drug Abuse. It is the first center for the socio-behavioral study of drug use and HIV in the United States. The Center is dedicated to increasing the understanding of the drug use-HIV/AIDS epidemic, particularly among high-risk individuals. The goal of the Center is to advance knowledge regarding social-level and other influences on HIV-related risk behavior, prevention and transmission. In addition, the Center facilitates the development of timely new research efforts and disseminates information to researchers and service providers.

North American Syringe Exchange Network (NASEN)

Internet address: www.nasen.org

NASEN is dedicated to the creation, expansion and continued existence of syringe exchange programs as a proven method of stopping the transmission of blood borne pathogens in the injecting drug using community. Site contains numerous links to harm reduction information.

Substance Abuse and Mental Health Services Administration (SAMHSA)

Internet address: www.samhsa.gov
SAMHSA is an agency of the U.S. Department of Health and Human Services. SAMHSA's vision is a life in the community for everyone. SAMHSA's mission is to build resilience and facilitate recovery for people with or at risk for substance abuse and mental illness. The SAMHSA site has subsections including, but not limited to:
services for HIV/AIDS and hepatitis (www.samhsa.gov/Matrix/matrix_HIV.aspx)
buprenorphine for the treatment of opiate addiction (www.buprenorphine.samhsa.gov)
substance abuse treatment facility locator (findtreatment.samhsa.gov)
center for substance abuse treatment (csat.samhsa.gov)

INTERNET RESOURCES FOR INFORMATION ON HEALTH CARE PROVIDERS
A Note About Fee-Based Referral Services

Many referral services are fee-based, which means that while they may be free for you to access, health care providers pay a fee to be listed. Therefore, these services do not guarantee the experience level of the health care provider, they just provide general information. It is up to you to find out if a health care provider listed with these services has experience with hepatitis C.

Information and Referral Resources on the Internet for Western (Allopathic and Osteopathic) Healthcare Providers

American Board of Family Medicine (ABFM)

Internet address: www.theabfm.org
The mission of the ABFM is to promote excellence in medical care through educational and scientific initiatives. Through certification and maintenance of certification programs the ABFM pursues its mission by establishing, maintaining, and measuring high standards of excellence in the specialty of Family Medicine. The ABFM seeks to provide assurance to the public that certified family physicians possess the knowledge, skills and attitudes necessary to provide quality care to the individual, family and community through commitment to professional standing, continued competency in the specialty of Family Medicine, and lifelong learning.

American Board of Internal Medicine (ABIM)

Internet address: www.abim.org
For more than 70 years, Certification by the ABIM has stood for the highest standard in internal medicine and its 18 subspecialties and has meant that internists have demonstrated – to their peers and to the public – that they have the clinical judgment, skills and attitudes essential for the delivery of excellent patient care. ABIM is not a membership society, but a non-profit, independent evaluation organization. Our accountability is both to the profession of medicine and to the public.

American Board of Medical Specialties (ABMS)

Internet address: www.certifieddoctor.org
This site has a public education program, a physician locator, and information services. You can verify the board certification status, location by city and state, and specialty of any physician certified by one or more of the 24 member boards of the ABMS. This service is free to consumers but physicians have subscribed to be listed in this service.

American Medical Association

Internet address: www.ama-assn.org
The Doctor Finder link or AMA Physician Select allows you to search for a physician by name or medical specialty.

American Society of Clinical Hypnosis

Internet address: www.asch.net
The American Society of Clinical Hypnosis is the largest U.S. organization for health and mental health care professionals using clinical hypnosis. The site offers a free patient referral system.

National Association of County Veterans Service Officers
Internet address: www.nacvso.org
This site is for veterans who need to locate a local Veterans Service Officer.

Information and Referral Resources on the Internet for Non-Western Healthcare Providers

American Institute of Homeopathy
801 North Fairfax Street, Suite 306
Alexandria, VA 22314
Phone: 703-246-9501
E-mail: aih@bigplanet.com
Internet address: www.homeopathyusa.org

American Naturopathic Medical Association
P.O. Box 96273
Las Vegas, Nevada 89193
Phone: 702-897-7053
Internet address: www.anma.com
The American Naturopathic Medical Association will make referrals to naturopathic physicians and homeopathic practitioners.

HealthWorld On-Line
Internet address: www.healthy.net
This comprehensive site provides links to resources for help in finding a health care provider in several different disciplines.

Institute for Traditional Medicine (ITM)
Internet address: www.itmonline.org
This site has extensive information about CAM disciplines. There are also direct links to other sites on topics such as Chinese medicine, Tibetan medicine, Ayurvedic medicine, Native American medicine, western medicine, and others.

Healthfinder
Internet address: www.healthfinder.gov
This site is sponsored by the U.S. Department of Health and Human Services. In addition to a Health Library, the section entitled Health Care has extensive information about finding quality health care.

CONSUMER AND GOVERNMENT RESOURCES

Americans with Disabilities Act Information Line
Phone: 800-514-0301 (voice) or 800-514-0383 (TDD)

Centers for Disease Control and Prevention
Internet address: www.cdc.gov

Consumer Health Information Research
Phone: 816-228-4595

Department of Justice
Internet address: www.usdoj.gov

Equal Employment Opportunity Commission
For questions:
Phone: 800-669-4000 (voice) or 800-669-6820 (TDD)
To request documents:
Phone: 800-669-3362 (voice) or 800-800-3302 (TDD)

Food and Drug Administration (FDA)
Office of Special Health Issues
Parklawn Building, HF-12
5600 Fishers Lane
Rockville, MD
Phone: 800-FDA-1088
Internet address: www.fda.gov
Contact the FDA to report side effects or other problems with drug treatment.

Food and Nutrition Information Center
National Agricultural Library/USDA
10301 Baltimore Avenue, Room 304
Beltsville, MD 20705-2351
Internet address: www.nal.usda.gov/fnic/pubs/bibs/gen/dietsupp.html
This site provides a dietary supplement resource list.

National Center for Complementary and Alternative Medicine Clearinghouse
Phone: 888-644-6226
Internet address: www.nccam.nih.gov
You can request free information either on-line or by phone.

National Council Against Health Fraud
Phone: 909-824-4690

National Digestive Diseases Info Clearinghouse
Phone: 301-654-3810
Internet address: nddic@info.niddk.nih.gov
You can request free information either on-line or by phone.

National Foundation for Infectious Diseases
Phone: 301-656-0003
Internet address: www.nfid.org

National Institutes of Health
Phone: 301-496-1776
Internet address: www.nih.gov

National Library of Medicine
Internet address: www.nlm.nih.gov

Social Security Disability Line
Phone: 800-772-1213

U.S. Department of Health and Human Services
Internet address: www.healthfinder.com

PHARMACEUTICAL COMPANIES

Roche Patient Assistance Program
Roche Hotline: 877-734-2797
Internet address: www.pegassist.com

Schering "Be in Charge" Program
Phone: 888-437-2608
"Commitment to Care": 800-521-7157
Internet address: www.beincharge.com

Three Rivers Pharmaceuticals Infergen® Aspire Nursing and Reimbursement Program
Phone: 888-668-3393
Internet address: http://www.infergen.com

RECOMMENDED READING

Books on Hepatitis C

Healing Hepatitis C with Modern Chinese Medicine, Qingcai Zhang, M.D.,Sino-Med Institute, New York, NY 2000.

Hepatitis and Liver Disease; What You Need to Know, Melissa Palmer, MD, Avery. Vonore, TN 2000.

Hepatitis C, T. Liang, J. Hoofnagle, et al, Academic Press, San Diego, CA 2000.

Living with Hepatitis C: : A Survivor's Guide, Gregory T. Everson, Hedy Weinberg, John M. Vierling, Hatherleigh, Long Island City, NY 1999.

My Mom Has Hepatitis C, Hedy Weinberg, and Shira Shump, Hatherleigh, Long Island City, NY 2000.

The Hepatitis C Handbook, Matthew Dolan, Iain M. Murray-Lyon, John Tindall, North Atlantic Books, Berkeley, CA 1999.

The Hepatitis C Help Book: : A Groundbreaking Treatment Program Combining Western and Eastern Medicine for Maximum Wellness and Healing, Revised Edition, Misha Ruth Cohen, Robert G., M.D Gish, Kalia Doner (Contributor), St. Martins Griffin, New York, NY 2007.

Other Health Care Books

Alternative Medicine: : The Definitive Guide, Burton Goldberg Group, Future Medicine Publishing, Tiburon, CA 1994.

Between Heaven and Earth: A guide to Chinese Medicine, Harriet Beinfield, L.Ac. , Efrem Korngold, O.M.D., L.Ac., Ballantine Books, New York, NY 1991.

Chinese Herbal Medicine, Formulas and Strategies, Compiled and translated by Dan Bensky and Andrew Gamble, with Ted Kaptchuk, Eastland Press, Vista, CA 1986.

The Chinese Way to Healing:: Many Paths to Wholeness, Misha Cohen, O.M.D., L.Ac., Penquin Putnam, New York, NY 1996.

*Complete Drug Reference, United States Pharmacopeia 200*2. Rockville, MD 2002. (This is an annual publication.)

Discovering Homeopathy: Medicine for the 21st Century, Dana Ullman and Ronald W. Davey, North Atlantic Books, Berkeley, CA 1991.

Eat, Drink and be Wary, T. Graedon, Rodale Inc., Emmaus, PA 2000.

Eating Well for Optimum Health: The Essential Guide to Food, Diet, and Nutrition, Andrew Weil, Alfred A Knopf, New York, NY 2000.

The Encyclopedia of Natural Medicine, M. Murray and J. Pizzorno, Prima Publishing, Roseville, CA 1997.

The Green Pharmacy, J. Duke, St. Martin's Press New York, NY 1998.

Healing and The Mind, Moyers, Bill, Doubleday, New York, NY. 1993.

The HIV Wellness Sourcebook, Misha Cohen, Henry Holt and Company, New York, NY 1998.

Homeopathic Methodology: : Repertory, Case Taking, and Case Analysis: : An Introductory Homeopathic Workbook, M.D.,Todd Rowe, Todd Rowe, Roger Morrison, North Atlantic Books, Berkeley, CA 1998.

The Illustrated Encyclopedia of Healing Remedies; Over 1000 natural remedies for the prevention, treatment, and cure of common ailments and conditions. CN Shealy, Shaftsbury, Dorset, Elephant Books, Gilroy, CA 1998.

Love, Medicine, and Miracles, Siegel, Bernie, MD., HarperCollins Publishers. New York, NY. 1986.

Natural Health, Natural Medicine: A Comprehensive Manual for Wellness and Self-Care, Andrew Weil, Houghton Mifflin Co., Boston, MA 1998.

PDR for Herbal Medicines, J. Gruenwald et al, Medical Economics Co., Montvale, NJ 1998.

The People's Pharmacy to Home and Herbal Remedies, J. Graedon and T. Graedon, St. Martin's Press, New York, NY 1999.

Physicians' Desk Reference (PDR®), Medical Economics Co., Montvale, NJ 2004. (This is an annual publication.)

Pocket Manual of Meterica Medica with Repertory, Boericke, William, M.D., Jain, 1982.

Quantum Healing, Deepak Chopra, Bantam Books, New York, NY 1989.

Repertory of the Homoeopathic Materia Medica, J.T. Kent , South Asia Books, Columbia, MO 1994.

Return of the Rishi, Deepak Chopra, Houghton Mifflin Co., Boston, MA 1988.

The Web That Has No Weaver, Ted Kaptchuk, Contemporary Books, Chicago, IL 1983.

Why People Don't Heal and How they Can, Myss, Caroline, Ph.D., Three Rivers Press, New York NY. 1997.

abstinence – the act or practice of refraining from something such as a food or alcohol

acetaldehyde – a compound produced in the body from the breakdown of alcohol

acetaminophen – an over-the-counter pain reliever; also known by the trade names Tylenol®, Anacin-3®, Datril®, Liquiprin®, Panadol®, Tempra®, and Valadol® and the generic term APAP; acetaminophen is found in many over-the-counter cold and sinus medicines

activated B cell – see plasma cell

acute hepatitis – a course of hepatitis (liver inflammation) that resolves in six months or less

adjuvant – a substance that enhances the effect of a drug or treatment; a substance added to a vaccine to increase the immune response to the vaccine

advocate – a person who works for the benefit and rights of others

AFP – see alfa-fetoprotein

alanine aminotransferase (ALT) – an enzyme found in liver cells and other cells of the body; measuring blood levels is an indicator of liver cell damage and/or death

albumin – a protein made by the liver; blood levels are used to check liver function

alcohol – the intoxicating substance in beer, wine, and hard liquors; also found in some over-the-counter products such as mouthwashes and cold remedies; also known as ethanol

alk phos – see alkaline phosphatase

alkaline phosphatase – an enzyme found in nearly every tissue of the body but found in the highest concentrations in the liver and bones; elevated levels often indicated blocked bile flow either inside or outside the liver; also known as ALP

ALP – see alkaline phosphatase

ALP isoenzymes

alfa-fetoprotein – a protein produced by liver cells normally found in only trace amounts in the body; the blood test for this substance is used to screen for liver cancer (hepatocellular carcinoma)

alfa glucosidase inhibitors – drugs that delay the digestion of sugars (carbohydrates); used to treat type II or adult onset diabetes mellitus

ALT – see alanine aminotransferase

amantadine – a drug used to prevent cells from being infected by a virus by interfering with the virus' ability to enter the cell

amino acid – one of a group of substances that are the building blocks of proteins

aminopyrine clearance test – test used to determine how well the liver is metabolizing and detoxifying substances; a test of liver function

aminotransferase – see alanine aminotransferase and aspartate aminotransferase

ammonia – a chemical normally found in very low levels in the blood that comes from the normal breakdown of proteins in the body; elevated levels are present in severe liver failure and hepatic encephalopathy

ANA – see anti-nuclear antibodies

analogue – a molecule or substance that closely resembles another substance and may act like the original substance in some ways; sometimes called an isomer

anasarca – generalized swelling (edema) of the body due to an abnormal accumulation of fluid in the tissues; can be seen in severe liver failure

anecdotal – referring to an anecdote (see below)

anecdote – in medicine, an account of one person's experience usually with a particular treatment

anemia – a condition in which the blood is deficient in red blood cells and/or hemoglobin; a condition that reduces the blood's ability to carry oxygen to the tissues

antibody (pl. antibodies) – a protein produced by the immune system usually in response to infecting organisms such as bacteria or viruses; antibodies are one way the immune system tries to rid the body of infection

antifibrosis – in liver disease, refers to the slowing of scar tissue in the liver that forms as a result of ongoing inflammation

antigen – a protein that stimulates the immune system to produce antibodies; derived from the words "antibody generator"

anti-HCV antibody – any of a number of antibodies produced by the immune system in response to the hepatitis C virus; the presence of these antibodies in the blood indicate that the person has been exposed to the hepatitis C virus; the screening test for hepatitis C (the anti-HCV test) detects these antibodies in the blood

anti-liver-kidney microsomal antibodies – an autoantibody; see autoantibodies for additional details

anti-LKM – see anti-liver-kidney microsomal antibodies

anti-nuclear antibodies (ANA) – an autoantibody; see autoantibodies for additional details

antioxidant – a substance that inhibits the chemical process called oxidation; in hepatitis C, antioxidants are used to limit damage done by high levels of free radicals present because of ongoing inflammation caused by the virus

antiproliferative – having the effect of decreasing the ability of something to rapidly grow and increase in number

antisense – in drug development, a small molecule that binds to part of the genetic material of a target substance (such as the hepatitis C virus) to stop specific metabolic (life sustaining) functions; in hepatitis C, researchers are trying to develop antisense drugs that will prevent HCV replication (reproduction)

anti-SMA – see anti-smooth muscle antibodies

anti-smooth muscle antibodies – an autoantibody; see autoantibodies for additional details

antiviral – an agent that kills viruses or suppresses their replication (reproduction)

apoptosis – process of programmed cell death, which causes the cell to die within a specific timeframe

APTT – see partial thromboplastin time

arthralgia – pain in one or more joints

ascites – abnormal accumulation of fluid in the abdomen; a common complication of portal hypertension

aspartate aminotransferase (AST) – an enzyme found in liver cells and other cells of the body; measuring blood levels is an indicator of liver cell damage and/or death

AST – see aspartate aminotransferase

asymptomatic – without symptoms

autoantibody (pl. autoantibodies) – abnormal antibodies that act against the body's own tissues because it has mistaken them for foreign; more than half of all people with chronic hepatitis C have one or more autoantibodies in their blood

autoimmune – a condition characterized by the production of abnormal antibodies that attack the body's own tissues

B cell – an immune cell that when activated produces antibodies; the cells responsible for the body's humoral (antibody) immune response; also known as B lymphocyte

B cell lymphoma – a form of B cell cancer

b-DNA – see branched DNA test for HCV

B lymphocyte – see B cell

bicarbonate – a charged particle called an electrolyte; blood level may be abnormal in liver failure and a variety of other diseases

bile – a yellowish green fluid made by the liver from bile salts, bilirubin (broken-down red blood cells), cholesterol, and other substances; the fluid stored in the gallbladder; the fluid released from the gallbladder into the intestine to help fat digestion

bile acids – a group of chemicals produced by the breakdown of cholesterol; levels are often abnormal with liver and/or gallbladder disease

bilirubin – a yellow-orange substance generated in the liver from the breakdown of hemoglobin from old red blood cells; the substance that causes jaundice when blood levels are abnormally high; blood levels are one indicator of liver function

> **conjugated bilirubin (direct bilirubin)** – bilirubin that is attached to another chemical called glucuronic acid in a process called conjugation. Conjugation takes place inside liver cells. Conjugated bilirubin is excreted in the bile. Normally, conjugated bilirubin makes up less than 10% of the total bilirubin.

> **total bilirubin** – the sum of both the conjugated and unconjugated bilirubin

> **unconjugated bilirubin (indirect bilirubin)** – Unconjugated bilirubin has not undergone the conjugation process in the liver. Normally, unconjugated bilirubin makes up over 90% of the total bilirubin.

biofeedback – a way of monitoring small changes in the body with the aid of sensitive machines; a technique used to teach people to control bodily functions such as blood pressure, temperature, blood flow, gastrointestinal functioning, and brain wave activity

bleeding esophageal varices – see varix

blood serum – the liquid part of blood; the liquid that separates from blood when it clots completely

blood sugar – see glucose

blood urea nitrogen – a chemical produced by the liver in the process of breaking down proteins; blood levels are used to monitor kidney function and to a lesser extent, liver function

body mass index (BMI) – a measure of a person's weight in proportion to height; an indicator of being over or underweight; calculated by dividing your weight (in kilograms) by your height in meters squared; a healthy BMI for adults is between 18.5 and 24.9

bone marrow suppression – inhibition of the body's ability to produce blood cells that are normally produced in the bone marrow

branched DNA test for HCV (b-DNA) – test used to check for the presence of the hepatitis C virus in the blood; test used to check viral load

BUN – see blood urea nitrogen

caffeine – the stimulating chemical in coffee, black teas, colas, chocolate, and other foods; processed (metabolized) by the liver; caffeine metabolism reflects the adequacy of the liver's metabolic functions

calcium – a charged particle called an electrolyte; needed for many important functions of the body including bone formation and muscle contractions; can be abnormally high or low in various types of liver disease

CAM – see complementary and alternative medicine

caput medusae – enlarged, visible veins that start at the navel and spread out and up over the abdomen; caused by portal hypertension

carbohydrate – a sugar (simple carbohydrate) or starch (complex carbohydrate); a food component found in sugars, certain vegetables, grains, and beans

carbon tetrachloride-induced hepatotoxicity – liver damage resulting from exposure to carbon tetrachloride (CCl4); liver damage caused by exposure to any of a number of substances containing CCl4 such as dry cleaning fluid, solvents, rubber waxes, and resins

carcinogenic – capable of causing cancer

cardinal signs – signs that indicate the presence of a specific disease or condition

cardiovascular – relating to the heart and blood vessels

CBC – see complete blood count

CD4 cell – an immune cell that participates in the body's cellular immune response; the cell that is the main target of the human immunodeficiency virus; immune cells that help turn on the body's immune response; also known as T4 cell or T helper cell (sometimes called Th1 and Th2 cells) *Th1 and Th2 cells*)

CD4 count, absolute – the number of T helper cells in a cubic millimeter of blood; also called a T4 count

CD8 cell – an immune cell that participated in the body's cellular immune response; cells that destroy virus infected cells and cause transplant rejection; also known as T8 cell, T suppressor cell, and cytotoxic T cell)

CD81 – a protein on the surface of cells including liver cells; another term for TAPA-1 molecule (target of an antiproliferative antibody); may be a binding site for the hepatitis C virus that allows it to enter cells

cell-mediated immunity – one of the two branches of the immune system that defends the body through the actions of specialized immune cells such as cytotoxic T cells

chemotherapy – the use of chemical agents to treatment or control disease; commonly refers to drugs used to kill cancer cells

chloride – a charged particle called an electrolyte; one of the four major electrolytes in the body; levels may be abnormal in advanced liver failure

cholestasis – slowed or blocked bile flow; may be associated with elevated bilirubin levels

cholesterol – a lipid or fat that is both absorbed from the food we eat and manufactured by the liver; blockage of bile flow either inside or outside the liver increases the amount of cholesterol in the blood

chronic hepatitis – a course of hepatitis (liver inflammation) that lasts more than six months

cirrhosis – scarring of the liver that has progressed to the point that the structure of the liver is abnormal; the stage of liver disease that follows if there is progressive fibrosis

cis – a chemical prefix that refers to a specific arrangement of chemical bonds; the opposite of this chemical arrangement is known as trans

Cl – see chloride

clearance – see spontaneous clearance

clinical – in medicine, anything related to disease that can be observed or diagnosed in a patient

clinical trial – process used to evaluate the effectiveness and safety of new medications, procedures, or medical devices by monitoring their effects on large groups of people; the testing usually required by the Food and Drug Administration before approving a new drug, procedure or medical device

> **phase I trial** – This is the first clinical trial for studying an experimental drug or treatment in humans. Phase I trials are usually small (10-100 people) and are used to determine safety and the best dose for a drug. These trials provide information about side effects, and how the body absorbs and handles the drug. People in these trials usually have advanced disease and have already received the best available treatment.

> **phase II trial** – Phase II trials examine whether a drug or therapy is active against the disease it is intended to treat. Side effects are studied. A phase II trial is a noncomparative study, meaning the therapeutic effects and side effects of the experimental treatment are not compared to another drug or a placebo.

> **phase III trial** – Phase III trials are conducted to find out how well a drug or therapy works compared to standard treatment or no treatment. Phase III trials are large studies and usually involve several hundred to thousands of patients.

> **controlled clinical trial** – A controlled clinical trial divides participants into study groups to determine the effectiveness and safety of a new treatment. One group receives the experimental treatment; the other group receives placebo (an inactive substance) or the standard therapy. This group is called the control group. Comparison of the experimental group with the control group is the basis of determining the safety and effectiveness of the new treatment.

> **randomized clinical trial** – A randomized clinical trial involves patients who are randomly (by chance) assigned to receive either the experimental treatment or the control treatment (placebo or standard therapy).

CMV – see cytomegalovirus

collagen – fibrous protein that is one of the main components of scar tissue (fibrotic tissue); a component of bones, cartilage, tendons, and other connective tissues

combination therapy – therapy that involves two or more components that can be drugs, procedures, or other specific treatments

complementary and alternative medicine (CAM) – medical practices that are not routinely taught at western medical schools; medical disciplines other than allopathic medicine including traditional Chinese medicine, acupuncture, Ayurvedic medicine, naturopathy, homeopathy, chiropractic medicine, massage therapy, aromatherapy, and others

complete blood count (CBC) – a blood test that includes measurements of white blood cells, red blood cells, hemoglobin, hematocrit, platelets, and possibly others

conjunctiva – the lining of the inner surfaces of the eyelid and the exposed surface of the eyeball

conjunctival capillaries – the tiny blood vessels of the conjunctiva

contraindicate –in medicine, a condition or other reason not to use a particular drug or treatment

contraindication – see contraindicate

controlled clinical trial – see clinical trial

coproporphyrin – a substance produced in the liver and bone marrow during the process of making a chemical called heme; blood levels reflect how well the liver is performing its job of making heme

creatinine – a waste product of muscle cell metabolism; used to check for hepatorenal syndrome in people with cirrhosis and liver failure

cryoglobulin – abnormal blood protein formed when several antibody molecules (gamma globulins) clump together; protein in the condition cryoglobulinemia that can cause abnormal blood clots in the brain (stroke), eyes, and/or heart

cryoglobulinemia – the presence of abnormal antibodies called cryoglobulins in blood; the condition may lead to kidney damage, kidney failure, and a variety of other symptoms; this condition is commonly found in people with chronic hepatitis C

cure – in hepatitis C, sustained viral clearance is considered a cure; undetectable hepatitis C virus in the blood for six or more months after the completion of treatment

cytokine – a small protein released by cells that has specific effects on other cells; proteins that carry the signals for many of the immune system responses

cytomegalovirus (CMV) – any of a group of viruses in the herpes virus family that cause infections in humans and animals; a virus that usually does not cause disease in healthy adults, but can cause disease in people with immune suppression such as those with HIV/AIDS or transplant recipients

cytopathic – relating to disease or deterioration of cells; direct damage to cells

cytotoxic T cell – a member of the T lymphocyte family of white blood cells; acts to destroy cells marked for destruction by the immune system as part of the body's cellular immune response

decoction – in traditional Chinese medicine, a strong tea made by combining herbs with cold water, bringing the mixture to a boil, and simmering it for 10-20 minutes

decompensation – in the liver, the inability of the liver to regenerate itself and compensate for damage it has sustained; liver damage that has progressed to the point that the liver functions begin to deteriorate

dehydration – in medicine, the condition when the body is deficient in water

delta hepatitis – see hepatitis, hepatitis D

deoxyribonucleic acid (DNA) – the type of molecule that human genes are made of; the molecule that carries all genetic information in humans

depression – a mental condition characterized by apathy, lack of emotional expression, social withdrawal, changes in eating and sleep patterns, and fatigue; a mental condition that can accompany any life-changing event including being diagnosed with a chronic illness; a possible side effect of interferon/ribavirin therapy

dextrose – see glucose

direct bilirubin – see bilirubin, conjugated bilirubin

distend – to swell out or expand from internal pressure; in hepatitis C, ascites causes distension of the abdomen

DNA – see deoxyribonucleic acid

durable response – see sustained response

dyspnea – difficult or labored breathing

edema – swelling due to an excess fluid (water) in the body; most often seen in the lower legs and feet, but also seen in the hands

EIA – see enzyme immunoassay

electrolyte – in medicine, a dissolved chemical that carries either a positive or negative charge; commonly refers to sodium, potassium, chloride, bicarbonate, calcium, and phosphate

emaciation – extreme thinness; generally the result of starvation or severe illness

encephalopathy – see hepatic encephalopathy

endogenous interferon - a naturally-occurring protein produced by the immune system in response to attack by a virus that helps protect other healthy cells from attack

endorphin – a substance produced in the brain, spinal cord, and other parts of the body that causes elevated mood, reduced pain, and reduced stress; the body's natural pain killer; a substance released by the body during exercise

enzyme – a protein that starts and/or propels a specific chemical reaction; commonly tested liver enzymes include ALT, AST, and GGT

enzyme immunoassay (EIA) – one of the tests used to detect antibodies to HCV (anti-HCV antibody)

epitope – specific amino acid sequence of a foreign antigen, such as the hepatitis C virus, that an antibody recognizes, binds to, and reacts against

erythema nodosum – a type of skin inflammation that results in reddish, tender lumps most commonly located in the front of the legs below the knees

esophageal varices – see varix

ethanol – see alcohol

exogenous – derived or produced outside the body

extracellular – outside of a cell

extrahepatic – situated or originating outside the liver

fatigue – the state of extreme tiredness that is usually not relieved by rest or sleep

fatty liver – a condition in which the liver cells contain an abnormal amount of fat

Fe – see iron

ferritin – a protein that binds iron; tested to check the amount of iron in the body

fibrinogen – a protein that when activated by the clotting (coagulation) system turns into fibrin, an essential component of a blood clot; measured in liver disease to check the liver's protein-making ability; a test of liver function

fibroblastic – referring to cells or cell activities that lead to the formation of fibrous tissue or scarring

fibrocatalytic

fibrosis – in liver disease, the laying down of scar tissue in the liver; usually the result of ongoing inflammation

FIBROSpect™ – a proprietary set of blood tests used together to differentiate no/mild liver fibrosis from severe fibrosis; this is not a substitute for liver biopsy but can possibly provide some useful information for people who cannot or do not wish to have a liver biopsy

fibrous – composed of or containing fibers; scar-like

flatulence – excess gas in the lower intestinal tract

flavinoid – a vitamin A-like substance found in many fruits and vegetables; many flavinoids are powerful antioxidants

free radical – a highly reactive chemical that oxidizes other chemicals in the body; the chemicals that cause oxidative stress in the body; the chemicals that cause oxidative damage in the body; chemicals normally produced in the body and neutralized by antioxidants; chemical produced in excessive amounts by chronic infection and/or inflammation

fulminant liver failure – severe and rapidly progressive liver cell death

galactosamine – a compound made in the body consisting of sugar and protein molecules that is used in the production of certain types of tissue; can be toxic to the liver; used in animal experiments to cause liver damage

gamma globulin – see immune globulin

gamma-glutamyl transferase (GGT) – a liver enzyme (protein); blood GGT levels are measured to check for liver damage associated with slow or blocked bile flow; GGT is elevated in all forms of liver disease

gastroenterologist – a doctor who specializes in diagnosing and treating diseases of the digestive system including the liver

gastroesophageal varices – see varix

gastrointestinal – having to do with the digestive tract, which includes the mouth, esophagus, stomach, and intestines

gene – the material that encodes for all inherited traits and characteristics of a living thing; a piece of DNA (deoxyribonucleic acid) the carries the message for a particular trait or characteristic

genetic – having to do with the digestive tract, which includes the mouth, esophagus, stomach, and intestines

genome – all the genetic information of a particular organism

genotype – in hepatitis C, one of several different species of the hepatitis C virus; different genotypes have different responses to interferon-based therapy; different genotypes have some differences in the genes they contain

genotype test – a test to identify the specific genotype of the HCV virus

GGT – see gamma-glutamyl transferase

GGTP – see gamma-glutamyl transferase

glomerulonephritis – a kidney disease in which the filtering units of the kidney (the glomeruli) are damaged; the disorder is characterized by edema (swelling), elevated blood pressure, and excess protein in the urine

glossitis – inflammation of the tongue; usually accompanied by redness and uncomfortable soreness

glucose – the form of sugar found in the blood; the breakdown product of simple and complex carbohydrates that can be used by the body; also known as dextrose or blood sugar

glutamate oxaloacetate transaminase (GOT or SGOT) – see aspartate aminotransferase

glutamate pyruvate transaminase (GPT or SGPT) – see alanine aminotransferase

glutathione – a protein formed in the liver that plays an important role in the immune system; the body's most abundant natural antioxidant (protects against free radical damage)

glycemic index – a scale for evaluating foods, based on the rate at which sugar is absorbed into the bloodstream after eating a specific food

glycemic load – a ranking system for carbohydrate content in food portions based on their glycemic index and the portion size

glycogen – a large molecule made up of smaller glucose molecules; the storage form of glucose primarily formed in the liver

glycoprotein – a compound made of protein and carbohydrate (sugar); also known as glucoprotein

GOT – see aspartate aminotransferase

GPT – see alanine aminotransferase

grade – in liver biopsy, a term used to describe the amount of inflammation in the liver; the higher the grade, the greater the inflammation

HAV – see hepatitis, hepatitis A

HBcAg – hepatitis B core antigen; a blood marker of active hepatitis B infection

HbeAg – hepatitis B e antigen; a blood marker of active hepatitis B infection

HbsAg – hepatitis B surface antigen; a blood marker of active hepatitis B infection

HBV – see hepatitis, hepatitis B

HCC – see hepatocellular carcinoma

HCT – see hematocrit

HCV – see hepatitis, hepatitis C

HCV antibody – see anti-HCV antibody

HCV-EIA – see anti-HCV antibody

HCV PCR – see HCV polymerase chain reaction

HCV polymerase chain reaction (PCR) – test to check for the presence of the hepatitis C virus in the blood; a qualitative HCV PCR test determines the presence or absence of virus in the blood; a quantitative HCV PCR test measures the amount of detectable HCV in the blood

HCV RNA – hepatitis C virus ribonucleic acid; the genetic material of HCV

HCV TMA – see transcription mediated amplification

helicase – an enzyme used in viral replication; it enables the genetic material to uncoil so it can be replicated

hematemesis – vomiting of blood

hematocrit – the percentage of the blood made up by red blood cells

heme – the iron-containing portion of hemoglobin, the substance in red blood cells that enables them to carry oxygen

hemochromatosis – a hereditary disease caused by increased absorption and excessive storage of iron in the tissues, especially the liver; the untreated disorder can lead to cirrhosis of the liver, heart disease, diabetes mellitus, testicular atrophy, and arthritis

hemoglobin – the protein in red blood cells that carries oxygen

hemoglobinopathy – a group of hereditary disorders characterized by abnormal hemoglobin structure; sickle cell anemia is an example

hemolytic anemia – anemia due to increased destruction of red blood cells; can be a side effect of ribavirin therapy

hemorrhoids – enlarged, fragile veins found around the anus (the opening through which bowel movements pass); can lead to bleeding, discomfort, and itching; may be associated with portal hypertension

hepatic – relating to the liver

hepatic cell – see hepatocyte

hepatic encephalopathy – a complication of liver failure that results from large amounts of ammonia that accumulate in the brain; symptoms include euphoria, depression, confusion, slurred speech, abnormal sleeping patterns, incoherent speech, tremors, rigid muscles, and eventually coma

hepatitis – inflammation of the liver

hepatitis A – a disease caused by the hepatitis A virus (HAV); transmitted by food or drink that has been contaminated by an infected person; symptoms include nausea, fever, and jaundice (yellowing of the skin and/or eyes); hepatitis A does not progress to chronic hepatitis

hepatitis B – a disease caused by the hepatitis B virus (HBV); transmitted sexually or by contact with infected blood; hepatitis B may progress to chronic hepatitis and can be fatal

hepatitis C – a disease caused by the hepatitis C virus (HCV) C; transmitted by contact with infected blood via contaminated needles and transfusion of infected blood products; rarely transmitted sexually; hepatitis C becomes chronic in 85% of people infected and can be fatal in a small percentage of cases

hepatitis D, delta hepatitis – a disease caused by the hepatitis D virus; transmitted via infected blood, contaminated needles, or sexual contact with an infected person; the virus only causes disease in patients who already have HBV

hepatitis E – a disease caused by the hepatitis E virus; transmitted via food or drink handled by an infected person, or through infected water supplies in areas where fecal matter may get into the water; more common in tropical and subtropical regions of the world than in the United States and Canada

hepatitis C screening test – see anti-HCV antibody

hepatocellular carcinoma (HCC) – the most common malignant tumor of the liver; chronic hepatitis B and C are risk factors for this cancer especially in those with cirrhosis; also known as liver cancer, hepatoma, and HCC

hepatocyte – liver cell; also known as hepatic cell

hepatologist – a doctor whose practice is limited to diseases and disorders of the liver

hepatoma – see hepatocellular carcinoma

hepatomegaly – liver enlargement

hepatoprotective – protective of the liver

hepatotoxic – toxic to the liver

herbicide – a substance used to kill plants

histologic – pertaining to study of the microscopic structure, composition, and function of tissues; sometimes written as histological

histological – see histologic

histology – the study of the form of cells and tissues that can only be seen with the microscope; also called microscopic anatomy

HIV – see human immunodeficiency virus

hives – see urticaria

hormone – a substance produced in the body that controls and regulates the activity of other cells or organs; most hormones are secreted by specialized glands such as the thyroid gland; they control digestion, metabolism, growth, reproduction, mood and other essential body functions

human immunodeficiency virus (HIV) – the virus that causes AIDS (acquired immunodeficiency syndrome); HIV infection weakens the body's immune defenses by destroying CD4 lymphocytes (T cells)

humoral immunity – one of the two branches of the immune system that protects the body from infections through the use of antibodies

hyperglycemia – high amounts of glucose (sugar) in the blood

hypertension – high blood pressure

hyperthyroidism – a condition caused by excess production of thyroid hormone resulting from an overactive thyroid gland

hypoactivity – abnormally reduced activity

hypochondrium – area of the upper abdomen below the ribs

hypothyroidism – deficiency of the thyroid hormone from the thyroid gland

ibuprofen – a non-steroidal anti-inflammatory drug (NSAID) commonly used to treat pain, swelling, and fever. Common brand names for Ibuprofen include Advil®, Motrin®, and Nuprin®

IFN – see interferon

Ig – see immunoglobulin

IL-10 (interleukin 10) – an anti-inflammatory and immunosuppressive cytokine; normally produced in the body at sites of injury and inflammation; controls the degree of inflammation

immune globulin – a concentrated preparation of gamma globulins (antibodies) taken from a large group of human donors that is given by injection for the treatment of specific diseases; used to treat hepatitis A in people already infected with HBV and/or HCV; also known as gamma g

immune system – a complex group of cells and organs that collectively protect the body from bacterial, parasitic, fungal, and viral infections and from the growth of tumor cells; includes T-helper cells (CD4 cells), T-suppressor cells, natural killer cells, B cells, granulocytes (polymorphonuclear leukocytes), macrophages, dendritic cells, the bone marrow, the thymus gland, the spleen, and the lymph nodes

immunity – the condition of being protected from an infectious disease either by the action of the immune system or immunization (vaccines)

immunodeficiency – a defect in the functioning of the immune system which renders the body more susceptible to illness

immunogen – see antigen

immunoglobulin – proteins that act as antibodies in the body; produced by plasma cells and B lymphocytes; part of the humoral immune response; antibodies that attach to foreign substances such as bacteria and viruses and assist in destroying them; also known as Ig

immunologist – a person who studies or practices medicine in the area of immunology

immunomodulator – a chemical agent that modifies the immune response or the functioning of the immune system

immunopathic – substances or processes that are harmful to the immune system

immunopathologic – see immunopathic

immunosuppressive – substances or processes that decrease the immune response

immunotherapy – treatment to stimulate or restore the ability of the immune system to fight infection and disease; a treatment that acts by stimulating or working with the immune system

indirect bilirubin – see bilirubin, unconjugated bilirubin

inference – the act of drawing logical conclusions from known facts or facts assumed to be true

inflammation – a localized tissue reaction to irritation, injury, or infection; usually characterized by swelling, redness, pain, and sometimes loss of function; abnormally intense inflammation can cause tissue damage as in chronic hepatitis C

insulin – the hormone that controls the level of glucose in the blood; allows glucose to move from the blood into cells; produced in the pancreas by specialized cells called beta cells

integrative medicine – an approach to medicine that combines aspects of many medical disciplines; usually includes western medicine and any number of complementary and/or alternative medicine (CAM) approaches

interferon – any of a group of glycoprotein cytokines that occur naturally in the body; they can have antiviral, and antibacterial actions; synthetic interferons are used to treat a number of diseases; interferons on the basis for current western therapy for chronic hepatitis C

interferon-based therapy – any therapy that uses interferon as the main component; interferon-based therapy is currently the standard treatment of chronic hepatitis C in western (allopathic) medicine

interleukin 10 – see IL-10

interstitial – in biology, pertaining to the small, narrow spaces between tissues or parts of an organ

intracellular – inside the cell; HCV and HIV are intracellular viruses

in vitro – literally means in glass; something that is observed in a laboratory setting (as opposed to observations made in animals or people)

in vivo – something that is observed in a living organism, either animals or people

iron – a metal found in red blood cells; helps red blood cells carry oxygen to all the cells of the body

jaundice – yellowish discoloration of the skin and whites of the eyes caused by abnormally high amounts of bilirubin in the body

lactate dehydrogenase – an enzyme found in many cells of the body but highly concentrated in liver, heart, and muscle cells; elevated blood levels may indicate liver cell damage

lassitude – weariness, listlessness, or reduced energy

LDH – see lactate dehydrogenase

lethargy – a state of sluggishness, inactivity, and apathy

LFT – see liver function test(s)

lichen planus – a recurrent skin rash characterized by small, flat-topped, many-sided (polygonal) bumps that can grow together into rough, scaly patches on the skin; may occur in the lining (mucous membrane) of the mouth or vagina

LIPA assay – see genotype test

lipid – fat; there are many different types of fats in the diet and in the body such as cholesterol and triglyceride; some fats are healthful and necessary for good health; some fats are harmful and play a role in various diseases including hepatitis C; includes fatty acids, neutral fats, and waxes

lipodystrophy – any of a group of conditions due to defective metabolism of fat that results in loss or redistribution of fat; believed to be a side effect of some HIV medications although the virus itself may also contribute to this condition; fat is usually redistributed from the face, arms, and legs into the abdomen and back

lipoprotein – a lipid-protein complex; the form in which fats are transported in the blood; responsible for transporting cholesterol and triglycerides and other fats from the liver to other parts of the body

liver biopsy – the removal and subsequent microscopic examination of small samples of liver tissue; the only reliable method to determine the amount of damage done to the liver by the hepatitis C virus; performed by inserting a long needle through the skin into the liver

liver cancer – see hepatocellular carcinoma

liver enzyme – any of the many enzymes present in liver cells including ALT, AST, GGT, LDH, alkaline phosphatase, and others; liver enzymes are monitored in chronic hepatitis C to determine the amount of ongoing damage occurring in the liver

liver failure – a state in which the liver is unable to adequately perform its many functions; usually the result of end-stage cirrhosis; characterized by clotting abnormalities, protein abnormalities, abnormal electrolytes, and many other signs and symptoms

liver function test(s) (LFT) – any of a number of tests used to check for liver function; includes bilirubin, albumin, prothrombin time, total protein, and many others.

living donor liver transplantation – a new procedure involving the transplantation of a portion of a liver from a living donor to replace a failed liver; both livers can grow to normal size

loins – the region of the hips, groin, and lower abdomen

lymph – see lymphatic fluid

lymph node – small clusters of immune cells, especially lymphocytes, located throughout the body along the channels of the lymphatic system; found in the underarms, groin, neck, chest, abdomen, and other areas throughout the body; also called lymph glands

lymph system – see lymphatic system

lymphatic fluid – the colorless slightly opaque fluid that travels through vessels called lymphatics that connect the lymph nodes in the body; carries immune cells that help fight infection and disease

lymphatic system (lymph system) – the network of lymph nodes and lymph vessels (lymphatics) in the body; lymph nodes are small, tightly packed collections of lymphocytes that filter, attack, and destroy organisms that cause infection; organs and tissues involved in the lymphatic system include bone marrow, thymus gland, liver, spleen, and collections of lymphatic tissue in the throat and small intestine

lymphocyte – a specific type of white blood cell; a type of immune cell that specializes to perform different immune system activities; types of lymphocytes include T cells, B cells, NK cells (natural killer cells), and others

macrophage – a type of white blood cell that specializes in ingesting (eating) foreign matter and debris; these cells often ingest invading bacteria

malabsorption – impaired or inadequate absorption of nutrients from the digestive tract; also known as maldigestion

maldigestion – see malabsorption

melena – the passage of dark, tarry stools containing decomposing blood; an indication of bleeding in the upper part of the digestive tract (the esophagus, stomach, and first part of the small intestine)

manipulation – the application of manual force for healing; describes the techniques used in osteopathy, chiropractic medicine, massage, and other bodywork therapies

meditation – any of many practices in which the mind is inwardly focused and quieted; the practice is a spiritual practice for many but is also used for stress reduction; meditation is known to lower levels of cortisol (a hormone released in response to stress), and is believed to enhance the immune system

melanosis – gradual darkening of those areas of skin that are exposed to the sun

membranoproliferative glomerulonephritis (MPGN) – an inflammatory condition of the kidneys in which immune deposits in the tiny blood vessels of the kidneys cause damage and impair their filtering capability

memory B cell – a member of the B lymphocyte family of white blood cells; these cells hold the memory of exposures to microbes that have entered the body in the past; they can be reactivated to quickly begin producing antibodies if the body is invaded by the same microbe at a later date

memory T cell – a member of the T lymphocyte family of white blood cells; these cells hold the memory of exposure to microbes that have entered the body in the past; they can be reactivated to unleash a cell-mediated immune response if the body is invaded by the same microbe at a later date

meridians – in traditional Chinese medicine, the specific pathways through which vital energy (qi) and blood flow; acupuncture points are located along these meridians

meta-analysis – statistical analysis that allows the results of several different studies of the same subject to be combined and analyzed

metabolism – the collective biochemical processes that occur in a living organism; involves the balanced process of anabolism (building up or creating substances) and catabolism (breaking down or using substances); commonly used to refer the breakdown of food and its transformation into energy

microcirculation – the flow of blood in smallest blood vessels in the body; the part of the circulation where oxygen and nutrients pass into the tissues, and waste products are passed out of the tissue

microbe – a microscopic organism; includes bacteria, viruses, algae, fungi, protozoa, and some parasites; also known as a microorganism

microorganism – a microscopic organism; includes bacteria, viruses, algae, fungi, protozoa, and some parasites

modality – a form of therapy; usually refers to physical forms of therapy such as acupuncture, massage, chiropractic adjustments, etc.

monocyte – see peripheral blood mononuclear cell

monogamous – having only one sexual partner

monotherapy – the use of a single drug to treat a particular disorder or disease

moxibustion – a technique that involves the stimulation of acupuncture points by burning a small cone of dried moxa (mugwort) leaves on the end of the needle, directly on protected skin, or above the body

mutation – a permanent change in a gene or chromosome of an organism creating a new characteristic or trait not previously found; mutations can lead to new resistance to treatment; mutated versions of HCV are known as quasispecies

myalgia – pain or ache in muscle(s)

mycophenolate mofetil – drug marketed with trade name Cellcept®; given to organ transplant recipients to prevent rejection of the new tissue; an immune system inhibitor

NAFL – abbreviation for nonalcoholic fatty liver

NAFLD – abbreviation for nonalcoholic fatty liver disease

NASH – abbreviation for nonalcoholic steatohepatitis

natural killer cell – a member of the lymphocyte family of white blood cells; part of the cell-mediated immune system; an important immune cell that kills invading microbes and attacks tissues it sees as foreign; also called an NK cell

necrosis – death of cells or tissues

neurochemical – chemical that naturally occurs in the nervous system and plays a part in its functioning

neurological – of, or pertaining to the nervous system and the diseases that affect it

neuropathy – a condition that involves damage to the peripheral nerves (those nerves outside of the brain and spinal cord); many neuropathies affect those nerves most distant from the spinal cord, that is those of the hands and feet; sensation is altered with neuropathy and patients may experience any of several symptoms including numbness, tingling, and pain

neutrophil – a type of granular white blood cell that attacks microorganisms such as bacteria

NK cell – see natural killer cell

non-Hodgkin's lymphoma – a form of cancer of the lymphatic system

nonresponder – a person who does not respond to therapy at all or a person who initially responds to therapy, then experiences a relapse or has abnormal liver enzyme tests during therapy

nonspecific – not due to any single known cause, such as a specific pathogen

nonsteroidal analgesic – of, or pertaining to, a substance that is not a steroid but has similar effects, such as the anti-inflammatory, ibuprofen

nontoxic – does not contain substances that are harmful, poisonous, or destructive

5'NT – see 5'-nucleotidase

nucleocapsid – the coat (capsid) of a virus plus the enclosed nucleic acid genome

nucleoside – a subunit of DNA or RNA; To form a DNA or RNA molecule, thousands of nucleotides are joined in a long chain

nucleoside reverse transcriptase inhibitor (NRTI) – a group of drugs used primarily in the treatment of HIV/AIDs; these drugs are incorporated into the viral DNA and block viral replication; examples include AZT (Retrovir®), 3TC®, ddC (Hivid®), ddI (Didanosine®), and d4T (Zerit®)

5'-nucleotidase (5'NT) – an enzyme found in many tissues throughout the body including the liver; increased 2-6 times above the normal amount when bile flow is blocked either inside or outside the liver

nucleotide – see nucleoside

nutritional supplement – any product such as a vitamin, mineral or other substance that is taken to augment the amount of nutrients in the diet; used to improve overall health and/or to help correct specific health problems

OSHA – Occupational Safety and Health Administration, U.S. Department of Labor

osteoporosis – thinning of the bones with reduction in bone mass due to depletion of calcium and bone protein; a condition that predisposes to bone fractures that are often slow to heal and/or heal poorly; more common in older adults, particularly postmenopausal women and people taking steroidal drugs

oxidative stress – a condition that occurs when an overabundance of free radicals are present in the body; chronic infection and inflammation cause increased oxidative stress; high levels of free radicals can lead to tissue damage

oxygenation – the chemical process of adding oxygen to something

palpation – the act of feeling with the hand; the application of light pressure to the surfaces of the body to determine the consistency of the body parts as part of a physical diagnosis

palpitations – involuntary awareness of one's heart beat; can be experienced as feeling the heart is beating harder or faster than usual, or that it is beating irregularly

partial thromboplastin time (PTT) – a test to see how quickly blood is able to form a clot

pathogen – an agent that causes disease, particularly a living microorganism such as a virus or bacterium

pathogenesis (pl. pathogeneses) – the development of a disease or illness

pathological – relating to or caused by disease

PBMC – see peripheral blood mononuclear cell

PCR – see HCV polymerase chain reaction

PCT – see porphyria cutanea tarda

pedal edema – swelling of the feet caused by an excess accumulation of fluid in the body

peginterferon – see pegylated interferon

pegylated interferon – a form of interferon in which polyethylene glycol molecules have been bound to the interferon molecule; pegylated interferon has a slower rate of breakdown and clearance from the body than standard interferon

peptide – a compound containing two or more amino acids; groups of peptides form proteins

peripheral blood mononuclear cell (PBMC) –a large white blood cell found in the blood; one of the cell types of the immune system; also known as monocyte

pesticide – a chemical preparation used to kill insects or other plant/animals pests

petechia – tiny, flat, round, purplish-red spots on the skin caused by bleeding between the layers of the skin or in the mucosal membranes

pharmacology – the study of drugs; includes study of drug sources and their properties; also the study of the body's metabolism of and reaction to drugs

phosphatidylcholine – a compound consisting of glycerol, fatty acids, and phosphorus; as a nutritional supplement, this compound has been shown to have a hepatoprotective effect

phospholipid – the major form of lipids in the body; a principal structural material of living cells; the main component of cell membranes (the outer layer of cells)

physiologic – see physiological

physiological – normal; not pathologic; characteristic of the normal functioning or state of the body, or a tissue or organ

phytopharmacology – the study of compounds that are found in plants that have medicinal uses; the related terms phytochemical and phytonutrient are used interchangeably to describe those plant compounds that are thought to have medicinal properties

pituitary (gland) – the main endocrine gland that controls endocrine functions in the body; called the master gland because it produces hormones that control other glands and many body functions

placebo – an inactive substance, or dummy medication, or sugar pill; widely used in clinical trials to test if an observed effect is truly due to the experimental drug; for a drug to be considered effective, it must show significantly better results than that produced by the placebo

plasma cell – a member of the B lymphocyte family of white blood cells; this cell is responsible for antibody production; also known as an activated B cell

platelet – an irregular, disc-shaped element of the blood that assists in blood clotting; during normal blood clotting, platelets group together (aggregate); platelets are fragments of larger cells called megakaryocytes; liver disease can cause a shortage of platelets

polyarteritis nodosa – a disorder of small and medium sized arteries characterized by inflammation and possible death of the blood vessel cells; usually affects adult males; can be associated with hepatitis C infection; the kidneys are most commonly involved, but muscles, the intestine, and the heart can also be affected

polymer – a compound created by joining smaller molecules called monomers

polymerase – any enzyme that catalyzes polymerization, the successive joining together of smaller monomers to make a polymer

polymyalgia – pain or aching in many muscles; sometimes short for polymyalgia rheumatica (PMR), a disorder of the muscles and joints of older persons characterized by pain and stiffness

porphyria cutanea tarda (PCT) – an inherited disorder of porphyrins metabolism; the liver uses porphyrins to make hemoglobin, the iron-containing portion of the red blood cells; PCT can be acquired with certain types of chemical poisoning

porphyrin – pigmented (colored) compounds that are found in heme (the iron containing molecule in hemoglobin), bile, and cytochromes; blood levels of the various porphyrins can be affected by liver failure

portal hypertension – increased blood pressure in the portal vein that brings blood into the liver; usually occurs because scarring in the liver resists the free flow of blood into the liver; the increased pressure in the portal vein also causes increased pressure in the veins of the abdomen, intestines, stomach, and esophagus; portal hypertension causes many of the complications associated with liver cirrhosis

portal vein – the large vein that carries blood from the intestines to the liver for processing before returning it to circulation via the hepatic veins

potassium – a charged particle called an electrolyte; one of the four major electrolytes in the body; blood levels may be abnormal in cirrhosis and a variety of other diseases

prealbumin – see transthyretin

prodromal symptom – symptom that starts just before the onset of an illness

prognosis – the probable outcome or course of a disease; a person's chance of recovery from a disease or injury

protease – see proteinase

protease inhibitor – any of a class of anti-HIV drugs designed to inhibit the HIV protease enzyme; protease inhibitors prevent the replication of viruses

protein – a large molecule composed of one or more chains of amino acids (peptides); proteins are required for the structure, function, and regulation of the body's cells, tissues, and organs; the liver is responsible for making many of the body's proteins

proteinase – any enzyme that breaks down proteins by splitting them into chains of peptides; also called protease

prothrombin time (PT) – the time it takes for blood to form a clot; monitored in liver disease to assess liver function; many of the proteins needed for clotting are produced in the liver

protocol – a detailed plan for medical treatment or an experiment

pruritus – intense itching of the skin

psoriasis – a reddish, scaly rash often located on the elbows, knees, scalp, and around or in the ears, navel, genitals or buttocks; caused by the body making too many skin cells; some cases are believed to be autoimmune conditions

psychosocial – having aspects of social and psychological behavior

PT – see prothrombin time

PTT – see partial thromboplastin time

purpura – dark red to purple lesions on the skin that typically lose their color when pressed upon; this skin rash can be seen with a wide variety of disorders including cryoglobulinemia

qi – in traditional Chinese medicine, the energy that flows through everything and is the organizing force of the universe; the most important substance circulating through the body

qi gong – qi means energy, and gong means skill; a self-healing art that combines movement and meditation; visualizations are employed to enhance the mind/body connection and assist healing

quasispecies – species of viruses that are very similar but have differences; quasispecies are the result of a virus mutation; mutation can cause several quasispecies to exist in the same person

RA factor – a specific antibody present in the blood of 60-80% of people with rheumatoid arthritis

randomized clinical trial – see clinical trial

Raynaud's phenomenon – intermittent episodes when the arteries of the fingers or toes suddenly go into spasm causing the skin to become very pale, cold, and numb; attacks are usually brought on by exposure to the cold or emotional stress and are commonly relieved by warming the affected body part

RBC – see red blood cell

Rebetron® – a combination of interferon alfa-2b and ribavirin used to treat hepatitis C infection; ribavirin is taken by mouth and interferon alfa-2b is administered subcutaneously (beneath the skin)

recombinant immunoblot assay (RIBA) – a sensitive testing method used to detect the presence of anti-HCV antibodies in the blood; most often used to confirm a positive result on an EIA (enzyme immunoassay) screening test for anti-HCV antibodies

red blood cell – cells that carry oxygen from the air we breathe to all the organs and tissues of the body; supply may be decreased in people with liver disease

relapse – the return of signs and symptoms of a disease following a period of remission (absence of the disease; in hepatitis C, a relapse is the reappearance of the virus after an period of it being undetectable; less frequently used to mean a spike in the liver enzymes after a period of being normal

relapser – someone who has experienced a relapse (see relapse)

remission – the resolution of the signs and symptoms of a disease; can be temporary or permanent

renal – relating to the kidneys

replication – process of duplicating or reproducing; viral reproduction is called replication

replication rate – the rate at which a virus or other microbe is able to reproduce itself

reservoir – in chronic viral illnesses (such as HIV) a place in the body where the virus exists but is not detectable by usual medical means; some researchers believe there is a possibility there is one or more reservoirs of HCV in the body, at least in some people with the infection

retinol – see vitamin A

retrovirus – an RNA virus; a virus with an RNA genome instead of a DNA genome

rheumatoid arthritis – an autoimmune disease that causes chronic inflammation of the joints, the tissue around the joints, and other organs in the body

rheumatoid factor – an autoantibody; see autoantibodies for additional details

RIBA – see recombinant immunoblot assay

ribavirin – a nucleoside analogue drug; it has no activity against HCV when used alone, but is effective in some people when used in combination with interferon; ribavirin is believed to act against HCV not as antiviral but as an immune enhancer

ribonucleic acid (RNA) – one of two types of molecules that encode genetic information (the other is DNA)

ribozyme – an RNA molecule that also acts as an enzyme; ribozymes bind to RNA and cut (cleave) it

RNA – see ribonucleic acid

secondary condition – condition that develops as a consequence of another condition that preceded it

serum – see blood serum

SGOT – see aspartate aminotransferase

SGPT – see alanine aminotransferase

short interfering RNA (siRNA) – small pieces of double-stranded RNA produced when larger pieces of are cut (cleaved); siRNA molecules bind with proteins to form a unit called the RNA-induced silencing complex (RISC) that suppresses the expression of the gene it corresponds to in the viral genome silencing the gene from which the siRNA is derived

shortness of breath – see dyspnea

Sicca syndrome – see Sjögren's syndrome

sign – in medicine, any objective (observable) evidence of a disease

Sjögren's syndrome – an autoimmune disease characterized by dry eyes and mouth, purple spots on the face or inside the mouth, and swollen salivary glands; a condition sometimes seen in people with chronic hepatitis C; also known as Sicca syndrome

sodium – a charged particle called an electrolyte; one of the four major electrolytes in the body; blood levels may be abnormal in cirrhosis and a variety of other diseases

sonography – see ultrasonography

spontaneous clearance – in hepatitis C, the ability to rid the body of virus without treatment; this occurs in 15-20% of people infected with HCV

stage – in hepatitis C, the degree of fibrosis present on liver biopsy; the higher the stage, the more fibrosis present

steatohepatitis – the presence of fat in the liver cells with inflammation

steatorrhea – passing fat in bowel movements; fatty stools are usually accompanied by a particularly bad odor and excessive intestinal gas; stool containing high amounts of fat often floats in the toilet bowl

steatosis – accumulation of fat in the liver that can cause inflammation and lead to fibrosis and/or cirrhosis

stellate cells – in the liver, the main cell type responsible for making fibrous connective tissue

sustained responder – in hepatitis C, a person who has no detectable virus in his or her blood and whose liver enzyme tests continue to be normal six months after completing therapy

sustained response – see sustained responder

symptom – any subjective change (something experienced by the patient) that may indicate a disease process such as fatigue, pain, thirst, etc.

T3 – see triiodothyronine

T4 – see thyroxin

T4 cell – see CD4 cell

T4 count – see CD4 count

T8 cell – see CD8 cell

tai chi – a system of gentle, flowing exercises designed to keep the body's qi (energy) moving

T cell – a type of white blood cell that is a crucial part of the immune system; they activate the rest of the immune system and directly attack invading organisms; also known as T lymphocyte

T helper cell – see CD4 cell

T suppressor cell – a member of the T lymphocyte family of white blood cells that are part of the body's immune system; these cells act to blunt the immune response

thymus gland – the organ in which T lymphocytes (such as CD4 and CD8 T cells) mature; part of the immune system

thyroid gland – the organ that produces thyroid hormones that control the metabolic rate of every cell in the body

thyroid stimulating hormone (TSH) – protein produced by the pituitary gland that acts on the thyroid gland to cause it to produce the two thyroid hormones

thyroiditis – inflammation of the thyroid gland; can cause the release of excess of thyroid hormones into the blood stream

thyroxin – one of two hormones produced by the thyroid gland

TIA – see transient ischemic attack

TIBC – see total iron binding capacity

tinnitus – ringing in the ears; can be caused by certain medications (such as aspirin and other anti-inflammatory drugs), aging, trauma, and other disorders

total bilirubin – see bilirubin

total iron binding capacity (TIBC) – a measurement of how much iron the blood is able to capture

total protein (TP) – a measurement of all proteins in the blood; used to determine how well the liver is performing its job of making proteins

toxic – poisonous; capable of causing injury or harm, especially by chemical means

toxicity – the quality of being toxic

toxin – a poisonous substance, particularly a protein produced by living cells or organisms; certain toxins are capable of inducing the immune system to produce neutralizing antibodies called antitoxins

TP – see total protein

trans – a chemical prefix that refers to a specific arrangement of chemical bonds; the opposite of the trans chemical arrangement is known as cis

transcription mediated amplification (TMA) – a testing technique used to measure the amount of HCV in the blood

transient ischemic attack (TIA) – also called a mini-stroke; a neurological event that has the signs and symptoms of a stroke but that resolve in a short period of time; due to a temporary lack of adequate oxygen (ischemia) in the brain

transthyretin – a small protein made by the liver in the process of making the larger protein albumin; a sensitive indicator of how well the liver is able to produce proteins

triglyceride – a form of fat that exists in many foods and in the body; triglycerides in blood come from fats in foods and can also made in the body

triiodothyronine (T3) – one of two hormones produced by the thyroid gland

TSH – see thyroid stimulating hormone

tui na – Chinese massage therapy

tumor – an abnormal mass of tissue that can be either benign (noncancerous) or malignant (cancerous)

ultrasonography –diagnostic imaging technique that uses sound waves to construct a picture (sonograph) of an internal organ or body structure; also known as sonography

ultrasound – high-frequency sound waves; an ultrasound test (sonography) bounces sound waves off internal organs of the body to construct images of the target organ; liver ultrasound is used to screen for liver cancer

urticaria – raised, itchy areas of skin that are usually a sign of an allergic reaction; also known as hives

vaccination – the introduction of vaccine into the body for the purpose of inducing immunity to a specific disease or group of diseases

vaccine – a suspension of weakened or killed microorganisms, or other substances that are introduced into the body to induce an immune reaction; the immune reaction is intended to protect the recipient from getting the illness associated with a specific microorganism; newer vaccines are being developed to alter the course of infectious diseases

varices – see varix

varix (pl. varices) – an abnormally dilated or swollen vein; portal hypertension can cause esophageal varices that can rupture and cause vomiting of large amounts of blood; bleeding esophageal varices are a medical emergency

vascular – relating to the blood vessels of the body

vasculitis – a general term for a group of diseases that feature inflammation of the blood vessels

vertigo – the sensation of dizziness or spinning

viral clearance – elimination of a virus or reducing it to the point that it cannot be detected in the blood

viral load – the amount of virus present in the blood

virologist – a scientist who specializes in the study of viruses

virology – the branch of microbiology that is concerned with viruses and viral diseases

vitamin – an organic substance that acts as a coenzyme and/or regulator of metabolic processes and is crucial for many bodily functions

vitamin A – a fat-soluble vitamin; may be deficient with severe liver disease leading to night blindness, dry skin, and brittle hair and nails

vitamin B – a complex of several important vitamins including B1 (thiamine), B2 (riboflavin), B3 (niacin), B6 (pyridoxine), B9 (folic acid), and B12 (cobalamin). As a group, the B vitamins are required for the metabolism of carbohydrates, fats, and amino acids; for proper neural functioning and mood regulation

vitamin D – a fat-soluble vitamin; may be deficient with severe liver disease leading to softening of the bones and bone pain

vitamin E – a fat-soluble vitamin; may be deficient with severe liver disease leading to a shortage of red blood cells and muscle loss

vitamin K – a fat-soluble vitamin; may be deficient with severe liver disease leading to easy bruising and bleeding problems

WBC – see white blood cells

white blood cells – part of the body's immune system; different kinds of white blood cells include neutrophils, lymphocytes, and macrophages; a change in white blood cell count may indicate a change in hepatitis C disease status

xanthelasma – small deposits of fat just under the surface of the skin around the eyes; appear as small, raised, yellowish bumps on the skin

xanthomas – small deposits of fat just under the surface of the skin over the joints and/or tendons; appear as small, raised, yellowish nodules

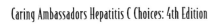

Terry Baker
Executive Director, Veterans Aimed Toward Awareness
Middletown, Delaware
Terry Baker is an advocate for military veterans and Executive Director of Veterans Aimed Toward Awareness (VATA). Terry advocates for veterans' rights regarding hepatitis C and other illnesses related to military service. Terry works to educate veterans about the need to be tested for viral hepatitis. VATA represents the interests of a large portion of the hepatitis C population in the United States.

Misha Cohen, OMD, LAc
Clinical Director, Chicken Soup Chinese Medicine
San Francisco, California
Misha R. Cohen is a doctor of oriental medicine and a licensed acupuncturist. She is an internationally recognized practitioner, lecturer, and leader in the field of traditional Chinese medicine. Dr. Cohen is the author of The Chinese Way to Healing: Many Paths to Wholeness (Perigee 1996, iUniverse 2007), The HIV Wellness Sourcebook (Holt 1998), and The Hepatitis C Help Book (St. Martin's Press 2000, 2007). She has also authored numerous professional articles and book chapters on Chinese medicine and research subjects. Dr. Cohen is Clinical Director of Chicken Soup Chinese Medicine, Research and Education Chair of Quan Yin Healing Arts Center, Research Specialist at the University of California Institute for Health and Aging, and Research Consultant to the University of California, San Francisco School of Medicine Cancer Center. She contributes regular columns to *Liver Health* magazine and NuMedx.com magazine. POZ Magazine named her one of the "Top 50 AIDS Researchers in the Country" in 1997. She currently sits on the Board of Directors and is the 2004 Conference Chair for the Society for Acupuncture Research.

Stewart Cooper, MD
Director of Liver Research, California Pacific Medical Center
San Francisco, California
Dr. Cooper is an expert in immunology and hepatology with special clinical and research interests in viral hepatitis. He has been a pioneer in liver immunology research for more than a decade. At California Pacific Medical Center, Dr. Cooper oversees the Liver Immunology Laboratory. His research investigates hepatic immunity, focusing on the determinants of HCV clearance. Dr. Cooper has served as Assistant Professor of Medicine, Microbiology & Immunology at University of California San Francisco and as a Research and Gastroenterology Fellow at Stanford University School of Medicine. He has an international reputation in viral hepatitis research and management, and is listed in *Who's Who of Medical Science Educators*.

Randy Dietrich
Patient Advocate
Centennial, Colorado
Randy Dietrich was diagnosed with hepatitis C in January 1999 following a routine physical examination. Randy is a successful executive in the finance arena. As a result of his diagnosis, Mr. Dietrich, together with his employer Republic Financial Corporation, founded the Caring Ambassadors Hepatitis C Program.

Gregory T. Everson, MD
Professor of Medicine and Director of Hepatology, University of Colorado Health Sciences Center
Aurora, Colorado
Dr. Everson received his medical degree from Cornell Medical College in New York, New York. He is currently a Professor of Medicine and the Director of Hepatology in the Division of Gastroenterology and Hepatology, Department of Internal Medicine at the University of Colorado. Dr. Everson is a recipient of both NIH and industry sponsored research grants and contracts to study and treat patients with hepatitis C. He was a principal investigator of the HALT C trial. Dr. Everson

is an author and contributor to many scientific and clinical publications related to hepatitis C and liver disease. He and his coauthor Hedy Weinberg have written four editions of Living with Hepatitis C: A Survivor's Guide, one edition of My Mom has Hepatitis C, one edition of Living with Hepatitis B: A Survivor's Guide, and the new book Hemochromatosis: Answers to Your Questions About Iron Overload. Dr. Everson is a fellow of the American College of Physicians, and a member of the American Gastroenterologic Association, the American Association for the Study of Liver Disease, and the American Society of Transplantation. He is the Associate Editor of the journal Liver Transplantation, and a reviewer for numerous scientific and medical journals.

Sylvia Flesner, ND
Denver, Colorado

Dr. Flesner is a naturopathic doctor, a graduate of the former American Holistic College of Nutrition (now the Clayton School of Natural Healing). She has maintained clinical practices in Houston, Texas and Denver, Colorado for the past 23 years. Her training as a doctor of naturopathy included the study of several alternative medical disciplines including homeopathy, nutrition, pressure points, herbology, massage, acupressure, reflexology, iridology, psychology, degenerative diseases, allergic diseases, immune deficiency problems, and techniques for survival in the 21st century. Dr. Flesner is also certified in psychoneuroimmunology. She is a member of the American Naturopathic Medical Association and the American Holistic Medical Association. Currently, Dr. Flesner is participating in research at the Duke University Rhine Research Center correlating medical records of patients using intuitive diagnostics. She is also working on alternative treatment approaches for cancer and other illnesses. Dr. Flesner has lectured at the School of Public Health and MD Anderson Methodist Hospital in Texas.

Robert Gish, MD
Medical Director of the Liver Transplant Program, California Pacific Medical Center
San Francisco, California

Dr. Gish is Medical Director of the Liver Transplant Program at California Pacific Medical Center in San Francisco. He is an associate professor at the University of California, San Francisco and the University of Nevada, Reno. He earned his medical degree from the University of Kansas and received his training in internal medicine at the University of California, San Diego. Dr. Gish has conducted extensive research on treatments for hepatitis B and C, and has authored more than 100 original articles, review articles, abstracts, and book chapters. Along with being a co-principal investigator or sub-investigator on a number of grants from the National Institutes of Health (NIH), Dr. Gish has also received the NIH physician scientist award. He is actively involved in numerous professional societies including the American Association for the Advancement of Science, the American Society of Transplant Physicians, and is a fellow of the American College of Physicians and the American Association for the Study of Liver Disease. Dr. Gish collaborated with Dr. Misha Cohen to author The Hepatitis C Helpbook, which examines the use of Chinese medicine in combination with conventional western biomedical therapies.

Peter Hauser, MD
Professor, Departments of Behavioral Neurosciences, Internal Medicine & Psychiatry at Oregon Health and Science University
Associate Director, NW Hepatitis C Resource Center
Portland, Oregon

Dr. Peter Hauser lives in Portland, Oregon with his wife and three children. He is a Professor in the departments of Behavioral Neurosciences, Internal Medicine and Psychiatry at Oregon Health and Science University and Associate Director of the NW Hepatitis C Resource Center. His primary research and clinical focus is the psychiatric and substance use co-morbidities in patients with hepatitis C, the development of educational products for patients with hepatitis C and the treatment of interferon-induced depression. He has edited two books, authored several chapters, and published over 80 articles and letters in journals such as *Molecular Psychiatry, New England Journal of Medicine, Journal of Affective Disorders* and *Proceedings of the National Academy of Sciences*; the primary focus of his publications has been hepatitis c, mood disorders and psychoneuroendocrinology.

Randy Horwitz, MD, PhD
Medical Director, Program in Integrative Medicine, University of Arizona
Tucson, Arizona
Dr. Horwitz is the Medical Director of the Program in Integrative Medicine and assistant professor of Clinical Medicine at the University of Arizona. He earned his medical degree from the University of Illinois and a PhD in immunology and molecular biology from the University of Florida. Dr. Horwitz did his postdoctoral training at the National Institutes of Health, and completed a three-year fellowship in Allergy and Clinical Immunology at the University of Wisconsin. Dr. Horwitz also completed a two-year integrative medicine fellowship at the University of Arizona, which focused on mind-body approaches to illness. He is board certified in internal medicine, and allergy and clinical immunology.

David W. Indest, PsyD
Psychology Training Director, Portland VA Medical Center
Program Manager of the Northwest Hepatitis C Resource Center (NWHCRC).
Portland, Oregon
David Indest, PsyD, is a Supervisory Clinical Psychologist at the Portland VA Medical Center where he serves as the Psychology Training Director and as the Program Manager of the Northwest Hepatitis C Resource Center (NWHCRC). He is an Assistant Professor in Psychiatry at Oregon Health & Science University. He develops programs assisting veterans with hepatitis C and HIV. While emphasizing the total care of the person, Dr. Indest integrates his work with ongoing research studies to develop best clinical practices. Dr. Indest's commitment to integrated care comes from two decades of working in the prevention and treatment of HIV. His specialties are behavioral medicine, mind-body disorders, public health, behavior change, human sexuality, and applied clinical research.

Jessica Irwin, PAC
Physician Assistant
San Francisco, California
Jessica Irwin is a Physician Assistant working in the field of hepatology and liver transplant. Ms. Irwin completed her Master's in Physician Assistant Studies and Public Health at Touro University in California. Her continuing education through the AASLD Hepatology Physician Assistant fellowship was completed at the University of California, San Francisco under the preceptorship of Norah Terrault, MD.

Julia Jernberg, MD
Clinical Assistant Professor of Medicine, University of Wisconsin
Tucson, Arizona
Dr. Jernberg is a board-certified internist and a clinical assistant professor of medicine at the University of Wisconsin. She received her medical degree from the University of Illinois, and completed her internal medicine training at Case Western Reserve University in Cleveland, Ohio. She has a keen interest in basic science and clinical research, and previously performed postdoctoral research at the National Institutes of Health. Dr. Jernberg's work has been published in numerous professional journals. She currently practices in Wisconsin and Arizona.

Joyce S. Kobayashi, MD
Psychiatrist
Denver, Colorado
Dr. Kobayashi is a renowned Psychiatrist who works with people living with hepatitis C. She was an Associate Professor of the Department of Psychiatry, University of Colorado Health Sciences Center and staff psychiatrist at Denver Health Medical Center where she was a consultant to the Hepatitis C Clinic. Dr. Kobayashi received the 2007 "Outstanding Achievement Award" from the Colorado Psychiatric Society. Dr. Kobayashi served on the Institute of Medicine Board on Population Health and Public Health Practice, as the Board liaison to the Committees on HIV Prevention Strategies, Public Financing of HIV Care. as well as a number of components of the American Psychiatric Association, including the Commission on AIDS and the Committee of Asian-American Psychiatrists.

Douglas LaBrecque, MD
Professor and Director of Liver Services, University of Iowa Hospitals and Clinics
Iowa City, Iowa
Dr. LaBrecque received his medical degree from Stanford Medical School, Stanford, CA. He is currently a Professor in the Department of Internal Medicine at the University of Iowa College of Medicine. Dr. LaBrecque was Chief of Gastroenterology-Hepatology at the Veterans Administration hospital in Iowa City, IA from 1982 to 2001. He has won a number of awards including the Lange Book Award, the J. D. Lane Research Award, and the Medical Residents Teaching Award at the University of Iowa. Dr. LaBrecque is recognized nationally and internationally for his expertise in liver diseases, particularly the field of hepatitis. Dr. LaBrecque has built a nationally recognized program in liver diseases at the University of Iowa with an over 1000% increase in patients over the past 15 years, five full-time faculty members, and a liver transplant program. He has written key chapters on clinical subjects in standard internal medicine and hepatology textbooks, and co-edited a textbook on liver diseases.

Lark Lands, PhD
Medical Writer and Editor
Georgetown, Colorado
Lark Lands is a contributing medical writer and editor for the American Academy of HIV Medicine, AIDS Treatment News, www.AIDSmeds.com, CATIE's The Positive Side, CATIE's Practical Guides, and the Houston Buyers Club. She is a long-time HIV treatment activist, journalist, and educator. A former think tank scientist, she was a pioneer in bringing attention to the need for an integrated approach to HIV disease. Her articles, many of which are available at www.larklands.net, have been widely printed and reprinted in AIDS newsletters and on the Internet. She is a frequent speaker at international, national, state, and local HIV/AIDS conferences.

Shri K. Mishra, ABMS, MD, MS, FAAN, FNAAM
Professor of Neurology and Coordinator of the Integrative Medicine Program
University of Southern California, Keck School of Medicine
Los Angeles, California
Dr. Mishra is a professor of neurology and Coordinator of the Integrative Medicine Program at the University of Southern California School of Medicine. He graduated from Banaras Hindu University Ayurveda Charya with an ABMS (bachelor of medicine and surgery) from the Institute of Medical Sciences. He holds an MS degree in anatomy from Queens University, Canada and an MD from the University of Toronto, Canada. He also holds an MBA in Health Systems from the University of Wisconsin. He is a neurologist with a special interest in neuromuscular diseases. He served as medical director at the Veterans Administration Outpatient Clinic and Associate Dean at the University of Southern California. He is a member of many neuroscience societies and serves on editorial boards of many neurological and integrative medicine journals. Dr. Mishra has been very active in the field of integrative medicine and serves on various committees in this field. He is a practicing Ayurvedist, and yoga teacher and practitioner. Dr. Mishra's goals are to develop evidence-based, cost-effective, quality clinical care education and research in integrative medicine. He is president of the American Academy of Ayurvedic Medicine (AAAM).

Sharon D. Montes, MD
Physician, Private Practice
Baltimore, Maryland
Dr. Montes received her degree from the University of Colorado. She is an Assistant Professor at the University of Maryland Medical School, and Board certified in Family medicine and in Holistic Medicine with a certificate in Geriatrics. Dr. Montes has extensive experience in tending to women's health and conditions associated with aging. She has a particular interest in acupuncture, herbal, energetic, and nutritional therapies.

Julie Nelligan, PhD
Portland, Oregon
Julie Nelligan received her doctorate from Ohio State University in Clinical Psychology with a specialty in Health Psychology. Her area of expertise is in brief interventions to address alcohol use in patients with hepatitis C. While working with the Hepatitis C

Resource Center at the Portland VA Medical Center she assisted in developing an intervention with a toolkit to enable specialty and primary care providers to address alcohol use in chronically-infected hepatitis C patients who continue to drink alcohol. She also has experience in evaluating substance use and relapse risk in patients being considered for liver transplant, conducting psychosocial assessments as part of a multidisciplinary chronic pain team, and facilitating support groups for veterans who are being treated with interferon for hepatitis C. Dr. Nelligan is currently in private practice in Portland, Oregon.

J. Lyn Patrick, ND
Private Naturopathic Physician
Hesperus, Colorado

Dr. Patrick graduated from Bastyr University in 1984 and was in private practice as a state-boarded naturopathic physician in Tucson, Arizona for 17 years. She is currently in private practice in Durango, Colorado and specializes in chronic hepatitis C and environmental medicine. She is a member of the American College for Advancement in Medicine, the American Association of Naturopathic Physicians, and the Colorado Association of Naturopathic Physicians. She has provided care for HIV positive and HIV/HCV coinfected patients through federally funded programs that incorporate complementary medicine in a primary care treatment model. She is currently a Contributing Editor for Alternative Medicine Review, a peer-reviewed journal. She has published over 20 scientific reviews in the field of complementary and alternative medicine. Dr. Patrick has presented information on CAM and hepatitis C at numerous medical meetings.

Bharathi Ravi, BAMS
Private Ayurvedic Practitioner
Los Angeles, California

Dr. Bharathi Ravi graduated from the University of Bangalore, India. She is a chief ayurvedic practitioner at the Ayurvedic Center in Southern California. Dr. Ravi specializes in pancha karma, diet, and lifestyle. She volunteers and conducts research at the University of Southern California in the Integrative Medicine Program. She regularly lectures on CAM and healthy living through Ayurveda. Dr. Ravi is an active participant in numerous medical conferences to help raise awareness about natural living and healing. She is also a consultant at the Local Charity Health Care Center. Her areas of interest include chronic fatigue, fibromyalgia, hepatitis, skin diseases, and gynecological disorders.

Aparna Roy MD, MPH
Senior Research Clinical Trials Coordinator
Division of Pediatric Gastroenterology and Nutrition
Baltimore, Maryland

Dr. Roy received her medical degree from Grant Medical College, Mumbai, India. She then completed her clinical internship at the Sir J.J. Group of Hospitals, Mumbai, India. She has a Master of Public Health from the Johns Hopkins School of Public Health with an area of focus on infectious diseases and international health. Dr. Roy works as the Senior Research Clinical Trials Coordinator in the Pediatric Liver Center at Johns Hopkins. She works on NIH-funded grants in a variety of pediatric liver diseases including biliary atresia, acute liver failure, hepatitis C and hepatitis B. She has initiated and coordinated several community projects in India. Dr. Roy currently sees research patients in the Johns Hopkins David M. Rubenstein Pediatric Subspecialty Clinic and the Pediatric Clinical Research Unit.

Lorren Sandt
Hepatitis C Program Director, Caring Ambassadors Program
Vancouver, Washington

Ms. Sandt has managed the hepatitis C division of the Caring Ambassadors Program since its inception in 1999. She is responsible for the oversight and implementation of all program activities and spearheads its ongoing mission. Ms. Sandt is the liaison to the program's Medical Brainstorming Team, which is comprised of hepatitis C health care professionals from the different disciplines and the program's research staff. Ms. Sandt regularly participates in state-of-the-art medical conferences to stay abreast of cutting-edge information in hepatitis C clinical and applied research. She is a frequent participant and presenter at conferences and symposia, interacting with those living with hepatitis C as well as with their families, patient advocates, representatives of hepatitis C organizations, physicians, and other health care workers. Ms. Sandt is the founder and past President of the National Hepatitis C Advocacy Council, vice-chair on the Board of Directors of the National Viral Hepatitis Roundtable (NVHR), and a member of the Hepatitis C Appropriations Partnership (HCAP), and the Oregon State Hepatitis Advisory Group (HAG). In 2001, The Hepatitis C Global Foundation honored Ms. Sandt with the Ronald Eugene Duffy Memorial Award for Patient Activism: for leadership and mentoring of patients, making them advocates for their own health.

Kathleen B. Schwarz, MD
Professor of Pediatrics,
Division of Pediatric Gastroenterology and Nutrition
Baltimore, Maryland

Dr. Schwarz received her medical degree from Washington University. She then completed her residency in pediatrics and fellowship in pediatric gastroenterology at St. Louis Children's Hospital, Washington University School of Medicine. Dr. Schwarz is Director of the Pediatric Liver Center at Johns Hopkins in which there are over 1,000 patients who receive medical care. She focuses on liver disorders of childhood with a particular emphasis on biliary atresia, metabolic liver disorders, autoimmune liver disease, and viral hepatitis B and C. Dr. Schwarz is the Medical Director of the Pediatric Liver Transplant Program at Johns Hopkins and directs NIH-funded grants in a variety of pediatric liver diseases including biliary atresia (BARC), cholestatic liver diseases of childhood (CLIC), acute liver failure, pediatric liver transplantation, cystic fibrosis liver disease and hepatitis C. Baltimore Magazine named her as one of the top 25 pediatricians in Baltimore and she has won teaching awards at both St. Louis University and Johns Hopkins. In 2005 she received the Distinguished Service Award of the North American Society of Pediatric Gastroenterology, Hepatology, and Nutrition and, since 2001, has been named one of the Castle Connolly Top Doctors in America. Dr. Schwarz currently sees patients in the Johns Hopkins David M. Rubenstein Pediatric Subspecialty Clinic.

Amy E. Smith, PAC
Physician Assistant
Organization to Achieve Solutions in Substance-Abuse (O.A.S.I.S.)
Oakland, California

Amy E. Smith, PA-C obtained a BA degree from California State University at Long Beach, and a Physician Assistant Certificate from Stanford-Foothill Primary Care Associate Program in Palo Alto, CA. She is currently employed by O.A.S.I.S., Inc (Organization to Achieve Solutions in Substance-Abuse), a non-profit organization located in Oakland, CA. The clinic and research has focused on hepatitis C access and outcomes in marginalized populations, including those with substance abuse and mental illness.

Tina M. St. John, MD
Executive Director and Medical Director
Caring Ambassadors Program
Vancouver, Washington

Dr. St. John is a graduate of Emory University School of Medicine in Atlanta, Georgia; she is an epidemiologist, medical writer, editor, educator, and clinical research consultant. She was formerly a senior medical officer with the Centers for Disease Control and Prevention (CDC). At CDC, Dr. St. John designed and conducted epidemiological and practice-based research, and oversaw continuing medical education activities sponsored by CDC and the Agency for Toxic Substances and Disease Registry (ATSDR). She worked in the private sector as a medical director and medical editor before launching her own company in 2000. She is a member of the American Public Health Association, the American Medical Women's Association, the American Medical Writers Association, and the Alpha Omega Alpha Medical Honor Society. She has published extensively in the peer-reviewed literature, is the author of With Every Breath: A Lung Cancer Guidebook, and has been an invited author in a number of professional texts. Dr. St. John is the Executive Director and Medical Director of the Caring Ambassadors Program.

Diana L. Sylvestre, MD
Executive Director and Founder
Organization to Achieve Solutions in Substance-Abuse (O.A.S.I.S.)
Oakland, California

Diana L. Sylvestre, MD obtained a BS degree from the University of Florida, and her MD from Harvard Medical School. She trained in Internal Medicine at the Brigham and Women's Hospital in Boston, MA, and underwent fellowship training in Biochemical Genetics at the Sloan Kettering Institute in New York, NY. She is currently an Assistant Clinical Professor of Medicine at the University of California, San Francisco, and Executive Director and Founder of O.A.S.I.S. (Organization to Achieve Solutions in Substance-Abuse), a non-profit organization located in Oakland, CA. Her research has focused on hepatitis C access and outcomes in marginalized populations, including those with substance abuse and mental illness.

Norah Terrault, MD, MPH
Hepatologist, UCSF Medical Center
San Francisco , California

Dr. Norah Terrault is Associate Professor of Medicine and Director of Viral Hepatitis Research in Liver Transplantation at the University of California San Francisco and recognized nationally and internationally for her work related to viral hepatitis and liver transplantation. She has authored over 100 original articles, reviews and book chapters on viral hepatitis, and serves on the editorial boards for Liver Transplantation and Clinical Gastroenterology and Hepatology. She is an investigator on several clinical studies funded by National Institutes of Health in special populations infected with hepatitis C, and an investigator on several ongoing clinical trials of antiviral therapy in patients with chronic hepatitis B and C.

Sivarama Prasad Vinjamury
Ayurvedic Practitioner
Los Angeles, California

Dr. Sivarama Prasad Vinjamury graduated from University of Kerala, South India. He is in private practice as a licensed Ayurvedic physician. He is currently studying for his master's degree in acupuncture and oriental medicine at the Southern California University of Health Sciences at Los Angeles. He volunteers and conducts research at the University of Southern California in the Integrative Medicine Program. He is also involved in part-time research at Southern California University of Health Sciences. Dr. Vinjamury is the former Director of Product Development for Venkat Pharma, Hyderabad, South India, and a former consultant Ayurvedic physician at Apollo Hospitals, Hyderabad, South India. For the past eight years, he has been treating various chronic ailments with Ayurvedic medicines at his clinic and at Apollo hospitals. His areas of interest include HIV, hepatitis B and C, and rheumatology. Dr. Vinjamury is a member of the American Association of Alternative Medicine Practitioners.

Qing-Cai Zhang, LAc, MD (China)
Zhang's Clinic
New York, New York

Dr. Qing-Cai Zhang graduated from Shanghai Second Medical University. He worked as a clinician at Reijing Hospital of the medical university. Dr. Zhang conducted clinical work and research to integrate Chinese and western medicine. In 1980, he was awarded a World Health Organization scholarship, which supported his two-year fellowship at Harvard Medical School and Massachusetts General Hospital. He worked as a research fellow at the Wakai Clinic in Nagoya, Japan. Dr. Zhang received a one-year appointment from the University of California, Davis as a visiting professor. Since 1986, Dr. Zhang has been the primary researcher at the Oriental Healing Arts Institute where he conducts research on treating HIV/AIDS with Chinese medicine. He has published two books on this topic. Dr. Zhang went into private practice in 1990, first in Cypress, California, and now in New York City. He focuses on treating chronic infectious diseases such as viral hepatitis, HIV/AIDS, Lyme disease, and autoimmune diseases. He is the author of Healing Hepatitis C with Modern Chinese Medicine.

Susan L. Zickmund, PhD
Assistant Professor of Medicine, University of Pittsburgh
Pittsburgh, Pennsylvania
Susan Zickmund is an Assistant Professor in the Departments of Medicine at the University of Pittsburgh and at the VA Pittsburgh Healthcare System at the Center for Health Equity Research and Promotion (CHERP) where she directs the Qualitative Research Core. She has a PhD in Communication Arts at the University of Wisconsin-Madison. Subsequently she studied inter-ethnic conflict at the University of Bielefeld, Germany and was a Gastprofessorin at the University of Dortmund, Germany. She was a Visiting Faculty member in the Program in Biomedical Ethics and Medical Humanities and was the Certificate Director for the Project on the Rhetoric of Inquiry at the University of Iowa (UI). There she was the Primary Investigator of the Patient Narrative Study, a psychosocial study examining quality of life and health outcomes of patients with hepatitis C, heart failure, and cancer. At the UI she also completed a three-year post-doctoral training in the Cardiovascular Center exploring the impact of communication problems on health outcomes in patients with congestive heart failure. At the University of Pittsburgh she now focuses her research on barriers to initiating antiviral therapy for patients with hepatitis C and has completed a career development award in the VA Medical Center on that topic. Her VA Medical Center study, entitled the Patient/Provider Attitude toward Hepatitis Study (PATHS) explores patient as well as provider barriers that HCV positive veterans can experience when deciding to enter antiviral treatment.

Authors' Disclosures

All of the authors of <u>Hepatitis C Choices</u> submitted a voluntary disclosure form indicating financial and/or collaborative affiliations with organizations that may have an interest in hepatitis C. While we do not believe that these voluntarily disclosed interests or affiliations bias the material presented, in the spirit of transparency, we are making the contents of the disclosures available to our readers.

Terry Baker
None

Misha Cohen, OMD, LAc
Health Concerns - Consultant

Stewart Cooper, MD, MB, ChB, MRCP
Genentech - Consultant

Randy Dietrich
None

Gregory Everson MD
Hoffman-LaRoche - Research Grants
Schering Plough Corp. - Speakers Bureau
Intermune - Advisory Board

Sylvia Flesner, ND
None

Robert Gish, MD
Akros Pharma, Inc. - Grants, Research, and/or Support
Amgen - Grants, Research, and/or Support
Bayer Pharmaceuticals - Grants, Research, and/or Support
Bristol Myers Squibb - Grants, Research, and/or Support
Celera Diagnostics - Grants, Research, and/or Support

Chiron Corporation - Grants, Research, and/or Support
Gilead Sciences - Grants, Research, and/or Support
Glaxo - Grants, Research, and/or Support
Hoffman-LaRoche – Grants, Research, and/or Support
Intermune - Grants, Research, and/or Support
Matrix Pharmaceuticals - Grants, Research, and/or Support
Ortho Biotech Products, LP - Grants, Research, and/or Support
Ribapharm, Inc. - Grants, Research, and/or Support
Schering Plough Corp. – Grants, Research, and/or Support
SciClone Pharmaceuticals - Grants, Research, and/or Support
Triangle Pharmaceuticals - Grants, Research, and/or Support
United Therapeutics - Grants, Research, and/or Support

Peter Hauser, MD
None

Randy Horwitz, MD, PhD
None

David W.Indest, PsyD
None

Jessica Irwin, PAC
None

Julia Jernberg, MD
None

Joyce S. Kobayashi, MD
None

Douglas R. LaBrecque
Schering Plough - Research Grants, Speakers Bureau
Hoffman-LaRoche - Research Grants, Speakers Bureau
Ortho McNeil Pharmaceuticals - Speakers Bureau
Axian Scandipharm - Speakers Bureau

Lark Lands, PhD
None

Shri K. Mishra
None

Sharon D. Montes, MD
None

Julie Nelligan, PhD
None

Lyn Patrick
None

Aparna Roy, MD, MPH
Hoffman-LaRoche –Research - Study Coordinator – PEDS C Trial, Johns Hopkins site

Bharathi Ravi
None

Lorren Sandt
None

Kathleen B. Schwarz, MD
Hoffman-LaRoche –Research - Principal Investigator – PEDS C Trial

Amy E. Smith, PAC
None

Tina M. St. John, MD
None

Diana L. Sylvestre, MD
None

Norah Terrault, MD, MPH
None

Sivarama Prasad Vinjamury
None

Qing-Cai Zhang, LAc, MD (China)
Tai Hi Company – Partner
HepaPro Corporation - Consultant

Susan L. Zickmund, PhD
None